Vascular and Endovascular Complications

Vascular and Endovascular Complications
A Practical Approach

Edited by

Sachinder Singh Hans, MD, FACS

Medical Director
Vascular and Endovascular Services
Henry Ford Macomb Hospital
Clinton TWP, MI
and
Clinical Assistant Professor of Surgery
Wayne State University School of Medicine
Detroit, MI

Mark F. Conrad, MD, MMSc, RPVI, FACS

Director of Clinical Research
Division of Vascular and Endovascular Surgery
Massachusetts General Hospital
and
Associate Professor of Surgery
Harvard Medical School
Boston, MA

CRC Press
Taylor & Francis Group
Boca Raton London New York

CRC Press is an imprint of the
Taylor & Francis Group, an **informa** business

Access the Support Material: www.routledge.com/9780367698430

First edition published 2021
by CRC Press
6000 Broken Sound Parkway NW, Suite 300, Boca Raton, FL 33487-2742
and by CRC Press
2 Park Square, Milton Park, Abingdon, Oxon, OX14 4RN

Library of Congress Cataloging-in-Publication Data

Names: Hans, S. S. (Sachinder Singh), editor. | Conrad, Mark F., editor.
Title: Vascular and endovascular complications : a practical approach / edited by Sachinder Singh Hans, Mark F. Conrad.
Description: First edition. | Boca Raton, FL : CRC Press, 2021. | Includes bibliographical references and index. | Summary: "Avoiding and minimizing the impact of complications after vascular and endovascular procedures is important for all vascular surgeons. Clinical success is achieved through a combination of careful patient selection, thoughtful pre-procedure planning, and surgical execution with meticulous operative and endovascular technique. However, despite best efforts, complications do occur and need to be recognized and treated in a timely fashion. The early diagnosis of complications, followed by prompt action and intervention, are the keys to improving clinical outcomes. This well illustrated, concise and practical book ensures that vascular and endovascular surgeons will be able to optimize clinical results and patient care"-- Provided by publisher.
Identifiers: LCCN 2020039009 (print) | LCCN 2020039010 (ebook) | ISBN 9781138352933 (hardback) | ISBN 9780429434464 (ebook)
Subjects: MESH: Vascular Surgical Procedures | Endovascular Procedures | Postoperative Complications--prevention & control
Classification: LCC RD598.5 (print) | LCC RD598.5 (ebook) | NLM WG 170 | DDC 617.4/13--dc23
LC record available at https://lccn.loc.gov/2020039009
LC ebook record available at https://lccn.loc.gov/2020039010

ISBN: 9781138352933 (hbk)
ISBN: 9780367698430 (pbk)
ISBN: 9780429434464 (ebk)

Typeset in Minion Pro
by KnowledgeWorks Global Ltd.

Contents

Access the Support Material: www.routledge.com/9780367698430

Preface

The practice of vascular surgery has evolved over the last 20 years. The rise in surgeon comfort with and sophistication for endovascular procedures has expanded the number of patients who can be offered an intervention, even in a population of advancing age and increasing comorbidities. Indeed, we perform complex vascular procedures on patients with multiple comorbid conditions and expect them to recover without complication. However, complications do occur, and early recognition and treatment can ultimately reduce the impact on our patients. It has been some time since a textbook was created, that is devoted to the avoidance and minimization of complications. The chapters herein detail popular open repair and endovascular procedures while highlighting the most frequently incurred adverse advents with tips for avoidance and amelioration. We are extremely thankful and appreciative of the contributions of Miranda Bromage, Samantha Cook and Linda Leggio from the Taylor & Francis/CRC Press. Meeta Singh of KGL and her team were diligent in getting the correction of the proofs at a fast pace and are well deserving of our gratitude in completion of this project. We hope you enjoy the text. With every best wish.

Sachinder Singh Hans, MD, FACS
Mark F. Conrad, MD, MMSc, RPVI, FACS

Contributors

Daniyal Abbas
Henry Ford Hospital
Detroit, Michigan

Monica Abdelmasih
Department of Surgery
University of Toronto
Toronto, Ontario, Canada

Christopher J. Abularrage
Division of Vascular Surgery and Endovascular Therapy
The Johns Hopkins Hospital
Baltimore, Maryland

Robert Acho
Henry Ford Macomb Hospital
Clinton Township, Michigan

Nathan J. Aranson
Non-Invasive Vascular Lab
Maine Health Vein Center
Portland, Maine

Elizabeth A. Blazick
Maine Medical Center
Portland, Maine

Laura T. Boitano
Massachusetts General Hospital
Harvard Medical School
Boston, Massachusetts

Paul G. Bove
Oakland University
William Beaumont School of Medicine
Royal Oak, Michigan

Dawn M. Coleman
Pediatric Renovascular Hypertension Center
Integrated Vascular Surgery
Section of Vascular Surgery
Department of Surgery
University of Michigan
Ann Arbor, Michigan

Robert Cuff
Spectrum Health
Michigan State University
Grand Rapids, Michigan

Frank M. Davis
Section of Vascular Surgery
Department of Surgery
University of Michigan
Ann Arbor, Michigan

Collin Gandillon
Vascular Surgery
Michigan State University/Michigan Vascular Center
Flint, Michigan

Karem C. Harth
HHVI Vascular Laboratories
Department of General Surgery
Division of Vascular Surgery and Endovascular Therapy
Harrington Heart and Vascular Institute
Cleveland, Ohio

Mounir J. Haurani
Division of Vascular Diseases and Surgery
The Ohio State University Wexner Medical Center
Columbus, Ohio

Nicole Heidt
Maine Medical Center
Portland, Maine

Peter K. Henke
Section of Vascular Surgery
Department of Surgery
University of Michigan
Ann Arbor, Michigan

Kara Hessel
Vascular Surgery
The Ohio State University Wexner Medical Center
Columbus, Ohio

Maen Aboul Hosn
Department of Vascular Surgery
University of Iowa Hospitals and Clinics
Iowa City, Iowa

Prakash Jayanthi
Ascension Providence Hospital/Michigan State
University College of Human Medicine
Southfield, Michigan

Vikram S. Kashyap
Division of Vascular Surgery and Endovascular Therapy
Cardiovascular Surgery
Vascular Center, Harrington Heart & Vascular Institute
University Hospitals Cleveland Medical Center
and
Case Western Reserve University
Cleveland, Ohio

Ahmed Kayssi
Division of Vascular Surgery
Department of Surgery
University of Toronto
Toronto, Ontario, Canada

Daniel Kim
Massachusetts General Hospital
Harvard Medical School
Boston, Massachusetts

Gloria Y. Kim
University of Michigan
Ann Arbor, Michigan

Thomas W. Wakefield
University of Michigan
Ann Arbor, Michigan

Christopher A. Latz
Massachusetts General Hospital
Harvard Medical School
Boston, Massachusetts

Jason T. Lee
Division of Vascular Surgery
Stanford University School of Medicine
Stanford, California

Mary Lee
Henry Ford Macomb Hospital
Clinton Township, Michigan

Srihari K. Lella
Vascular and Endovascular Surgery
Massachusetts General Hospital
Harvard Medical School
Boston, Massachusetts

Judith C. Lin
Division of Vascular Surgery
Henry Ford Health System
Detroit, Michigan

Graham W. Long
Oakland University
William Beaumont
School of Medicine
Royal Oak, Michigan

Joyce Lu
Spectrum Health
Michigan State University College of Human
Medicine
Grand Rapids, Michigan

Junaid Malek
Department of Surgery
Massachusetts General Hospital
Boston, Massachusetts

M. Ashraf Mansour
Department of Surgery
Spectrum Health
Michigan State University College of Human
Medicine
Ann Arbor, Michigan

Hazel L. Marecki
Division of Vascular and Endovascular Surgery
University of Massachusetts Medical School
Worcester, Massachusetts

Matthew T. Major
William Beaumont Hospital
Royal Oak, Michigan

Imani McElroy
Department of Surgery
Massachusetts General Hospital
Boston, Massachusetts

Mia Miller
University of Minnesota
Minneapolis, Minnesota

Farah Mohammad
Henry Ford Hospital
Detroit, Michigan

Jahan Mohebali
Vascular and Endovascular Surgery
Massachusetts General Hospital
Harvard Medical School
Boston, Massachusetts

Robert G. Molnar
Michigan Vascular Center
Department of Surgery
Michigan State University
and
McLaren Regional Medical Center
Flint, Michigan

Dipankar Mukherjee
INOVA Fairfax Hospital
Falls Church, Virginia

William Oppat
Ascension Providence Hospital
Wayne State University
Detroit, Michigan

Chloé A. Powell
Department of Surgery
Section of Vascular Surgery
University of Michigan
Ann Arbor, Michigan

Mahmood K. Razavi
Department of Clinical Trials
St. Joseph Heart and Vascular Center
Orange, California

Vikram Reddy
Henry Ford Macomb Hospital
Clinton Township, Michigan

Kaitlyn Rountree
General Surgery
Henry Ford Macomb Hospital
Clinton Township, Michigan

Samuel Schwartz
Division of Vascular and Endovascular Surgery
Massachusetts General Hospital
Boston, Massachusetts

Mel J. Sharafuddin
Division of Vascular Surgery
University of Iowa Hospitals and Clinics
Iowa City, Iowa

Kush Sharma
Department of Vascular Surgery at Spectrum Health
Michigan State University College of Human Medicine
Grand Rapids, Michigan

Jessica P. Simons
Division of Vascular and Endovascular Surgery
University of Massachusetts Medical School
Worcester, Massachusetts

Renganaden Sooppan
Division of Vascular Surgery and Endovascular Therapy
Department of Surgery
The Johns Hopkins Hospital
Baltimore, Maryland

Jordan R. Stern
Division of Vascular and Endovascular Surgery
Stanford University School of Medicine
Stanford, California

David H. Stone
Geisel School of Medicine at Dartmouth
Section of Vascular Surgery
Dartmouth-Hitchcock Medical Center
Lebanon, New Hampshire

Bjoern D. Suckow
Geisel School of Medicine
Section of Vascular Surgery
Dartmouth-Hitchcock Medical Center
Lebanon, New Hampshire

Truc M. Ta
Maine Medical Center
Portland, Maine

Adam Tanious
Department of Surgery
Division of Vascular and Endovascular Surgery
Massachusetts General Hospital
Boston, Massachusetts

Robert W. Thompson
Center for Thoracic Outlet Syndrome
Washington University and Barnes-Jewish Hospital
St. Louis, Missouri

Michael Trpkovski
Vascular and Interventional Radiology
Henry Ford Macomb Hospital
Clinton Township, Michigan

Mitchell R. Weaver
Division of Vascular Surgery
Henry Ford Hospital
Detroit, Michigan

1

Preoperative risk assessment

JUNAID MALEK AND IMANI MCELROY

As the prevalence of vascular disease increases within the population, one can expect a rise in the number of vascular interventions performed with a subsequent increase in the absolute number of complications that occur. Negative outcomes after vascular interventions can be categorized into three general categories: systemic, nonvascular, and vascular, and occur in direct proportion to the severity of patient comorbidities and complexity of the procedure.[1] Vascular procedures can be stratified into emergent, urgent, and elective, and each level carries a different level of risk for the patients. Emergent procedures usually involve the arterial circulation and can include hemorrhage from aneurysm rupture or trauma, thromboembolic events leading to acute ischemia of the limbs or visceral organs, and malperfusion secondary to dissection of the arterial wall. Patients who require urgent procedures can present with venous thromboembolic events, stroke in evolution, symptomatic aneurysms, and infected extremities that require amputation or drainage. Both emergent and urgent problems limit the surgeon's ability to perform an adequate preoperative risk assessment and medial optimization, and, in these cases, a thorough history and physical in addition to optimization of medical comorbidities is ideal though may not always be feasible. Indeed, for these patients, the bulk of medical management occurs after completion of the procedure and is aimed at managing comorbidities rather than risk factor reduction and optimization. For patients undergoing elective vascular surgery, the best outcomes are enjoyed when the patient is medically optimized and operative risk is minimized. One strategy for achieving this goal is discussed in this chapter.

INITIAL WORKUP

For patients who do not require urgent or emergent interventions, a thorough history and physical should be performed with particular focus on significant cardiac, pulmonary, renal, endocrine, neurologic, vascular, or hematologic history. An understanding of the patient's activities of daily living, degree of independence, and exercise tolerance is critical. The cardiac history should take special note of any prior interventions, review of any previous electrocardiograms (ECG), echocardiograms, and/or any stress testing that may be available. A preoperative ECG should be performed within 90 days of any elective procedures. Noninvasive stress testing is recommended for any patients with significant clinical risk factors such as coronary artery disease, congestive heart failure, diabetes, or chronic renal insufficiency.

Many vascular patients have some history of smoking with resultant underlying lung disease, so it is important to have a good understanding of the patient's baseline pulmonary functional status prior to any major procedure. The use of bronchodilators or need for home oxygen should be noted. Basic chemistries should be reviewed to evaluate for any underlying renal dysfunction, and any history of renal replacement therapy or transplant should be noted. A recent A1c should also be obtained given the relationship between postoperative complications and poor glycemic control. A thorough social history should also be obtained to evaluate for any lifestyle modifications such as smoking cessation and alcohol or drug misuse.

The history should also include any previous vascular interventions that the patient has undergone, including a review of previous operative notes. The identification of scars can help give insight into previous vascular procedures, which can be particularly helpful in patients who present without documentation or are unable to give a full surgical history. A baseline pulse exam should also be performed, and the absence of pedal pulses should lead to arterial noninvasive testing of the lower extremities. Any neurologic deficits should also be noted. Finally, a review of any hematologic disorders within the patient and immediate family should be identified as it could change management of anticoagulation status in the perioperative period.

PERIOPERATIVE IMAGING

The best imaging study for evaluation of specific vascular disease processes is addressed in their respective chapters. Indeed, the importance of obtaining appropriate perioperative imaging cannot be overemphasized as it provides insight into the degree of vascular disease, identifies variant anatomy, and is the first step toward avoiding perioperative complications through sound case planning. Computed tomography (CT) angiography is most useful for rapid identification of suspected pathology of the aorta and major vessels of the neck, thorax, and abdomen. However, it may have limitations in its ability to accurately characterize the patency or severity of stenosis of the smaller and more peripheral vessels. MR angiography is another option for patients with a contrast allergy or higher creatinine as vessel definition can be obtained without contrast with time of flight imaging. However, MR angiography can be time consuming and is contraindicated in patients that have certain metallic implants.[3] Ultrasonography is a useful adjunct for evaluation of vascular pathology of the neck and extremities that can be used for surveillance and case planning. In addition, it can provide rapid evaluation of pseudoaneurysm, dissection, thrombosis, or stenosis.

CARDIAC COMORBIDITIES

The extent to which the heart must be evaluated prior to a vascular procedure is dependent upon the overall procedural risk, patient risk factors, and their exercise capacity. For instance, a patient who is undergoing a low risk percutaneous intervention may be sufficiently cleared by a history that is negative for chest pain and shortness of breath while those who will require general anesthesia at minimum will require a 12-lead electrocardiogram prior to surgery. In addition, patients who are undergoing high risk surgeries, including open aortic repair and lower extremity bypass, and any patient with significant cardiac disease, including unstable angina, known arrhythmias, severe valvular disease, or decompensated heart failure should be evaluated by a cardiologist prior to any major vascular procedure (Figure 1.1). It is also recommended that patients with evidence of myocardial infarction, unstable angina, or stable angina involving the left main coronary artery or three vessel disease undergo coronary revascularization prior to any major elective endovascular intervention.[2] When patients who have reconstructible coronary disease who need more urgent (within 12 months) intervention, existing coronary artery disease should be treated with balloon angioplasty or bare metal stent placement followed by dual antiplatelet therapy for 4 to 6 weeks. If patients are unable to wait 4–6 weeks, then it is possible to undergo intervention at 30 days post stenting. Beta-blockade, when medically mandated, should be initiated well before surgery and should be continued in the perioperative period.

PULMONARY COMORBIDITIES

Pulmonary complications are common after major vascular procedures, especially those involving a thoracic or thoracoabdominal incision. Active smokers are counseled to stop smoking for at least 2 weeks prior to moderate and high-risk procedures to decrease the risk of pulmonary complications. However, the risk continues to decrease with longer abstinence from tobacco use. Indeed, patients are at highest risk for complications within the first 2 months of quitting smoking and their risk becomes similar to a non-smoker after 6 months. For patients with long standing tobacco use, chronic obstructive pulmonary disease (COPD), or poor baseline respiratory function (unable to walk 1 flight of stairs), preoperative pulmonary function tests are recommended in addition to obtaining a baseline arterial blood gas. These patients should also be started on pulmonary bronchodilators for at least 2 weeks prior to intervention.[2]

CHRONIC RENAL INSUFFICIENCY

Non-dialysis dependent patients with chronic renal insufficiency should receive adequate preoperative hydration. For patients at risk of contrast-induced nephropathy, we recommend pre-hydration with normal saline or 5% dextrose/sodium bicarbonate. For patients with an estimated glomerular filtration rate (eGFR) of < 60 mL/min, withholding metformin is recommended at the time of contrast administration. In addition, for those with an eGFR of < 45 mL/min, metformin should be held for at least 48 hours prior to contrast administration. Euglycemia can be maintained with an insulin sliding scale in the peri-procedure period. Ideally a patient's glycemic control should be optimized prior to admission to the hospital to decrease the risk of perioperative glycemic crisis as well as the risk of wound complications.

MAINTENANCE MEDICATIONS

As with most other surgical procedures, angiotensin-converting enzyme (ACE) inhibitors and angiotensin receptor blockers should be held during the perioperative period. If patients are already on beta-blocker therapy, it is recommended they continue therapy throughout the perioperative period. Initiating beta-blocker therapy immediately before intervention should be avoided until

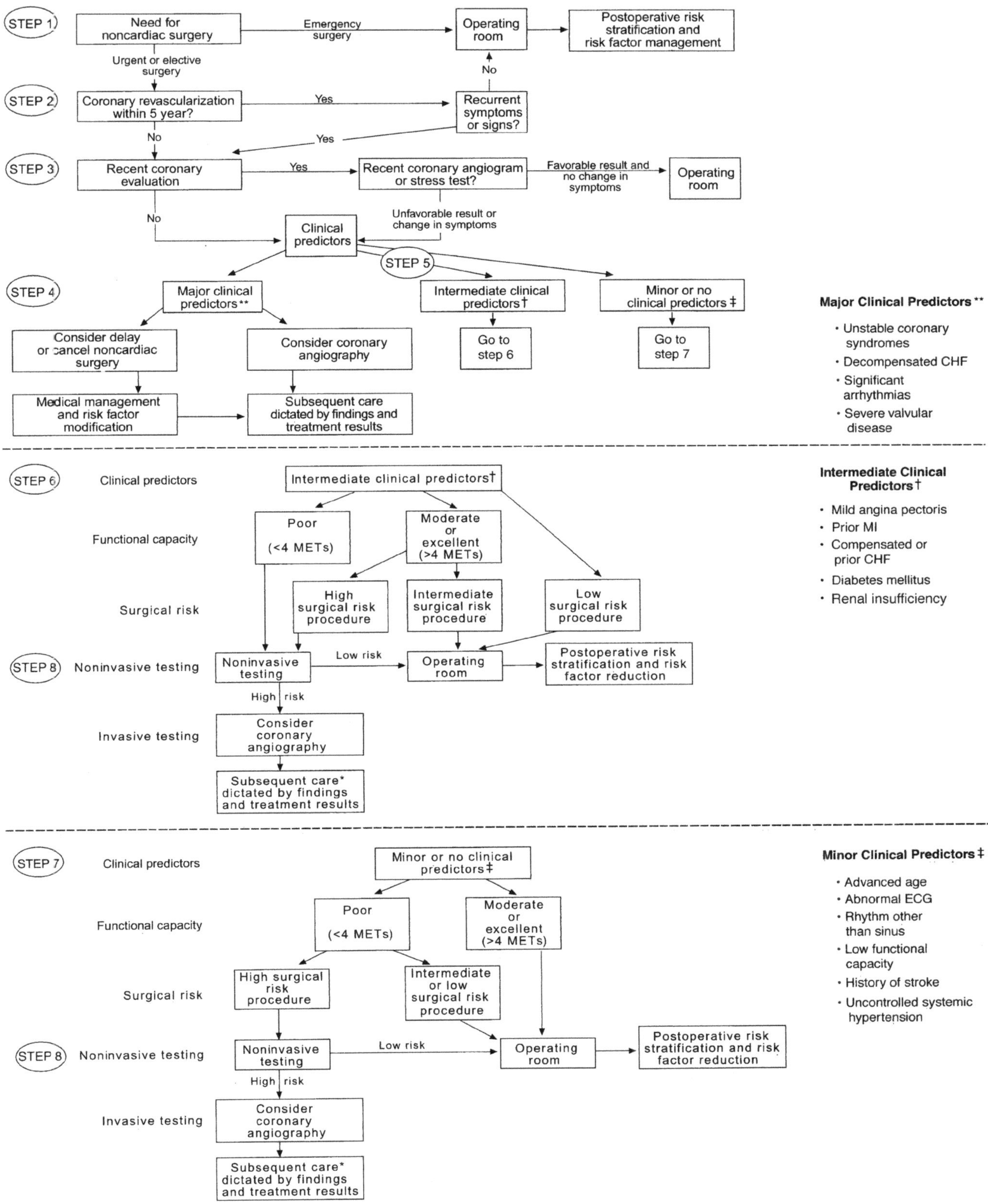

Figure 1.1 Approach to preoperative cardiac assessment. (Eagle, KA et. al. "ACC/AHA Guideline Update for Perioperative Cardiovascular Evaluation for Noncardiac Surgery – Executive Summary" Journal of the American College of Cardiology. 2002; 39(30):542–53.)

it is determined that the patient is tolerant of therapy. Initiating beta-blocker medications for the sole purpose of reducing aneurysm expansion or rupture is not recommended.[2] Moreover, there is little evidence to support the use of statins to reduce aneurysm expansion or risk of rupture in the surveillance period, and thus considerations for use should be strictly for cardiac benefit.[2] Despite evidence of decreased rates of aneurysm expansion in mouse models with the use of ACE inhibitors and angiotensin receptor blockers, this has not been replicated in human populations, and thus empiric administration during the surveillance period is not recommended.[2] Randomized controlled trials have shown there is no effect on aneurysmal expansion with the use of empiric azithromycin and doxycycline, and thus such treatment is currently not recommended.[2] In summary, patients should be maintained on their maintenance therapies for management of comorbid conditions during surveillance periods. Standard preoperative guidelines should be followed in stopping medications (e.g., ACEi/ARBs), and there are currently no recommendations for initiation of empiric therapies.

HEMATOLOGIC OPTIMIZATION

In the event of thrombotic complications, heparin is often the first-line agent for management. Heparin and other anticoagulants help reduce the risk of additional thrombus formation. Initial dosing begins with a 5,000 unit intravenous bolus that is followed by a maintenance dose of 30,000–40,000 units per 24 hours by continuous intravenous infusion.[4] Patients with a known history of heparin-induced thrombocytopenia (HIT) or those who develop HIT should be anticoagulated with alternative medications. Argatroban is the most commonly used agent in these circumstances.[5] For patients on therapeutic anticoagulation such as Coumadin, heparin, low molecular weight heparin (LMWH), or thrombin inhibitors, reversal prior to an intervention may be necessary in the emergent setting. Both heparin and LMWH are readily reversible with protamine sulfate. Vitamin K antagonists like warfarin can be reversed with the administration of oral or intravenous vitamin K or prothrombin complex concentrate. Fresh frozen plasma (FFP) may also be used to correct coagulopathy. However, there are several important limitations with such administration. Most commonly, use of FFP can be associated with risk of hypervolemia in addition to limitations with lowering the International Normalized Ratio (INR) below 1.5. For these reasons, it is often used as an adjunct in the acute setting. Thrombin inhibitors like dibigatran (Pradaxa) can be reversed with idarucizumab (Praxbind), while rivaroxaban/apixaban can be reversed with recombinant factor Xa (Andexxa).[6]

Patients taking antiplatelet agents such as aspirin or clopidogrel may benefit from discontinuation of these agents prior to intervention, though one must carefully weigh the risks of bleeding versus thrombosis or embolism. As platelet inhibition can continue for days, urgent correction can be achieved in the acute setting with administration of desmopressin or platelet transfusion. The use of desmopressin and cryoprecipitate can also be helpful in patients with underlying renal dysfunction or failure, as uremia can result in significant platelet dysfunction.[7]

Given the high rate of comorbidities in most vascular patients as well as the nature of the interventions, it is not uncommon for patients to require transfusion of blood products in the perioperative period. For patients presenting with chronic iron deficiency anemia, if time allows, iron supplementation is advantageous during the preoperative period.[8] The use of intraoperative cell-saver is becoming increasingly common as an adjunct to minimize the need for allogeneic red cell transfusion. It also has been proven to be a safe and cost effective way to reduce burden on limited resources when used with the appropriate indications.[9] In the perioperative setting, most patients can be managed with standard transfusion triggers for hemoglobin < 7. The main exception to this rule are patients with significant cardiac history, who should be maintained with hemoglobin > 8.[10] If significant intraoperative blood loss is encountered during the procedure, a massive transfusion protocol should be initiated with resuscitation carried out in a 1:1:1 or 2:1:1 ratio per individual institution protocol.[11] Last, for patients that are chronically thrombocytopenic (platelets < 150,000) prior to intervention, hematology may be consulted for assistance in perioperative management.[2]

REFERENCES

1. Diener H., et al. Postoperative Komplikationen in Der Gefäßchirurgie. Der Chirurg. 2009; 80(9): 814–826. doi:10.1007/s00104-009-1692-1.
2. Chaikof E, Dalman R, Eskandari M, Jackson B, Lee W, Mansour M et al. The Society for Vascular Surgery Practice Guidelines on the Care of Patients With an Abdominal Aortic Aneurysm. Journal of Vascular Surgery [Internet]. 2018 [cited 6 May 2020]; 67(1): 2–77.e2. Available from: https://www.jvascsurg.org/article/S0741-5214(17)32369-8/fulltext
3. Wu, Timothy. "Computed Tomography Angiography (CTA) and Magnetic Resonance Angiography (MRA) Tests." *CTA and MRA Tests | Society for Vascular Surgery*, vascular.org/patient-resources/vascular-tests/computed-tomography-angiography-cta-and-magnetic-resonance.
4. Raskob GE, et al. Heparin Therapy for Venous Thrombosis and Pulmonary Embolism. Blood Reviews. 1988; 2(4): 251–258. doi:10.1016/0268-960x(88)90014-8.

5. Ahmed I, et al. Heparin-Induced Thrombocytopenia: Diagnosis and Management Update. Postgraduate Medical Journal. 2007; 83(983). 575–582. doi:10.1136/pgmj.2007.059188.
6. Thomas S, Michael M. The Reversal of Anticoagulation in Clinical Practice. Clinical Medicine. 2018; 18(4). 314–319. doi:10.7861/clinmedicine.18-4-314.
7. Yeung LYY, et al. Surgeon's Guide to Anticoagulant and Antiplatelet Medications Part Two: Antiplatelet Agents and Perioperative Management of Long-Term Anticoagulation. Trauma Surgery & Acute Care Open. 2016; 1(1). doi:10.1136/tsaco-2016-000022.
8. American Society of Anesthesiologists Task Force on Perioperative Blood Management. Practice Guidelines for Perioperative Blood Management. Anesthesiology. 2015; 122(2): 241–275. doi:10.1097/aln.0000000000000463.
9. Esper SA, Waters JH. Intra-operative Cell Salvage: A Fresh Look at the Indications and Contraindications. Blood Transfusion = Trasfusione del sangue. 2011; 9(2): 139–47. doi:10.2450/2011.0081-10
10. Franchini M, et al. Red Blood Cell Transfusion Policy: A Critical Literature Review. Blood Transfusion = Trasfusione del sangue. 2017; 15(4): 307–317. doi:10.2450/2017.0059-17.
11. Patil V, Shetmahajan M. Massive Transfusion and Massive Transfusion Protocol. Indian Journal of Anaesthesia. 2014; 58(5): 590–5. doi:10.4103/0019-5049.144662.

SUGGESTED READINGS

Chaikof E, Dalman R, Eskandari M, Jackson B, Lee W, Mansour M et al. The Society for Vascular Surgery practice guidelines on the care of patients with an abdominal aortic aneurysm. Journal of Vascular Surgery. 2018; 67(1):2–77.e2.

Zhan. HT, Purcell ST, Bush RL. Preoperative Optimization of the Vascular Surgery Patient. Vascular Health Risk and Management. 2015; 11: 379–385.

2

Systemic complications following vascular reconstruction

SRIHARI K. LELLA AND MARK F. CONRAD

Most vascular surgery procedures are classified as moderate to high risk regardless of individual patient factors. However, with the added preoperative medical comorbidities that are quite common in this population, operative risk for an individual patient can rise substantially. In addition, the intraoperative flow of the procedure and condition of surrounding tissues can have a significant impact on the postoperative course and development of complications. As a result, it is important for vascular surgeons to anticipate the possible negative outcomes for a given procedure, triage patients to the appropriate care unit, and institute measures to reduce the risk of postoperative complications.

The most appropriate level of care for patients after vascular surgery is determined by a number of factors including their medical comorbidities, the complexity of the procedure, intraoperative factors such as ischemic time and blood loss, and, their immediate perioperative acuity. There are several scoring systems that have been developed to assist in the decision making for immediate postoperative destination. However, variation exists in local practice patterns, and the admission criteria for the intensive care unit (ICU) vary based upon hospital acuity. This makes it challenging to create a universal guide for appropriate triage after vascular surgery. Despite this, there are certain high-risk procedures, such as open aortic aneurysm repair, that always require a higher level of postoperative management and should routinely be admitted to the ICU directly from the operating room.

Some hospitals have developed step-down units (SDU) that act as a bridge between the ICU and floor where certain patients who do not require ICU resources may go for close monitoring. Selective admission of patients to these units can reduce the number of utilized resources without significantly increasing mortality. Indeed, at some high volume centers with protocolled pathways, high-risk surgical procedures such as open infrarenal abdominal aortic aneurysm repair (AAA) can be managed in a step-down unit rather than an ICU setting.[1] Lawlor et al. showed that direct ICU admission after open infrarenal AAA repair was decreased by up to 90% if strict criteria were used for ICU admission.[2] This included patients who required continued ventilator support, suffered significant perioperative cardiac ischemia or arrhythmias, sustained significant perioperative hypotension, had transfusion requirements > 3 L, or were hypothermic (< 35°C).[2]

Importantly, unplanned admission to the ICU of postsurgical patients may sometimes be necessary due to unexpected or adverse events. Patients who required an unplanned ICU admission, when compared to patients with direct ICU admission, were shown to have a greater severity of illness on ICU admission, longer ICU length of stay, increased requirements for ventilation and other organ support, and higher risk of perioperative and long-term mortality.[3,4] While surgeons may have little control over these unforeseen events, the proper triaging of patients can help avoid unnecessary healthcare utilization and provide the intensive monitoring and care for the patients who require it.

Once a patient has been triaged to the appropriate setting for postoperative care, they can begin the process of recovery from surgery. Unfortunately, vascular patients are inherently at higher risk for complications even after minor procedures. The remainder of this chapter addresses common complications seen after vascular surgery by system.

NEUROLOGIC

PAIN CONTROL

Postoperative pain control can be difficult to gauge in critically ill patients, especially when they are sedated and/or intubated. Historically, postoperative pain has been poorly controlled with prior studies showing that it was inadequately managed in as high as 80% of patients.[5] This, of course, is highly dependent upon the extent of surgery performed and type of analgesia used. Other independent predictors of severe postoperative pain are younger age, female sex, preoperative pain, and incision size.[6] Pain management is important because inadequate postoperative pain control can drive a number of negative outcomes. For instance, there are a range of organ systems that can be compromised by acute, inadequately managed pain, including cardiovascular (myocardial ischemia/infarction), pulmonary (hypoventilation, pneumonia), gastrointestinal (decreased motility with nausea/vomiting), renal (urinary retention and oliguria), and overall immune function.[7–10] These complications can often be avoided and have been shown to increase hospital length of stay with a resultant increase in healthcare costs.[8] Finally, early inadequate pain control can have a negative impact on patient physical functioning, recovery, and quality of life, and leads to an increased risk of developing chronic postoperative pain.[11–14]

Recently there has been significant progress in the understanding of this complex topic, and a number of strategies have been developed for appropriate postoperative analgesia (see Figure 2.1). In general, for awake, non-sedated patients, patient-controlled analgesia (PCA) is preferred to the intermittent breakthrough pain control method. When able, use of non-opioid analgesia has also been shown to be effective. This can include NSAIDs, N-methyl-D-aspartate (NMDA)-receptor antagonist (e.g., ketamine), and local and regional anesthesia (e.g., lidocaine and epidural), among others.[15,16] This thinking differs from some areas of medicine where poly-pharmacy is avoided by maximizing the dose of one medication before adding another. For postoperative pain, it is better to use lower doses of several medications with different mechanisms of action than to escalate dosing of a single drug. Through this type of multimodal approach to pain control, there is the potential for decreased need for opiates with a resultant reduction in their risk of side effects from prolonged use (Figure 2.1).

DELIRIUM

Given that the majority of vascular surgery patients are over 65-years of age, delirium is a common postoperative complication that is often overlooked. Studies have shown that the incidence is as high as 80–90%, depending on the patient population, operations performed, and overall clinical stress experienced by the patient.[17] Several risk factors that have been associated with postoperative delirium include: older age (> 65-years), baseline dementia or other forms of cognitive impairment, poor vision or hearing, poor preoperative functional status, the presence of infection, and multiple significant co-morbidities (see Figure 2.2).[18,19] Additionally, the operative stress can be an additive risk for developing delirium.[20]

There are three types of delirium: hypoactive, hyperactive, and mixed. Hypoactive delirium is the most common of the three, with some studies reporting it to be two-thirds as common as the other two presentations combined.[21] This problem often goes unrecognized because the patient may show a quiet, calm, and non-disruptive demeanor. After the diagnosis of delirium is made, the Mini-Mental State Examination or the Confusion Assessment Method-Intensive Care Unit can be used to rule out organic causes.[22,23] This includes laboratory evaluation, a workup for common infectious, medication review, and potential imaging if warranted.[24] If an organic cause is found, then targeted treatment can be implemented (Figure 2.2).

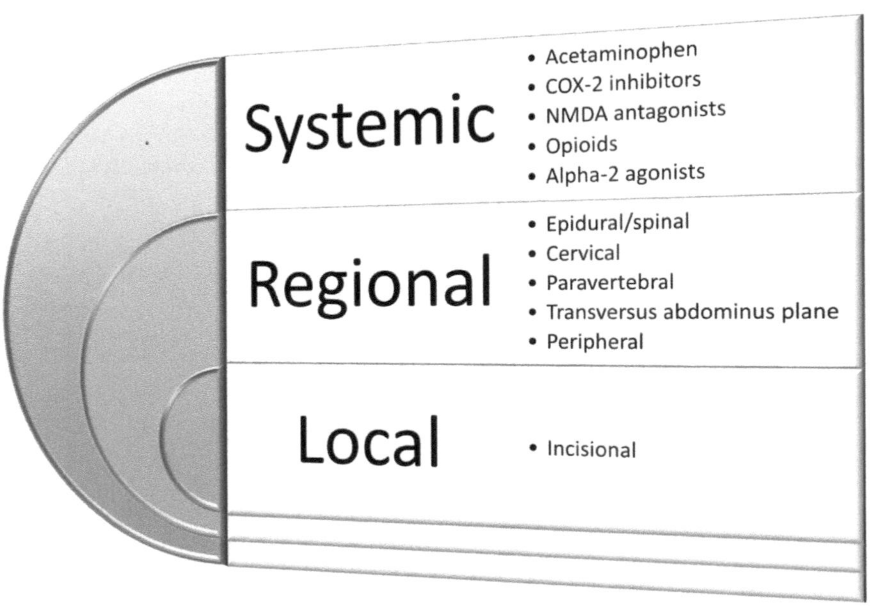

Figure 2.1 Multimodal approach to pain control.

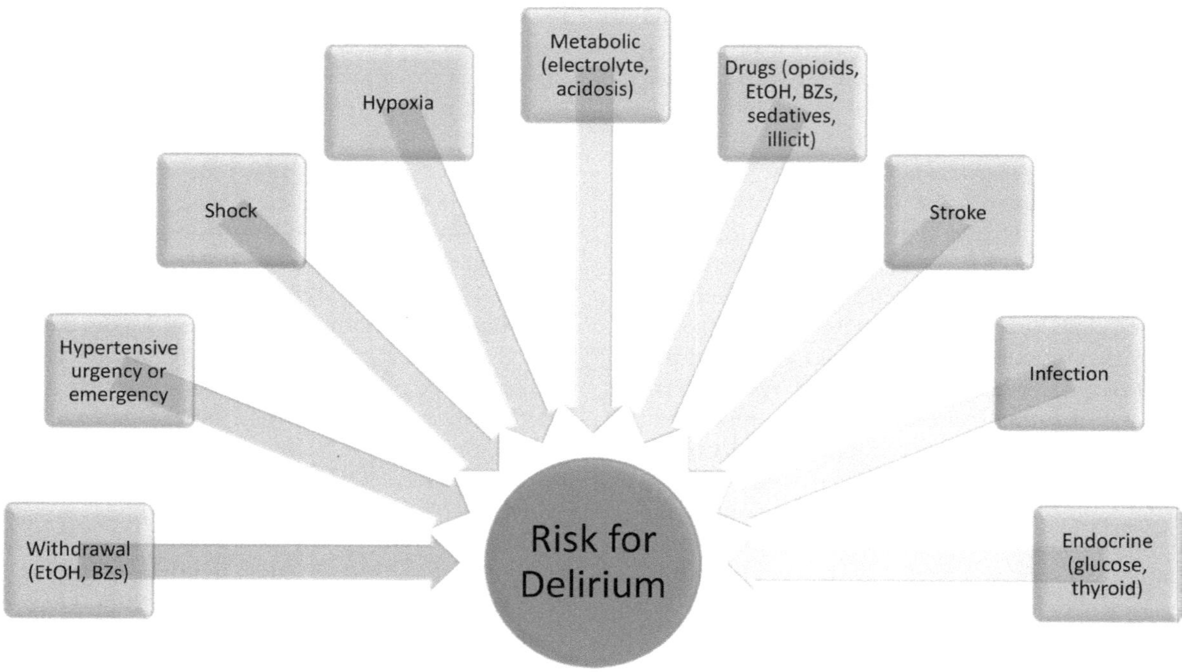

Figure 2.2 Causes of delirium. EtOH – alcohol; BZs – benzodiazepines.

However, nonspecific postoperative delirium is often more difficult to correct. Prevention of this begins in the operating room with maintenance of hemodynamic stability, providing adequate tissue oxygenation, and limiting acidosis, all of which can be difficult in select vascular surgical operations.[25] Postoperative preventive measures that have been shown to reduce delirium include: repeated orientation to surroundings and care team, uninterrupted night time sleep, early mobilization with daily ambulation, removal of catheters and lines when appropriate, and visual/hearing protocol for easy access to visual/hearing aids.[26] With acute agitation and/or with disruption of care, chemical and non-chemical restraints may be necessary. Recognition and treatment of postoperative delirium is critical as it could result in further perioperative complications, longer hospital length of stay, and higher mortality.[24,27]

CARDIOVASCULAR

MYOCARDIAL ISCHEMIA/INFARCTION

The patient's cardiac evaluation should begin preoperatively with variable workup from an electrocardiogram (EKG) to a stress test and/or left heart catheterization depending on the patient's severity of symptoms and the expected degree of stress from the type of operation. In urgent/emergent situations, preoperative optimization generally cannot be performed and related complications are dealt with as they present.

Advanced age, presence of angina (currently or prior), and a history of cardiac or cerebral events were found to be the most important clinical predictors of perioperative myocardial infarction (MI).[28–32] In addition, patients who

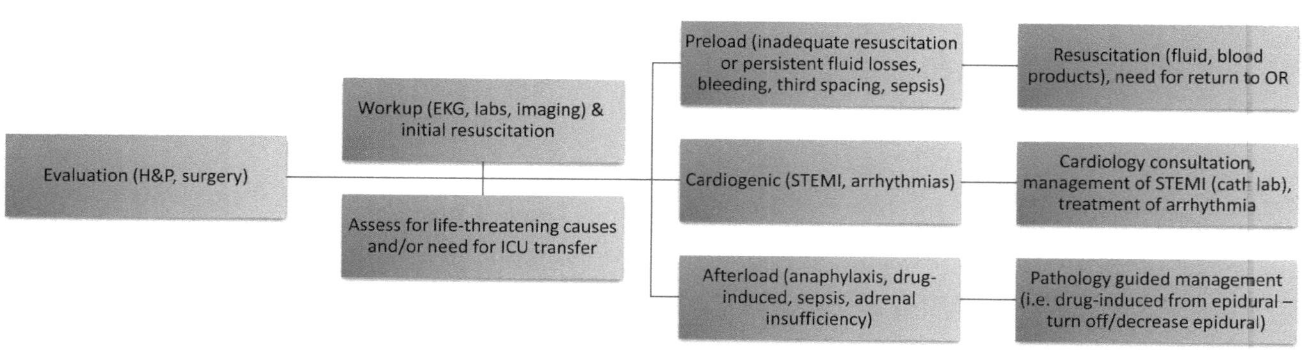

Figure 2.3 Evaluation and management of postoperative hypotension. H&P – history and physical; EKG – electrocardiogram; ICU – intensive care unit; OR – operating room; STEMI – ST segment elevation myocardial infarction.

have a positive dobutamine stress echocardiogram are at high risk for adverse cardiac outcomes.[28,33–37] Indeed, patients who have a new wall motion abnormality, generally considered a hallmark of myocardial ischemia, had up to a 40% increased risk of cardiac death or myocardial infarction within 30 days of surgery.[36,38,39] Studies have also shown that perioperative beta-adrenergic blockade can reduce the risk of 30-day complications in patients with new wall motion abnormalities to the levels of those observed in patients without wall motion abnormalities.[40,41] However, this alone is not entirely sufficient, and some patients will benefit from coronary revascularization.

Myocardial ischemia presents in a variety of ways. Patients may exhibit symptoms of chest pain, shortness of breath, diaphoresis, nausea and vomiting among others. A patient who experiences an MI event intraoperatively or while sedated may not show any outward symptoms. In that event, there is a high index of suspicion secondary to episodic hypotensive episodes or EKG changes, and the patient would need to undergo cardiac evaluation with serial cardiac enzymes such as creatine kinase-MB isozyme and cardiac-specific troponin I. This workup is important even in a seemingly asymptomatic patient as Kim et al. showed that patients with elevated troponin I levels postoperatively, even in the absence of clinical symptoms, had an increased risk of perioperative MI and 6 months mortality compared to those who did not.[42]

Patients who experience a postoperative MI may or may not have EKG changes such as ST-segment elevations. These changes in the EKG are thought to be driven by the presence of thrombotic occlusion of the coronary arteries from plaque rupture, while those without EKG changes should not have had a thrombotic event. Indeed, the management strategy for these patients differs based upon the EKG findings and cardiology should be involved early. For patients with an ST-segment elevation myocardial infarction (STEMI), treatment begins with aspirin, supplemental oxygen, sublingual of intravenous nitroglycerin (permitting hemodynamics), oral or intravenous beta-blockers, morphine as the analgesia of choice or other anxiolytics, and urgent/emergent reperfusion therapy.[43] Angiotensin converting enzyme inhibitor or angiotensin receptor blockers should be initiated within 24 hours of the event, and a high intensity statin should also be started if patient is not already on it.[43] Reperfusion strategies include percutaneous coronary intervention (PCI), fibrinolytic therapy, or emergent surgical revascularization. PCI is generally the preferred option when compared to fibrinolysis as it has been shown to have lower short-term mortality rates, less nonfatal reinfarction, and less risk of hemorrhagic stroke.[43] In addition, fibrinolytic therapy is contraindicated in many post-surgical patients but can be considered in select cases. Anticoagulation is generally used as an ancillary adjunct to PCI, but the method of dosing (bolus vs hourly rate) should be based upon the bleeding risk of the patient. Urgent/emergent coronary artery bypass grafting (CABG) should be considered for patients who have failed or are not candidates for PCI and fibrinolytic therapy.[43] Post-infarction complications such as ventricular septal rupture or papillary muscle rupture with mitral valve insufficiency also mandate surgical repair, at which time CABG may be performed.[43] Non-ST-segment elevation myocardial infarction (NSTEMI) is generally medically managed as above, although revascularization can be considered on an individual patient basis depending on the extent and complexity of coronary artery disease as well as other medical comorbidities (Figure 2.3).[44]

ATRIAL FIBRILLATION

Arrhythmias are common in the postoperative setting. These can range from mild sinus brady or tachycardia to significant ventricular fibrillation. Causes of such arrhythmias include: electrolyte imbalances, sudden fluid shifts, and myocardial ischemia. Prompt recognition is necessary to implement correction measures to counteract and prevent recurrence.

Atrial fibrillation (AF) is one of the more common postoperative arrhythmic complications, with an incidence nearing 10% after open aortic operations.[45] Factors that place patients at higher risk for AF include older age, hypertension, cardiac diseases (e.g., coronary artery disease, valvular heart disease, and cardiomyopathies), previous history of atrial fibrillation, and chronic obstructive pulmonary disease (COPD).[45,46] When AF occurs, there is a loss of the atrial kick during systole and an increase in the ventricular rate without full ventricular contractions that leads to a significant reduction in left ventricular filling.[47] Symptomatic patients will endorse chest palpitations, lightheadedness, fatigue, and shortness of breath.[47] However, in many instances, AF is asymptomatic and identified through an abnormal pulse examination.

Treatment centers around controlling the heart rate and reducing the risk of embolic events.[47] While there is still controversy regarding rate control versus rhythm control, no mortality benefit has been seen in patients with a solitary rhythm control strategy.[47] As such, for hemodynamically stable patients, restoration of a normal heart rate with beta-blockers, calcium channel blockers, amiodarone, and digoxin is often implemented.[48] In hemodynamically unstable patients, electrical cardioversion is the treatment of choice. As atrial fibrillation persists, there is a high risk of intra-cardiac thrombus development, which most frequently occurs in the left atrial appendage where blood can be static.[47] If atrial fibrillation persists for longer than 48 hours, anticoagulation with intravenous heparin should be considered while in the hospital and oral anticoagulation for outpatient long-term management.

HEMODYNAMIC MANAGEMENT

Postoperative hypotension should be avoided as it will result in end-organ ischemia. In the critically ill patient, this can manifest as myocardial ischemia, stroke, mesenteric ischemia, renal failure, paraplegia and graft thrombosis.[49] When a patient develops hypotension, it is important to determine the root cause as this will drive therapy (see Figure 2.3). In the immediate perioperative period, sudden hypotension should prompt the surgeon to exclude bleeding as the primary cause. Indeed, if the patient does not respond appropriately to fluid resuscitation, there should be a low threshold for re-exploring the patient as delay in a bleeding patient will yield catastrophic results. While recommendations regarding postoperative blood pressure parameters will vary depending on the type of operation performed, typically mean arterial pressure (MAP) of at least 60 mm Hg is required to maintain adequate tissue perfusion. Fluid administration and vasopressors are the mainstay of therapy for these patients. The Frank-Starling curve must be considered when making decisions to administer fluids. If the patient is on the plateau or the downslope of the curve, fluids will cause edema with no improvement in the cardiac output.[50] Vasopressors should be used as needed for satisfactory perfusion. However, it is important to consider the fact that these are not without adverse effects and should be used cautiously in patients at risk for arrhythmias.[46] Additionally, when there is a concern for cardiogenic shock, inotropic support may be necessary for maintenance of cardiac output. In more severe instances with cardiogenic shock secondary to MI, further cardiac optimization may be necessary (as discussed above), and intra-aortic balloon pump or other forms of mechanical circulatory support may be required.

Postoperative hypertension may be caused by pain, hypothermia, hypoxia, hypercarbia, intravascular volume overload, and discontinuation of preoperative antihypertensive medications.[51] If left untreated, patients are at increased risk of developing myocardial infarction, cerebrovascular events, and bleeding.[52] After exclusion of the other causes, antihypertensive medications should be administered. Patients should resume their home antihypertensive medications or a hospital equivalent as soon as possible after surgery. If systolic blood pressure (SBP) remains elevated ≥ 180 and/or diastolic blood pressure ≥ 110, then further treatment is recommended to reduce the risk of hypertensive crisis. Intravenous short-acting medications are generally preferred in this instance. However, if the blood pressure remains persistently elevated, it can be controlled with a combination of an intravenous drip, increased dosing of prior oral medications, or the addition of ones. Once again, it is important to consider the potential adverse effects of the different medications and possible interactions when used concurrently with regard to the patients' history and surgery. It is also best to involve the patient's cardiologist or primary care provider (PCP) who has been managing their hypertension as medication needs may change after discharge and outpatient adjustment will be necessary.

PULMONARY

Postoperative pulmonary complications result in added morbidity and mortality of surgical patients. They can range from mild atelectasis to severe acute respiratory distress syndrome (ARDS), COPD exacerbation and pneumonia. Some type of pulmonary complication has been identified in up to 80% of postoperative patients depending on the definition of complication and type of surgery performed.[53] Risk factors for pulmonary issues include: advanced age, male gender, current or recent history of smoking, history of COPD, acuity of procedure, more complex operations, and higher American Society of Anesthesiologists classification.[54] Importantly, the reduction in lung volumes perioperatively as a result of both the surgical incision and the induction of general anesthesia renders the patient susceptible to the development of a variety of pulmonary complications.[55]

Hypoxemia can occur after major surgical insults due to an abnormal alveolar to arterial oxygen difference. The functional residual capacity of the lung reaches its lowest value in the postoperative period and may take up to a week to return to normal levels.[56] Poor pain control can lead to shallow breathing or splinting that will further impact the already reduced functional vital capacity, forced expiratory volume, and peak expiratory flow rate.[57] In addition, anesthetic agents may cause weakness or dis-coordination of the respiratory and abdominal muscles that can further depress respiratory function.[58] Indeed, respiratory control may be impaired for several weeks post-surgery, which may cause a blunted response to hypercapnic and hypoxic episodes.[59] The combination of the above factors and pre-existing pulmonary conditions places the patient in a vulnerable state that makes them more susceptible to postoperative pulmonary complications.

Acute respiratory failure can be caused by a problem with oxygenation that leads to hypoxemia, a problem with ventilation that leads to hypercapnia, or a combination of both. Management includes identification and correction of any underlying cause (e.g., pneumothorax, aspiration, airway occlusion). Hypoxemia is managed by increasing the positive end expiratory pressure (PEEP) and/or fraction of inspired oxygen (FiO_2). Improvement in minute ventilation by increasing the tidal volumes or respiratory rate will reduce the CO_2 retention seen in hypercapnia. With the persistence of respiratory failure and a significant underlying systemic inflammatory response, the patient may develop ARDS.

Controversy exists regarding the definition of ARDS, but the Berlin Definition significantly improved the

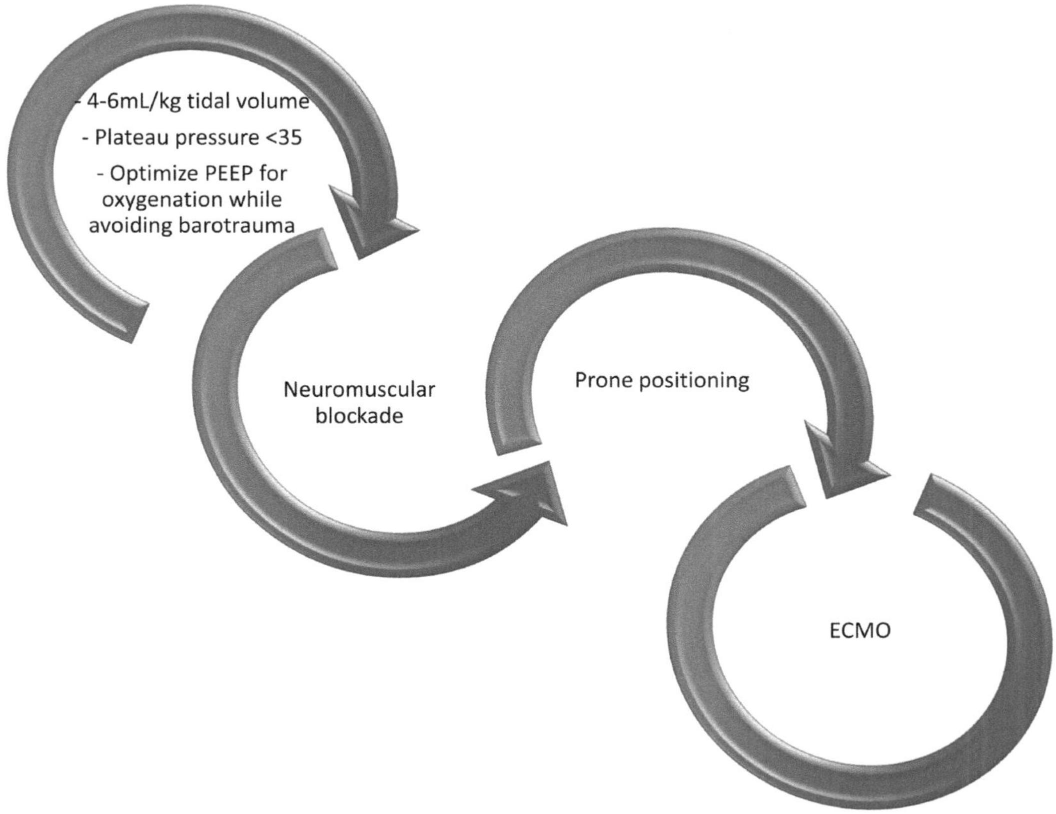

Figure 2.4 Stepwise management of acute respiratory distress syndrome (ARDS) presented in a cyclical fashion to emphasize the importance of regular assessment to escalate/de-escalate care. PEEP – positive end expiratory pressure; ECMO – extracorporeal membrane oxygenation.

predictive validity for mortality and is currently most often used. It includes acute onset within 1 week, bilateral lung opacities not explained by other causes seen on chest imaging, pulmonary edema with exclusion of cardiogenic and hydrostatic edema, and the severity of lung injury. This final parameter is graded based on the ratio of partial pressure of oxygen in arterial blood to FiO_2 and PEEP requirement ≥ 5 cm H_2O.[60] As the severity of ARDS worsens, there are increased ventilation requirements and mortality.[60] Management of ARDS revolves around protective lung ventilation with decreased tidal volumes (4–6 mL/kg) and limitation of plateau pressure (< 35 cm H_2O) allowing for maximization of alveolar recruitment and reducing inflammation (see Figure 2.4). Implementation of these strategies has shown to decrease the rate of barotrauma and reduce mortality (Figure 2.4).[61–63]

RENAL FAILURE

Renal impairment is frequently seen after major vascular surgical procedures. For instance, after open infrarenal abdominal aortic aneurysm repair, renal dysfunction (RD) has been shown to occur in as many as 1 in 5 patients postoperatively.[64] In the endovascular era, the vascular patient population is becoming older with more comorbidities and open procedures are becoming more complex, so it is likely that the incidence of postoperative RD after open aortic repair will continue to rise. RD can range from a mild increase in the patient's creatinine to complete kidney failure requiring dialysis. Patients who have preoperative chronic kidney disease have the highest risk of postoperative renal failure.[65] Other important risk factors include perioperative hypotension, prolonged renal ischemia, need for blood transfusion, use of iodinated contrast, and rhabdomyolysis.[66] Overall, the course of the surgical procedure has an enormous bearing over the risk of developing RD.[64,66–71] Patients who develop RD have been shown to have an increased risk of developing other organ dysfunction, with longer ICU lengths of stay and increased overall mortality.[64]

With acute renal ischemia, large accumulations of cytosolic and mitochondrial calcium develop that result in renal vasoconstriction, especially in the afferent arterioles of the glomerulus. Secondarily, the outer medulla of the kidney develops significant congestion with worsening of the hypoxia and a proposed resultant worsening of endothelial damage from increased oxidant injury. Following reperfusion, the proximal tubules lose their polarity and brush border. Reactive oxygen species develop with resulting cell death, and these dead cells are then shed into the tubular lumen. This creates the formation of casts that causes tubular obstruction and reduces the glomerular filtration rate (GFR).[72]

Prevention of postoperative RD begins preoperatively with appropriate planning to maximize renal protection. Patients who are deemed to be at high risk of RD should be given adequate intravenous fluid hydration prior to any procedure. Continued fluid resuscitation and adequate replacement of blood products intraoperatively and postoperatively is important to prevent transient hypotension and to support continued renal blood flow. Limiting renal warm ischemia time with open aortorenal procedures is also vital to decrease the renal metabolic requirements. While there is conflicting evidence, intraoperative use of mannitol with aortic cross clamping has been shown to improve urine flow rate, attenuate renal cortical blood flow reduction, and scavenge oxygen-free radicals.[73,74] Diuresis postoperatively, specifically with loop diuretics, is used in oliguric RD patients to improve volume overload and reduce accumulation of toxins. Additionally, dopamine has historically been used as a renal vasodilator to increase the renal perfusion and GFR.[75–77] However, dopamine has not been shown to reduce RD or death.[78] Another option is fenoldopam, a dopamine type 1 receptor agonist, that has specifically been shown to have a reno-protective effect during and after aortic cross-clamping.[79] Importantly, while theoretically calcium channel blockers should decrease the intracellular calcium accumulation in patients with acute renal ischemia, they can cause unwanted systemic vasodilation and hypotension and increase sympathetic tone by activating the renin-angiotensin system.[80] Finally, hemodialysis should be considered for patients with significant acidosis, electrolyte accumulation (e.g., hyperkalemia), volume overload, and uremic symptoms.

HEMATOLOGIC

BLEEDING

All vascular surgical procedures carry some risk of blood loss due to the nature of the operations and the common use of systemic anticoagulation. However, there are other patient-related factors that need to be considered prior to vascular procedures. Many vascular patients have a history of cardiovascular disease and are routinely on single or dual antiplatelet therapy or some form of chronic systemic anticoagulation. These medications must be identified and appropriately managed based upon the procedure. For example, many surgeons will stop clopidogrel for abdominal operations but will keep their patients on dual antiplatelet therapy for carotid or lower extremity interventions. Patients who present with some degree of preoperative renal impairment are also at higher risk of bleeding during a procedure as they may have some degree of platelet dysfunction from uremia. Finally, sustained intraoperative tissue injury and hypotension can also trigger an acute coagulopathy. Specifically, shock promotes coagulopathy due to activation of the immune and complement system, platelet degranulation, endothelial disruption, and increased activities of both thrombomodulin and protein C.[81–83] Indeed, tissue hypoperfusion and the resulting acidosis causes an impairment in coagulation factor complexes as well as a significant reduction in the production and activity of factors that promote clotting.[84]

Ensuring adequate hemostasis during the initial dissection is the first step towards reducing the risk of high-volume blood loss and need for transfusion. If heparin is used for anticoagulation, protamine may be used for reversal once the clamps have been removed and distal flow is restored. Additionally, for suture hole and anastomotic bleeding, a number of topical hemostatic agents are available. Importantly, for vascular trauma, a damage control approach is favored in the patients with significant coagulopathy, hypothermia, and acidosis.

Postsurgical bleeding assessment begins with a complete examination of the patient. Hemoglobin/hematocrit, prothrombin time/international normalized ratio (PT/INR), activated partial thromboplastin time (aPTT), and fibrin split products/fibrinogen levels are part of the basic lab testing performed for these patients. If there is a concern for further underlying coagulopathy that cannot be explained by the procedure or medication administration, additional workup for bleeding disorders should be considered (e.g., von Willebrand's disease, hemophilia, protein C/S deficiency). Depending on the stability of the patient and whether a clear source of the bleeding is known, further imaging can be pursued or the surgeon can return to the operating room for control of bleeding.

TRANSFUSION

The need for transfusion will vary based on the overall clinical status of the patient and the risk due to comorbidities. Restrictive transfusion strategies (hemoglobin 7 g/dL vs 10 g/dL) have become popular to decrease infection risk, and some have been shown to decrease blood requirements without increasing the 30-day mortality or rate of organ dysfunction.[85] Indeed, a recent Cochrane review of 19 trials showed similar results with an improved in-hospital mortality in patients who were transfusion restricted.[86] However, Fominskiy et al. performed a systematic review that focused on surgical and critically ill patients and found that perioperative patients had a lower all-cause mortality when a liberal transfusion strategy was utilized.[87] While evidence is conflicting, it is generally accepted that healthy patients with hemodynamic stability should not be transfused until their hemoglobin drops below 7 g/dL, but in higher risk patients, transfusion should be guided by the patient's degree of blood loss, presence of significant coronary artery disease, and signs of organ ischemia rather than adhering to restrictive protocols. In fact, the best transfusion threshold for such patients may be closer to 8–9 g/dL.

Platelet transfusion thresholds are not well defined in the surgical patient. There has not been a specific platelet count that consistently correlates with increased bleeding in surgical patients. While there is strong evidence for a 1:1 transfusion of platelets and red blood cells in trauma patients, there are no guidelines in the non-trauma surgical patients or those who are on antiplatelet therapy. Although currently the decision to transfuse platelets is dependent on the patient's risk factors and surgery as well as surgeon preference, stable non-bleeding patients are maintained above platelet counts of 10,000/mm^3. Patients with high risk of bleeding or who are actively bleeding are typically transfused to a level above 50,000/mm^3.

Similarly, guidelines for the administration of fresh frozen plasma (FFP) have not been well established in the surgical patient. FFP is commonly used for reversal of an elevated INR or when there is a known coagulation factor deficiency and no recombinant factor is available. In addition, it is accepted that massive transfusions of red blood cells, platelets, and FFP could cause fibrinogen deficiency with dilutional coagulopathy.[84] A systematic review comparing administration of fibrinogen concentrate vs FFP in the perioperative and massive trauma setting found FFP to have inconsistent outcomes while fibrinogen was shown to have consistently positive outcomes (blood loss, transfusion requirement, length of stay, and survival).[88] Specifically, three studies directly compared fibrinogen to FFP in surgical patients with perioperative bleeding requiring transfusion.[89–91] While the evidence is still insufficient to draw definitive conclusions, fibrinogen may be a safer and more effective alternative to FFP.

DEEP VENOUS THROMBOSIS

Deep venous thrombosis (DVT) is a common, preventable complication after surgery. Multiple studies have established the association between surgery and DVT. Historically, vascular surgery, and specifically aortic surgery, was thought to have a lower incidence of DVT due to the use of systemic heparin during the procedure. Indeed, perioperative prophylaxis against DVT in vascular patients has been controversial because of planned heparin use intraoperatively, which is believed to provide sufficient protection for development of DVT. There is also the concern that additional use of postoperative heparin or other forms of anticoagulation could increase the risk of hemorrhagic complications.

While large-scale data are limited, previous studies have reported that the incidence of DVT in vascular surgery patients is somewhere between 2–20%.[92–95] More recently, Aziz et al. showed that when compared to general surgical procedures, patients undergoing vascular procedures have a 1.5 times greater risk of developing a DVT during the postoperative period.[96] Despite the intraoperative anticoagulation, vascular surgery patients have multiple factors that predispose them to DVT development including: advanced age, higher number of comorbidities, limb ischemia, operative trauma, risk of venous injury, and long duration of operations.[96] As such, intraoperative anticoagulation is not necessarily protective against the development of postoperative DVT, and stricter guidelines should be used for prophylaxis.

HEPARIN-INDUCED THROMBOCYTOPENIA

Heparin-induced thrombocytopenia (HIT) is a rare condition that may be encountered in vascular surgery due to the common exposure to heparin in these patients. It involves the formation of immunoglobulin antibodies against heparin-platelet factor 4 complex. These complexes coat platelets, activate them, and cause them to be removed by macrophages. This results in thrombocytopenia. There is generally a 30–50% decline in platelet count 5–10 days after the initiation of heparin, but this isolated thrombocytopenia is not usually associated with significant bleeding complications. Indeed, with HIT, thrombosis is the more severe complication that leads to increased morbidity and mortality. Venous thrombotic complications are most common, but HIT may affect any vascular bed. Interestingly, not all patients with seropositivity progress to the severe form with thrombosis. Management of HIT-positive patients begins with immediate discontinuation of all heparin products (i.e., unfractionated and low molecular weight heparin) on suspicion. If there is a need for anticoagulation, direct thrombin inhibitors are generally the preferred agents. Vitamin K antagonists are avoided with the acute phase of thrombocytopenia due to the increased risk of warfarin-induced skin necrosis and venous limb gangrene in the absence of a heparin bridge.[97] Anticoagulation is recommended for 1 month for non-thrombotic HIT while it may be continued for 3–6 months for those patients with thrombotic HIT.[98]

HIT was found to have an incidence of 0.3% in patients undergoing vascular and cardiovascular procedures.[99,100] Patients specifically undergoing thoraco-subclavian and vein reconstruction procedures were found to have the highest incidences at 0.74% and 0.67%, respectively. Additionally, patients undergoing endovascular procedures had a higher incidence versus those undergoing open procedures (0.39% vs 0.25%, respectively).[99] Medical comorbidities that may predispose a patient to the development of HIT include: congestive heart failure, atrial fibrillation, endocarditis, chronic renal failure, liver disease, and obesity.[99,100] The most encountered complications included venous thrombosis, pulmonary embolism, renal failure, and respiratory failure, and there was an associated threefold increase in mortality in patients with HIT.[99]

CONCLUSION

Given the relative higher risk of vascular procedures, becoming familiar with the common systemic complications is crucial. Patient comorbidities, preoperative optimization, and intraoperative course can have a tremendous impact on such complications. In addition to the complications listed above, there are a number of procedure-specific complications that will be described in the coming chapters. Recognizing, and subsequently, managing all of these complications appropriately is imperative in providing proper postoperative patient care and improving patient outcomes.

REFERENCES

1. Vandy FC, Campbell D, Eliassen A, et al. Specialized Vascular Floors After Open Aortic Surgery: Cost Containment While Preserving Quality Outcomes. Annals of Vascular Surgery. 2013;27(1): 45–52. doi:10.1016/j.avsg.2012.09.002.
2. Lawlor DK, Lovell MB, DeRose G, Forbes TL, Harris KA. Is Intensive Care Necessary After Elective Abdominal Aortic Aneurysm Repair? Canadian Journal of Surgery. 2004;47(5): 359–363.
3. Gillies M, Harrison E, Pearse R, et al. Intensive Care Utilization and Outcomes After High-risk Surgery in Scotland: A Population-based Cohort Study. British Journal of Anaesthesia. 2017;118(1): 123–131. doi:10.1093/bja/aew396.
4. Haller G. Indirect Admission to Intensive Care After Surgery: What Should be Considered? British Journal of Anaesthesia. 2017;118(2): 153–154. doi:10.1093/bja/aew433.
5. Relieving Pain in America: A Blueprint for Transforming Prevention, Care, Education, and Research. 2011. doi:10.17226/13172.
6. Kalkman JC, Visser K, Moen J, Bonsel JG, Grobbee ED, Moons MK. Preoperative Prediction of Severe Postoperative Pain. 2003;105(3): 415–423. doi:10.1016/s0304-3959(03)00252-5.
7. Breivik H. Postoperative Pain Management: Why is it difficult to Show that it Improves Outcome? European Journal of Anaesthesiology. 1998;15(6): 748–751. doi:10.1097/00003643-199811000-00022.
8. Carr DB, Goudas LC. Acute Pain. Lancet. 1999;353(9169): 2051–2058.
9. Joshi GP, Ogunnaike BO. Consequences of Inadequate Postoperative Pain Relief and Chronic Persistent Postoperative Pain. Anesthesiology Clinics of North America. 2005;23(1): 21–36. doi:10.1016/j.atc.2004.11.013.
10. Kehlet H. Multimodal Approach to Control Postoperative Pathophysiology and Rehabilitation. British Journal of Anaesthesia. 1997;78(5): 606–617. doi:10.1093/bja/78.5.606.
11. Macrae WA. Chronic Pain After Surgery. Br J Anaesth. 2001;87(1): 88–98.
12. Johansen A, Romundstad L, Nielsen CS, Schirmer H, Stubhaug A. Persistent Postsurgical Pain in a General Population: Prevalence and Predictors in the Tromsø Study. Pain. 2012;153(7): 1390–1396. doi:10.1016/j.pain.2012.02.018.
13. Vandenkerkhof EG, Hopman WM, Reitsma ML, et al. Chronic Pain,Healthcare Utilization, and Quality of Life Following Gastrointestinal Surgery. Canadian Journal of Anesthesia/Journal canadien danesthésie. 2012;59(7): 670–680. doi:10.1007/s12630-012-9712-x.
14. Peters ML, Sommer M, Rijke JMD, et al. Somatic and Psychologic Predictors of Long-term Unfavorable Outcome After Surgical Intervention. Annals of Surgery. 2007;245(3): 487–494. doi:10.1097/01.sla.0000245495.79781.65.
15. Andreae MH, Andreae DA. Local Anaesthetics and Regional Anaesthesia for Preventing Chronic Pain after Surgery. Cochrane Database of Systematic Reviews. 2012. doi:10.1002/14651858.cd007105.pub2.
16. Dolin SJ. Effectiveness of acute postoperative pain management: I. Evidence from published data. British Journal of Anaesthesia. 2002;89(3): 409–423. doi:10.1093/bja/aef207.
17. Demeure MJ, Fain MJ. The elderly surgical patient and postoperative delirium. Journal of the American College of Surgeons. 2006;203(5): 752–757. doi:10.1016/j.jamcollsurg.2006.07.032.
18. Dasgupta M, Dumbrell AC. Preoperative Risk Assessment for Delirium After Noncardiac Surgery: A Systematic Review. Journal of the American Geriatrics Society. 2006;54(10): 1578–1589. doi:10.1111/j.1532-5415.2006.00893.x.
19. Chow WB, Rosenthal RA, Merkow RP, Ko CY, Esnaola NF. Optimal Preoperative Assessment of the Geriatric Surgical Patient: A Best Practices Guideline from the American College of Surgeons National Surgical Quality Improvement Program and the American Geriatrics Society. Journal of the American College of Surgery. 2012;215(4): 453–466. doi: 10.1016/j.jamcollsurg.2012.06.017.
20. Marcantonio ER. A Clinical Prediction Rule for Delirium After Elective Noncardiac Surgery. JAMA: The Journal of the American Medical Association. 1994;271(2): 134. doi:10.1001/jama.1994.03510260066030.
21. Marcantonio E, Ta T, Duthie E, Resnick NM. Delirium Severity and Psychomotor Types: Their Relationship with Outcomes after Hip

Fracture Repair. Journal of the American Geriatrics Society. 2002;50(5): 850–857. doi:10.1046/j.1532-5415.2002.50210.x.

22. Ely EW, Inouye SK, Bernard GR, et al. Delirium in Mechanically Ventilated Patients: Validity and Reliability of the Confusion Assessment Method for the Intensive Care Unit. JAMA. 2001;286(21): 2703. doi:10.1001/jama.286.21.2703.
23. Folstein MF, Folstein SE, McHugh PR. "Mini-mental state": A Practical Method for Grading the Cognitive State of Patients for the Clinician. Journal of Psychiatric Research. 1975;12(3): 189–198.
24. Robinson T. Postoperative Delirium in the Elderly: Diagnosis and Management. Clinical Interventions in Aging. 2008;Volume 3:351–355. doi:10.2147/cia.s2759.
25. Jin F, Chung F. Minimizing Perioperative Adverse Events in the Elderly. British Journal of Anaesthesia. 2001;87(4): 608–624.
26. Inouye SK, Bogardus ST, Charpentier PA, et al. A Multicomponent Intervention to Prevent Delirium in Hospitalized Older Patients. The New England Journal of Medicine. 1999;340(9): 669–676. doi:10.1056/NEJM199903043400901.
27. Ely EW. Delirium as a Predictor of Mortality in Mechanically Ventilated Patients in the Intensive Care Unit. JAMA. 2004;291(14): 1753. doi:10.1001/jama.291.14.1753.
28. Boersma E. Predictors of Cardiac Events After Major Vascular Surgery: Role of Clinical Characteristics, Dobutamine Echocardiography, and ß-Blocker Therapy. JAMA. 2001;285(14): 1865–1873.
29. Mangano DT, Goldman L. Preoperative Assessment of Patients with Known or Suspected Coronary Disease. N Engl J Med. 1995;333(26): 1750–1756.
30. Eagle KA, Brundage BH, Chaitman BR. et al. for the Committee on Perioperative Cardiovascular Evaluation for Noncardiac Surgery. Guidelines for Perioperative Cardiovascular Evaluation for Noncardiac Surgery: Report of the American College of Cardiology/American Heart Association Task Force on Practice Guidelines. Circulation. 1996;93:1278–1317.
31. L'Italien GJ, Paul SD, Hendel RC. et al. Development and validation of a Bayesian model for perioperative cardiac risk assessment in a cohort of 1,081 vascular surgical candidates. Journal of the American College of Cardiology. 1996;27:779–786.
32. Lee TH, Marcantonio ER, Mangione CM. et al. Derivation and Prospective Validation of a Simple Index for Prediction of Cardiac Risk of Major Noncardiac Surgery. Circulation. 1999;100:1043–1049.
33. Poldermans D, Fioretti PM, Forster T. et al. Dobutamine Stress Echocardiography for Asessment of Perioperative Cardiac Risk in Patients Undergoing Major Vascular Surgery. Circulation. 1993;87:1506–1512.
34. Poldermans D, Arnese M, Fioretti PM. et al. Improved Cardiac Risk Stratification in Major Vascular Surgery with Dobutamine-Atropine Stress Echocardiography. Journal of the American College of Cardiology. 1995;26:648–653.
35. Pellikka PA, Roger VL, Oh JK, Seward JB, Tajik AJ. Safety of Performing Dobutamine Stress Echocardiography in Patients with Abdominal Aortic Aneurysm > or = 4 cm in Diameter. American Journal of Cardiology. 1996;77:413–416.
36. Davila-Roman VG, Waggoner AD, Sicard GA, Geltman EM, Schechtman KB, Perez JE. Dobutamine Stress Echocardiography Predicts Surgical Outcome in Patients with an Aortic Aneurysm and Peripheral Vascular Disease. American Journal of Cardiology. J Am Coll Cardiol.1993;21:957–963.
37. Poldermans D, Bax JJ, Thomson IR. et al. Role of Dobutamine Stress Echocardiography for Preoperative Cardiac Risk Assessment before Major Vascular Surgery. Echocardiography. 2000;17:79–91.
38. Lalka SG, Sawada SG, Dalsing MC. et al. Dobutamine Stress Echocardiography as a Predictor of Cardiac Events Associated with Aortic Surgery. J Vasc Surg. 1992;15:831–840.
39. Langan EM, Youkey JR, Franklin DP, Elmore JR, Costello JM, Nassef LA. Dobutamine Stress Echocardiography for Cardiac Risk Assessment before Aortic Surgery. J Vasc Surg. 1993;18:905–911.
40. Poldermans D, Boersma E, Bax JJ. et al. The Effect of Bisoprolol on Perioperative Mortality and Myocardial Infarction in High-risk Patients Undergoing Vascular Surgery. N Engl J Med. 1999;341:1789–1794.
41. Lee TH. Reducing Risk in Noncardiac Surgery. N Engl J Med. 1999;341:1838–1840.
42. Kim LJ, Martinez EA, Faraday N, et al. Cardiac Troponin I Predicts Short-Term Mortality in Vascular Surgery Patients. Circulation. 2002;106(18): 2366–2371.
43. Antman EM, et al. ACC/AHA Guidelines for the Management of Patients with ST-Elevation Myocardial Infarction—Executive Summary. A report of the American College of Cardiology/American Heart Association Task Force on Practice Guidelines (Writing Committee to Revise the 1999 Guidelines for the Management of Patients with Acute Myocardial Infarction). Journal of the American College of Cardiology. 2004;44(3): 671–719. doi: 10.1016/j.jacc.2004.07.002.

44. Amsterdam EA, et al. 2014 AHA/ACC Guideline for the Management of Patients With Non–ST-Elevation Acute Coronary Syndromes: A Report of the American College of Cardiology/American Heart Association Task Force on Practice Guidelines. J Am Coll Cardiol. 2014;64(24): 139–228. doi: 10.1016/j.jacc.2014.09.017.
45. Valentine R, Rosen SF, Cigarroa JE, Jackson MR, Modrall J, Clagett G. The Clinical Course of New-onset Atrial Fibrillation after Elective Aortic Operations 1 No Competing Interests Declared. Journal of the American College of Surgeons. 2001;193(5): 499–504. doi:10.1016/s1072-7515(01)01028-6.
46. Heintz KM, Hollenberg SM. Perioperative Cardiac Issues: Postoperative Arrhythmias. Surgical Clinics of North America. 2005;85(6): 1103–1114. doi:10.1016/j.suc.2005.09.003.
47. Royster RL, Deng H, Whalen SP. Postoperative Atrial Fibrillation. Anesth Analg. 2017;125(1): 10–12. doi: 10.1213/ANE.0000000000002070.
48. Crawford TC, Oral H. Cardiac Arrhythmias: Management of Atrial Fibrillation in the Critically Ill Patient. Critical Care Clinics. 2007;23(4): 855–872. doi:10.1016/j.ccc.2007.06.005.
49. Choudhury M. Postoperative Management of Vascular Surgery Patients: A Brief Review. Clinics in Surgery. 2017;2:1584.
50. Marik PE, Baram M. Noninvasive Hemodynamic Monitoring in the Intensive Care Unit. Critical Care Clinics. 2007;23(3): 383–400. doi:10.1016/j.ccc.2007.05.002.
51. Varon J. Perioperative Hypertension Management. Vascular Health and Risk Management. 2008;4(3): 615–627.
52. Goldberg Me, Larijani GE. Perioperative Hypertension. Pharmacotherapy. 1998;18(5): 911–914.
53. Shander A, Fleisher LA, Barie PS, Bigatello LM, Sladen RN, Watson CB. Clinical and Economic Burden of Postoperative Pulmonary Complications: Patient safety Summit on Definition, Risk-reducing Interventions, and Preventive Strategies*. Critical Care Medicine. 2011;39(9): 2163–2172. doi:10.1097/ccm.0b013e31821f0522.
54. Johnson RG, Arozullah AM, Neumayer L, Henderson WG, Hosokawa P, Khuri SF. Multivariable Predictors of Postoperative Respiratory Failure after General and Vascular Surgery: Results from the Patient Safety in Surgery Study. Journal of the American College of Surgeons. 2007;204(6): 1188–1198. doi:10.1016/j.jamcollsurg.2007.02.070.
55. Rosenberg J, Rasmussen GI, Wojdemann KR, Kirkeby LT, Jorgensen LN, Kehlet H. Ventilatory pattern and associated episodic hypoxaemia in the late postoperative period in the general surgical ward. Anaesthesia. 1999;54(4): 323–328. doi:10.1046/j.1365-2044.1999.00744.x.
56. Craig DB. Postoperative Recovery of Pulmonary Function. Anesth Analg. 1981;60(1): 46–52.
57. Liu S, Carpenter RL, Neal JM. Epidural Anesthesia and Analgesia. Anesthesiology. 1995;82(6): 1474–1506. doi:10.1097/00000542-199506000-00019.
58. Sasaki N, Meyer MJ, Eikermann M. Postoperative Respiratory Muscle Dysfunction. Anesthesiology. 2013;118(4): 961–978. doi:10.1097/aln.0b013e318288834f.
59. Nieuwenhuijs D, Bruce J, Drummond G, Warren P, Wraith P, Dahan A. Ventilatory responses after major surgery and high dependency care. British Journal of Anaesthesia. 2012;108(5): 864-871. doi:10.1093/bja/aes017.
60. Ferguson ND, Fan E, Camporota L, et al. The Berlin definition of ARDS: an expanded rationale, justification, and supplementary material. Intensive Care Medicine. 2012;38(10): 1573–1582. doi:10.1007/s00134-012-2682-1.
61. Amato MB, et al. Effect of a Protective-Ventilation Strategy on Mortality in the Acute Respiratory Distress Syndrome. N Engl J Med. 1998;338(6): 347–354.
62. Ventilation with Lower Tidal Volumes as Compared with Traditional Tidal Volumes for Acute Lung Injury and the Acute Respiratory Distress Syndrome. The Acute Respiratory Distress Syndrome Network. N Engl J Med. 2000;342(18): 1301–1308.
63. Brower RG, et al. Higher versus Lower Positive End-Expiration Pressures in Patients with the Acute Respiratory Distress Syndrome. N Engl J Med. 2004;351(4): 327–336. doi: 10.1056/NEJMoa032193.
64. Ryckwaert F, Alric P, Picot M-C, Djoufelkit K, Colson P. Incidence and Circumstances of Serum Creatinine Increase after Abdominal Aortic Surgery. Intensive Care Medicine. 2003;29(10): 1821–1824. doi:10.1007/s00134-003-1958-x.
65. Wijeysundera DN, Karkouti K, Beattie WS, Rao V, Ivanov J. Improving the Identification of Patients at Risk of Postoperative Renal Failure after Cardiac Surgery. Anesthesiology. 2006;104(1): 65–72. doi:10.1097/00000542-200601000-00012.
66. Ellenberger C, Schweizer A, Diaper J, et al. Incidence, risk factors and prognosis of changes in serum creatinine early after aortic abdominal surgery. Intensive Care Medicine. 2006;32(11): 1808–1816. doi:10.1007/s00134-006-0308-1.
67. Sugawara Y, Sato O, Miyata T, Deguchi J, Kimua H, Namba T, Furuya T, Shirakawa M, Makuuchi M. Surgical Results of Abdominal Aortic Aneurysm Repair in Patients with Chronic Renal Dysfunction. Jpn Circ J. 1997;61(9): 762–766.

68. Wald R, Waikar SS, Liangos O, Pereira BJ, Chertow GM, Jaber BL. Acute renal failure after endovascular vs open repair of abdominal aortic aneurysm. Journal of Vascular Surgery. 2006;43(3). doi:10.1016/j.jvs.2005.11.053.
69. Braams R, Vossen V, Lisman B, Eikelboom B. Outcome in Patients Requiring Renal Replacement Therapy After Surgery for Ruptured and Non-ruptured Aneurysm of the Abdominal Aorta. European Journal of Vascular and Endovascular Surgery. 1999;18(4): 323–327. doi:10.1053/ejvs.1999.0893.
70. Norwood MG, Polimenovi NM, Sutton AJ, Bown MJ, Sayers RD. Abdominal Aortic Aneurysm Repair in Patients with Chronic Renal Disease. Eur J Vasc Endovasc Surg. 2004;27(3): 287–291.
71. Welten GM, Schouten O, Chonchol M, et al. Temporary Worsening of Renal Function after Aortic Surgery Is Associated with Higher Long-Term Mortality. American Journal of Kidney Diseases. 2007;50(2): 219–228. doi:10.1053/j.ajkd.2007.04.002.
72. Schrier RW, Wang W, Poole B, Mitra A. Acute renal failure: definitions, diagnosis, pathogenesis, and therapy. Journal of Clinical Investigation. 2004;114(1): 5–14. doi:10.1172/jci200422353.
73. Abbott WM, Austen WG. The reversal of renal cortical ischemia during aortic occlusion by mannitol. Journal of Surgical Research. 1974;16(5): 482–489. doi:10.1016/0022-4804(74)90073-0.
74. Hanley MJ, Davidson K. Prior mannitol and furosemide infusion in a model of ischemic acute renal failure. American Journal of Physiology-Renal Physiology. 1981;241(5). doi:10.1152/ajprenal.1981.241.5.f556.
75. Denton MD, Chertow GM, Brady HR. "Renal-dose" dopamine for the treatment of acute renal failure: Scientific rationale, experimental studies and clinical trials. Kidney International. 1996;50(1): 4–14. doi:10.1038/ki.1996.280.
76. Girbes AR, Lieverse AG, Smit AJ, et al. Lack of specific renal haemodynamic effects of different doses of dopamine after infrarenal aortic surgery. British Journal of Anaesthesia. 1996;77(6): 753–757. doi:10.1093/bja/77.6.753.
77. Baldwin L, Henderson A, Hickman P. Effect of Postoperative Low-Dose Dopamine on Renal Function after Elective Major Vascular Surgery. Survey of Anesthesiology. 1994;38(6): 341. doi:10.1097/00132586-199412000-00039.
78. Friedrich JO, Adhikari N, Herridge MS, Beyene J. Meta-Analysis: Low-Dose Dopamine Increases Urine Output But Does Not Prevent Renal Dysfunction or Death. Annals of Internal Medicine. 2005;142(7): 510. doi:10.7326/0003-4819-142-7-200504050-00010.
79. Halpenny M, Rushe C, Breen P, Cunningham AJ, Boucher-Hayes D, Shorten GD. The effects of fenoldopam on renal function in patients undergoing elective aortic surgery. European Journal of Anaesthesiology. 2002;19(1): 32–39. doi:10.1097/00003643-200201000-00005.
80. Schrier RW, Wang W. Acute Renal Failure and Sepsis. N Engl J Med. 2004;351(2): 159–169.
81. Cap A, Hunt BJ. The pathogenesis of traumatic coagulopathy. Anaesthesia. 2014;70. doi:10.1111/anae.12914.
82. Maegele M, Schöchl H, Cohen MJ. An Update on the Coagulopathy of Trauma. Shock. 2014;41:21–25. doi:10.1097/shk.0000000000000088.
83. Brohi K, Cohen MJ, Ganter MT, Matthay MA, Mackersie RC, Pittet J-F. Acute Traumatic Coagulopathy: Initiated by Hypoperfusion. Annals of Surgery. 2007;245(5): 812–818. doi:10.1097/01.sla.0000256862.79374.31.
84. Chee Y, Liu S, Irwin M. Management of bleeding in vascular surgery. British Journal of Anaesthesia. 2016;117:ii85–ii94. doi:10.1093/bja/aew270.
85. Hébert PC, Wells G, Blajchman MA, et al. A Multicenter, Randomized, Controlled Clinical Trial of Transfusion Requirements in Critical Care. New England Journal of Medicine. 1999;340(6): 409–417. doi:10.1056/nejm199902113400601.
86. Carson JL, Carless PA, Hebert PC. Transfusion thresholds and other strategies for guiding allogeneic red blood cell transfusion. Cochrane Database of Systematic Reviews. 2012. doi:10.1002/14651858.cd002042.pub3.
87. Fominskiy E, Putzu A, Monaco F, et al. Liberal transfusion strategy improves survival in perioperative but not in critically ill patients. A meta-analysis of randomised trials. British Journal of Anaesthesia. 2015;115(4): 511–519. doi:10.1093/bja/aev317.
88. Kozek-Langenecker S, Sørensen B, Hess JR, Spahn DR. Clinical effectiveness of fresh frozen plasma compared with fibrinogen concentrate: a systematic review. Critical Care. 2011;15(5). doi:10.1186/cc10488.
89. Rahe-Meyer N, Solomon C, Winterhalter M, et al. Thromboelastometry-guided administration of fibrinogen concentrate for the treatment of excessive intraoperative bleeding in thoracoabdominal aortic aneurysm surgery. The Journal of Thoracic and Cardiovascular Surgery. 2009;138(3): 694–702. doi:10.1016/j.jtcvs.2008.11.065.
90. Rahe-Meyer N, Pichlmaier M, Haverich A, et al. Bleeding management with fibrinogen concentrate targeting a high-normal plasma fibrinogen level: a pilot study. British Journal of Anaesthesia. 2009;102(6): 785–792. doi:10.1093/bja/aep089.

91. Karlsson M, Ternström L, Hyllner M, et al. Prophylactic fibrinogen infusion reduces bleeding after coronary artery bypass surgery. Thrombosis and Haemostasis. 2009;102(07): 1137–1144. doi:10.1160/th08-09-0587.
92. Fletcher JP, Batiste P. Incidence of deep vein thrombosis following vascular surgery. Int Angiol. 1997;16(1): 65–68.
93. Eagleton MJ, Grigoryants V, Peterson DA, et al. Endovascular treatment of abdominal aortic aneurysm is associated with a low incidence of deep venous thrombosis. Journal of Vascular Surgery. 2002;36(5): 912–916. doi:10.1067/mva.2002.128640.
94. Killewich LA. A Randomized, Prospective Trial of Deep Venous Thrombosis Prophylaxis in Aortic Surgery. Archives of Surgery. 1997;132(5): 499. doi:10.1001/archsurg.1997.01430290045007.
95. Olin JW, Graor RA, Ohara P, Young JR. The incidence of deep venous thrombosis in patients undergoing abdominal aortic aneurysm resection. Journal of Vascular Surgery. 1993;18(6): 1037–1041. doi:10.1016/0741-5214(93)90559-5.
96. Aziz F, Patel M, Ortenzi G, Reed AB. Incidence of Postoperative Deep Venous Thrombosis Is Higher among Cardiac and Vascular Surgery Patients as Compared with General Surgery Patients. Annals of Vascular Surgery. 2015;29(4): 661–669. doi:10.1016/j.avsg.2014.11.025.
97. Arepally GM. Heparin-Induced Thrombocytopenia. Blood. 2017:129(21): 2864–2872.
98. Lamuraglia GM, Houbballah R, Laposata M. The identification and management of heparin-induced thrombocytopenia in the vascular patient. Journal of Vascular Surgery. 2012;55(2): 562–570. doi:10.1016/j.jvs.2011.10.082.
99. Chaudhry R, Wegner R, Zaki JF, et al. Incidence and Outcomes of Heparin-Induced Thrombocytopenia in Patients Undergoing Vascular Surgery. Journal of Cardiothoracic and Vascular Anesthesia. 2017;31(5): 1751–1757. doi:10.1053/j.jvca.2017.05.024.
100. Seigerman M, Cavallaro P, Itagaki S, Chung I, Chikwe J. Incidence and Outcomes of Heparin-Induced Thrombocytopenia in Patients Undergoing Cardiac Surgery in North America: An Analysis of the Nationwide Inpatient Sample. Journal of Cardiothoracic and Vascular Anesthesia. 2014;28(1): 98–102. doi:10.1053/j.jvca.2013.07.021.

SUGGESTED READING

Sidawy AN, Perler BA. Rutherford's Vascular Surgery and Endovascular Therapy, 9th Edition. 2018. Section 7 Complications; Chapters 42–52; 530–652.

3

Complications of stenting for occlusive disease of aortic arch branches

CHRISTOPHER A. LATZ AND MARK F. CONRAD

Percutaneous interventions have become first-line therapy for treatment of arterial occlusive disease. This is especially true for lesions in the branches of the aortic arch where open repair often requires complex and maximally invasive operative approaches. When performed by a well-trained operator, these procedures carry a low risk of morbidity and mortality; however, the consequences of poor planning or poor technique can be devastating. It is imperative that anyone performing these procedures is aware of possible complications associated with each arterial bed and has a sophisticated understanding of the nuances of diagnosis and management of occlusive disease of the arch branches. This chapter details endovascular approaches to treating occlusive disease of the aortic arch vessels including perioperative medical management, procedural steps, options for access, and stent selection. It will also focus on the most commonly encountered complications and their management. The complications reviewed include stroke, dissection, restenosis, perforation/rupture, as well as complications specific to arm access.

PATIENT SELECTION

IMAGING

The aortic arch gives rise to three arterial branches: the brachiocephalic (innominate) artery, the left common carotid artery, and the left subclavian artery. Arterial occlusive disease can occur in each of these branches caused by a range of etiologies including atherosclerosis (most common), radiation-induced injury, dissection, aneurysm, and arteritis.[1] The distribution of disease favors the left subclavian artery, most commonly followed by the innominate and then the left common carotid artery.[2] The less invasive nature of an endovascular approach to occlusive lesions of the aortic arch branches has made it the first choice of therapy at most institutions. The technical or anatomic factors that could increase the risks associated with a catheter-based approach can often be identified on preoperative axial imaging in the form of computed tomographic angiography (CTA) or magnetic resonance angiography (MRA). In particular, the detection of mural atherosclerotic disease within the aortic arch or a high burden of ostial calcification of the arch vessels may make conventional arteriography less likely to succeed and may lead the surgeon to consider an alternate approach to repair. Additional considerations that may preclude endovascular therapy include excessive vessel tortuosity, total occlusions, ulcerated plaques, and aberrant arch anatomy. Indeed, up to 20% of patients will have a bovine arch where the left common carotid artery originates from the innominate artery, around 5% will have a left vertebral artery origin on the arch, and 0.5–2% will have an aberrant origin of the right subclavian artery[3,4] (Figure 3.1).

GENERAL PRINCIPLES OF TREATMENT

PERIOPERATIVE MEDICAL MANAGEMENT

There is a paucity of data available to inform a recommendation for the most effective antiplatelet strategy after endovascular intervention of the arch vessels. However, based upon the carotid and peripheral endovascular literature, it is likely that the safest approach is for patients to at least be taking an aspirin prior to any supra-aortic branch vessel endovascular intervention. In addition, assuming no patient-specific contraindications, dual antiplatelet therapy in the form of aspirin and

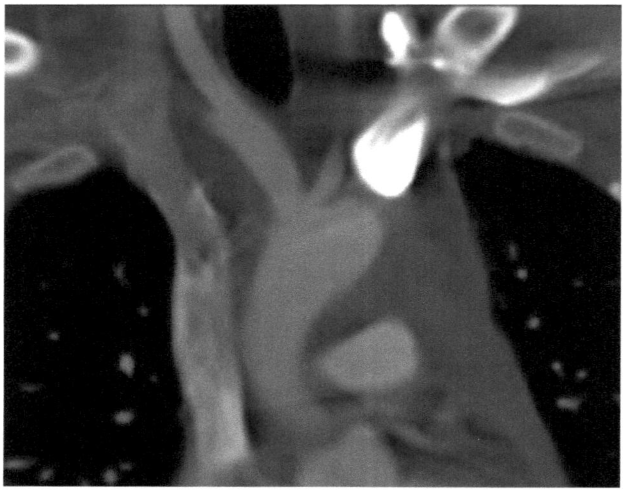

Figure 3.1 Bovine arch.

clopidogrel is recommended for all patients undergoing arch interventions to reduce the risk of embolic events.[5] Intra-procedural anticoagulation with heparin should be used in all arch branch interventions for occlusive disease assuming no patient-specific contraindications [i.e., documented heparin-induced thrombocytopenia (HIT)]. In that case, an alternative anticoagulation strategy should be employed. Intermittent boluses should be given to target an activated clotting time (ACT) of 250–300 seconds to decrease the risk of intraprocedural embolic phenomena, especially during wire manipulation in the arch. Indeed, it is prudent for the operator to wait at least 3 minutes after original bolus and confirm that the patient has a therapeutic ACT prior to crossing the arch with wires and catheters. Postoperative protamine sulfate reversal may be administered at the operator's discretion.

ACCESS

Arterial access is typically obtained via the transfemoral or the transbrachial route depending on the planned intervention. The transfemoral approach has traditionally been preferred to reach the carotid arteries; however, with severe ostial lesions, there is no room to place a sheath in the artery which can lead to an unstable system. In this situation, access via open exposure of the carotid artery may be the best way to treat a proximal lesion and protect the brain from an embolic shower during angioplasty and stenting. This is especially true when the patient has tandem severe lesions at the ostia of the common carotid and at the carotid bifurcation.[6] Brachial access provides an attractive alternative for treating subclavian and innominate lesions, especially flush occlusions, which would be difficult to select from the aorta. For brachial access, the arm is placed straight out with the hand supinated. The artery can be accessed just above the antecubital fossa. Here it passes under the bicipital aponeurosis and traverses the medial aspect of the arm just below the long head of the biceps brachii muscle and can be compressed against the humerus once the procedure is complete. Access is best obtained under ultrasound guidance with a micropuncture needle to avoid injury to the median nerve, which lies in close proximity to the brachial artery. Finally, radial access for supra-aortic trunk intervention has also been described and is becoming more popular due to a perceived decrease in complications.[7]

ARCH ANGIOGRAPHY

Once access is obtained, an angled catheter such as a Kumpe (Cook Medical) can be used to pass a wire into the aortic arch for angiography, and this is usually followed by a pigtail catheter. Straight flush catheters should be avoided, especially in a diseased arch, due to the risk of dissection with a power injection. The image intensifier is rotated in the left anterior oblique position (often 30–45 degrees) to open the arch to best visualize the arch vessel origins. This can be done with the catheter in place to identify the correct angle. Conversely, the right anterior oblique (20–30 degrees) angle facilitates visualization of the origin of the innominate artery. Catheter and wire manipulation should be minimized in the arch to decrease the risk of distal embolization from loose atherosclerotic and thrombotic debris. It is also important to avoid the introduction of air into the system as a distal air embolus in this region can lead to stroke symptoms.

CHOICE OF STENT

Early experience with endovascular management of occlusive lesions of the arch vessels was favorable with initial success rates over 80% and 1–2 year recurrence rates that ranged from 8–25%.[8] These outcomes were achieved with balloon angioplasty alone, and the addition of stenting to the procedure has shown improved patency rates in some series and primary stenting is favored by many authors, especially in cases involving highly calcified and complex lesions. A Cochrane review comparing primary angioplasty vs stenting for subclavian artery stenosis concluded that there was insufficient evidence to determine whether stenting was more effective.[9] However, a meta-analysis of 8 studies with 544 patients that compared angioplasty alone to angioplasty and stenting found that the 1 year patency was superior with stent placement without additional complication rates.[10] Ostial lesions tend to be an extension of aortic disease with heavy calcification, and balloon-expandable stents are favored over self-expanding stents here because of their higher radial force and more precise deployment. Conversely, self-expanding stents are useful when treating tortuous lesions away from the ostium and in vessels that have a variable diameter. The choice of a bare metal stent versus a covered stent graft remains controversial. Proponents of bare metal stents argue that they allow coverage of branch vessels without exclusion, especially in the innominate that branches early. Conversely, covered stents offer the theoretical advantage of complete decreased embolic potential by trapping all atherosclerotic debris and preventing future intimal hyperplasia, but to date, studies have had mixed results.[11,12]

CEREBRAL PROTECTION STRATEGIES

Endovascular procedures cause micro-emboli that can be deleterious to the down-stream vascular bed; this is of particular concern when the brain is the end-organ. For patients with carotid or innominate lesions, distal cerebral protection is the standard of care. Indeed, the Centers for Medicare and Medicaid Services (CMS) do not cover carotid or innominate artery stenting without embolic protection. Therefore, the method of embolic protection must be considered as part of the preoperative planning for these lesions and will differ depending on which artery is being treated. Options include placement of a distal embolic filter or clamping of the proximal common carotid artery during hybrid procedures.

ENDOVASCULAR APPROACH BY ARTERY

LEFT SUBCLAVIAN ARTERY

The left subclavian artery is the most frequently treated of the arch branches because it is most commonly affected by atherosclerotic disease and is also the easiest to access. Lesions of the left subclavian artery can be approached from either a retrograde transfemoral or via retrograde left brachial access, the latter serving an important role in treating proximal left subclavian arterial occlusions. An in-depth discussion of the catheters used to select each artery is beyond the scope of this text, but the left subclavian artery can usually be selected from the arch with a mild angled catheter.

A 6-French sheath system is established proximal to the lesion, and the lesion is usually crossed with a hydrophilic wire. The imaging system can be adjusted to center the disease and minimize parallax. Once beyond the lesion, a hand injection arteriogram is performed to confirm that the catheter is intra-luminal and a wire with an atraumatic tip is placed for treatment. The authors favor the platinum-tipped wires, but surgeons should choose to use wires with which they are most familiar. If the artery is tortuous, it may be difficult for sheaths, balloons, or stents to track over the wire. In this situation, it is prudent to obtain brachial and transfemoral access and snare the wire for through and through access, which will facilitate advancement of the sheath and balloon and stent placement. Most operators will pre-dilate the lesion with an undersized angioplasty balloon. This practice began when stents were not firmly fixed to their delivery systems, and a tight lesion could dislodge the stent prior to deployment. This is still possible with some covered stents and it is good practice to cross the lesion with the sheath after pre-dilation if a covered stent is to be used. Imaging should confirm the take-off locations of the vertebral and internal mammary arteries, as these must be preserved during stent placement, especially in patients who have had prior coronary bypass grafting. A balloon-expandable stent should then be deployed to match the size of the normal artery. Every effort should be made to avoid covering the vertebral artery origin; even with a bare metal stent. In addition, although embolic protection of the vertebral artery has been described, it is likely rarely for the treatment of subclavian lesions and should be reserved for specific circumstances such as a symptomatic ulcerative lesion.[13] Finally, if the proximal aspect of the stent protrudes into the aorta, it is advantageous to flare it open with a larger balloon to facilitate vessel selection in the future, if necessary (Figure 3.2).

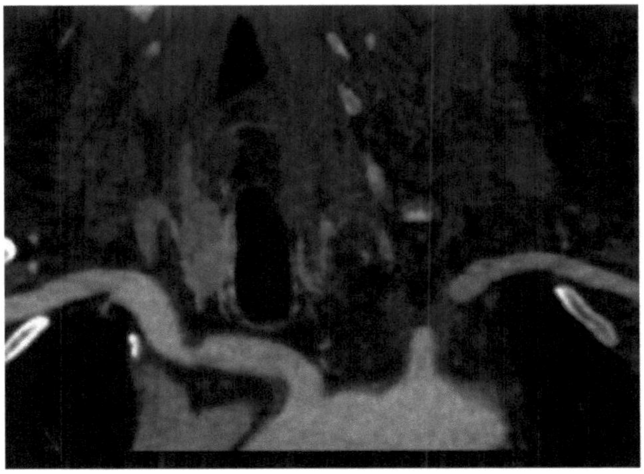

Figure 3.2 Left subclavian artery occlusion.

INNOMINATE ARTERY

The endovascular treatment of atherosclerotic lesions of the innominate artery can be challenging secondary to the potential for embolization of debris to both the carotid and vertebral arteries and the risk of creating a plaque shift potentially compromising blood flow to the carotid or subclavian artery. The innominate artery can be approached from a retrograde transfemoral access, retrograde transbrachial access, retrograde from the common carotid, via a cut-down, or with any combination of the three. Imaging of the vessel in the left anterior oblique projection allows accurate identification of the innominate origin, but the right anterior oblique projection with a degree of cranial or caudal angulation is necessary to see the origins of the right subclavian and right common carotid arteries. This view is especially important prior to stent placement to avoid inadvertently jailing one of the branches.

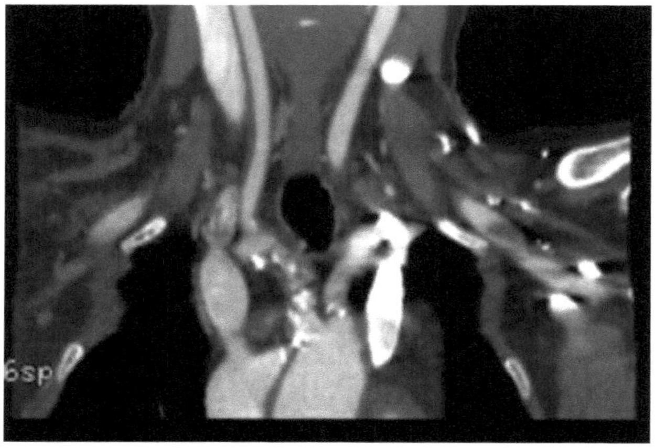

Figure 3.3 Innominate artery occlusive disease.

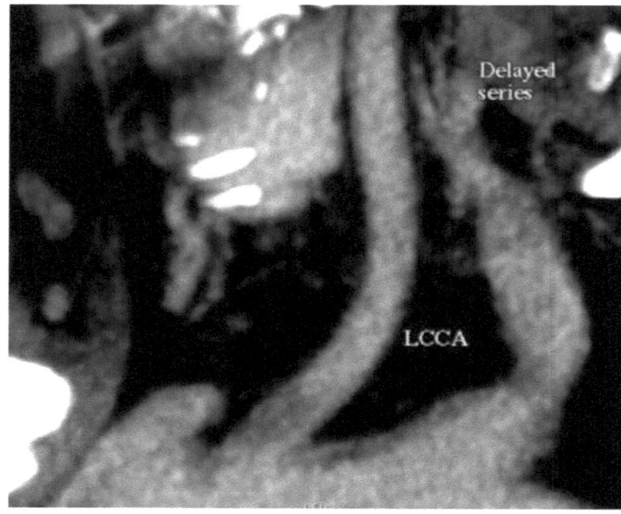

Figure 3.4 Left common carotid artery occlusive disease.

There is controversy regarding the need for distal neuroprotection during endovascular treatment of the innominate artery. Paukovits et al. reported a series of 72 patients with symptomatic innominate lesions who underwent angioplasty with or without stenting without the use of neuroprotection with no peri-procedural strokes and a 2.6% rate of ipsilateral TIA.[14] Their argument against neuroprotection is that it is technically difficult to use neuroprotection devices and their benefit is unproven. However, if distal protection is desired, Ryer et al. described a two-wire technique that can be utilized. This involves snaring a wire from the arm for through and through support, allowing a sheath or guide to be held in place. The protection device is then placed in the right carotid artery, and the innominate lesion is treated from the groin over the protection device wire, so that the protection device is not jailed by the stent.[15] A final approach to carotid protection during innominate intervention involves cutting down on the right common carotid artery and crossing the lesions through retrograde access from the common carotid with a clamp on the internal carotid artery. This is especially useful when tandem lesions are present.[16]

There are instances when the disease extends beyond the innominate artery into the origins of the right common carotid and subclavian arteries. In this situation, it is often necessary to stent both arteries, and this should be performed in a kissing fashion. This is best accomplished with dual access from the right brachial artery and the groin. From the right brachial artery, the subclavian lesion can be crossed, and the right common carotid lesion can be crossed from the femoral approach. With this system in place, stents can be deployed simultaneously to prevent plaque shift and preserve the patency of the ostia of each vessel[17] (Figure 3.3).

LEFT COMMON CAROTID ARTERY

Disease in the left common carotid artery is most likely to occur at the ostium of the vessel, as it is usually an extension of disease from the aortic arch. In its normal anatomic position, the common carotid can be approached from the groin in a manner similar to the left subclavian artery with angioplasty and stenting delivered via a guiding catheter or a sheath. Access to the origin of the vessel is aided, and the access sheath or guide can be stabilized, by a "buddy-wire" placed in the left external carotid artery. A protection device can be deployed in the left internal carotid artery, and the wire used to deploy the protection device is also the wire over which the intervention is performed. The need for neuroprotection during angioplasty and stenting of lesions of the left common carotid arteries remains controversial. In a study of 147 patients with 153 lesions, neuroprotection was not used for isolated ostial lesions and they reported a 2% ipsilateral stroke rate and 2.6% rate of TIA.[18] Indeed, a recent update in the European Society for Vascular Surgery guidelines for the management of atherosclerotic disease recommended against the use of protection devices in the endovascular treatment of common carotid lesions[19] (Figure 3.4).

COMBINED INTERNAL AND COMMON CAROTID DISEASE

Multilevel disease involving the carotid bifurcation and the proximal common carotid artery or innominate artery is rare and occurs in about 5% of patients with severe internal carotid stenosis. Although a total endovascular approach to tandem lesions is possible, it imposes technical limitations that may lead to a higher stroke risk. Therefore, a hybrid approach wherein a carotid endarterectomy is performed followed by retrograde stenting of the common carotid artery has been promoted because of the ease of neuroprotection by clamping of the endarterectomized distal common carotid artery.[20] With this technique, the carotid endarterectomy (CEA) is performed first and then the retrograde stenting is performed through the side of the patch with tourniquet control of inflow over the sheath, or the patch can be completed and then accessed. In both instances, the proximal lesion is crossed with a wire, angioplastied, and stented with a clamp on the internal or common carotid to prevent embolic complications to the brain. Early results with this approach were promising. A meta-analysis of 13 studies that included 133 patients, of whom 83% were symptomatic, showed that the 30-day stroke and death rate was 1.7%, essentially equal to that of treatment of isolated disease.[21] However, a multi-institutional series of 62 patients treated over 14 years reported an ipsilateral stroke rate of 6.5% and a combined 30-day stroke and death rate of 11.3%.[22] Additionally, a review of the Vascular Quality Initiative identified 404 patients who underwent CEA combined with an ipsilateral proximal intervention and showed a combined stroke and death rate that was double that of isolated CEA.[23] Based upon these studies, asymptomatic common carotid lesions should be left alone when performing CEA and the combined procedure should be reserved for symptomatic patients.

PROCEDURE-RELATED COMPLICATIONS

Fortunately, the endovascular treatment of atherosclerotic lesions of the branches of the aortic arch is safe, with high technical success rates and a low associated morbidity and mortality. The complication rates from multiple studies range from 0–20% and the most commonly seen are access-related problems which are discussed below. The neurologic complication rate has been low despite a variable use of neuroprotection. The main complications from the literature are addressed herein.

EMBOLIC/THROMBOTIC STROKE

The dreaded complication of endovascular management of atherosclerotic disease of the arch branches is stroke, but fortunately it rarely occurs. In the acute setting, stroke symptoms are usually caused by reduction of cerebral flow due to embolization, thrombosis, or dissection, with embolization being the most common. The routine use of preoperative dual antiplatelet therapy and intra-procedural anticoagulation reduces the risk of micro-emboli by stabilizing plaque prior to intervention. Several of the largest studies have reported stroke rates of 0–2.6% without the routine use of neuroprotection.[13,18,24] Although there is potential for angioplasty of the arch branches to cause emboli to the brain through both the carotid and vertebral arteries, in practice, it is not common. Indeed, a recent meta-analysis noted a 30-day stroke rate of 3.1% following endovascular repair of common carotid artery stenosis or occlusion.[25] Technique is important for the prevention of stroke during this procedure as inaccurate deployment of a stent risks covering the ostium of the carotid or vertebral origins. If this occurs with a covered stent, it can lead to thrombosis of the artery, but a bare metal stent may also serve as a nidus for micro-emboli or promote intimal hyperplasia. Subclavian stenting is particularly vulnerable to inadvertent coverage if the stent encroaches on the origin of the vertebral artery.

The management of embolic or thrombotic stroke following an endovascular intervention of the arch branches should be driven by the goals of expeditious recognition and early treatment. It is good practice to start all procedures with imaging of the intracerebral circulation to establish a baseline prior to any intervention. The evaluation and management of an acute embolic stroke will depend on the timing of symptom development. For example, if a patient exhibits signs of neurologic compromise during the procedure, an intracerebral angiogram should be performed. If an acute occlusion or change from baseline is seen, an interventionalist with expertise in neuro-interventional treatment should be emergently consulted for consideration of a neuro-rescue procedure. Options for neuro-rescue continue to develop but include mechanical retrieval with proximal devices such as aspiration catheters or distal devices including baskets or spiral wires, fragmentation of the embolus, or thrombolysis.[26] If the stroke symptoms occur after the patient is in the recovery room, a CT angiogram is usually the quickest modality by which to obtain an accurate diagnosis. This will show the vessels involved in the intervention as well as the intra-cerebral vessels. If the etiology is stent thrombosis, the patient should be taken emergently back to the operating room for endovascular repair salvage. In addition, if an embolus is identified on CTA, the neuro-rescue techniques described above should be instituted as soon as possible. The results of neuro-rescue are mixed, but the carotid stenting literature shows that patients who experience a periprocedural stroke have a three-fold increase in 4 year mortality regardless of any degree of recovery after the event.[27]

DISSECTION

Dissection is a rare complication of endovascular interventions. A review of iatrogenic dissections that occurred during cerebral angiogram showed an incidence of 0.39%.[28] Dissections can be caused by catheter or wire trauma to the arterial wall and is associated with tortuous and diseased arteries. They can also occur within the lesion after angioplasty. Flow-limiting dissections after angioplasty are best treated with stenting. However, most identified dissections are treated conservatively with medical therapy alone. There are some cases where intervention is warranted. For instance, there was a case report of a patient who developed a dissection of the left subclavian artery that was found to be flow-limiting to a left internal mammary bypass graft to the coronary vessels. This was treated with bare metal stent coverage of the dissection entry tear, which then caused the dissection to lay down against the wall and re-established flow.[29] If a dissection appears to be flow-limiting, it should be addressed. This can be proven by transducing the aortic pressure and the pressure beyond the dissection flap. It is important not to lose wire access across a dissection flap because it can be difficult to re-establish intra-luminal access. An 0.014 wire can be placed, and pull-back pressure measurements can be obtained over the wire through a Tuohy Borst (Cook Medical) adapter attached to the end of the catheter. As in the above case report, management consists of deployment of a stent over the dissection entry tear. After deployment, a second pull back can be performed to demonstrate resolution of flow limitation.

RESTENOSIS

Early reports of endovascular repair showed that the primary patency was inferior to open surgical repair, and long-term studies are rare. In a recent report of 411 patients with long-term follow-up, restenosis occurred in 15% of patients, and most of these presented with symptom recurrence. The primary patency in this cohort was 92% at 1 year and 82.6% at 5 years, and patients with innominate interventions were more likely to present with recurrent stenosis.[30] Follow-up after intervention usually consists of a clinic visit and noninvasive imaging at 6 weeks and then yearly thereafter. Most patients who developed restenosis experienced a return of symptoms as well. If a change is noted on noninvasive imaging, the anatomy can be further defined with axial imaging via a CTA or MRA. If a patient has restenosis but remains asymptomatic, they should be treated with medical therapy and monitoring with serial imaging. However, symptomatic patients should undergo re-intervention. Repeat intervention is usually endovascular, and open repair is rarely required. Indeed, in the previously noted study, the secondary patency at 5 years was 96%.[30]

PERFORATION/RUPTURE

Vessel perforation following endovascular intervention is a rare but potentially deadly complication. This usually occurs following angioplasty with an oversized balloon within a calcified vessel.[31] Wire perforation may also occur, but this is usually less severe and usually can be managed expectantly. Suspicion for acute perforation/rupture should be high following sudden onset of pain in an awake patient during or immediately following angioplasty. Any intraprocedural hemodynamic instability should also raise concern for vessel perforation or rupture. In cases of perforation and rupture, it is important to identify the source with angiography, maintain wire access and then perform balloon occlusion for control while definitive treatment is planned. Definitive management can include balloon occlusion for 3–5 minutes for small perforations, stent grafting across the rupture or, in extreme cases, vessel occlusion and conversion to open repair.

COMPLICATIONS RELATED TO ARM ACCESS

Upper extremity access via the brachial artery is commonly used in endovascular interventions of the arch branches. However, brachial artery access is known to be associated with a higher complication rate than femoral access.[32] This is likely secondary to the smaller caliber of the vessel and its proximity to important neurological structures (i.e., the median nerve). The brachial artery can be accessed either percutaneously under ultrasound guidance or via surgical exposure. There are reports that support an open approach for all brachial access because percutaneous access is associated with a higher rate of complications.[32,33] Kret et al. looked at 732 patients who underwent a procedure through brachial access in the Vascular Quality Initiative (VQI) and noted a 9% complication rate compared to 3.3% for femoral access. In addition, the complication rate after brachial cut-down was significantly lower than ultrasound-guided percutaneous access (4.1% vs 11.8%).[32] Conversely, Franz et al. reviewed their experience with 265 percutaneous brachial access cases and found only 1.9% had complications that required a further intervention.[34] They concluded that the percutaneous approach leads to similar complication rates to femoral access when a standardized protocol is followed.[34] One of the main disadvantages of surgical exposure of the brachial artery is that it leaves a wound that requires more time to heal than a percutaneous approach and leads to more scar tissue secondary to the surgical dissection, which can make future access difficult.[35] Unlike femoral access, where closure devices are often used to control the artery after sheath removal, the standard of care for percutaneous brachial artery access remains manual compression. There have been isolated case reports detailing the use of closure devices successfully in the brachial artery, but this practice remains off label.[36]

The most common complication seen after brachial access is hematoma development. This has been reported to occur in 2.5–7% of cases.[32,34] Hematoma formation usually begins during the procedure through vessel trauma upon initial access and a lack of arterial control during sheath exchanges. Both of these can be reduced or prevented through the use of ultrasound guidance for access and meticulous manual compression when upsizing the sheath. Finally, appropriate manual compression after the sheath is removed is important for prevention of hematoma formation. Local bleeding quickly creates pressure in the brachial sheath which contains the brachial artery, paired veins, and median nerve, and these structures have little tolerance for hematoma formation. The first symptoms related to brachial hematomas are usually neurologic secondary to median nerve compression. Therefore, any postprocedure paresthesia or motor paresis in the median nerve distribution needs to be taken extremely seriously after a brachial sheath pull, as delayed recognition can leave the patient with a permanent median nerve palsy.

Management of a symptomatic brachial sheath hematoma requires emergent surgical decompression. Once a neuro deficit is identified, the hematoma can be confirmed with ultrasound, but delays in surgical decompression should be avoided. The access point should be used to guide the incision point; once encountered, the brachial sheath should be opened, and all blood should be drained from the sheath. In most cases, a pseudoaneurysm is encountered in the acute setting and the artery access point should be closed primarily, to prevent further bleeding.

Thrombosis following brachial access occurs around 2% of the time, and usually is the result of aggressive manual compression after the sheath pull. The small vessel size and relatively easy compressibility compared to the femoral artery render this artery more prone to thrombosis. The technique for compression that can reduce thrombosis is to place a pulse oximeter finger-probe to monitor digital waveforms while pressure is applied. When the pressure becomes too aggressive, the waveform will blunt, and the operator can release pressure until the waveform returns. This allows the surgeon to apply the perfect amount of pressure to prevent hematoma formation without occluding the artery. Patients who thrombose their brachial artery will present with some combination of the six P's of limb ischemia (pain, pallor, pulselessness, paresthesia, paresis and poikilothermia) but will only have all six later in the presentation. It is common for the first symptoms to be pain and pulselessness after the sheath pull, and it is important to document the status of the radial pulse prior to accessing the brachial artery. Thrombosis can be confirmed with duplex ultrasound, but is not necessary if there is an obvious pulse deficit after the sheath is pulled. Management of brachial arterial thrombosis is surgical with exploration of the artery and thrombectomy. After the brachial artery is exposed, a transverse arteriotomy is extended at the site of puncture, and a fogarty catheter is passed until no more thrombus is retrieved and there is pulsatile inflow and adequate backflow bleeding. Most of the time, the thrombus is focal and this can be a limited procedure. However, if more extensive clot is encountered, it may be necessary to dissect out the origins of the radial and ulnar arteries and arteriography may be warranted. Finally, in cases of severe intimal disruption or arterial destruction, segmental resection with or without an interposition graft is required.[37]

Nerve palsy following percutaneous intervention is rare but occurs most commonly in association with brachial or axillary artery access. Impairment usually results from nerve compression from a hematoma or pseudoaneurysm. More rarely, injury due to direct needle injury or neuropraxic/cautery injury during dissection or via ischemic injury following thrombosis of the access vessel has been described. The most commonly injured nerve with brachial access is the median nerve, and symptoms can include difficulty with forearm pronation, finger flection, or opposition of the thumb. Management is based on the cause and a duplex ultrasound of the affected area can help make the diagnosis. For minor hematomas, compression to stop expansion can be enough, but once neuro compressive symptoms develop, open surgical decompression is usually necessary. If a pseudoaneurysm is identified, this should be repaired surgically as well. It is important not to delay diagnosis or intervention in these patients as decompression beyond 48 hours from symptom development is associated with improvement in only 50% of patients, while almost all who are treated early show improvement in symptoms.[38]

REFERENCES

1. Wiley EJ, Effeney DJ. Surgery of the Aortic Arch Branches and Vertebral Arteries. Surgical Clinics of North America. 1979 Aug; 59(4): 669–80. PMID:382406
2. Hass WK, Fields WS, North RR, Kircheff II, Chase NE, Bauer RB. Joint Study of Extracranial Arterial Occlusion. II. Arteriography, Techniques, Sites and Complications. JAMA. 1968 Mar; 203(11): 961–968. PMID 5694318
3. Choi Y, Chung SB, Kim MS. Prevalence and Anatomy of Aberrant Right Subclavian Artery Evaluated by Computed Tomographic Angiography in a Single Institution in Korea. J Korean Neurosurg Soc. 2019 Mar; 62(2): 175–182. PMID 30840972
4. Ahn SS, Chen SW, Miller TJ, Chen JF. What is the True Incidence of Anomalous Bovine Left Common Carotid Artery Configuration? Ann Vasc Surg. 2014 Feb; 28(2): 381–385. PMID 2427527.
5. CAPRIE Steering Committee. A randomised, Blinded, Trial of Clopidogrel Versus Aspirin in Patients at Risk of Ischaemic Events (CAPRIE). Lancet. 1996 Nov; 348: 1329–39. PMID 8918275
6. Makaloski V, von Deimling C, Mordasini P, Gralla J, Do DD, Schmidi J, Wyss TR. Transcarotid Approach for Retrograde Stenting of Proximal Innominate and Common Carotid Artery Stenosis. Ann Vasc Surg. 2017 Aug; 43: 242–248. PMID: 28478176.
7. van Dijk LJD, Bijdevaate DC, Moelker A. Rupture of the Radial Artery after Brachiocephalic Stent Placement per Transradial Access. Journal of vascular and interventional radiology: JVIR. 2018 Sep; 29(9): 1281–1283. PMID: 30146195.
8. Wilms G, Baert A, Dewaele D, Vermylen J, Nevelsteen A, Suy R. Percutaneous Transluminal Angioplasty of the Subclavian Artery: Early and Late Results. Cardiovasc Intervent Radiol. 1987; 10(3): 123–128. PMID 2955895.
9. Lared W, Mourano JE, Puchnick A, Soma F, Shigueoka DC. Angioplasty Versus Stenting for Subclavian Artery Stenosis. Cochrane Database of Systematic Reviews 2014, Issue 5. Art No: CD008461.

10. Chatterjee S, Nerella N, Chakravarty S, Shani J. Angioplasty Alone Versus Angioplasty and Stenting for Subclavian Artery Stenosis – A Systematic Review and Meta-Analysis. Am J Ther. 2013 Sept-Oct; 205(5): 520–523.
11. Ice D, Ierovante N, Signarovitz D. Outcomes of Covered Versus Bare Metal Stents in the Treatment of Subclavian Artery Stenosis. Journal of the American College of Cardiology. 2019 Oct; 74(13 Supplement): B559.
12. Ammi M, Henni S, Du Mont LS, Settembre N, Loubiere H, Sobocinski J, Goueffic Y, Feugier P, Duprey Am Martinez R, Bartoli M, Coscas R, Chaufour X, Kaladji A, Rosset E, Abraham P, Picquet J. Lower Rate of Restenosis and Reinterventions with Covered vs Bare Metal Stents Following Innominate Artery Stenting. J Endovasc Ther. 2019 Jun; 26(3): 385–390. PMID 30935282.
13. Canyigit M, Peynicioglu B, Metin Y, Cil BE, Cekirge S. Subclavian Artery Stenting with Vertebral Artery Embolic Protection via Brachial Approach Complicated by Transient Cortical Blindness. European J of Rad Extra. 2008 Mar; 65(3): 109–112.
14. Paukovits TM, Lukacs L, Berczi V, Hirschberg K, Nemes B, Huttl K. Percutaneous Endovascular Treatment of Innominate Artery Lesions: A Single-Centre Experience on 77 Lesions. European J of Vasc and Endovasc Surg. 2010;40: 35–43.
15. Ryer EJ, Oderich GS. Two-wire (0.014 and 0.018-inch) Technique to Facilitate Placement of an Embolic Protection Device and Innominate Artery Stenting. J Endovasc Ther. 2010;17: 652–656.
16. Clouse WD, Ergul EA, Cambria RP, Brewster DC, Kwolek CJ, LaMuraglia GM, Patel VI, Conrad MF. Retrograde stenting of proximal lesions with carotid endarterectomy increases risk. J Vasc Surg. 2016 Jun; 63(6):1517–23. doi: 10.1016/j.jvs.2016.01.028.PubMed PMID: 27106249.
17. Sahsamanis G, Vourliotakis G, Pirgakis K, Lekkas A, Kantounakis L, Terzoglou A, Tzilalis V. Primary Stenting of Right-Sided Subclavian Artery Stenosis Presenting as Subclavian Steal Syndrome: Report of 3 Cases and Literature Review. Annals of Vasc Surg. 2018 Apr; 48: 245e1–e5.
18. Paukovits TM, Haasz J, Molnar A, Szeberin Z, Nemes B, Varga D, Huttl K, Berczi V. Transfemoral Endovascular Treatment of Proximal Common Carotid Artery Lesions: A Single-Center Experience on 153 Lesions. J Vasc Surg. 2008 Jul; 48(1): 80–87.
19. Eckstein HH. European Society for Vascular Surgery Guidelines on the Management of Atherosclerotic Carotid and Vertebral Artery Disease. European J of Vasc and Endovasc Surg 2017 Aug; 55(1): 1–2.
20. Moore JD, Schneider PA. Management of Simultaneous Common and Internal Carotid Artery Occlusive Disease in the Endovascular Era. Semin Vasc Surg. 2011;24: 2–9.
21. Sfyroeras GS, Karathanos C, Antoniou GA, Salptsis V, Giannoukas AD. A Meta-Analysis of Combined Endarterectomy and Proximal Balloon Angioplasty for Tandem Disease of the Arch Vessels and Carotid Bifurcation. J Vasc Surg. 2011;54: 534–540. PMID: 21684709
22. Clouse WD, Ergul EA, Wanken ZJ, Kleene J, Stone DH, Darling RC, Cambria RC, Conrad MF. Risk and Outcome Profile of Carotid Endarterectomy with Proximal Intervention is Concerning in Multi-Institutional Assessment. J Vasc Surg. 2018;68: 760–769.
23. Wang LJ, Ergul EA, Conrad MF, Malas MB, Kashyap VS, Goodney PP, Patel VI, Clouse WD. Addition of Proximal Intervention to Carotid Endarterectomy Increases Risk of Stroke and Death. J Vasc Surg. 2019 Apr; 69(4): 1102–1110.
24. Ahmed SB, Benezit M, Hazart J, Brouat A, Daniel G, Rosset E. Outcomes of the Endovascular Treatment for the Supra-Aortic Trunks Occlusive Disease: A 14-Year Monocentric Experience. Ann Vasc Surg. 2016; 33: 55–66.
25. Zhang X, Ma H, Li L, Zou J, Jiao Y, Zhang X, Yang H. A Meta-Analysis of Transfemoral Endovascular Treatment of Common Carotid Artery Lesions. World Neurosurg. 2019 Mar; 123: 89–94. PMID: 30453085.
26. van den Berg JC. Neuro-Rescue During Carotid Stenting. Eur J Endovasc Surg. 2008; 36: 627–636.
27. Hill MD, Brooks W, Mackey A, Clark WM, Meschia JF, Morrish WF, Mohr JP, Rhodes JD, Popma JJ, Lal BK, Longbottom ME, Voeks JH, Howard G, Brott TG, and the CREST Investigators. Stroke After Carotid Stenting and Endarterectomy in the Carotid Revascularization Endarterectomy Versus Stenting Trial (CREST). Circulation. 2012;126: 3054–3061.
28. Groves AP, Kansagra AP, Cross DT, Moran CJ, Derdeyn CP. Acute Management and Outcomes of Iatrogenic Dissections During Cerebral Angiography. J Neurointerv Surg. 2017 May; 9(5): 499–501.
29. Spies C, Fergusson D. Treatment of an iatrogenic subclavian artery dissection. Catheterization and Cardiovascular Interventions. 2010 Jul 1;76(1): 35–8. PMID: 20578187.
30. Przewlocki T, Wrotniak L, Kablak-Ziembicka A, Pieniazek P, Roslawiecka A, Rzeznik D, Misztal M, Zajdel W, Badacz R, Sokolowski A, Trystula M, Musialek P, Zmudka K. Determinants of long-term outcome in patients after percutaneous stent-assisted management of symptomatic

subclavian or innominate artery stenosis or occlusion. EuroIntervention: journal of EuroPCR in collaboration with the Working Group on Interventional Cardiology of the European Society of Cardiology. 2017 Dec 20;13(11): 1355–1364. PMID: 28846540.
31. Broadbent LP, Moran CJ, Cross DT, 3rd, Derdeyn CP. Management of ruptures complicating angioplasty and stenting of supraaortic arteries: report of two cases and a review of the literature. AJNR (American journal of neuroradiology). 2003 Nov-Dec; 24(10): 2057–61. PMID: 14625233.
32. Kret MR, Dalman RL, Kalish J, Mell M. Arterial cutdown reduces complications after brachial access for peripheral vascular intervention. J Vasc Surg. 2016 Jul; 64(1): 149–54. PMID: 27021376.
33. Madden NJ, Calligaro KD, Zheng H, Troutman DA, Dougherty MJ. Outcomes of Brachial Artery Access for Endovascular Interventions. Ann Vasc Surg. 2018 Oct 19. PMID: 30347242.
34. Franz RW, Tanga CF, Herrmann JW. Treatment of peripheral arterial disease via percutaneous brachial artery access. J Vasc Surg. 2017 Aug; 66(2): 461–465. PMID: 28433335.
35. Buck DB, Karthaus EG, Soden PA, Ultee KH, van Herwaarden JA, Moll FL, Schermerhorn ML. Percutaneous versus femoral cutdown access for endovascular aneurysm repair. J Vasc Surg. 2015 Jul; 62(1): 16–21. PMID: 25827969.
36. Giordano A, Messina S, Maresca G, Bondi-Zoccai G. Hemostasis After Brachial Artery Access With the MynxGrip Device: A Case Report. Clin Med Insights Cardiol. 2018;12: 1179546818759298. PMID 29497342.
37. Kitzmiller JW, Hertzer NR, Beven EG. Routine surgical management of brachial artery occlusion after cardiac catheterization. Archives of Surgery. 1982 Aug; 117(8): 1066–71. PMID: 7103726.
38. Kuo F, Park J, Chow K, Chen A, Walsworth MK. Avoiding Peripheral nerve Injury in Arterial Interventions. Diagn Interv Radiol. 2019 Sep; 25(5): 380–391.

SUGGESTED READINGS

Chatterjee S, Nerella N, Chakravarty S, Shani J. Angioplasty Alone Versus Angioplasty and Stenting for Subclavian Artery Stenosis - A Systematic Review and Meta-Analysis. Am J Ther 2013 Sept-Oct; 205(5): 520–523.

Clouse WD, Ergul EA, Cambria RP, Brewster DC, Kwolek CJ, LaMuraglia GM, Patel VI, Conrad MF. Retrograde stenting of proximal lesions with carotid endarterectomy increases risk. J Vasc Surg. 2016 Jun;63(6):1517–23. doi: 10.1016/j.jvs.2016.01.028. PubMed PMID: 27106249.

4

Complications of endovascular therapy for aneurysmal disease of splanchnic arteries including renal arteries

MAEN ABOUL HOSN AND MEL J SHARAFUDDIN

Splanchnic artery aneurysms are rare and comprise less than 2% of all aneurysms. These encompass visceral arteries and their branches as well as the renal arteries.[1] Despite their rarity, such aneurysms are being diagnosed more frequently due to the increased utilization of advanced imaging modalities. The most common underlying etiology remains atherosclerotic degeneration. However, other associated causes include medial degeneration, trauma, connective tissues disorders, portal hypertension and pregnancy.[2] Given their rarity, their natural history is unclear with most aneurysms being asymptomatic at the time of diagnosis. Conversely, they can sometimes present with vague nonspecific symptoms depending on their size, location, and underlying cause. Although small aneurysms can often be safely observed, aneurysm rupture is the most feared complication associated with high mortality and morbidity rates.[3] Several factors are weighed when devising the ideal treatment approach, including urgency of the intervention, anatomic factors such as the size, location, and accessibility to the aneurysm, as well as patients' clinical status and comorbidities. Open surgical repair has historically been the gold standard for treating such aneurysms with options including ligation, aneurysmectomy, and interposition grafting. However, over the past years, endovascular therapy has become the preferred treatment approach when feasible, owing to its minimally invasive nature and ability to treat otherwise inaccessible vessels effectively via embolization or exclusion using covered stents. Although access site complications including bleeding, dissection, vessel thrombosis, and distal embolization are commonly seen in all endovascular procedure, endovascular management of splanchnic aneurysms can result in an additional set of complications pertaining to the specific type of aneurysm being treated as well as the end organ the treated vessel supplies.

SPLENIC ARTERY ANEURYSMS

Splenic artery aneurysms account for over 60% of all splanchnic aneurysms with an incidence of 0.8%.[4] They are often found in multiparous women with a female to male ratio of 4 to 1. The majority are located in the distal third portion of the splenic artery. While the rupture risk is estimated to be around 3%, this risk is higher in the setting of pregnancy, portal hypertension, liver transplant, and vasculitis. Intervention is currently indicated in all symptomatic patients or those with high rupture risk due to the aforementioned factors as well as those with an aneurysm diameter larger than 2.5 cm.[5]

ENDOVASCULAR OPTIONS

Endovascular treatment options for splenic artery aneurysm have significantly lower associated morbidity and mortality when compared to open repair. They include transcatheter embolization of the aneurysm sac, exclusion of the aneurysm neck with a covered stent, or a combination of both. The size and location of the aneurysm typically dictates the ideal approach and treatment option, with the main objective being exclusion of the aneurysm while preserving collateral flow to the spleen via the gastric, pancreatic and omental branches. The aneurysm can be excluded by accessing it with a microcatheter and packing it with embolic agents such as coils or detachable balloons. Alternatively, coils can be deployed in the splenic artery just distal and proximal to the aneurysm, effectively excluding the aneurysm is what is termed the "sandwich technique." A third option is the placement of a self-expanding covered stent to exclude the aneurysm and maintain flow in the artery. Although the technical success rate of endovascular treatment is around 90%, vessel tortuosity, presence of multiple branches at the site of the aneurysm, as well as hilar location of the aneurysm can make endovascular treatment more challenging and increase failure rate.[6]

COMPLICATIONS

Complications associated with endovascular treatment of splenic artery aneurysms can be divided into access site complications or intervention-related complications. Access site complications include arterial injury, bleeding or hematoma formation, and these can be minimized by using ultrasound guided access. Other access-related complications include arterial dissection, thrombosis or distal embolization, and these can be avoided by utilizing proper access as well as careful wire manipulation.

Intervention associated complications can occur at any stage of the intervention. If the celiac artery takeoff is significantly angulated, access into the splenic artery from a femoral approach may be challenging and may require a combination of reverse curved catheters, microcatheters and microwires. Forceful wire or sheath manipulation can result in loss of access or even dissection or thrombosis of the vessel (Figure 4.1a,b). In cases of multiple failed attempts at celiac artery cannulation using femoral access, brachial artery access may be a better alternative. If access to the splenic artery is successful and embolization of the aneurysm is contemplated, care must be taken

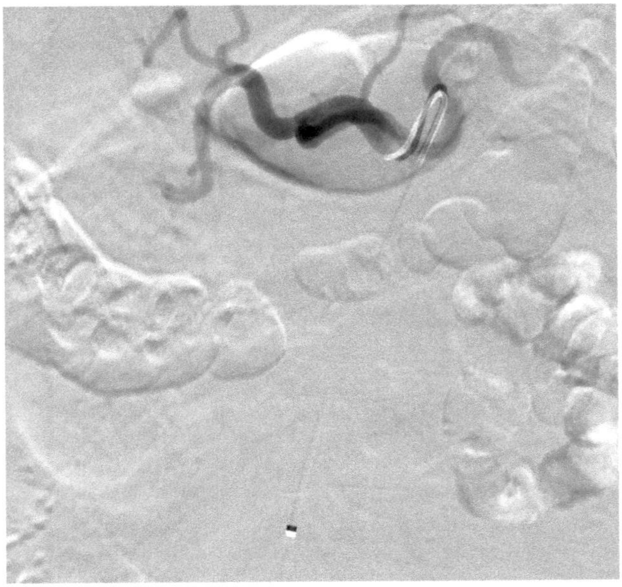

Figure 4.1a Celiac artery angiogram showing the takeoff of the celiac and hepatic arteries.

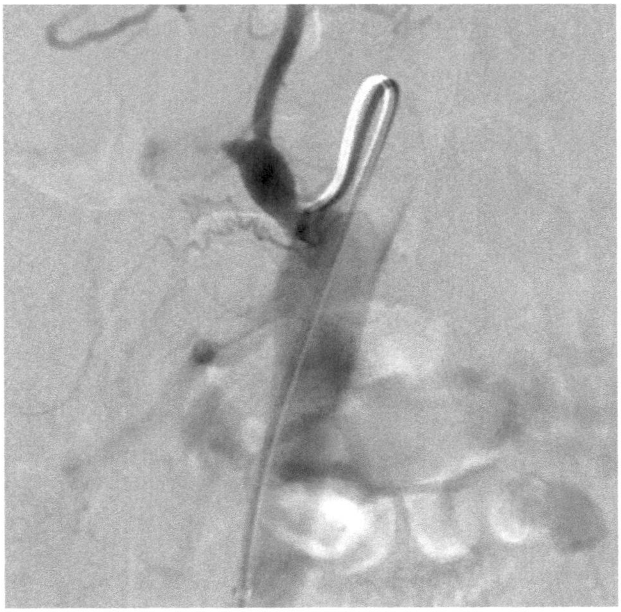

Figure 4.1b Follow-up angiogram after wire manipulation showing dissection and thrombosis of the splenic artery shortly after takeoff.

while advancing the wire and catheter into the aneurysm to avoid aneurysm rupture. Moreover, the tip of the catheter should be confirmed to be in the desired location and with no underlying torque to avoid improper coil deployment and distal dislodgement. In such an instance and depending on the size of the coil and where it lodges, the patient may develop a splenic infarct postoperatively. Post-embolization syndrome, characterized by fever and abdominal pain, ileus, and pancreatic inflammation, can also be commonly encountered after the procedure. Another less common complication seen days after the procedure is splenic abscess formation and may necessitate percutaneous drainage or even splenectomy.

Case Example 1

A 45-year-old female with a distal splenic artery 2 cm aneurysm was planned for an attempted coil embolization of the aneurysm via a sandwich technique versus a covered stent placement. Transfemoral access was obtained, and a 5F Ansel sheath was advanced for support. Given the acute angle of the celiac artery takeoff, an Sos Omni catheter was used to maneuver a Glidewire into the splenic artery. However, while attempting to cannulate the splenic artery and follow with the catheter, the wire went into a subintimal plane and a dissection flap occurred, causing thrombosis of the artery (Figure 4.1a,b). Multiple attempts at reentering the true lumen failed and the patient later required open exclusion of the aneurysm due to continued filling from collaterals.

HEPATIC ARTERY ANEURYSMS

Hepatic artery aneurysms are the second most common visceral aneurysms, and the majority are extrahepatic and occur in the common hepatic artery. As with other splanchnic aneurysms, atherosclerotic degeneration is the most common etiology with less common causes including fibromuscular dysplasia, polyarteritis nodosa, mycotic degeneration, and inflammatory aneurysms in the setting of pancreatitis or cholecystitis. In addition, traumatic pseudoaneurysms account for almost half of the intrahepatic aneurysms encountered.[7] They are often asymptomatic and diagnosed in the sixth decade of life. If they reach large sizes, patients can sometimes present with vague right upper quadrant discomfort or epigastric pain. Rupture rate can be as high as 20%, with intrahepatic aneurysms having even higher rupture rates.[8] As such, intervention is indicated for all symptomatic hepatic artery aneurysms as well as asymptomatic ones in the setting of vasculitis or larger than 2.5 cm.

ENDOVASCULAR OPTIONS

Endovascular treatment of hepatic aneurysms is often reserved for high risk patient and those with inaccessible aneurysms such as intrahepatic aneurysms and pseudoaneurysms. In such instances, embolization using microcatheters and coils may spare the patient a major hepatic resection. Embolization of the common hepatic artery can also be considered only if the portal vein supplies adequate flow to the liver thus avoiding fulminant hepatic necrosis and failure. Alternatively, if there are adequate seal zones proximal and distal to the aneurysm, a covered stent may be deployed across the aneurysm neck to exclude it. The location of the gastroduodenal artery relative to the aneurysm should be considered to avoid back filling of the aneurysm. In an instance when such a scenario is likely, such as with hepatic artery proper aneurysms in proximity to the gastroduodenal artery, embolization of the latter may be required to prevent persistent flow into the aneurysm sac.

COMPLICATIONS

As with splenic artery aneurysms, endovascular treatment of hepatic artery aneurysms carries similar access and vessel cannulation complication risks. The hepatic artery is often fragile especially in the setting of inflammatory or traumatic aneurysms and aggressive wire/catheter manipulation can results in arterial dissection or thrombosis. If such a scenario occurs, thrombolytic therapy may be required to recanalize the vessel and care should be taken to maneuver the wire into the true lumen and confirm its location prior to any subsequent interventions. Moreover, the wire tip should be observed at all time to avoid iatrogenic intrahepatic arterial injury and pseudoaneurysm formation. In addition, the angulation of the hepatic artery should be taken into consideration if deployment of a covered stent is anticipated since kinking of the stent graft can result in thrombosis and liver ischemia. Treatment of such a complication depends on the patient's clinical presenting and time from surgery. Early thrombosis may require catheter-directed thrombolysis and thrombectomy in addition to addressing the cause of thrombosis. Chronic occlusions in the absence of significant liver ischemia may be observed. Other complications include liver failure, cholecystitis, abscess formation and massive hemorrhage.

Case Example 2

A 74-year-old male with severe pancreatitis found to have a common hepatic artery pseudoaneurysm. The origin of the pseudoaneurysm appeared to be in the middle of the artery based on his computed tomography (CT) scan so he was taken to the operating room for an attempted covered stent placement. Brachial access was utilized, and a 75 cm 7F Ansel sheath was used for support. Angiography delineated the celiac bifurcation and a Glidewire was successfully maneuvered into the gastroduodenal artery (GDA). Two overlapping 7 mm × 2.5 cm Viabahn stents were then deployed across pseudoaneurysm but the follow-up angiogram showed kinking of the stents with no flow distally. A third 7 mm × 5 cm Viabahn was then deployed across both previous stents and profiled resolving the kinking and restoring flow (Figure 4.2a,b). Wire access to the GDA ensure, that it was not covered and allowed the option of coiling of the vessel should there be any backfilling into the aneurysm from it.

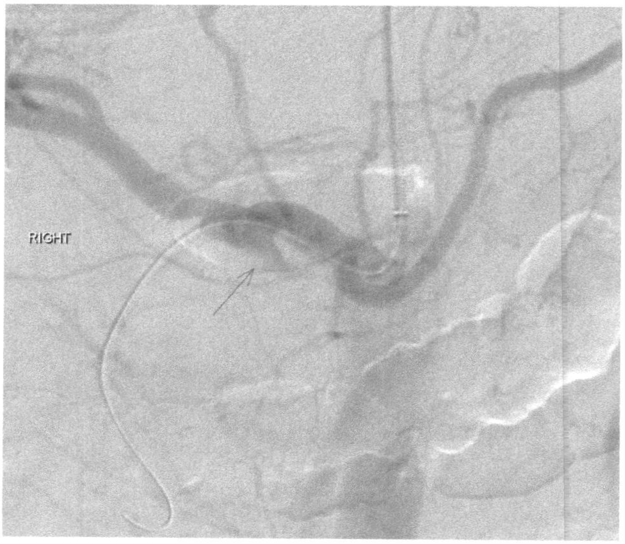

Figure 4.2a Hepatic artery pseudoaneurysm in the setting of severe pancreatitis.

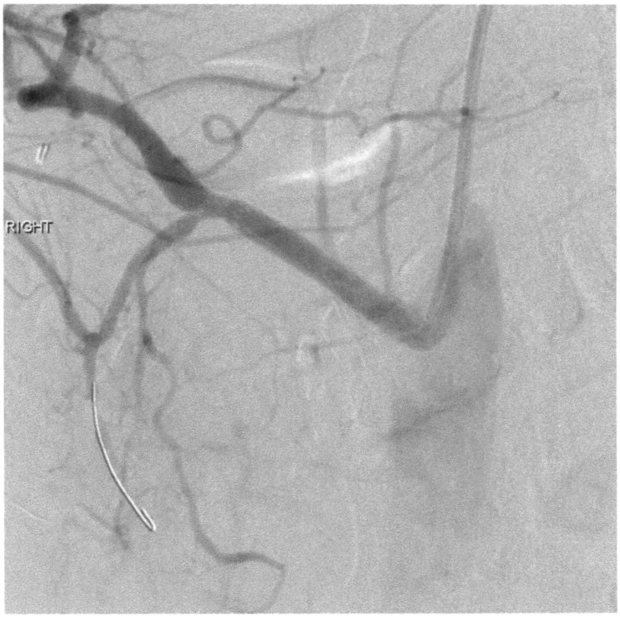

Figure 4.2b Exclusion of the pseudoaneurysm with covered stents while maintaining flow to the gastroduodenal artery.

SUPERIOR MESENTERIC ARTERY ANEURYSMS

Aneurysms of the superior mesenteric artery and its branches are rare, accounting for less than 7% of all visceral aneurysms.[9] Historically, the majority of such aneurysms had an underlying infectious etiology but in the current age, most are associated with atherosclerotic degeneration.[10] A small portion can also form as a result of post stenotic dilation. They are often located within the first 5 cm of the vessel. Careful evaluation of the location of these aneurysms is essential in order to differentiate them from an aneurysm affecting the pancreaticodudenal arcade as those are often the result of pancreatitis and have a worse prognosis when left untreated.[11] While small aneurysms can often be followed, symptomatic aneurysms and those larger than 2 cm in diameter are typically indicated for repair.

ENDOVASCULAR OPTIONS

Treatment options of superior mesenteric artery aneurysms vary depending on their underlying etiology, location and mode of presentation. Unruptured mycotic aneurysms often can be managed conservatively with antibiotics and serial imaging to assess for growth. If an intervention is contemplated, aneurysm location, size and proximity to major branches should be assessed as those will dictate the type of endovascular approach needed. The affected SMA segment can be embolized using coils or plugs without further revascularization if the pancreaticoduodenal artery branches are patent and the gastroduodenal artery is robust. Alternatively, a stent graft can be used to exclude the aneurysm if there are adequate proximal and distal seal zones. Attention should be given to any jejunal branches arising from the aneurysm itself as those may need to be embolized prior to a stent graft deployment to avoid continued back filling of the aneurysm sac.

COMPLICATIONS

In addition to access site complications, endovascular treatment of superior mesenteric artery aneurysms carries its own specific risk and complications. The angle of the vessel takeoff may prove challenging when approached using femoral access, especially in the setting of concomitant atherosclerotic occlusive disease. Forceful wire and catheter manipulation can result in vessel dissection or thrombosis and may necessitate thrombolysis to restore flow or even open conversion. In cases when difficult cannulation is anticipated, brachial artery access is recommended taking into consideration sheath and catheter length. After the vessel is accessed, it is imperative to keep the wire in a main branch to allow enough support and avoid loss of access. The wire tip should be seen at all times as unsupervised advancement may result in vessel injury, pseudoaneurysm formation and bleeding. If the main vessel is to be embolized, it is recommended to use long detachable coils that can be accurately deployed without risking dislodgement distally. Alternatively, detachable plugs can be used in a similar fashion. When using covered stents, it is important to ensure the absence of a replaced right hepatic artery as covering it may result in liver ischemia. Major small bowel branches should also be avoided to minimize the risk of bowel ischemia as well as continued filling of the aneurysm. Other complications include distal embolization, early stent thrombosis and bowel ischemia. Long-term complications include recanalization of the aneurysm, stent stenosis or occlusion.

Case Example 3

A 45-year-old female with known Marfan syndrome who had previously had a covered stent placed in her superior mesenteric artery at an outside hospital for a reported small aneurysm, presented with symptoms of chronic mesenteric ischemia. Vascular studies and CT imaging confirmed the presence of instent stenosis and she was taken for an attempted balloon angioplasty and possible re-stenting. Right femoral access was stylized and a 5F Ansel sheath was used for support. A flush catheter was used to cannulate the vessel and a glide wire was maneuvered distally. The sheath would not follow into the vessel, so a balloon was advanced and inflated in the stent and the sheath was then advanced over it as it was being deflated.

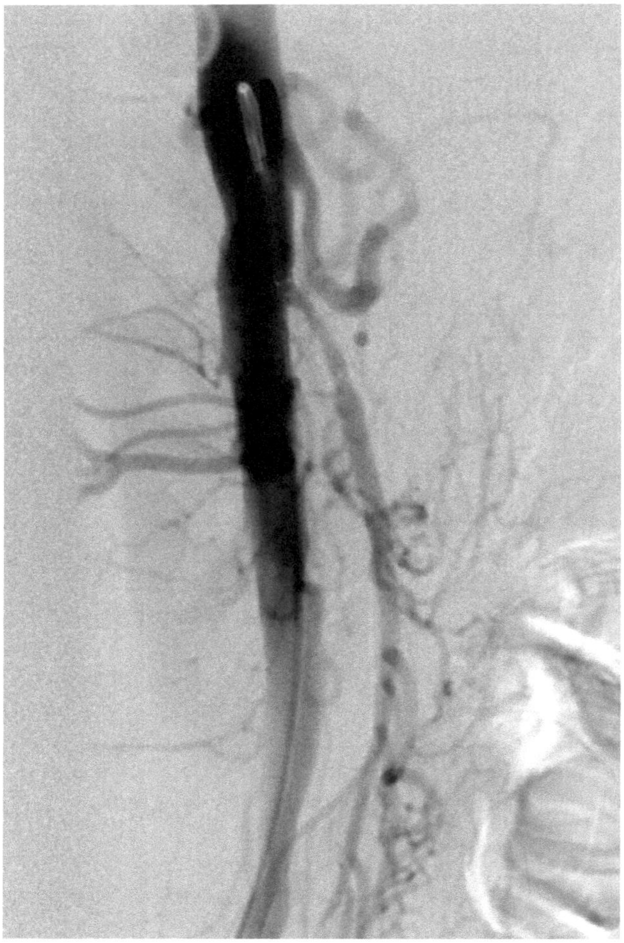

Figure 4.3a Aortoiliac angiogram showing stenosis at the site of a previously placed covered stent.

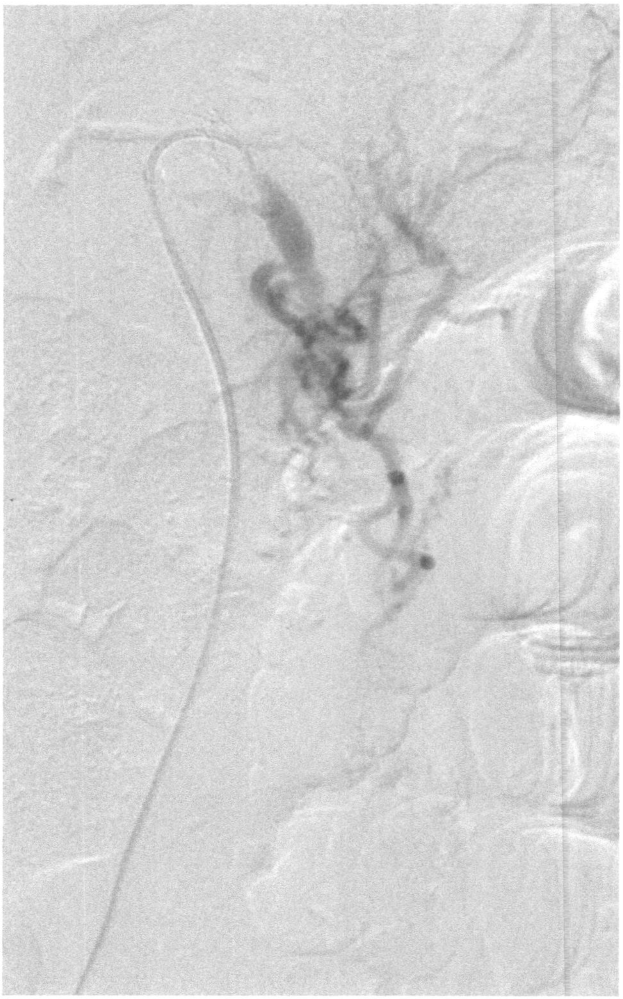

Figure 4.3b Iatrogenic dissection of the mesenteric artery following balloon angioplasty necessitating urgent open revascularization.

Follow-up angiography showed a flow-limiting dissection in the mesenteric artery distal to the stent with no flow seen in the distal branches (Figure 4.3a,b). Catheter directed thrombolytics and vasodilators failed to recanalize the true lumen and the patient subsequently underwent open exploration, mesenteric thrombectomy and revascularization.

RENAL ARTERY ANEURYSMS

Renal artery aneurysms are rare with a reported incidence of 0.01 to 1% in the general population.[12] Given their rarity, their natural history remains unclear with studies suggesting a more benign course compared to visceral aneurysms. As such, the indications for surgical intervention remain controversial and there is no consensus regarding treatment guidelines for renal artery aneurysms. Currently, interventions on renal artery aneurysms are performed for aneurysm diameter > 2 cm, aneurysm rupture or dissection, concomitant renovascular hypertension and in females in the child bearing age.[13] More recent studies on the natural history of these aneurysms confirm the extremely low rupture rates and slow growth rates suggesting that a size threshold of 2 cm in asymptomatic nonpregnant women may be too aggressive.[14,15] When they do occur, however, complications of renal artery aneurysms can be devastating. These include rupture, dissection, renal infarction, kidney failure, hypertension and arteriovenous fistula formation.

ENDOVASCULAR OPTIONS

Historically, open repair was the main treatment modality for renal artery aneurysms with surgical options including aneurysmectomy with primary or patch repair, resection with interposition graft placement, extracorporeal reconstruction with autotransplantation and even nephrectomy.[16] In select patients, endovascular therapy offers less invasive treatment options with demonstrated low morbidity and mortality. These mainly include coil embolization and stent graft placement. The choice of endovascular treatment depends on the anatomic location and characteristics of the aneurysm, proximity to a branching point, vessel tortuosity, elective or emergent repair and hemodynamic status of the patient. Covered stents are preferred aneurysms in the main renal artery and first division branches in the presence of adequate proximal and distal seal zones. Coil embolization is used for saccular aneurysms or pseudoaneurysms involving smaller segmental branches and the renal hilum. Occasionally, a combination of both may be utilized in which embolization is performed first followed by stent deployment to avoid retrograde filling from efferent vessels.

COMPLICATIONS

Although endovascular intervention on renal artery aneurysms carry a low morbidity with a high technical success rate, they are associated with minor and major complications. Minor complications include access site hematoma, hematuria, small arteriovenous fistula formation, minor renal infarct and transient renal insufficiency not requiring dialysis. Major early complications include aneurysm rupture or arterial dissection especially in the setting of an underlying connective tissue disorder. Major renal infarct can also occur if multiple branches are inadvertently coiled or covered with possible renal failure necessitating dialysis. Stent graft kinking and thrombosis can occur if the vessel is tortuous or if the stent is deployed across an acute branching point. Delayed complications include progressive renal function decline, recanalization of the aneurysm, stent graft stenosis or thrombosis and renal atrophy.

Case Example 4

A 38-year-old female with a suspected underlying connective tissue disorder presented with an apparent spontaneous isolated renal artery dissection with a hypovascularized right kidney. Given her worsening clinical symptoms despite medical management as well as the threatened status of her kidney, she was taken for attempted revascularization. A 6F Ansel sheath was used for support and an 0.018 wire was maneuvered successfully into the true lumen. Two 6 mm × 2.5 cm overlapping Viabahns stents were then deployed up to the level of the first bifurcation point favoring the true lumen and restoring flow to the kidney (Figure 4.4a,b).

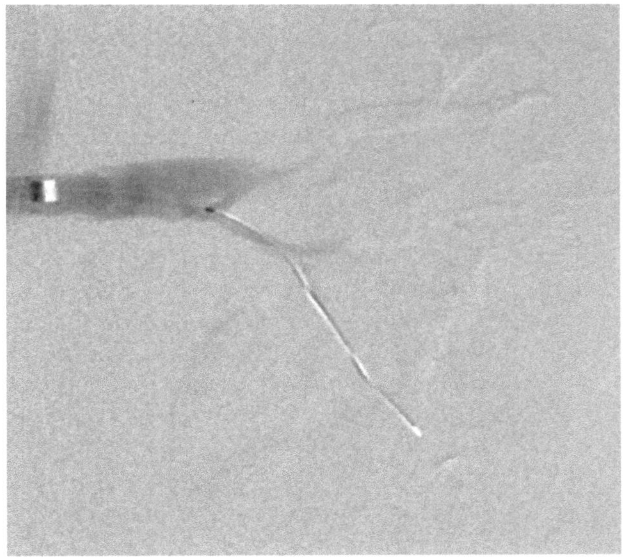

Figure 4.4a Flow-limiting dissection of the right renal artery.

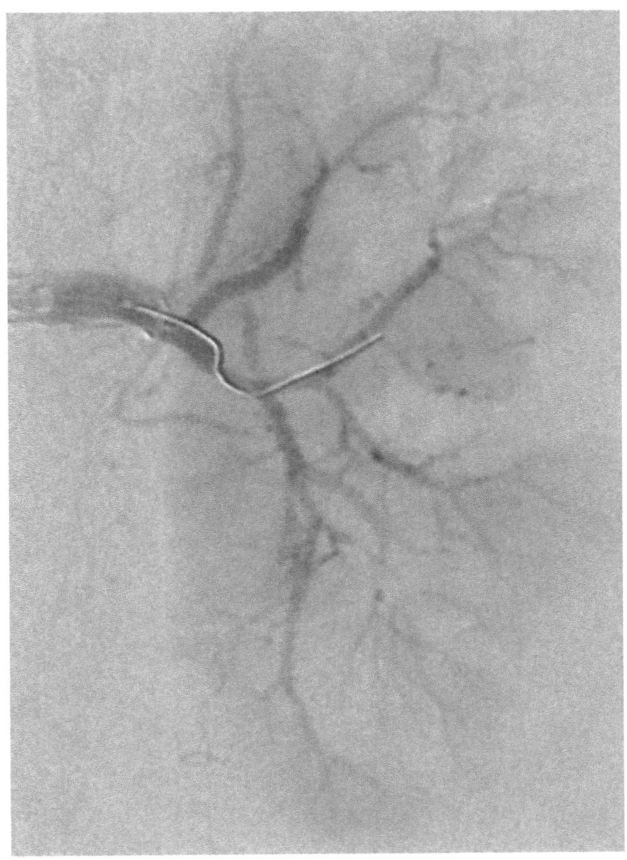

Figure 4.4b Management of the dissection with covered stent placement favoring the true lumen.

REFERENCES

1. Erben Y, Brownstein AJ, Rajaee S et al. Natural history and management of splanchnic artery aneurysms in a single tertiary referral center. J Vasc Surg. 2018;68(4): 1079–1087.
2. Pitton, MB, Dappa E, Jungmann F et al. Visceral artery aneurysms: Incidence, management, and outcome analysis in a tertiary care center over one decade. Eur Radiol. 2015; 25(7): 2004–2014.
3. Tulsyan, N, Kashyap VS, Greenberg RK et al., The endovascular management of visceral artery aneurysms and pseudoaneurysms. J Vasc Surg. 2007;45(2): 276–283.
4. Barrionuevo P, Malas MB, Nejim B et al. A systematic review and meta-analysis of the management of visceral artery aneurysms. J Vasc Surg. 2019; 70(5): 1694–1699.
5. Berceli, SA. Hepatic and splenic artery aneurysms. Semin Vasc Surg. 2005;18(4): 196–201.
6. Madoff DC, Denys A, Wallace MJ, et al. Splenic arterial interventions: anatomy, indications, technical considerations, and potential complications. Radiographics. 2005;25 Suppl 1: S191–211.
7. Abbas MA, Fowl RJ, Stone WM et al. Hepatic artery aneurysm: factors that predict complications. J Vasc Surg. 2003;38(1): 41–45
8. Shukla AJ, Eid R, Fish L et al. Contemporary outcomes of intact and ruptured visceral artery aneurysms. J Vasc Surg. 2015;61(6): 1442–1447.
9. Stone WM, Abbas M, Cherry KJ et al. Superior mesenteric artery aneurysms: is presence an indication for intervention? J Vasc Surg. 2002;36(2): 234–237.
10. Sharma G, Semel ME, McGillicuddy EA et al. Ruptured and unruptured mycotic superior mesenteric artery aneurysms. Ann Vasc Surg. 2014;28(8): 1931.e5–8.
11. van Rijn MJ, Ten Raa S, Hendriks JM et al. Visceral aneurysms: Old paradigms, new insights? Best Pract Res Clin Gastroenterol. 2017;31(1): 97–104.
12. Tham G, Ekelund L, Herrlin K et al. Renal artery aneurysms. Natural history andprognosis. Ann Surg. 1983;197: 348–352.
13. Henke PK, Cardneau JD, Welling TH et al. Renal artery aneurysms: a 35-year clinical experience with 252 aneurysms in 168 patients. Ann Surg. 2001;234: 454–462.
14. Klausner JQ, Harlander-Locke MP, Plotnik AN et al. Current treatment of renal artery aneurysms may be too aggressive. J Vasc Surg. 2014;59: 1356–1361.
15. Brownstein AJ, Erben Y, Rajaee S et al. Natural history and management of renal artery aneurysms in a single tertiary referral center. J Vasc Surg. 2018;68(1): 137–144.
16. Robinson WP 3rd, Bafford R, Belkin M et al. Favorable outcomes with in situ techniques for surgical repair of complex renal artery aneurysms. J Vasc Surg. 2011;53: 684–691.

5

Complications of endovascular therapy for occlusive disease of splanchnic arteries including renal arteries

ROBERT G. MOLNAR AND COLLIN GANDILLON

Management of atherosclerotic occlusive disease of the splanchnic vessels and renal arteries has evolved over the years, especially with the increased utilization of endovascular therapies across all aspects of vascular disease. Historically, open surgical revascularization has been the treatment of choice for both chronic mesenteric ischemia (CMI) and renal artery stenosis (RAS). Open surgical repair, however, has been associated with significant morbidity for both CMI (2–33%)[1–4] and RAS (15–43%),[5–8] as well as elevated mortality rate, 1–17% for CMI[1–4] and 2–26% for RAS.[5–8]

Endovascular therapy, using percutaneous transluminal angioplasty with or without stenting, sought to minimize the morbidity and mortality associated with open surgical repair while maintaining the clinical efficacy of open revascularization. Cai et al. showed that in-hospital complications were significantly lower in those treated with endovascular therapy compared to open surgery for chronic mesenteric ischemia with no differences noted in mortality.[9] Similarly, Patel et al. demonstrated significantly less peri-procedural complications in those with renal artery atherosclerotic disease treated with endovascular therapy compared to those who underwent open surgery.[6]

As the treatment paradigm for atherosclerotic occlusive disease of the splanchnic and renal vessels has shifted to an endovascular therapy first approach, the interventionalist must be cognizant of the potential complications associated with endovascular interventions. The aim of this chapter is to highlight some of these complications and to suggest techniques to help prevent these complications when performing splanchnic and renal interventions.

INDICATIONS

The indications for both renal and splanchnic interventions are fully covered in a previous chapter. For purposes of clarity, the following are generally accepted indications for intervention in each of these vascular beds. Indications for renal angioplasty with stenting are poorly controlled hypertension on four or greater blood pressure medications and flash pulmonary edema with severe renal artery stenosis. A relative indication is worsening renal function in the presence of one functioning kidney with severe atherosclerotic disease in an attempt to preserve renal function. Renal artery angioplasty without stenting is indicated in symptomatic hypertensive patients with fibromuscular dysplasia characterized by the classic "string of beads" appearance.

(CMI) is the most frequent indication for celiac or mesenteric angioplasty with or without stenting. While three vessels contribute to the splanchnic circulation (celiac, superior mesenteric and inferior mesenteric arteries), the superior mesenteric is the most commonly treated artery for CMI. Patients with progressive CMI usually present with post-prandial abdominal pain, significant weight loss and food fear. Most patients classically present with cachexia and significant weight loss over a 3–6 month period. While many patients will present with a previous gastro-intestinal workup, including EGDs and colonoscopies, most will never have had an evaluation of their mesenteric circulation.

DIAGNOSIS

The diagnosis of severe renal and mesenteric artery stenosis is fully covered in the previous chapter dedicated to the identification and treatment of these vascular beds. The diagnostic approach can, however, aid in developing a safe and effective endovascular approach that can limit potential complications. The first test to be considered should be a duplex evaluation as this test can often rule in or rule out hemodynamically significant occlusive disease. Skilled vascular technologists in certified vascular laboratories are best suited to evaluate both renal and mesenteric occlusive disease processes. Many patients with CMI will have had multiple previous tests as the diagnosis of CMI requires a high index of suspicion. These patients might have seen a number of physicians who had formulated a varied differential diagnosis with ancillary testing but did not include vascular insufficiency on their lists of potential diagnoses. Renal artery stenosis is frequently evaluated in patients with refractory hypertension as well as renal insufficiency.

Computerized Tomography (CT) scans and radiographic studies obtained during a patient's workup might suggest significant aortic and branch vessel calcifications, but will not provide an accurate assessment of the severity of disease. If a duplex examination confirms severe disease, a CT angiogram (CTA) can be obtained. A CTA will allow a thorough evaluation of the renal and splanchnic circulation and provide additional information that can be helpful in planning the endovascular approach.

ENDOVASCULAR INTERVENTION

It is acceptable to proceed with an angiogram with intent to treat with patients clearly having appropriate symptoms associated with duplex documentation of severe occlusive disease. However, prior to any intervention, it is helpful to obtain a CTA or magnetic resonance angiogram (MRA) to fully assess the disease process and the anatomy. A thorough review of these noninvasive images will significantly help with planning the appropriate approach to endovascular intervention. While most renal interventions are easily achieved from a trans-femoral approach, our approach to most mesenteric interventions is a brachial approach. The renal arteries originate from the aorta at a near 90-degree angle in most patients and allows for fairly straightforward endovascular intervention from the retrograde femoral approach. However, some renal arteries have a more acute aortic angle and are best approached by a brachial artery access. Most mesenteric artery interventions, while clearly possible from a trans-femoral approach, are usually much more easily accessed from an upper extremity arterial approach given a more consistent acute angle off of the aorta.

Any opportunity to plan the approach prior to the intervention will save time and also protect from potential complications. Once a retrograde or antegrade approach is selected, obtain either femoral or brachial artery access using ultrasound and a micro-puncture system. Some prefer to perform a cut down on the brachial artery to allow for artery repair at completion and to lessen the risk of postprocedural hematoma. We use a 6FR sheath, the length and shape of which should allow the tip to be in close proximity to the vessel to be treated. A coaxial system of a guiding catheter with a selective catheter is then used to select the vessel, obtain wire access, and complete the intervention. Completion angiograms are performed to assess for optimized treatment. A more complete description of the technique for endovascular treatment is highlighted in previous chapters, however our descriptive approach to the intervention allows for safe planning and eliminates many potential complications.

COMPLICATIONS

Complications are most commonly access-related, including access site hematomas (Figure 5.1), retroperitoneal bleeding or hematoma (Figure 5.2), pseudoaneurysm formation (Figure 5.3), access vessel dissection, or thrombosis. Distal embolization may occur to the vascular bed being treated but can also occur to any downstream territory in any arterial segment traversed by the sheath/catheter system. Renal or mesenteric artery dissection (Figures 5.4–5.6), perforation, or distal branch perforation with subsequent bleed are also possible. Contrast nephropathy can occur in patients with renal insufficiency and can be exacerbated in patients relatively dehydrated. Each of these will be addressed with attention to avoiding the complication using safe and effective techniques.

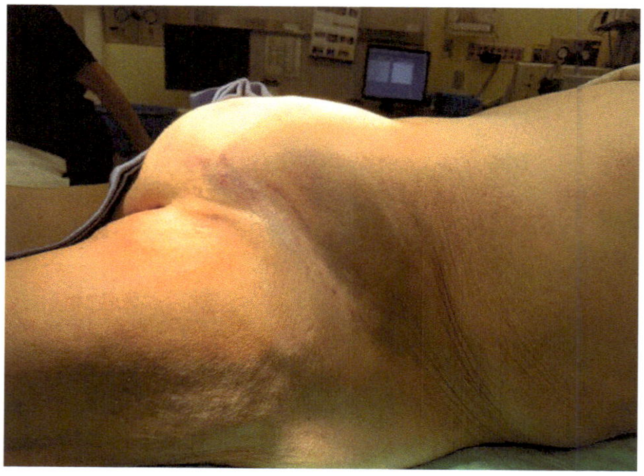

Figure 5.1 Large left femoral hematoma.

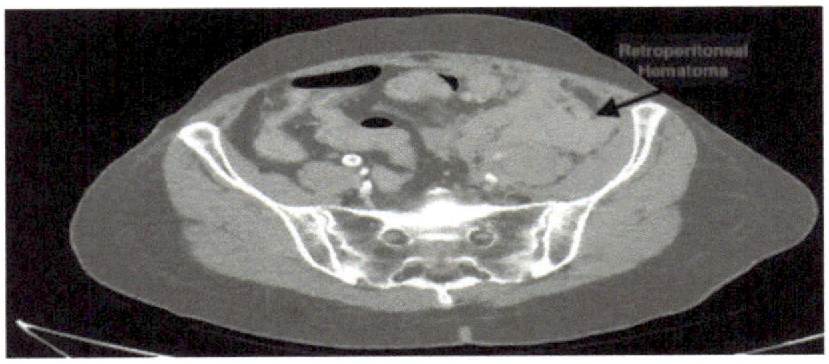

Figure 5.2 CT scan of large left retroperitoneal hematoma.

FEMORAL HEMATOMAS, PSEUDOANEURYSMS, DISSECTIONS, OCCLUSIONS, AND RETROPERITONEAL HEMATOMAS

As with any endovascular procedure using a femoral approach, attention to patient-specific characteristics and to the technical details of a safe and effective sheath placement is paramount. If the patient is obese and has a large pannus, it might be prudent to change to a brachial approach to avoid the more challenging femoral access. At times, in the morbidly obese, it is helpful to tape the pannus up toward the chest to allow unfettered access to the femoral artery.

Under fluoroscopy, the mid-femoral head should be located to ensure that femoral access is being performed in an area that can be compressed following the procedure. Ultrasound should be used to assess the common femoral artery, identify the femoral bifurcation, and identify a segment of the artery that is devoid of severe disease. Under direct ultrasound visualization, the artery should be accessed and the sheath placed via Seldinger technique. Should there be any resistance with wire advancement during access, fluoroscopy should be employed.

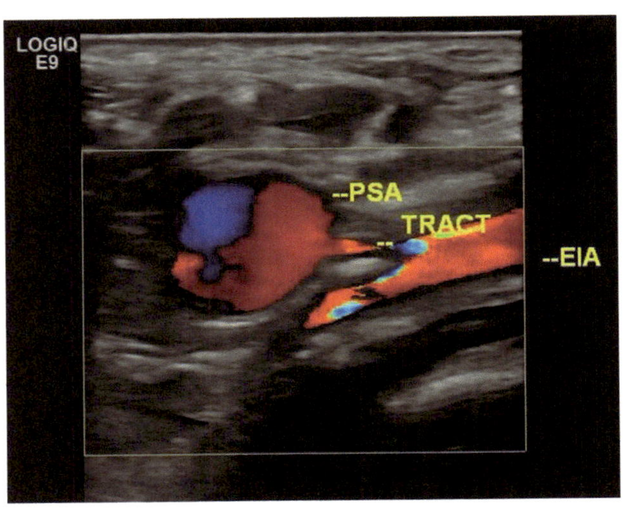

Figure 5.3 Duplex ultrasonography of common femoral artery pseudoaneurysm.

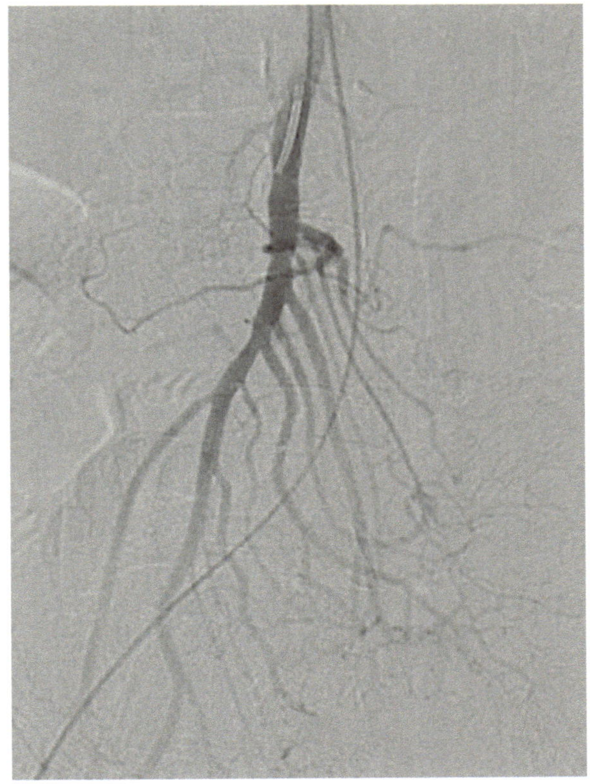

Figure 5.4 Selective superior mesenteric artery angiogram.

If continued resistance or failure of smooth wire passage is encountered, a retrograde angiogram should be obtained to assist in wire traversal, to ensure there is no arterial dissection, and to identify whether there is a contra-indication for sheath placement. Following the procedure, the femoral access site can be managed with a closure device per the device's instruction for use or with manual pressure by a trained member of the team.

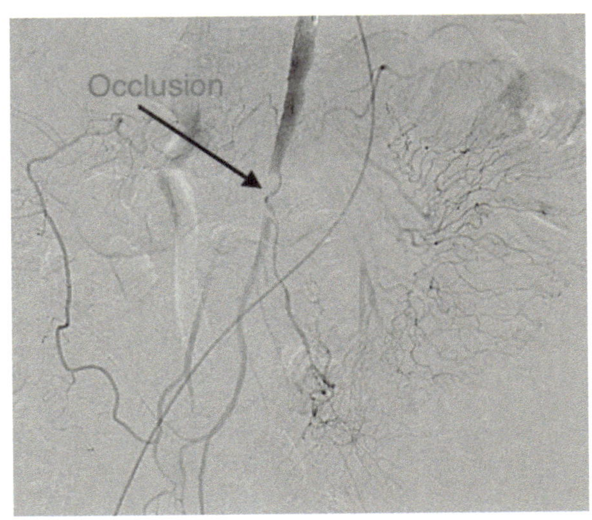

Figure 5.5 Occlusion of superior mesenteric artery secondary to dissection.

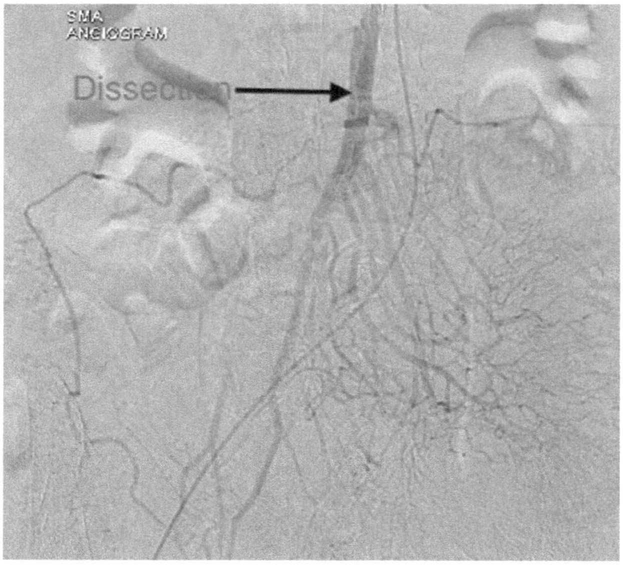

Figure 5.6 Dissection plane in superior mesenteric artery.

BRACHIAL ARTERY HEMATOMA WITH POTENTIAL NERVE COMPRESSION, DISSECTION, PSEUDOANEURYSM, OR OCCLUSION

While the brachial artery can certainly be accessed percutaneously, some patient characteristics would suggest that a surgical cut down be performed to manage the artery following the procedure. These characteristics would include a very obese arm, a brachial artery less than 3 mm or severe atherosclerotic disease. It is important to ensure that there is not a high brachial bifurcation in the access arm to avoid accessing a radial artery that is the dominant supply to the hand. If a percutaneous approach is utilized, it should be done in a healthy portion of the artery near the antecubital fossa to allow for compression on the underlying bony prominences following the procedure. A micropuncture sheath should be used first, then exchanged out over a j-tipped wire to the larger sheath. A small amount of diluted contrast can be used under fluoroscopy to ensure there is no dissection prior to intervention.

While either brachial artery can be utilized to gain access to the renal or mesenteric vessels, the left is generally preferred to avoid having the catheterization coursing across the origins of all great vessels. While there is still a risk of stroke, that risk is minimized by using the left brachial approach. Since the celiac and mesenteric images require a lateral or near-lateral view, standing cranial to the arm access allows the image intensifier to be rotated into a lateral abdominal position without competing for positioning with the interventionalist.

EMBOLIZATION

Embolization is a dreaded complication that can be identified following a technically successful angioplasty and stenting. Embolization can and will occur even with the most experienced and technically astute interventionalist. Some inherent risks arise from the "shaggy aorta," in reference to luminal irregularities of the aorta. These irregularities can include soft plaque, calcific lesions, and ectatic segments that are crossed with the balloon or stent delivery platform. Even with expert technical skills, those patients with this aortic pathology are at very high risk for distal embolization. To reduce the risk of such embolic events in these high-risk patients, it is particularly important to have adequate preprocedure planning so that the approach allows for the least catheter manipulation within the diseased aorta. Approaching a mesenteric vessel with a severe acute angle in a diseased aortic segment from a femoral approach can lead to increased risk of embolization. In this circumstance, approaching the intended artery from a brachial approach will be protective. On the contrary, if the descending thoracic aorta has severe disease, a retrograde femoral approach might be a safer approach. Pre-planning the approach and selecting appropriate sheaths and catheters can provide an important level of protection.

The recipient bed in either the renal or mesenteric outflow can also be subject to embolization. While there is a paucity of data on plaque morphology and the risk of embolization, filter options are available and should be used if it is felt the embolization risk is high. Predilatation of the target lesion should not be overly aggressive and should be performed to allow safe passage of the stent without stent dislodgement from the stent balloon. In addition, if there is inadequate anticoagulation or the working sheath/catheter is indwelling without periodic flushing, thrombus can form within the sheath/catheter and can embolize distally. Should embolization occur with significant distal flow reduction, aspiration embolectomy catheters can be used in an attempt to clear the embolic debris. One opportunity following stent deployment is to replace the obturator of the sheath, advance the large bore sheath as close as possible to the embolic debris, and perform a strong aspiration. If the sheath cannot be advance to the area of embolization, a 5Fr diagnostic catheter or an aspiration embolectomy catheter, such as the Export catheter (R-Medtronic Corporation, Santa Ana, California), can be used to advance to the embolic point and aspirate the debris.

If there is significant embolization that does not respond to aspiration, advancing the 0.014 wire past the blockage/occlusion can allow for positioning of a reference vessel diameter balloon that, once inflated, can break the embolic material into smaller pieces, allowing for more successful aspiration or preservation of some of the important distal branch vessels.

ARTERIAL DISSECTION, PERFORATION, AND OCCLUSION

Any intervention on an arterial segment can be complicated by a dissection (Figures 5.4–5.6). A meticulous technique with ensuring true luminal positioning of the crossing wire is fundamental in treating renal, mesenteric, or celiac vessels. Once a crossing catheter is confirmed in the true lumen, we generally place a 0.014 support wire and use 0.014 balloon-expandable stents. Balloon-expandable stents are necessary for these ostial lesions to provide additional radial force, allow for precise stent placement, and avoid mal-positioning of the stent. This platform allows for a lower-profile system, which can be advantageous with tortuosity or tight stenoses. For severely diseased segments, predilatation with a standard 0.014 balloon to approximately 75% of the reference vessel diameter will allow for safe placement of the stent at the target lesion. If this is not performed, the balloon-mounted stent might not cross the lesion without significant resistance, which can ultimately lead to the stent becoming dislodged from the balloon. If this were to occur, it might be necessary to deploy the stent not completely within the target lesion and extend into the aorta more than intended. It is critical that, should the stent become dislodged, the wire access is not lost. Losing wire access across the lesion with a dislodged stent can lead to stent embolization, which might not be successfully retrieved or deployed in another artery via endovascular techniques.

The stent size should be one to one with the reference vessel diameter to avoid vessel perforation, distal dissection, and under-sizing that can lead to malposition of the stent. Should the crossing wire not be within the true lumen, the stent will be deployed in a subintimal plane and likely lead to vessel occlusion. This is very difficult to correct without advanced endovascular skills and carries the potential of renal, mesenteric, or end-organ ischemia. Confirming that the crossing wire placement is within the true vessel distally is an essential part of any endovascular procedure and will almost certainly result in a complication if the wire is not in the true lumen.

One potential complication, that can occur given the inherent bias for the interventionalist to be fixated on the lesion, is distal small vessel perforation resulting in bleeding (Figure 5.7). This is due to failure to manage the distal tip of the crossing wire. Often times the crossing wire is confirmed in the true lumen distally, but increased magnification or a change in the orientation of the radiographic image leads to loss of visualization of the tip of the crossing wire. Inadvertent advancement of the wire during the intervention can lead to renal parenchymal perforation with retroperitoneal hemorrhage or mesenteric hematoma from perforation of a terminal vessel.

Other complications that can occur include contrast-induced nephropathy, cardiac events, and other bleeding complications due to anticoagulation and dual antiplatelet therapy. In patients with renal insufficiency (GFR 30–60), pre- and postprocedure hydration should be utilized with the judicious use of contrast – (i.e., less than 3 times the GFR). Intravascular ultrasound, CO_2 angiography of large vessels, and diluted contrast can be used to limit contrast administration. In patients with a GFR less than 30 ml/min, a nephrology consult should be obtained prior to procedures utilizing contrast to optimize renal function and reduce the risk of worsening renal insufficiency. Cardiac events can include hypotension, hypertension, arrhythmias, and even myocardial infarction. While these conditions are often due the patient's comorbidities, effective monitoring and appropriate medical treatment of these conditions are necessary to prevent cardiac-related complications, especially in those receiving moderate conscious sedation.

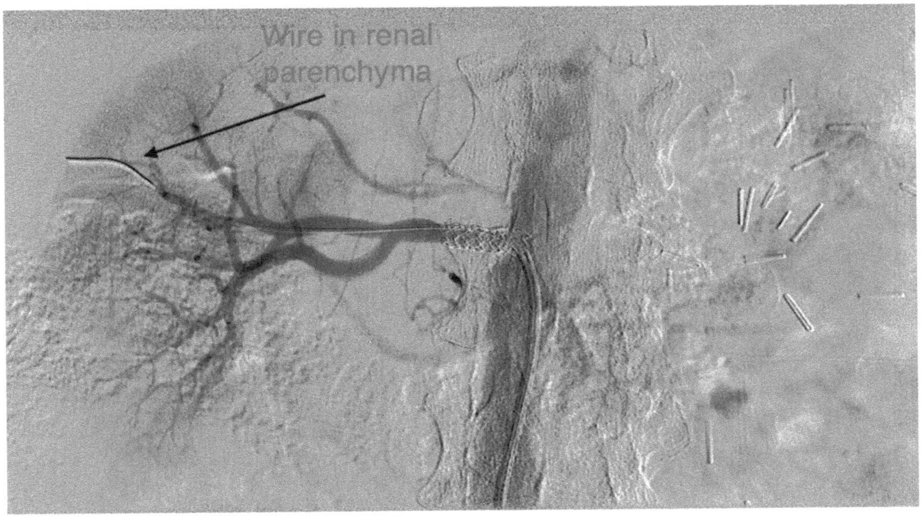

Figure 5.7 Guidewire in renal parenchyma.

CONCLUSION

Endovascular interventions in the renal and splanchnic vessels can be performed safely with minimal complications if appropriate and effective techniques are employed. Attention to detail with a thorough understanding of safe arterial access, target vessel cannulation, and pre-planning for the appropriate approach to the target vessel will help prevent potential complications. Anticipating the potential complications and having strategies to effectively treat the complications are essential for the competent and effective vascular interventionalist.

REFERENCES

1. Atkins, MD, Kwolek CJ, LaMuraglia GM, Brewster DC, Chung TK, Cambria RP. Surgical Revascularization Versus Endovascular Therapy for Chronic Mesenteric Ischemia: A Comparative Experience. J Vasc Surg. 2007 Jun; 45(6): 1162–1171.
2. Kasirajan K, O'Hara PJ, Gray BH, Hertzer NR, Clair DG, Greenburg RK, Krajewski LP, Beven EG, Ouriel K. Chronic Mesenteric Ischemia: Open Surgery Versus Percutaneous Angioplasty and Stenting. J Vasc Surg. 2001 Jan; 33(1): 63–71.
3. Tallarita T, Oderich GS, Gloviczki P, Duncan AA, Kaira M, Cha S, Misra S, Bower TC. Patient Survival After Open and Endovascular Mesenteric Revascularization for Chronic Mesenteric Ischemia. J Vasc Surg. 2013 Mar; 57(3): 747–755.
4. Lejay A, Georg Y, Tartaglia E, Creton O, Lucereau B, Thaveau F, Geny B, Chakfe N. Chronic Mesenteric Ischemia: 20 Year Experience of Open Surgical Treatment. Eur J Vasc Endovasc Surg. 2015 May; 49(5): 587–592.
5. Darling RC 3rd, Kreienburg PB, Chang BB, Paty PS, Lloyd WE, Leather RP, Shah DM. Outcome of Renal Artery Reconstruction: Analysis of 687 Procedures. Ann Surg. 1999 Oct; 230(4): 524–530.
6. Patel VI, Conrad MF, Kwolek CJ, LaMuraglia GM, Chung TK, Cambria RP. Renal Artery Revascularization: Outcomes Stratified by Indication for Intervention. J Vasc Surg. 2009 Jun; 49(6): 1480–1489.
7. Balzer KM, Pfeiffer T, Rossbach S, Voiculescu A, Modder U, Godehardt E, Sandmann W. Prospective Randomized Trial of Operative vs. Interventional Treatment for Renal Artery Ostial Occlusive Disease (RAOOD). J Vasc Surg. 2009 Mar; 49(3): 667–674.
8. Cambria RP, Brewster DC, L'Italien GJ, Gertier JP, Abbott WM, LaMuraglia GM, Moncure AC, Vignati J, Bazari H, Fang LT, Atamian S. Renal Artery Reconstruction for the Preservation of Renal Function. J Vasc Surg. 1996 Sep; 24(3): 371–380.
9. Cai W, Li X, Shu C, Qiu J, Fang K, Li M, Chen Y, Liu D. Comparison of Clinical Outcomes of Endovascular Versus Open Revascularization for Chronic Mesenteric Ischemia: A Meta-Analysis. Ann Vasc Surg. 2015 Jul; 29(5): 934–940.

6

Complications of endovascular management of aortoiliac occlusive disease

KAREM C. HARTH, SAIDEEP BOSE, AND VIKRAM S. KASHYAP

The second most common area of disease in patients with peripheral arterial disease, after the superficial femoral artery (SFA), is the aortoiliac segment.[1] Patients with aortoiliac occlusive disease (AIOD) have variable presentations ranging from asymptomatic to critical limb ischemia (CLI). Surgical management of the symptomatic patient has undergone a transformation with improving endovascular techniques shifting what was classically thought to be an open paradigm to one that is increasingly endovascular.

Historically, the aortobifemoral (ABF) bypass has been the gold standard. According to the Trans-Atlantic Inter-Society Consensus (TASC) II guidelines, patients with more severe disease, defined as C and D lesions, should be treated with open surgical reconstruction. A meta-analysis of studies published between 1970–1996 demonstrated a 10 year patency for ABF bypass of 86.8% in patients with claudication and 81.8% in patients with CLI. Furthermore, although the mortality associated with the procedure had decreased from 4.6% to 3.3%,[2] morbidity remained high with major systemic morbidity in up to 10% of patients and overall morbidity of 11–32%.[3]

With the rapid advancement of endovascular technology and experience since the publication of the TASC II guidelines, many vascular specialists have questioned whether those guidelines are applicable to current treatment modalities.[4] Although no large randomized trials exist that compare endovascular therapy to open repair for AIOD, it has become increasingly used as the initial treatment strategy in many centers. A review looking at 1711 AIOD patients treated with an endovascular approach found that clinical symptoms improved in 83–100% of patients with a 5 year primary patency rate of 60–86% and secondary patency rate of 80–98%.[5] Newer studies at high-volume centers provide 5 year secondary patency rates for endovascular treatment of AIOD that are similar to that of open surgical reconstruction, but with less associated morbidity. Importantly, limb salvage and survival are similar in the two groups.[6] Furthermore, the technical success rate of endovascular interventions is high, with most studies citing success rates > 90%. However, data also show that complications associated with an endovascular approach can be variable, ranging from 3–45% of patients, including distal embolization, hematoma, pseudoaneurysm, arterial rupture, and dissection.

One of the larger series looking at complications after aortoiliac intervention is a multicenter study from Japan that analyzed outcomes in 1995 consecutive patients who were followed for at least 30 days. The overall perioperative complication rate was 6.3%, with the three most common complications being distal embolization (1.6%), puncture site hematoma (1.6%), and acute kidney injury (0.9%). The rate of vessel perforation was 0.2%, and the rate of stent thrombosis was 0.3%. At an average of 5 years, the rate of major adverse cardiac events (MACE) was 14.3%, the rate of major adverse limb events (MALE) was 7.4%, the rate of any re-intervention was 6.7%, and the rate of surgical re-intervention was 1.4%. In a multi-variate model, the highest predictors for postoperative complications were age > 80, critical limb ischemia on presentation, and TASC C or D lesions.[7]

Another analysis of 223 patients undergoing interventions for either iliac artery occlusion or stenosis, found a combined intraoperative complication rate of 6.3%. The most common complication was thrombosis (3.1%) and rupture (1.8%). Dissection or distal embolization occurred in 0.4% patients.[8] Although performed in very different populations, the above results demonstrate that, in general, the rate of perioperative complications for endovascular intervention of AIOD is low. However, prompt recognition and intervention is key as they can lead to significant morbidity and mortality. Complications with AIOD intervention can be distinct from complications in the femoropopliteal area. This is related to the anatomy, distinct size changes at branch points including the aortic/iliac bifurcations, and risk of hemorrhage into the abdomen. We present a series of cases that provide examples of such complications, bail out techniques used for each case, and key learning points that can be drawn from each of these scenarios.

PATIENT CASES, LEARNING POINTS AND MANAGEMENT OF COMPLICATIONS

CASE 6.1: Dissection

The first patient is a 73-year-old female with isolated left leg lifestyle-limiting claudication. Her history is significant for severe chronic obstructive pulmonary disease (COPD) requiring continuous home oxygen, remote tobacco abuse, hypertension, and hyperlipidemia. She has had no prior revascularization procedures. She is unable to participate in her pulmonary rehab program secondary to her claudication. Preoperative evaluation included noninvasive studies suggestive of inflow disease of the left lower extremity and a preoperative CT angiogram (CTA) demonstrating an approximately 30 mm occlusion of her left common iliac artery (Figure 6.1). This CTA also demonstrated small, heavily calcified vessels.

She was taken electively to the interventional suite where ultrasound-guided access was obtained of her left radial artery, a 5 Fr Slender sheath was inserted, and an angle glide Navicross was used to perform an aortogram. Adequate heparinization with ACT checks was initiated. This confirmed occlusion of her left common iliac artery. The lesion was crossed with a 0.18 Gold Glidewire and Navicross catheter. True lumen entry and catheter positioning was confirmed with an angiogram at the level of the left common femoral artery prior to advancing our intervention wire. A long stiff Glidewire was advanced to her superficial femoral artery (SFA) and predilation was initiated with a 3 × 40 mm balloon. Angioplasty was then performed with a 4 × 100 mm radial to peripheral (R2P) balloon. Post-angioplasty angiogram showed no flow through the external iliac artery (Figure 6.2A), but it was unclear if this was due to thrombus or dissection. Wire access was never lost during these steps. Conversion to a more conventional transfemoral endovascular approach was adopted at this point to define the complication and treat her iliac occlusive disease.

Bilateral common femoral access was subsequently obtained, and it was clear from angiography that there was a dissection flap. Bilateral groin sheaths were upsized to 7Fr and kissing-balloon angioplasty with 6 × 80 mm balloons was performed in bilateral common iliac arteries after confirming successful retrograde recanalization (Figure 6.2B). Although this created a better angiographic result with inline flow from the aorta to the left common femoral artery, there was still a dissection flap present (Figure 6.3A). A self-expanding 9 × 80 Everflex stent was placed in the distal left iliac artery at the area of dissection with no luminal irregularities seen post-stent deployment. Bilateral 7 × 59 iCast stents were then deployed in the common iliac arteries as well as a 9 × 40 self-expanding stent to bridge the gap between the two stents on the left common and external iliac artery. Final angiogram showed arterial continuity with no flow-limiting lesions and inline flow down to the foot (Figure 6.3B). Protamine was given, sheaths were removed, and hemostasis was obtained with manual pressure. Postprocedure management included dual antiplatelet therapy and a high-intensity statin. The patient was seen in clinic at one and 6 months postprocedure with palpable pulses, resolved claudication symptoms, and full participation in her pulmonary rehabilitation.

KEY LEARNING POINTS: *DISSECTION*

There are several learning points from this complication.

1. Flow-limiting dissections need to be identified and treated at the index procedure. This can be achieved through a combination of using balloon dilation in an attempt to oppose the flap back to the arterial wall or placing a stent to tack the dissection flap in place. There is data to support that the severity of dissection (in terms of luminal compromise) is strongly correlated with restenosis, thrombosis, and need for target lesion revascularization.[9] Furthermore, in a study looking at the superficial femoral artery, dissections that were otherwise classified as mild (<1/3 vessel lumen) were nevertheless found to be significant predictors of restenosis if the dissection flap was long (>100 mm).[10] Another key point in identifying a dissection is that it can be missed using a retrograde injection of contrast (via a sheath) vs when doing an antegrade angiogram (flush catheter in the aorta). The latter is needed at the end of all interventions to prevent missing a flow-limiting dissection.

2. Choice of arterial access site for intervention is key. A radial first approach was chosen due to patient factors and surgeon choice. In this patient, the radial approach did not allow for a clear identification of the area of injury, and a change in approach was adopted to define the problem. In retrospect, this approach was not the ideal initial arterial access site given her extensive bilateral iliac disease and heavily calcified vessels with unilateral occlusion to the origin on the left. Bilateral transfemoral access with angioplasty provided the appropriate maneuver to treat the complicating flow-limiting dissection. While radial access technology is appealing and is undergoing rapid improvements, it is still in an early development stage and should be considered as a back-up or adjunct to a failed transfemoral approach.[11]

Despite the right side being asymptomatic for the patient, it was thought safest to treat both common iliac arteries in "kissing fashion" to avoid potentially compromising the right side via plaque shift. Finally, treatment of the dissection flap with a stent in the setting of more proximal occlusive disease was important to re-establishing inline flow. Given the location of the lesion at the distal left external iliac artery, overlapping stents from the area of dissection up to the common iliac arteries were performed in order to assure no residual focal flaps were left behind in the short interval segment of iliac artery between the two stented regions.

There is generally clinical equipoise regarding whether self-expanding (SE) or balloon-expandable (BE) stents performs better in the iliac vasculature. Large retrospective analyses have shown equivalent primary patency at 5 years (75% vs 79%).[12] However, the Efficacy Study of Iliac Stents to Treat Iliac Artery Lesions (BRAVISSIMO) data demonstrated an increased primary patency rate of SE (92.1%) vs BE (85.2%) stents at 2 years.[13] The randomized Iliac Artery Stents for Common or External Iliac Artery Occlusive Disease (ICE) trial also showed a decreased re-stenosis rate at 12 months for SE stents (6.1%) vs balloon-expandable stents (14.9%).[14] There is a belief that the common iliac artery and the external iliac artery behave very differently i.e., – the external iliac artery (EIA) is generally more tortuous and artificially straightening with a balloon expandable stent may increase sheer stress and enhanced neo-intimal proliferation.[15] Many have adopted a strategy of using covered stents in heavily calcified lesions in the common iliac artery and self-expanding stents in the external iliac arteries.

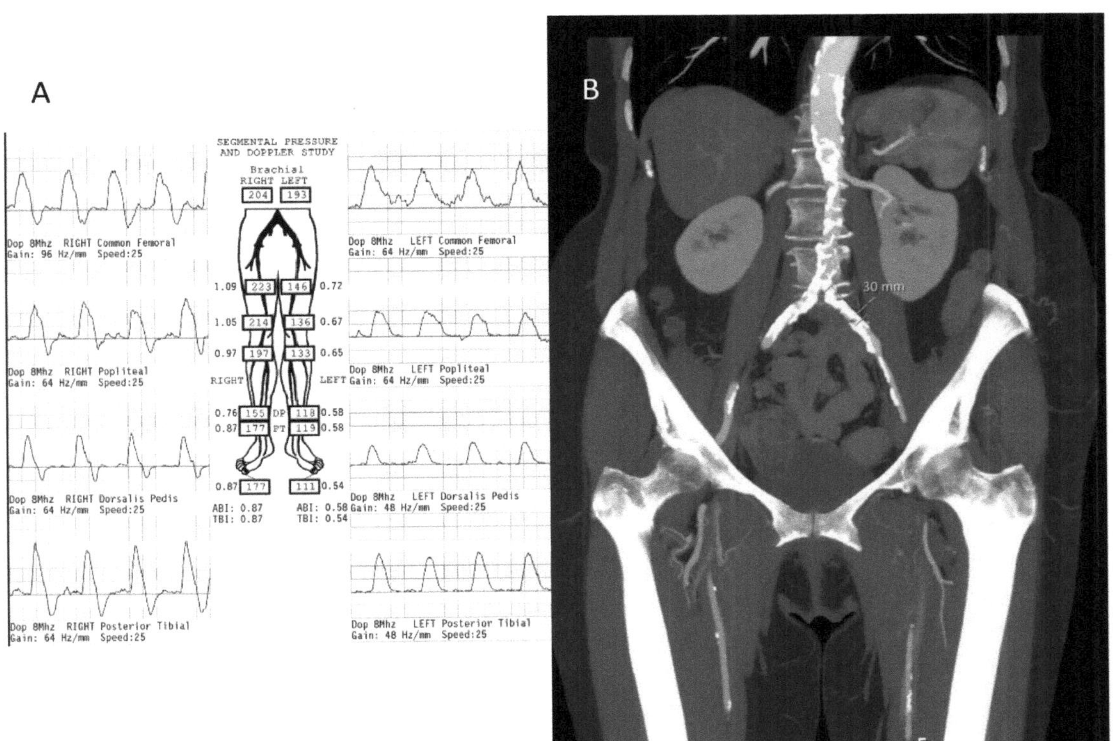

Figure 6.1 Preoperative imaging in patient presenting with lifestyle-limiting claudication of the left leg. (A) Non-invasive studies demonstrating inflow disease of the left leg. (B) CTA demonstrating severe aortoiliac disease with occlusion of the left common iliac artery.

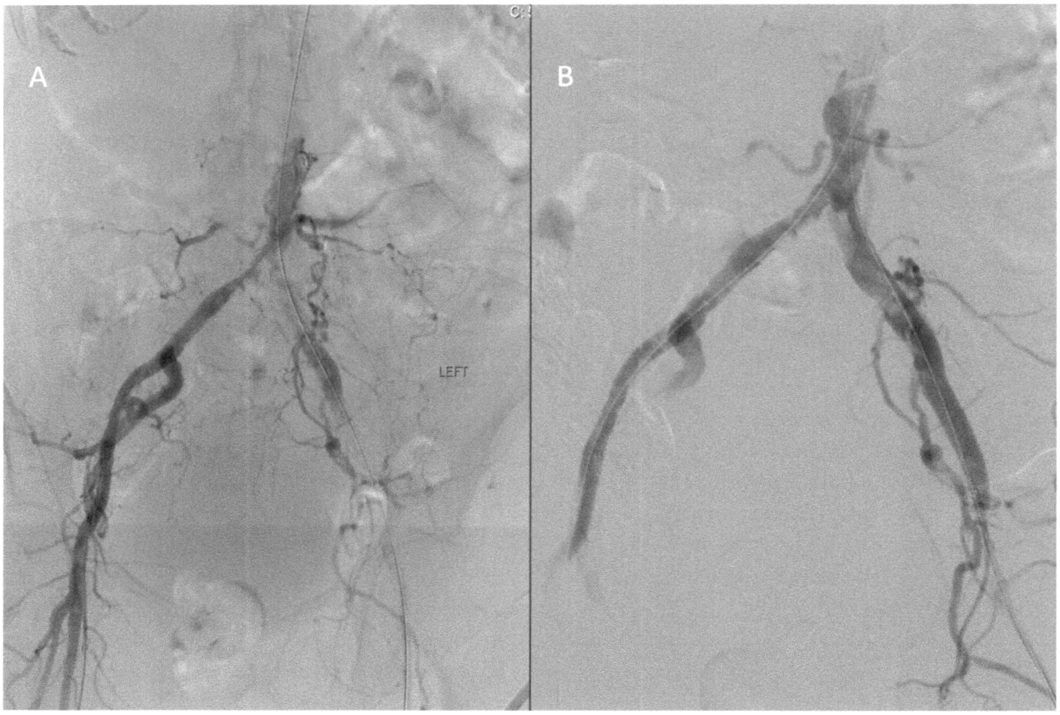

Figure 6.2 Angiography after transradial angioplasty of the left external iliac artery. (A) Initial angiogram demonstrating no flow through the external iliac artery. (B) Restored flow after retrograde recanalization and bilateral common iliac artery intervention.

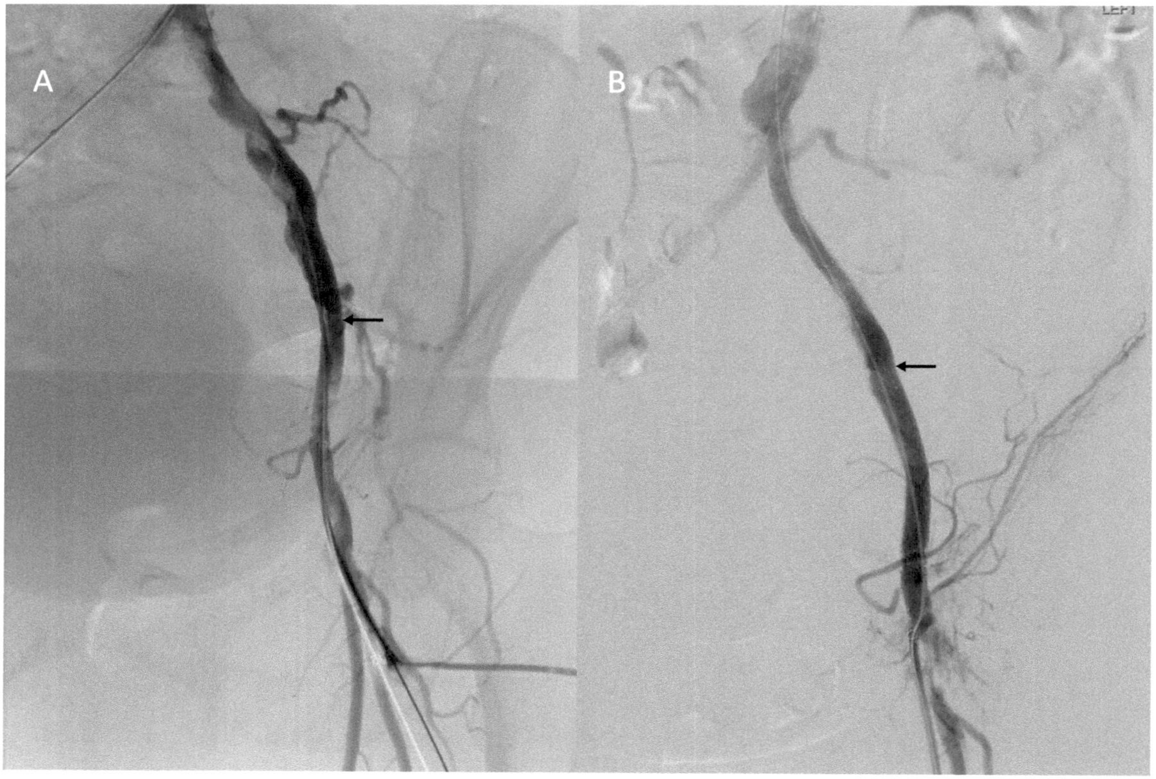

Figure 6.3 Dissection after angioplasty. (A) Demonstration of dissection on angiography via left common femoral artery access. (B) No residual dissection after deployment of self-expanding stent in the distal external iliac artery.

CASE 6.2: Thrombosis and Dissection

Patient is an 82-year-old male who presents with progressive lifestyle-limiting claudication of the left lower extremity. His medical history is significant for chronic obstructive pulmonary disease, pulmonary fibrosis, and hyperlipidemia. He has otherwise had no surgeries, no prior revascularizations, and stopped smoking more than 10 years ago.

The patient was electively brought to the interventional suite and ultrasound-guided right transfemoral access was obtained. Angiography revealed a focal distal left superficial femoral artery (SFA) lesion and a possible left iliac artery stenosis. The high-grade left SFA lesions was dilated with a 5 mm plain balloon angioplasty catheter. The left iliac lesion was evaluated further with pullback pressures demonstrating a systolic gradient > 40 mmHg with a mean gradient of 14 mmHg, indicating a hemodynamically significant lesion (Figure 6.4A). Balloon angioplasty was performed with a persistent gradient and a 9 mm × 60 mm Protégé self-expanding stent was deployed, which was post-dilated with a 9 mm balloon. The post-stent angiogram showed a significantly improved angiographic result with brisk flow. A non-flow-limiting dissection flap was noted at the distal external iliac artery (Figure 6.4B). No further intervention was undertaken; the patient was loaded with Plavix and sent home on a regimen of dual antiplatelet therapy.

The patient presented to clinic 5 days postprocedure complaining of increasing left foot numbness and an inability to dorsiflex. He had a cold pale foot with no left femoral pulse. Noninvasive studies showed flat waveforms at the ankle with monophasic flow at the high thigh indicative of iliac occlusion. The patient was taken urgently to the operating room where a right transfemoral aortogram was performed. This identified a left common, external, and internal iliac artery occlusion with reconstitution of the left common femoral artery via the circumflex vessels (Figure 6.5A).

Antegrade recanalization was first attempted with no success due to repeated entry into the subintimal plane distal to the stent. Retrograde access via the left common femoral artery was obtained, and recanalization was performed and successful. After angiography confirmed anatomic landmarks, lysis was initiated with a 10 cm long McNamara catheter (length of occlusion was about 15 cm). Sheaths were secured, and tissue plasminogen activator (tPA) was administered at a rate of 1 mg/hour with 500 units/hour of heparin via the sheath side port. This was carried out overnight.

Lysis check 24 hours later showed improved flow through the left iliac system with residual thrombus. This was treated with AngioJet pharmaco-mechanical thrombectomy through a 7Fr sheath for a total volume of 51 mL. Persistent proximal luminal irregularities on repeat angiography likely secondary to underlying calcific disease were treated with a covered stent (9 × 59 cm iCAST) to the left common iliac artery. A persistent dissection flap just beyond the originally placed stent in the external iliac artery—the likely culprit lesion leading to thrombosis—was treated with an 8 × 60 self-expanding stent (Figure 6.5B). Completion angiogram demonstrated brisk inline flow to the foot via the anterior tibial artery (AT). The patient had a femoral pulse on the left at this time.

The procedure was terminated, the sheaths were removed, and pressure was held. However, immediately after removal of the sheaths, it was noted that there was no left AT signal and no left femoral pulse once again. Given concern for persistent dissection, likely into the common femoral artery, the patient was taken back to the operating room and a left groin cutdown was performed. The left CFA was without thrombus and with a signal on Doppler but no pulse. Direct micro-puncture access was obtained at the distal CFA, and an angiogram demonstrated a persistent dissection flap to the level of the circumflex arteries. Through a 6Fr sheath, an 8 × 40 mmHg self-expanding stent was placed and was dilated with a 6 × 60 balloon to tack the remainder of the dissection flap, and a pulse returned. Completion angiogram once again showed brisk, in-line flow from the aorta to the AT. The wound was closed, and the rest of his hospital course was unremarkable. He has been seen in clinic more than 1 year postoperatively and he ambulates without difficulty, although he does have mild persistent numbness of the left foot.

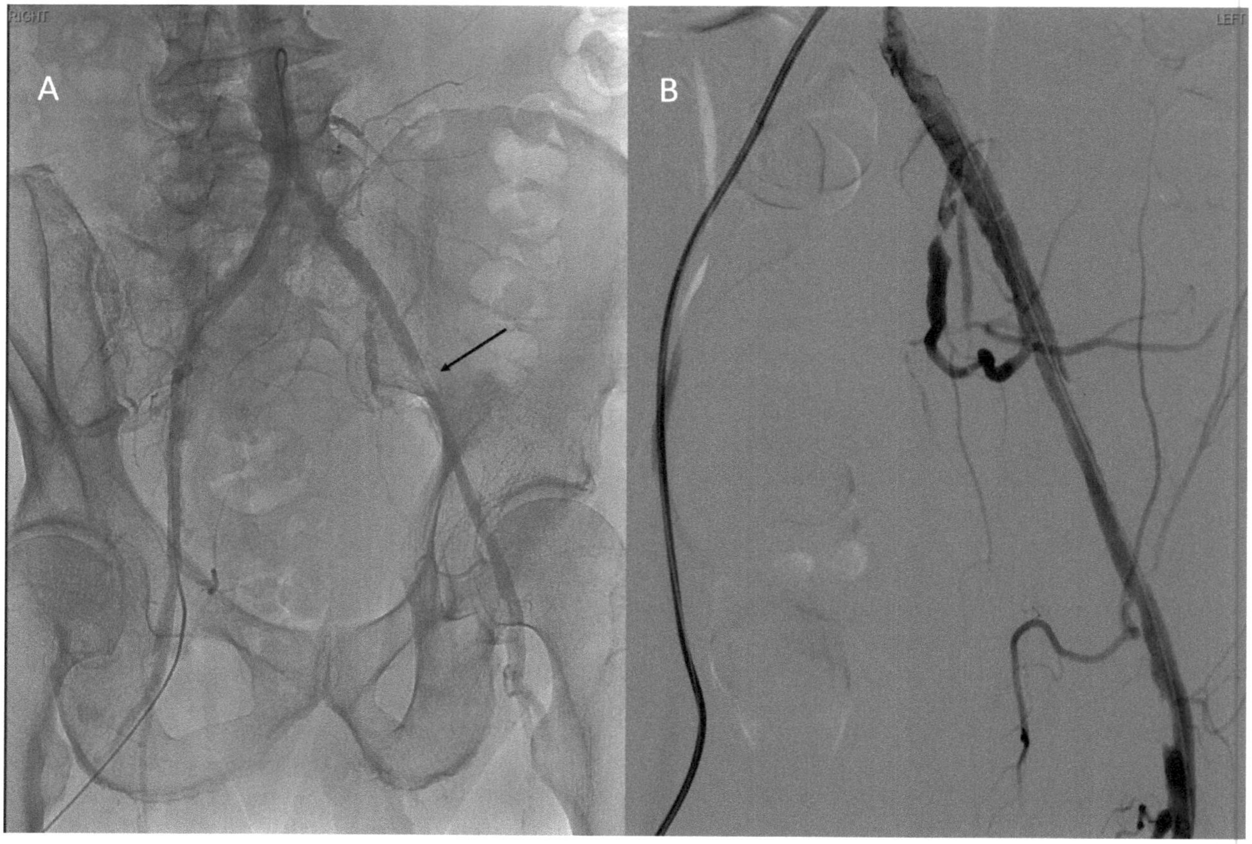

Figure 6.4 Angiogram demonstrating (A) Hemodynamically significant left external iliac artery stenosis. (B) Non-flow-limiting dissection flap post angioplasty and stenting.

KEY LEARNING POINTS: *THROMBOSIS AND DISSECTION*

There are several learning points from this series of complications.

1. Ensure complete treatment of a diseased area and identify plaque shift. As seen in this patient with persistent foot numbness more than a year after the index procedure, although thrombotic events are rare, they can lead to significant morbidity and hence their early recognition and treatment is important. At the index intervention, our pull-back pressures were key to deciding to treat the dissection flap with balloon angioplasty and a stent. A completion pull-back pressure may have led us to place additional stenting and tack what ultimately became a culprit lesion leading to thrombosis. On presentation 5 days following intervention, the patient was a Rutherford class IIb, and lysis was initiated expeditiously and successfully.
2. Always dissolve and remove thrombotic material prior to further angioplasty and/or stenting to mitigate embolization. There are multiple approaches to endovascular thrombectomy including percutaneous aspiration, thrombolysis, and mechanical thrombectomy. In this patient, a combination of thrombolysis with tPA and rheolytic thrombectomy with the AngioJet system were employed. Success of thrombolysis is based on the length of time from symptom onset to intervention[16] and the ability to recanalize the true lumen through the thrombus and not re-enter through a subintimal plane. Therefore, the AngioJet system is commonly used for *acute* thrombosis with excellent outcomes. One study of 18 patients demonstrated an amputation-free survival of 92.3% at 1 year,[17] and another study of 57 consecutive patients demonstrated amputation-free survival of 94.7% at 5 years.[18]

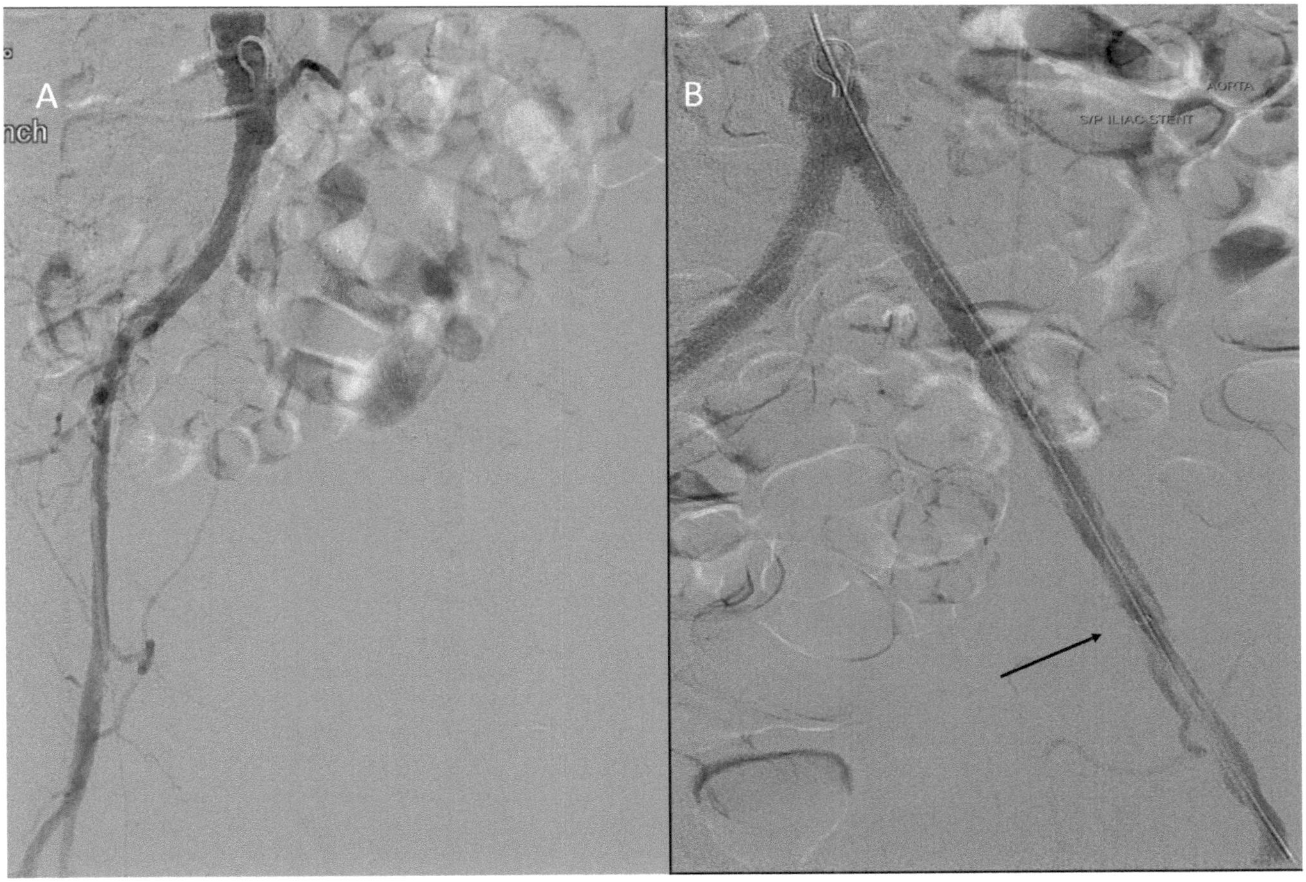

Figure 6.5 Patient presented 5 days after initial intervention with a cold foot and angiogram demonstrating (A) occluded left common, external, and internal iliac artery. (B) Brisk flow to the foot after overnight lysis, AngioJet, and stenting of the external iliac artery dissection. Arrow demonstrates likely dissection flap that was tacked up by sheath and became occlusive after sheath removal.

For patients who have had symptoms/thrombosis for longer periods of time, lysis is less successful. The Surgery versus Thrombolysis for Ischemia of the Lower Extremity (STILE) trial randomized 237 patients to thrombolysis or surgical revascularization and enrolled patients if they had symptoms for less than 6 months. After 1 year of follow-up, 43.8% of lysis patients experienced ongoing ischemia requiring intervention while only 20% of surgical patients did, and 28% experienced significant morbidity while only 5% of surgical patients did.[19] One additional explanation for the poor lysis outcomes in this trial is that only 21.8% of patients had AIOD, whereas more recent analysis demonstrate a higher success rate with endovascular interventions for AIOD when compared to femoropopliteal or tibial lesions.[20]

Overall, endovascular thrombectomy with or without thrombolysis can be an effective treatment for aortoiliac occlusion after intervention, especially in the acute/subacute setting. Even in the setting of acute limb ischemia, technical success can be as high as 82%, with a secondary patency rate of 65% at 2 years, and a limb salvage rate of 69%.[20]

The final learning point is that the persistent distal dissection at the level of the circumflex vessels was not identified on completion imaging. In hindsight, this is likely because the sheath in the left common femoral artery traversed through the distal dissection flap and helped to "tack up" the flap during the procedure. Once the sheath was removed, the unsupported flap became occlusive. If the etiology had been known in this case, additional stenting could have been accomplished endovascularly. However, if there was thrombosis instead of a flow-limited dissection, we would have proceeded with an open embolectomy. Open exploration to facilitate definitive treatment is an important approach to challenging cases.

CASE 6.3: Perforation

The patient is a 59-year-old male with debilitating claudication, with an absolute claudication distance of 75 m and unable to perform his assignments as a factory worker. His past medical history is significant for hypertension, hyperlipidemia, and ongoing smoking. Physical exam and noninvasive studies were consistent with bilateral inflow disease.

The patient was taken electively to the operating room where bilateral groin cutdowns were performed. An aortogram was performed that demonstrated occlusion of the right common iliac artery and significant stenosis of the left (Figure 6.6A). Retrograde recanalization of the right iliac was unsuccessful, so antegrade recanalization via the left side was successfully performed. A wire was passed, snared, and brought out through the right side. Bilateral true lumen access was achieved, through which long 6Fr sheaths were placed. Bilateral balloon angioplasty was performed with 8 mm balloons (Figure 6.6B). Antegrade injection showed a bilateral flow channels, however retrograde injection demonstrated a perforation of the right iliac system (Figure 6.7A). An 8 x 150 mm Viahban stent was then placed in the right iliac system with a post-stenting angiogram demonstrating no further extravasation (Figure 6.7B). Bilateral common femoral endarterectomies and profundoplasties were performed with great saphenous vein (GSV) patch closure, and a completion angiogram showed no significant stenosis with brisk flow down the leg.

KEY LEARNING POINTS: *PERFORATION*

Although iliac perforation in the setting of treatment of AIOD is rare, with a rate of < 1% in many studies,[21] preparation is key.

1. Meticulous preprocedural planning is key in avoiding a catastrophic outcome. When the clinical exam and noninvasive imaging reflect advanced iliac occlusive disease with suspicion of complete occlusion, consideration should be given to a preoperative CTA to better define the anatomy. Factors associated with rupture include heavily calcified vessels, occluded vessels, oversized balloons, recent endarterectomy, chronic steroid use, diabetes, female gender, and external iliac artery lesions.[22]
2. An iliac perforation can quickly lead to large volume blood loss and potentially death. Therefore, it is important to quickly identify it when it occurs. Any abrupt procedural hypotension or new-onset flank or back pain should prompt a thorough evaluation for active extravasation. Oftentimes, if the sheath is occlusive, this will not be noticed until the end of the procedure when the sheath is removed. Consideration should be given to continuous pressure monitoring through a manifold, peripheral arterial line, or frequent cuff pressures throughout an intervention.
3. Maintaining wire access and conservative angioplasty is of fundamental importance. In the case of recanalization, a small-caliber balloon (4 or 5 mm) should be used for predilation to minimize the risk of immediate injury and rupture. Larger balloons can then be used in tandem with appropriately sized stents. Furthermore, after angioplasty, the balloon can be left on the wire while hemodynamic checks are performed. In the presence of immediate hypotension or pain, the balloon can be quickly insufflated to prevent further bleeding. While performing any challenging iliac intervention, it is good practice to ensure that upsized sheaths and covered stents are available in the room. These can then be immediately opened and prepped while temporary hemostasis is achieved with balloon occlusion.

There is a higher risk of vessel rupture during dilation in heavily calcified lesions/arteries.[23,24] Because of this, the use of covered stents in heavily calcified AIOD has been advocated. Long-term follow-up of the randomized Covered versus Balloon Expandable Stent Trial (COBEST) demonstrated significantly higher patency of covered stents versus bare metal stents at 5 years, albeit with a small cohort that was followed for at least 60 months.[25] Covered stents may also decrease the risk of distal embolization in these calcified lesions.

If sheaths are pulled in the recovery area and hypotension occurs, a prompt return to the intervention suite or operating room should be made to evaluate for bleeding with re-intervention as needed. If the bleeding cannot be stopped endovascularly with a covered stent, then balloon occlusion can be used to control inflow while surgical

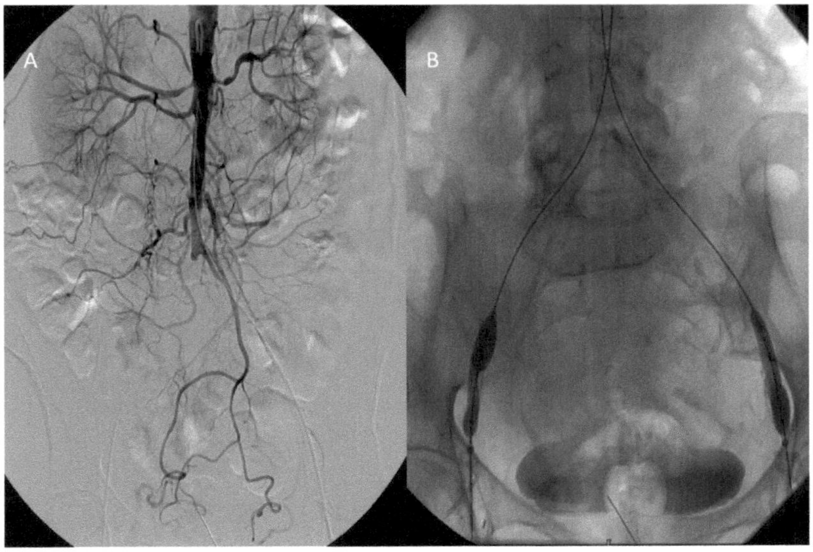

Figure 6.6 Patient with lifestyle-limiting claudication with (A) aortogram demonstrating occlusion of the right common iliac artery and significant stenosis of the left common iliac artery. (B) Balloon angioplasty of bilateral iliac system being performed.

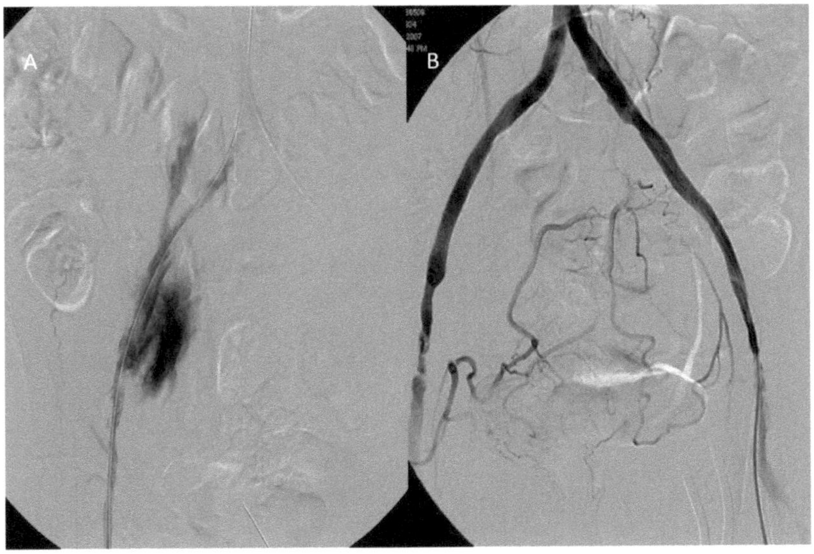

Figure 6.7 Post-angioplasty angiogram demonstrating (A) perforation of the right iliac system with contrast extravasation. (B) In-line flow with no further extravasation after placement of covered right iliac stent.

control is obtained. Repair of perforations closer to the common femoral artery are associated with high procedural success and low morbidity/mortality,[26] whereas perforations closer to the aorta are more treacherous affairs. Oftentimes a patient will experience some pain after intervention or after sheath removal without any corresponding hemodynamic changes. After access site complications are ruled out, development of a retroperitoneal hematoma can be evaluated with a non-contrasted CT scan. Stable physical exam, serial hemoglobins, and repeat imaging generally indicate a patient can be discharged safely without further intervention after an overnight observation.

CONCLUSION

Endovascular interventions for aortoiliac disease have a high rate of technical success as well as low rates of clinically significant complications. Certain anatomic and patient characteristics are associated with increased risk of complications. In general, the treatment of occlusions is the most challenging scenario. Case planning, patient preparation, and equipment preparedness are key components of successfully managing these difficult situations and avoiding significant morbidity and mortality.

Table 6.1 Associated complications, critical steps, and treatment options for aortolliac artery interventions

Complication		Critical Step	Treatment options
Access site complications	Retroperitoneal bleed	Clinical suspicion based on HD and symptoms	CTA v Repeat angiogram with intervention as needed vs operative intervention/hematoma evacuation
	Pseudoaneurysm	Dx with ultrasound	Thrombin injection vs surgical evacuation and primary repair
	Groin hematoma	Dx with ultrasound	If no pseudo, observe for 24 hours and check for expansion; use of closure device upfront
	AVF	Dx with ultrasound	Manage if symptoms develop
Dissection		Maintain wire access; antegrade and retrograde imaging to define anatomy	Prolonged balloon inflation and/or stenting as indicated
Rupture		Dx with prompt angiogram; maintain wire access and balloon-occlude for control	Reverse anticoagulants, balloon tamponade, and covered stents; open repair if persists
Distal embolization	Acute	On-table imaging to guide treatment; always do completion runoff to evaluate	Percutaneous thrombectomy, +/– lysis/ intervention vs open thrombectomy, be aware of compartment syndrome
	Subacute	Clinical Dx and angiogram	Evaluate for appropriateness of lysis and intervention vs surgical revascularization
Stent misadventures	Acute stent thrombosis	Assure no missed dissection, incomplete lesion coverage, maldeployment, poor runoff	Lysis if clinically able to and additional stenting of culprit lesions
	Balloon rupture with partial stent deployment	Identify tough lesions to cross	Advance sheath beyond lesion, place stent and balloon at desired location, pull-back sheath, deploy stent
	Stent migration	Assure controlled deployment of stent to avoid jailing contralateral iliac orifice	May require contralateral wire access and kissing iliac stents
	Stent compression of contralateral iliac	Obtain contralateral wire access if not already present	Kissing iliac stents
	Stent infection	Clinical suspicion with delayed presentation	Antibiotics, explant, reconstruction

Abbreviations: HD, hemodynamics; AVF, arteriovenous fistula; Dx , diagnosis;

REFERENCES

1. Weitz JI, Byrne J, Clagett GP, Farkouh ME, Porter JM, Sackett DL, Strandness DE, Taylor LM. Diagnosis and treatment of chronic arterial insufficiency of the lower extremities: a critical review. Circulation. 1996 Dec 1;94(11): 3026–49.
2. de Vries SO, Hunink MG. Results of aortic bifurcation grafts for aortoiliac occlusive disease: a meta-analysis. Journal of Vascular Surgery. 1997 Oct;26(4):558–69. doi: 10.1016/s0741-5214(97)70053-3.
3. Urayama H, Ohtake H, Yokoi K, Fujimori H, Kawaguchi M, Ishikawa T, Watanabe Y. Long-term results of endarterectomy, anatomic bypass and extraanatomic bypass for aortoiliac occlusive disease. Surgery Today. 1998;2(28):151–5.
4. Vascular surgery societies refuse to endorse TASC III. Vascular News. 2013 Nov. (60):1–2. Accessed 11.17.20 http:// https://vascularnews.com/vascular-news-60-november-2013/
5. Jongkind V, Akkersdijk GJ, Yeung KK, Wisselink W. A systematic review of endovascular treatment of extensive aortoiliac occlusive disease. Journal of Vascular Surgery. 2010 Nov 1;52(5):1376–83. doi: 10.1016/j.jvs.2010.04.080.
6. Kashyap VS, Pavkov ML, Bena JF, Sarac TP, O'Hara PJ, Lyden SP, Clair DG. The management of severe aortoiliac occlusive disease: endovascular therapy rivals open reconstruction. Journal of Vascular Surgery. 2008 Dec 1;48(6):1451–7.
7. Iida O, Soga Y, Takahara M, Kawasaki D, Yamauchi Y, Suzuki K, Hirano K, Koshida R, Kamoi D, Tazaki J,

Higashitani M. Perioperative complications after aorto-iliac stenting: associated factors and impact on follow-up cardiovascular prognosis. European Journal of Vascular and Endovascular Surgery. 2014 Feb 1;47(2):131–8.
8. Pulli R, Dorigo W, Fargion A, Innocenti AA, Pratesi G, Marek J, Pratesi C. Early and long-term comparison of endovascular treatment of iliac artery occlusions and stenosis. Journal of Vascular Surgery. 2011 Jan 1;53(1):92–8.
9. Fujihara M, Takahara M, Sasaki S, Nanto K, Utsunomiya M, Iida O, Yokoi Y. Angiographic dissection patterns and patency outcomes after balloon angioplasty for superficial femoral artery disease. Journal of Endovascular Therapy. 2017 Jun;24(3):367–75.
10. Kobayashi N, Hirano K, Yamawaki M, Araki M, Sakai T, Sakamoto Y, Mori S, Tsutsumi M, Honda Y, Ito Y. Simple classification and clinical outcomes of angiographic dissection after balloon angioplasty for femoropopliteal disease. Journal of Vascular Surgery. 2018 Apr 1;67(4): 1151–8.
11. Ruzsa Z, Tóth K, Nemes B, Édes IF, Nardai S, Berta B, Kovács N, Hüttl K, Merkely B. Transradial and transulnar access for iliac artery interventions using sheathless guiding systems: a feasibility study. Catheterization and Cardiovascular Interventions. 2016 Nov 15;88(6):923–31.
12. Soga Y, Iida O, Kawasaki D, Yamauchi Y, Suzuki K, Hirano K, Koshida R, Kamoi D, Tazaki J, Higashitani M, Shintani Y. Contemporary outcomes after endovascular treatment for aorto-iliac artery disease. Circulation Journal. 2012:CJ-12.
13. de Donato G, Bosiers M, Setacci F, Deloose K, Galzerano G, Verbist J, Peeters P, Setacci C. 24-Month Data from the BRAVISSIMO: A Large-Scale Prospective Registry on Iliac Stenting for TASC A & B and TASC C & D Lesions. Annals of vascular surgery. 2015 May 1;29(4):738–50. doi: 10.1016/j.avsg.2014.12.027.
14. Krankenberg H, Zeller T, Ingwersen M, Schmalstieg J, Gissler HM, Nikol S, Baumgartner I, Diehm N, Nickling E, Müller-Hülsbeck S, Schmiedel R. Self-expanding versus balloon-expandable stents for iliac artery occlusive disease: the randomized ICE trial. JACC: Cardiovascular Interventions. 2017 Aug 28;10(16):1694–704.
15. Feldman DN, Klein AJP. Stent Selection in the Iliac Arteries: Don't Fall Through the ICE! JACC Cardiovascular Interventions. 2017 Aug 28;10(16):1705–1707. doi: 10.1016/j.jcin.2017.05.056. PMID: 28838481.
16. Earnshaw JJ, Whitman B, Foy C. Thrombolysis Study Group. National Audit of Thrombolysis for Acute Leg Ischemia (NATALI): clinical factors associated with early outcome. Journal of vascular surgery. 2004 May 1;39(5):1018–25.
17. Spiliopoulos S, Katsanos K, Fragkos G, Karnabatidis D, Siablis D. Treatment of infrainguinal thromboembolic complications during peripheral endovascular procedures with AngioJet rheolytic thrombectomy, intraoperative thrombolysis, and selective stenting. Journal of vascular surgery. 2012 Nov 1;56(5):1308–16.
18. Ansel GM, Botti CF Jr, Silver MJ. Treatment of acute limb ischemia with a percutaneous mechanical thrombectomy-based endovascular approach: 5-year limb salvage and survival results from a single center series. Catheterization and Cardiovascular Interventions. 2008 Sep 1;72(3):325–330.
19. Weaver FA, Comerota AJ, Youngblood M, Froehlich J, Hosking JD, Papanicolaou G, STILE Investigators. Surgical revascularization versus thrombolysis for nonembolic lower extremity native artery occlusions: results of a prospective randomized trial. Journal of Vascular Surgery. 1996 Oct 1;24(4):513–23.
20. Kashyap VS, Gilani R, Bena JF, Bannazadeh M, Sarac TP. Endovascular therapy for acute limb ischemia. Journal of Vascular Surgery. 2011 Feb 1;53(2):340–6.
21. Allaire E, Melliere D, Poussier B, Kobeiter H, Desgranges P, Becquemin JP. Iliac artery rupture during balloon dilatation: what treatment? Annals of vascular surgery. 2003 May 1;17(3):306–14.
22. Ahmed MH, Laird JR. Complications After Iliac Artery Interventions. Endovascular today. 2005:55–7.
23. Björses K, Ivancev K, Riva L, Manjer J, Uher P, Resch T. Kissing stents in the aortic bifurcation--a valid reconstruction for aorto-iliac occlusive disease. European Journal of Vascular and Endovascular Surgery. 2008 Oct 1;36(4):424–31.
24. Chang RW, Goodney PP, Baek JH, Nolan BW, Rzucidlo EM, Powell RJ. Long-term results of combined common femoral endarterectomy and iliac stenting/stent grafting for occlusive disease. Journal of Vascular Surgery. 2008 Aug 1;48(2):362–7.
25. Mwipatayi BP, Sharma S, Daneshmand A, Thomas SD, Vijayan V, Altaf N, Garbowski M, Jackson M, Benveniste G, Denton M, Anderson J. Durability of the balloon-expandable covered versus bare-metal stents in the Covered versus Balloon Expandable Stent Trial (COBEST) for the treatment of aortoiliac occlusive disease. Journal of vascular surgery. 2016 Jul 1;64(1):83–94.
26. Stortecky S, Wenaweser P, Diehm N, Pilgrim T, Huber C, Rosskopf AB, Khattab AA, Buellesfeld L, Gloekler S, Eberle B, Schmidli J. Percutaneous management of vascular complications in patients undergoing transcatheter aortic valve implantation. JACC: Cardiovascular Interventions. 2012 May 1;5(5):515–24.

7

Complications of percutaneous intervention for femoral, popliteal, and infrapopliteal artery occlusive disease

RENGANADEN SOOPPAN AND CHRISTOPHER J. ABULARRAGE

Catheter-based revascularization of the lower extremity was first performed by Charles Dotter in 1964 and further refined by Andreas Gruentzig in 1974.[1,2] At that time, the mainstay of treatment was balloon angioplasty of stenotic lesions within calcified vessels performed via direct arterial cutdown. Endovascular therapy (EVT) has advanced significantly since that era, with the introduction of stent technology, smaller diameter sheaths, and lower profile balloons and stents. Along with incremental progress in catheter-based technologies, the majority of lower-extremity interventions are now performed via a percutaneous approach, obviating the need for an open cutdown. The outcomes associated with modern peripheral EVT are durable, safe, and reproducible.

EVT offers several basic advantages over open surgical revascularization. It can be performed under local anesthesia, thus avoiding general anesthesia for patients who are in a high-risk category due to their medical comorbidities.[3] EVT has a lower mortality and morbidity compared to bypass surgery. Patients are ambulatory on the same day of the procedure after EVT and can return to their normal activities within 48 hours after the procedure.[1]

From a clinician's standpoint, EVT has increased the number of ways that peripheral vascular disease can be addressed. Endovascular therapy offers minimally invasive options to better serve an aging population who have an increased prevalence of peripheral vascular disease. While EVT is the first-line treatment of peripheral artery disease (PAD) for TransAtlantic Inter-Society Consensus (TASC) II A-B localized atherosclerotic femoropopliteal lesions, questions remain regarding the durability of EVT for TASC II C-D lesions.[4] However, advancements in technology have improved the outcomes of EVT for TASC II C-D femoropopliteal lesions using EVT instead of traditional bypass surgery. Diabetic and end-stage renal disease patients on dialysis often suffer from critical limb ischemia due to infrageniculate arterial occlusive disease. This patient population is well known for its myriad of medical comorbidities, which often increases morbidity and mortality rates after open surgical bypass performed for limb salvage. Endovascular interventions on infrageniculate atherosclerotic lesions have offered this patient population an opportunity to attempt limb salvage with decreased rates of major amputations.[5] In fact, EVT may be associated with better primary patency rates compared to lower extremity bypass surgery in select populations.[6]

Nowadays, patients are increasingly savvy about the latest treatment options available to them, and it is inevitable that the number of percutaneous endovascular interventions performed for peripheral vascular disease will continue to rise. As such, it is important to revisit the complications that can arise from EVT to better counsel our patients and offer them the best treatment options. This chapter aims at discussing the complications of EVT for occlusive disease of the femoropopliteal and infrageniculate segments of the lower extremity, techniques to prevent these complications, and therapeutic approaches to treat them.

ACCESS COMPLICATIONS

Access site complications remain the most encountered complication in peripheral vascular intervention, with rates ranging from 3.5% to 8.9%.[7] Most of the data available for access complication is derived from percutaneous coronary intervention (PCI) registries. More recently, vascular surgery-specific registries, such as the Vascular Quality Initiative (VQI) database, have enabled the assessment of access complications specific to peripheral arterial intervention. Older age, extremely high or low body mass index, female sex, peripheral artery disease, hypertension, use of antithrombotic therapy, and prolonged procedure time are predictors of access site complications after PCI. These variables are comparable with predictors of access site complication in peripheral vascular interventions.[7–9]

Although the improvement in technology and equipment profiles have allowed complex endovascular procedures to be performed using radial, brachial, popliteal, and pedal arteries for access, the common femoral artery (CFA) remains the most commonly used artery for lower extremity vascular access.[10] Brachial and radial artery access may be warranted when a retrograde, up-and-over the bifurcation approach is not technically feasible. These instances include certain native aortoiliac occlusions, previous aortobifemoral bypass, previous modular stent grafts not positioned on the aortic bifurcation, and previous iliac stents with raised aortic bifurcation.[11]

Access complications can be avoided by understanding the anatomical landmarks and utilizing meticulous techniques to obtain arterial access. The CFA should be accessed below the inferior epigastric artery and above the point at which the CFA bifurcates into the deep femoral artery (profunda femoris) and the superficial femoral artery (SFA) (Figure 7.1). The CFA should be accessed over the femoral head to allow for eventual compression of the artery against the femoral head to facilitate hemostasis. It should be noted that in 35% of the population, the CFA bifurcates below the inferior border of the femoral head.[12] Accessing the CFA below the inferior border of the femoral head will result in an inability to apply optimal manual pressure, which can result in hematomas and pseudoaneurysms. Likewise, if the CFA is accessed above the level of the inferior epigastric, there is an increased risk of retroperitoneal hemorrhage.

The CFA can be accessed using bony landmarks, fluoroscopic guidance, and a micropuncture needle. The indirect fluoroscopy technique involves using a radio-opaque metallic object, such as the tip of a hemostat, to locate the inferior border of the femoral head in an anterior-posterior plane without any cranial or caudal angulation. Indirect fluoroscopic techniques are inaccurate because the amount of subcutaneous fat the needle is required to traverse before entering the artery can differ widely depending on patient body habitus. The point of access on the skin may appear to be exactly over the

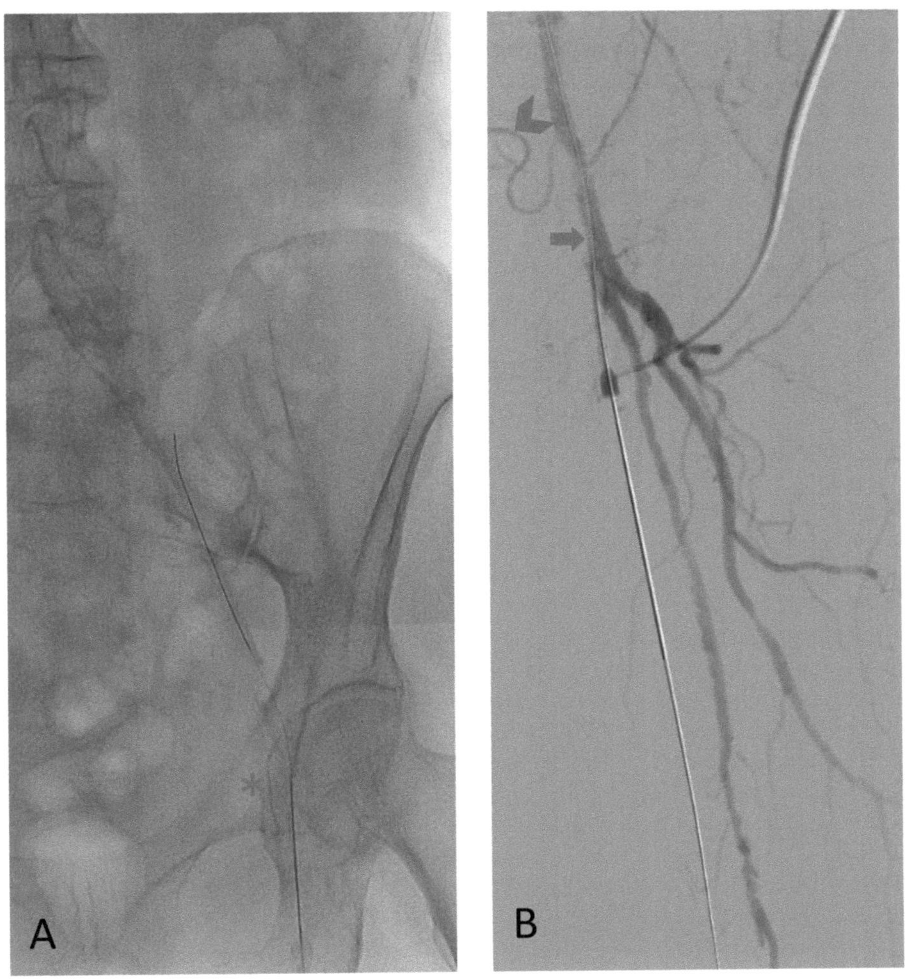

Figure 7.1 (a) CFA access with a micropuncture needle and wire over the mid-femoral head (asterisk). (b) Angiogram showing puncture of the CFA above the bifurcation (arrow) and below the inferior epigastric artery (arrowhead).

bony landmark, but the actual arteriotomy may be higher than anticipated. Moreover, the femoral bifurcation cannot be accurately identified using this technique. If a patient has a high femoral bifurcation, the arteriotomy may be in the SFA instead of the CFA. Direct fluoroscopy is used to access the CFA under live fluoroscopy. This technique does not increase accuracy and, thus, does not reduce the number of attempts required to access the CFA. It does, however, decrease the number of arteriotomies made below the inferior border of the femoral head.[10,13] Direct fluoroscopy exposes the patient and the physician to higher doses of radiation; hence, it is imperative to keep the fluoroscopy time to a minimum.

Once intraluminal access is obtained, the physician should follow the 0.018″ micropuncture wire up into the iliac system and aorta to avoid side branches and accidental perforation. Exchange for the micropuncture sheath is performed, and a femoral arteriogram should be done to identify the femoral bifurcation and the inferior epigastric artery. If the arteriotomy is unsatisfactory, the micropuncture sheath can be removed, pressure held until hemostasis in achieved, and the process repeated using the femoral angiogram as a road map.[10,12]

The technique that has been proven safest for accurately accessing the CFA utilizes ultrasound guidance in combination with the indirect fluoroscopy technique. Ultrasound-guided access has been proven to be superior to fluoroscopy alone to access CFA with high bifurcations in a randomized controlled trial.[14,15] Ultrasound guidance allows for direct visualization of the CFA such that diseased segments of the artery can be avoided. The physician can identify the bifurcation into the deep and superficial femoral arteries by scanning the patient in a cranio-caudal fashion. The CFA is accessed anteriorly under direct visualization, and it allows for fewer arteriotomy attempts, which significantly reduces access site complications by reducing inadvertent venipunctures and access site-related hematomas.[15]

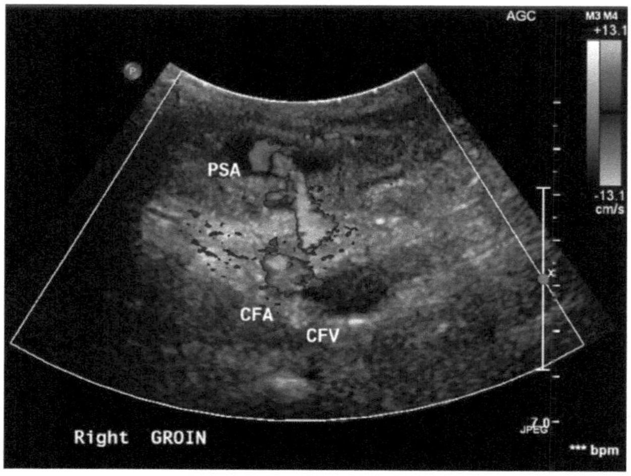

Figure 7.2 Right common femoral artery pseudoaneurysm (PSA).

PSEUDOANEURYSM

Arterial pseudoaneurysm (PSA) is a contained rupture that occurs when there is inadequate hemostasis at the arterial puncture site causing disruption of all three layers of the arterial wall by pulsatile blood flow. The blood forms a hematoma that surrounds the perivascular space and forms the wall of the PSA. The incidence of PSA in the literature varies widely. One prospective study of more than 1000 patients found a pseudoaneurysm in 3.8% of the patients on postprocedural arterial duplex.[16] The incidence may be as high as 8% after peripheral vascular intervention compared to 2% after a diagnostic study due to the use of larger caliber sheaths when interventions are warranted.[17] A pseudoaneurysm is suspected when the patient has pain out of proportion to the physical exam in instances where the PSA is small. Large PSAs present with swelling, pain, pulsatile mass, and an audible bruit on auscultation. They can compress structures in the femoral sheath causing neuropathy, deep vein thrombosis, claudication, and even critical limb ischemia in certain rare circumstances.[10] Large PSAs can also cause excessive soft tissue tension that can lead to skin ischemia and necrosis.

Ultrasound is the quickest and best modality for assessment of a suspected PSA. Due to the turbulent forward and backward flow, a characteristic "yin-yang" sign may be seen on color flow, while a "to-and-fro" pattern may be seen with spectral Doppler (Figure 7.2). Most PSAs smaller than 10 mm will resolve spontaneously, and it is recommended that the patient has biweekly ultrasound follow-up to assess the resolution or progression of the PSA. Larger PSAs > 20 mm often requires intervention. Historically, large PSA were treated surgically; however, surgical repair is invasive and has a higher rate of morbidity compared to minimally invasive techniques. Surgical repair of PSAs is reserved for patients with a rapidly expanding PSA, skin necrosis, limb ischemia, and nerve palsy.[10]

Ultrasound-guided compression emerged in 1991 as a noninvasive method to compress and thrombose PSAs.[18] This technique involves locating the PSA neck with ultrasound and then applying direct pressure with the probe to completely occlude blood flow within the PSA. However, this technique may be painful to the patient, time consuming, require moderate sedation, and has a success rate of 75% or less, especially if the patient is systemically anticoagulated.[19]

Ultrasound-guided thrombin injection was first described in 1998 and is now the preferred method to treat PSA.[20] This technique involves visualizing the PSA neck and sac under ultrasound and directly injecting the smallest amount of thrombin into the sac away from the neck, thereby inducing thrombosis of the sac contents and occluding flow into the PSA. Ideally, a long neck with a smaller diameter is preferred to avoid spilling thrombin into the artery. Its technical success is almost instantaneous compared to almost 30 to 45 minutes of compression and the results can be seen on ultrasound in real time. The procedure is relatively safe, with a 2% rate of distal embolization reported as the most common complication.[19,21] A repeat duplex is done 24 hours after the injection to verify that the pseudoaneurysm is completely thrombosed. Multilobular PSAs or patients on anticoagulation may require reinjection. Open surgical repair of a PSA is reserved for multiple failed attempts with thrombin injection.

RETROPERITONEAL HEMORRHAGE

Retroperitoneal hemorrhage (RPH) is an infrequent, but life-threatening complication of femoral artery access with an incidence of 0.15% to 6% in the literature. More recent studies are reporting a lower incidence of 0.5%.[22] Independent predictors of RPH are arterial access above the inferior epigastric artery, larger sheath size, low body weight, female sex, and the concomitant use of glycoprotein IIb/IIIa inhibitors.[23]

Hemorrhage into the retroperitoneum is insidious, and hemodynamic instability is usually a late sign of ongoing bleeding. The retroperitoneal space can accommodate a large volume of blood before the patient shows the typical signs and symptoms of hemorrhagic shock, including hypotension and tachycardia. Patients may complain of back or flank pain. If RPH is suspected and the patient is hemodynamically stable, a computerized tomography (CT) scan of the abdomen and pelvis with intravenous contrast should be obtained to assess the retroperitoneum for active extravasation from the external iliac artery (Figure 7.3). Clinical diagnosis and prompt resuscitation with blood and fluid is the most important lifesaving intervention. Anticoagulation should be stopped when possible and serial hemoglobin checks should be ordered.

Refractory hypotension and clinical sign of deterioration are clear indications that conservative management has failed and the patient will need either an open surgical repair or endovascular intervention. For arteriotomies in the distal external iliac artery proximal to the inferior epigastric artery, contralateral femoral access is obtained and the area of active contrast extravasation is identified with femoral angiography. Endovascular balloon tamponade or exclusion with a covered stent is then performed. For arteriotomies in the common femoral artery, open surgical repair is indicated due to the high rate of complications associated with common femoral stents.

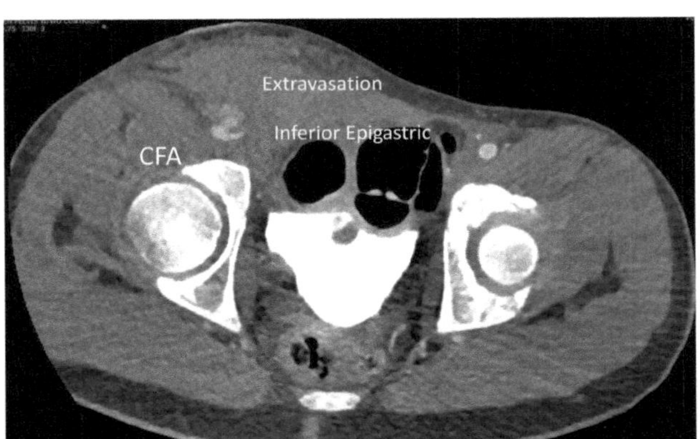

Figure 7.3 High stick proximal to the inferior epigastric artery resulting in contrast extravasation and retroperitoneal hemorrhage.

ACCESS-RELATED ARTERIAL DISSECTION/THROMBOSIS

Retrograde dissection of the CFA occurs when the micropuncture needle or guidewire enters a subintimal dissection plane at the time of femoral artery access. Alternatively, CFA or iliac artery dissection can occur when the working sheath is up against the arterial wall during power injection angiography. Entry into a dissection space is suspected when the guidewire tracks in an unusual fashion that does not correspond to common arterial anatomy. It is often difficult to advance, maneuver, and redirect the guidewire once it is within a dissection plane. Fortunately, most retrograde CFA dissections are asymptomatic because the dissection flap is compressed by the antegrade direction of blood flow. If a dissection is suspected, it is best to remove the guidewire, pull back the sheath and perform a femoral angiography to identify the point of entry and allow the operator to regain true lumen wire access. In rare occasions, the dissection flap will obstruct and occlude the CFA, which can result in arterial thrombosis and acute limb ischemia requiring open surgical intervention.

ACUTE LIMB ISCHEMIA

Acute limb ischemia results from thrombosis of the CFA or dissection. It may also be due to complications of vascular closure devices (e.g., embolization of the foot plate of the Angioseal closure device or circumferential back wall to anterior wall suturing of the CFA with the Perclose device).[24] In most instances, acute limb ischemia requires open surgical exploration of the artery, thrombectomy, endarterectomy, and direct repair of the blood vessel. Endovascular techniques using percutaneous mechanical thrombectomy have been described in the literature with variable success rates.

ARTERIOVENOUS FISTULA

Arteriovenous fistula (AVF) occurs when there is a direct connection between an artery and a vein. It is usually an iatrogenic complication of EVT when the artery and the vein are in close proximity and there is through-and-through access across the abutting walls of both structures. If a sheath is exchanged after micropuncture access, a larger common channel is formed, which allows for continuous flow from the artery into the vein. Multiple blind attempts with lateral and medial deviation of the needle from the CFA in the femoral sheath can lead to a combined venous and arterial puncture.[10] Another instance occurs when the CFA is accessed close to its bifurcation, and the proximal deep femoral artery or superficial femoral artery together with the lateral femoral circumflex vein can be accidentally punctured together resulting in an AVF.

Arteriovenous fistulae can be asymptomatic and painless, or can cause limb edema, ischemia secondary to steal, high-output cardiac failure, and aneurysmal degeneration of the arterial wall.[25,26] Duplex ultrasound is the imaging modality of choice to diagnose AVF, although some may also be identified incidentally on serial angiography. Small asymptomatic AVF typically thrombose spontaneously, whereas large, long-standing, symptomatic AVF will require intervention.

Surgical ligation and repair remains the gold standard, although endovascular exclusion with covered stents has been reported. Covered stents may be used to exclude the AVF in certain locations, such as the proximal SFA, but should be avoided in the CFA. Stents require regular interval surveillance for in-stent stenosis, stent migration, and occlusion, and one should weigh the risk to benefit aspect of endovascular exclusion versus open surgical repair.

BRACHIAL AND RADIAL ARTERY SPECIFIC COMPLICATIONS

Although the CFA is the most commonly used artery for EVT of the lower extremity, brachial and radial arterial access is warranted in select situations. Such situations include, but are not limited to, groin infection, recent CFA surgery, existing aortic stent grafts, bilateral kissing iliac stents, or otherwise artificially elevated aortic bifurcation from prior interventions. Radial and brachial artery access is limited in terms of the length of catheters and sheaths required to reach the infrageniculate arteries. In patients with a shorter stature, the distal SFA and popliteal artery can be reached using the brachial or radial arteries. Arterial tortuosity can also make catheter and wire manipulation more difficult, especially with radial access.[27]

Brachial and radial artery access is not without complications. The left brachial and radial artery are preferentially used because they avoid the need to place a sheath across the arch vessels and decrease the risk of thromboembolism to the intracranial circulation. Iatrogenic occlusion of the brachial artery due to dissection or thrombosis can cause acute upper extremity limb ischemia. The brachial artery courses close to the median nerve of the upper extremity in a relatively tight upper extremity fascia. Pseudoaneurysm, hematoma, or hemorrhage from the brachial artery can result in median nerve palsy or compartment syndrome requiring emergent surgical decompression and repair.[28]

The brachial artery should be accessed percutaneously using ultrasound guidance over the olecranon with the arm externally rotated to facilitate eventual application of pressure over the arteriotomy against the humerus. An oxygen saturation probe placed on the index finger can be used to assess distal perfusion and avoid complete occlusion of the artery while holding pressure. Intra-arterial injection of nitroglycerin can help reduce vasospasm and occlusion of the brachial artery.

Radial artery access is also safe for vascular access for EVT. Pseudoaneurysm or thrombosis of the radial artery rarely causes hand ischemia since the ulnar artery can sufficiently compensate for blood flow to the hand via extensive collateral channels. However, some patients have an incomplete palmar arch and inadequate communications between the radial and ulnar arteries. It is therefore important to assess the network of blood flow to the hand using the Allen's test in patients who are being considered for transradial access.[29]

PROCEDURAL-RELATED COMPLICATIONS

Peripheral endovascular interventions are relatively safe with a low incidence of procedural complications. In general, the burden of atherosclerotic disease and the complexity of the procedure undertaken determines the rate of complications. The majority of complications occur when attempting to recanalize chronic total occlusions and when crossing stenotic and heavily calcified lesions.[30] Some complications are self-limited, while others can have serious consequences such as major amputation.

PERFORATION

Arterial perforation can occur while advancing wires, catheters, balloons, and stents or other endovascular devices. It can be detected on angiography when extravasation of contrast is noted outside the vessel wall (Figure 7.4). If the perforation happens into an adjacent vein, a fistula with contrast flowing into the venous system is seen. Bleeding from perforation of blood vessels with the guidewire is usually self-limited and resolves spontaneously after the reversal of anticoagulation. However, if the perforation happens in a collateral or side branch of a larger caliber vessel and the arteriotomy is made wider by advancing a catheter over the wire, uncontrolled bleeding can result in hemodynamic instability, the need for blood transfusion, open repairs, and extended hospital stays.[31]

It is best to take the necessary precautions to avoid perforating an artery during a procedure. Road mapping should be used when attempting to cross any lesion, and any deviation from the normal course of the blood vessel should be treated as a perforation or side branch cannulation. Once the stenosis or occlusion is crossed, a catheter is advanced over the wire and angiography is performed to confirm that the wire and catheter combination is intraluminal and not in the extravascular space. If a perforation has occurred, the catheter should be pulled back into the true lumen and repeat angiography should be used to confirm the cessation of extravasation prior

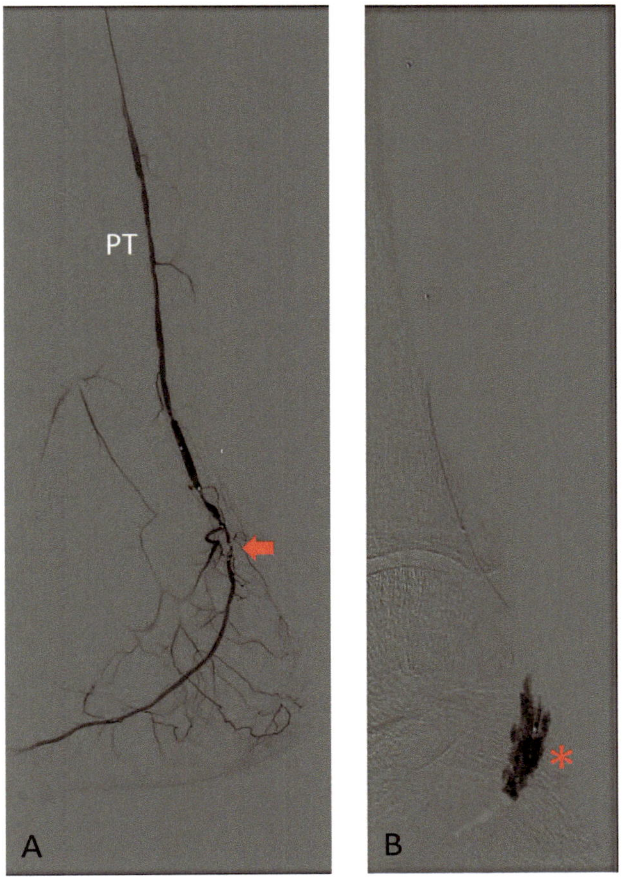

Figure 7.4 (A) Stenosis of the distal PT on selective angiography (arrow). (B) Perforation of the distal PT with hydrophilic guide wire with extravasation of contrast (asterisk).

to proceeding with the intervention. Balloon tamponade and cessation of anticoagulation may be required.

Perforation may also occur in heavily calcified blood vessels when higher endoflator pressures are required for angioplasty. The resulting dilatory effect can disrupt the plaque and perforate the adventitia of the artery. Progressive dilatation using smaller balloons and sequentially increasing the balloon diameter may prevent this complication. Alternatively, cutting and scoring balloons can be used with lower pressure, or the calcific burden of the vessel can be reduced by doing a debulking atherectomy procedure first, followed by a balloon angioplasty. If the desired technical result is not achieved and the use of higher-pressure angioplasty is absolutely warranted, the physician should be prepared to use balloon tamponade or a covered stent in the event of a perforation.[31]

Atherectomy has a relatively low rate of perforation in peripheral arteries. Atherectomy-related complications occur due to direct cutting or mechanical disruption of the adventitia. Directional atherectomy has a procedural perforation rate of 5.3%, laser atherectomy and rotational atherectomy have a perforation rate of 2%, and orbital atherectomy has a perforation rate between 0.5 and 2.2%.[31]

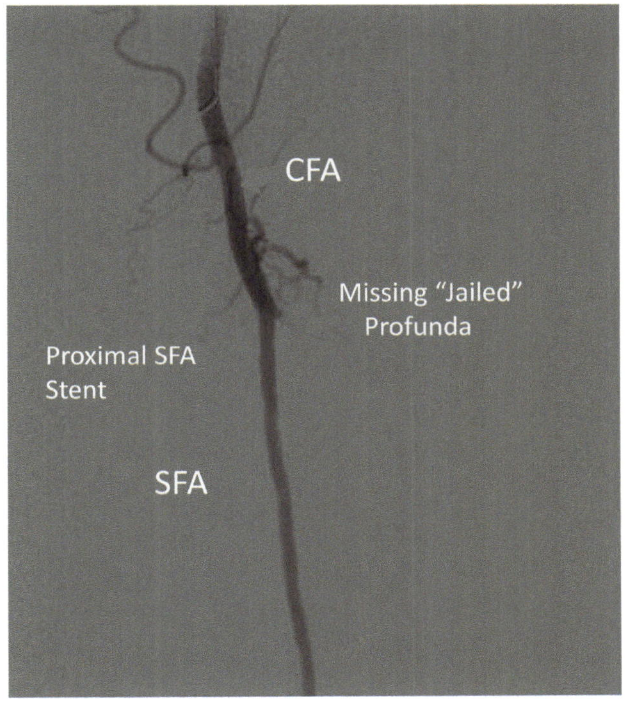

Figure 7.5 Deployment of a left proximal SFA stent causing occlusion ("jailing") of left profunda femoris artery.

BRANCH OCCLUSION

When a stent is deployed at or close to the bifurcation of an artery, the stent can occlude or "jail" the adjacent artery. For instance, the deep femoral artery ostia can be partially or completely occluded by the accidental incorrect deployment of a proximal SFA stent (Figure 7.5). Self-expanding nitinol stents do not deploy as accurately as balloon expandable stents. However, due to their flexibility, self-expanding stents are preferentially used in the femoropopliteal segment of the lower extremity. It is imperative for the physician to deploy self-expanding stents with precision to avoid jailing branch vessels due to a stent migrating or jumping out of position. The angiogram and road mapping should be performed perpendicular to the blood vessel and bifurcation (e.g., ipsilateral oblique projection in case of the CFA) to avoid parallax error when deploying the stent and inadvertently jailing the adjacent branch. It should also be noted that nitinol stents expand over time and may present with delayed jailing of a branch vessel.

STENT FRACTURE AND THROMBOSIS

The femoropopliteal artery crosses two joint structures (hip and knee joint) and courses through the adductor canal. This places the SFA at particularly increased risk for torsion, and longitudinal and radial compression forces. As such, stenting into the muscular adductor canal or behind the knee increases mechanical stress on the stent that leads to an increased rate of stent fracture, higher rate of stenosis, and decreased long-term primary patency rate

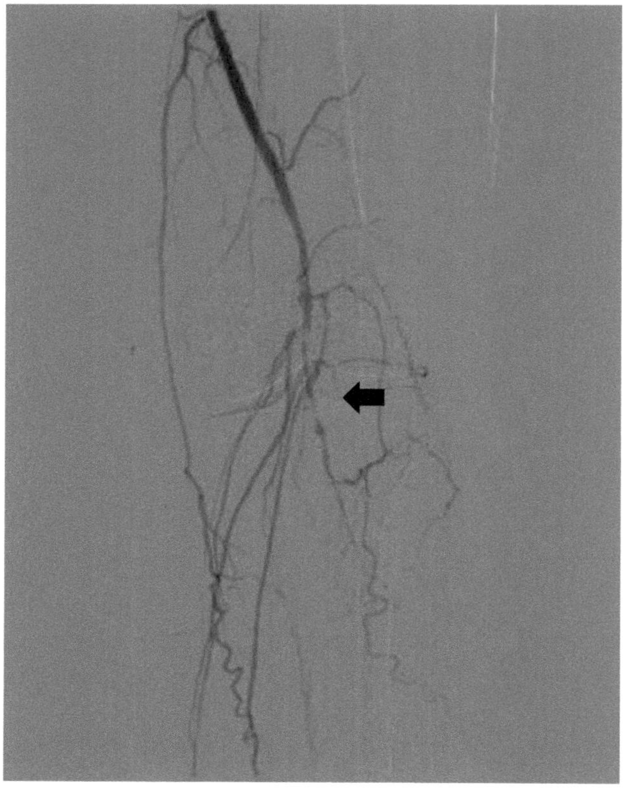

Figure 7.6 Thrombosis of a stent (arrow) in the popliteal artery behind the knee.

(Figure 7.6).[32] When treating the distal SFA, it is imperative to perform an angiogram in a perpendicular plane to the femur, with the patella centered on the femoral condyles, in order to visualize the distal SFA as it crosses the femur to enter the adductor canal. This will allow accurate distal SFA stenting, such that the distal end of the stent lands before the SFA crosses the femur and enters the adductor canal.

DISTAL EMBOLIZATION

Distal embolization (DE) occurs when a plaque or thrombus is dislodged further distally into the lower extremity arterial system during EVT (Figure 7.7). Its incidence is variable and depends on how embolization is measured and how often clinicians are diligent to look for them on angiography. Most studies report a low incidence of 1–5% that is mostly detected on angiography.[33] Distal embolization can be further categorized as micro- or macroembolization. Microembolization is mostly insignificant as it affects capillary perfusion only. Macroembolization, on the other hand, can lead to significant ischemia or worsening of an already compromised vascular bed especially if there is not enough collateral circulation.

The rate of DE is higher in patients treated for critical limb ischemia compared to those treated for claudication (3.2% vs 1.2%). DE is more likely to happen during infrainguinal vessel procedures compared to aortoiliac procedures. Patients who have femoropopliteal TASC II C

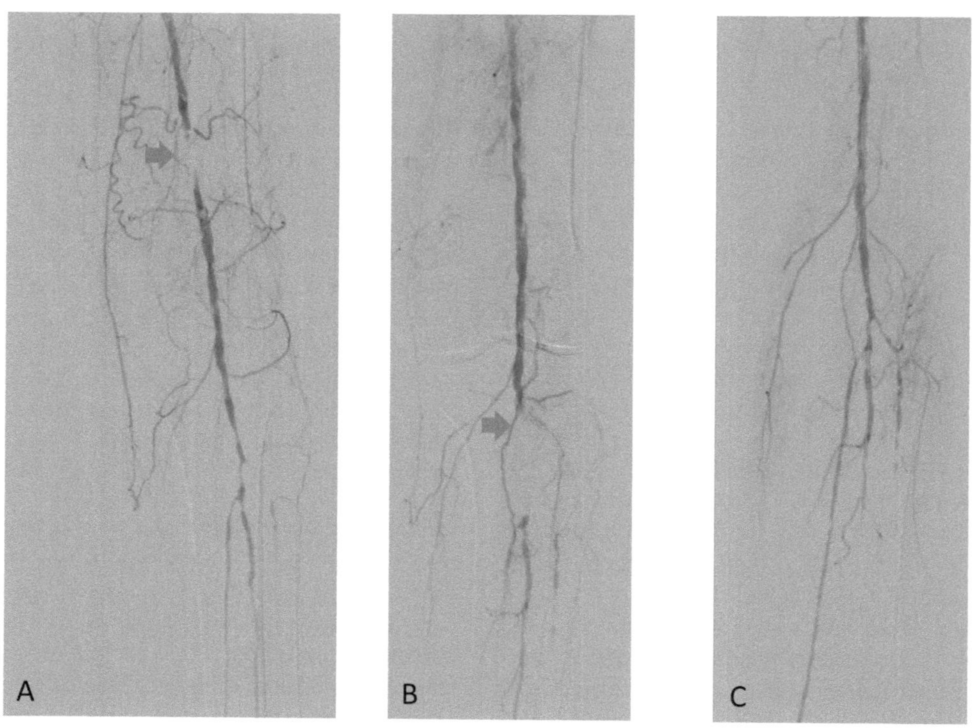

Figure 7.7 (A) Occlusion of the above-knee popliteal artery on angiography (arrow). (B) Occlusion of below-knee popliteal artery with limited flow distally due to embolization (arrow). (C) Recanalization with suction thrombectomy and balloon angioplasty.

and D lesions, and who undergo treatment of long-segment occlusions, have higher rates of DE. Atherectomy procedures carry a significantly higher incidence of DE as compared to other treatment modalities.[34] Patients who undergo urgent endovascular revascularizations have a higher rate of DE compared to patients who undergo elective revascularization. The rate of DE also increases with the number of arteries treated, treatment of chronic total occlusions, and treatment of in-stent restenosis. In one study, patients who had three or more arteries treated had a significantly higher incidence of DE compared with patients who had fewer than three arteries treated (3.4% vs 1.5%).[30]

Many studies have demonstrated that routine use of distal embolic protection devices or filters, especially during atherectomy procedures, with a decreased risk of symptomatic DE (Figure 7.8).[35] Debris that would otherwise embolize to the distal extremity can be captured by such devices and removed at the end of the intervention. These were small series, and no concrete evidence can be drawn from their conclusions. Moreover, it is difficult to assess the significance of these emboli in a vascular bed that is relatively resilient to deficient microperfusion. In the absence of practice guidelines, one should weigh the benefit of routinely using distal embolic protection devices with the risk that accompanies their use (i.e., perforation/embolization) and the added cost to the procedure.

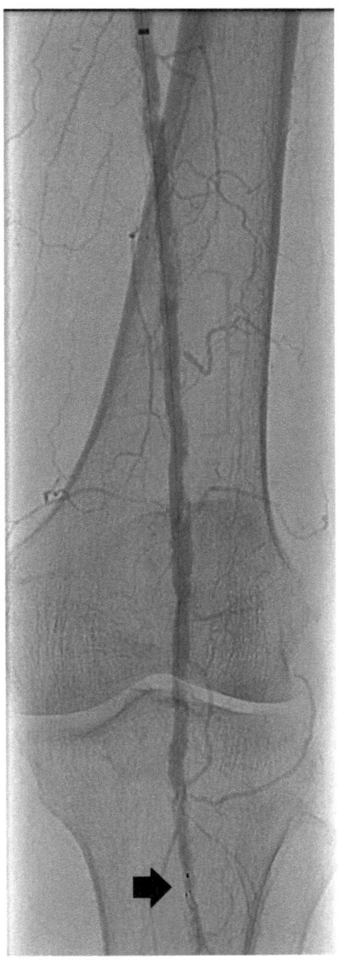

Figure 7.8 Post-atherectomy and drug-coated balloon angioplasty of the below-knee popliteal artery with distal embolic protection (arrow).

ARTERIAL DISSECTION

Arterial dissection is a separation of the arterial wall layers that may occur during EVT. This may occur as a consequence of balloon angioplasty, typically of heavily calcified lesions, or after subintimal recanalization of a chronic total occlusion (CTO). Dissections are further divided into those that are flow-limiting and those that are not. Non-flow-limiting lesions may be managed without further intervention, as they are not associated with thrombosis. However, they may lead to a decreased primary patency, which can be identified on serial outpatient duplex ultrasonography.

Flow-limiting dissections are associated with an increased rate of acute thrombosis and should be treated during the initial EVT (Figure 7.9). Prolonged balloon inflation or provisional stent placement are the most common treatment modalities, the latter of which should be avoided in areas subject to the previously described areas of the infrainguinal arterial tree susceptible to compressive and torsional forces.

Long-segment subintimal recanalization of CTOs are frequently associated with post-angioplasty dissections. These lesions are typically stented whether they are flow-limiting or not, based on the improved patency rates associated with primary stenting. Despite relatively low primary-assisted patency (68%) and secondary patency rates (70%) at 1 year, subintimal recanalization limb salvage rates are as high as 92%.[35] This technique, therefore, represents a good alternative to surgical bypasses in patients with critical limb ischemia, especially in the absence of a suitable vein or high surgical risk.

CONCLUSION

The advent of endovascular therapy has undoubtedly revolutionized the field of vascular surgery over the past few decades. Percutaneous lower extremity interventions have been shown to be both safe and efficacious. In many cases, EVT has proven to be an excellent alternative to open surgery, particularly for those patients who are at high risk for surgical morbidity and mortality. However, EVT is not without its own risks and complications. Endovascular interventions should only be performed after diligent, detailed planning and assessment of the pathology and indication for the procedure. Moreover, clinicians should master the procedural techniques, have a thorough understanding the endovascular devices they are using, and, most importantly, be prepared to identify and treat the complications of EVT for it to be an effective tool in saving limbs and lives.

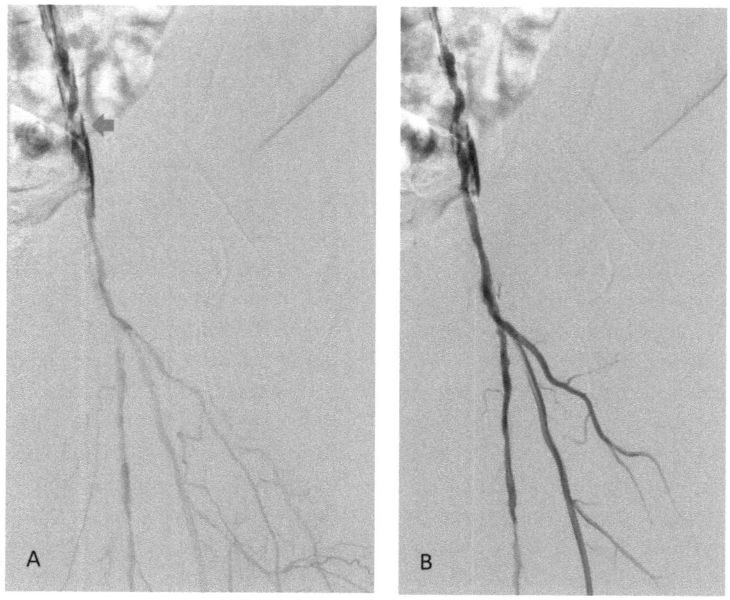

Figure 7.9 (A) Flow-limiting dissection of proximal common femoral artery (arrow). (B) Hemodynamic improvement with prolonged balloon inflation.

REFERENCES

1. White CJ, Gray WA. Endovascular Therapies for Peripheral Arterial Disease: An Evidence-Based Review. Circulation. 2007 Nov 6; 116(19): 2203–2215.
2. Barton M, Grüntzig J, Husmann M, Rösch J. Balloon Angioplasty – The Legacy of Andreas Grüntzig, M.D. (1939–1985). Front Cardiovasc Med [Internet]. 2014 Dec 29 [cited 2019 Feb 16]; 1. Available from: https://www.ncbi.nlm.nih.gov/pmc/articles/PMC4671350/
3. Isner JM, Rosenfield K. Redefining the treatment of peripheral artery disease. Role of percutaneous revascularization. Circulation. 1993 Oct; 88(4): 1534–57.
4. Norgren L, Hiatt WR, Dormandy JA, Nehler MR, Harris KA, Fowkes FGR. Inter-Society Consensus for the Management of Peripheral Arterial Disease (TASC II). J Vasc Surg. 2007 Jan; 45(1): S5–67.
5. Schamp KBC, Meerwaldt R, Reijnen MMPJ, Geelkerken RH, Zeebregts CJ. The Ongoing Battle Between Infrapopliteal Angioplasty and Bypass Surgery for Critical Limb Ischemia. Ann Vasc Surg. 2012 Nov; 26(8): 1145–1153.
6. Hicks CW, Najafian A, Farber A, Menard MT, Malas MB, Black JH, et al. Below-knee endovascular interventions have better outcomes compared to open bypass for patients with critical limb ischemia. Vasc Med. 2017 Feb 1; 22(1): 28–34.
7. Ortiz D, Jahangir A, Singh M, Allaqaband S, Bajwa TK, Mewissen MW. Access Site Complications After Peripheral Vascular Interventions: Incidence, Predictors, and Outcomes. Circ Cardiovasc Interv. 2014 Dec; 7(6): 821–828.
8. Fuchs S, Kornowski R, Teplitsky I, Brosh D, Lev E, Vaknin-Assa H, et al. Major bleeding complicating contemporary primary percutaneous coronary interventions-incidence, predictors, and prognostic implications. Cardiovasc Revascularization Med Mol Interv. 2009 Jun; 10(2): 88–93.
9. Sulzbach-Hoke LM, Ratcliffe SJ, Kimmel SE, Kolansky DM, Polomano R. Predictors of complications following sheath removal with percutaneous coronary intervention. J Cardiovasc Nurs. 2010 Jun; 25(3): E1-8.
10. Abu-Fadel M. Complications of Peripheral Arterial Interventions. In: Banerjee S, editor. Practical Approach to Peripheral Arterial Chronic Total Occlusions [Internet]. Singapore: Springer Singapore; 2017 [cited 2019 Feb 15]. p. 95–122. Available from: http://link.springer.com/10.1007/978-981-10-3053-6_7
11. Stone PA, Campbell JE. Complications Related to Femoral Artery Access for Transcatheter Procedures. Vasc Endovascular Surg. 2012 Nov 1; 46(8): 617–623.
12. Abu-Fadel MS, Sparling JM, Zacharias SJ, Aston CE, Saucedo JF, Schechter E, et al. Fluoroscopy vs. traditional guided femoral arterial access and the use of closure devices: a randomized controlled trial. Catheter Cardiovasc Interv Off J Soc Card Angiogr Interv. 2009 Oct 1; 74(4): 533–539.
13. Cilingiroglu M, Feldman T, Salinger MH, Levisay J, Turi ZG. Fluoroscopically-guided micropuncture femoral artery access for large-caliber sheath insertion. J Invasive Cardiol. 2011 Apr; 23(4): 157–161.
14. Gedikoglu M, Oguzkurt L, Gur S, Andic C, Sariturk C, Ozkan U. Comparison of ultrasound guidance with the traditional palpation and fluoroscopy

method for the common femoral artery puncture. Catheter Cardiovasc Interv Off J Soc Card Angiogr Interv. 2013 Dec 1; 82(7): 1187–1192.
15. Seto AH, Abu-Fadel MS, Sparling JM, Zacharias SJ, Daly TS, Harrison AT, et al. Real-time ultrasound guidance facilitates femoral arterial access and reduces vascular complications: FAUST (Femoral Arterial Access With Ultrasound Trial). JACC Cardiovasc Interv. 2010 Jul; 3(7): 751–758.
16. Stone PA, Campbell JE, AbuRahma AF. Femoral pseudoaneurysms after percutaneous access. J Vasc Surg. 2014 Nov; 60(5): 1359–1366.
17. Katzenschlager R, Ugurluoglu A, Ahmadi A, Hülsmann M, Koppensteiner R, Larch E, et al. Incidence of pseudoaneurysm after diagnostic and therapeutic angiography. Radiology. 1995 May; 195(2): 463–466.
18. Fellmeth BD, Roberts AC, Bookstein JJ, Freischlag JA, Forsythe JR, Buckner NK, et al. Postangiographic femoral artery injuries: nonsurgical repair with US-guided compression. Radiology. 1991 Mar 1; 178(3): 671–675.
19. Ehieli WL, Bozdogan E, Janas G, Jaffe TA, Miller CM, Bashir MR, Allen BC. Imaging-guided percutaneous thrombin injection for the treatment of iatrogenic femoral artery pseudoaneurysms. Abdom Radiol (NY). 2019 Mar;44(3): 1120–1126. doi: 10.1007/s00261-019-01923-6.
20. Kang SS, Labropoulos N, Mansour MA, Baker WH. Percutaneous ultrasound guided thrombin injection: A new method for treating postcatheterization femoral pseudoaneurysms. J Vasc Surg. 1998 Jun 1; 27(6): 1032–1038.
21. Paulson EK, Sheafor DH, Kliewer MA, Nelson RC, Eisenberg LB, Sebastian MW, et al. Treatment of Iatrogenic Femoral Arterial Pseudoaneurysms: Comparison of US-guided Thrombin Injection with Compression Repair. Radiology. 2000 May 1; 215(2): 403–408.
22. Sajnani N, Bogart DB. Retroperitoneal Hemorrhage as a Complication of Percutaneous Intervention: Report of 2 Cases and Review of the Literature. Open Cardiovasc Med J. 2013 Feb 28; 7: 16–22.
23. Ellis SG, Bhatt D, Kapadia S, Lee D, Yen M, Whitlow PL. Correlates and outcomes of retroperitoneal hemorrhage complicating percutaneous coronary intervention. Catheter Cardiovasc Interv Off J Soc Card Angiogr Interv. 2006 Apr; 67(4): 541–545.
24. Sprouse LR, Botta DM, Hamilton IN. The management of peripheral vascular complications associated with the use of percutaneous suture–mediated closure devices. J Vasc Surg. 2001 Apr 1; 33(4): 688–693.
25. Glaser RL, McKellar D, Scher KS. Arteriovenous fistulas after cardiac catheterization. Arch Surg Chic Ill 1960. 1989 Nov; 124(11): 1313–1315.
26. Kim D, Orron DE, Skillman JJ, Kent KC, Porter DH, Schlam BW, et al. Role of superficial femoral artery puncture in the development of pseudoaneurysm and arteriovenous fistula complicating percutaneous transfemoral cardiac catheterization. Cathet Cardiovasc Diagn. 1992 Feb; 25(2): 91–97.
27. Matsukage T, Masuda N, Ikari Y. Successful transradial intervention by switching from 6 French to 5 French guiding catheter. J Invasive Cardiol. 2011 Jun; 23(6): E153-155.
28. Treitl KM, König C, Reiser MF, Treitl M. Complications of Transbrachial Arterial Access for Peripheral Endovascular Interventions. J Endovasc Ther. 2015 Feb; 22(1): 63–70.
29. Greenwood MJ, Della-Siega AJ, Fretz EB, Kinloch D, Klinke P, Mildenberger R, et al. Vascular Communications of the Hand in Patients Being Considered for Transradial Coronary Angiography: Is the Allen's Test Accurate? J Am Coll Cardiol. 2005 Dec 6; 46(11): 2013–2017.
30. Wheatley BJ, Mansour MA, Grossman PM, Munir K, Cali RF, Gorsuch JM, et al. Complication Rates for Percutaneous Lower Extremity Arterial Antegrade Access. Arch Surg. 2011 Apr 1; 146(4): 432–435.
31. Swee W, Wang JY, Lee AC. Managing perforations of the superficial femoral artery. Endovascular Today. 2014 Oct. Pg 59–68.
32. Bishu K, Armstrong EJ. Supera self-expanding stents for endovascular treatment of femoropopliteal disease: a review of the clinical evidence. Vasc Health Risk Manag. 2015; 11: 387–395.
33. Ochoa Chaar CI, Shebl F, Sumpio B, Dardik A, Indes J, Sarac T. Distal embolization during lower extremity endovascular interventions. J Vasc Surg. 2017;66(1):143–1450.
34. Shrikhande GV, Khan SZ, Hussain HG, Dayal R, McKinsey JF, Morrissey N. Lesion types and device characteristics that predict distal embolization during percutaneous lower extremity interventions. J Vasc Surg. 2011 Feb; 53(2): 347–352.
35. Suri R, Wholey MH, Postoak D, Hagino RT, Toursarkissian B. Distal embolic protection during femoropopliteal atherectomy. Catheter Cardiovasc Interv Off J Soc Card Angiogr Interv. 2006 Mar; 67(3): 417–422.

SUGGESTED READINGS

White CJ, Gray WA. Endovascular Therapies for Peripheral Arterial Disease: An Evidence-Based Review. Circulation. 2007 Nov 6; 116(19):2203–15.
Norgren L, Hiatt WR, Dormandy JA, Nehler MR, Harris KA, Fowkes FGR. Inter-Society Consensus for the Management of Peripheral Arterial Disease (TASC II). J Vasc Surg. 2007 Jan; 45(1): S5–67.

8

Complications of endovascular repair of infrarenal abdominal aortic aneurysms

ROBERT CUFF AND JOYCE LU

Abdominal aortic aneurysm (AAA) is a pathologic dilation of the aorta defined as 50% greater than normal diameter. The etiology of this condition has been shown to be associated with medial weakening of the vessel wall through smooth muscle cell dysfunction and structural weaknesses related to connective tissues. The majority of AAA occur in the infrarenal aorta, but aneurysmal degeneration can occur along the entirety of the vessel. While there are many cardiovascular risk factors associated with AAA incidence, the strongest medical factors predisposing individuals to AAA are tobacco abuse and genetic connective tissue disorders. In the aging population, incidence of AAA has also been shown to rise by four fold from the fifth and sixth decades of life and it continues to rise further with increasing age. The natural history of AAA is continuous growth with increasing risk over time of aortic rupture. As the diameter increases, there is a direct relationship of the amount of tension experienced by the vessel wall, thus leading to further aneurysmal degeneration that magnifies as the aneurysm continues to grow. Given this predictable consequence of AAA pathology, elective repair is currently recommended once AAAs are 5.5 cm in diameter (sometimes 5.0 cm in women). Urgent and emergent repair is indicated for patients experiencing symptomatic and ruptured AAA that clinically manifests itself as severe abdominal or back pain which is often described as "stabbing" or "tearing" and, if ruptured, can give rise to hemodynamic changes of tachycardia and hypertension in response to the pain and hypotension in the setting of acute rupture.

Surgical repair has historically been either a transabdominal or retroperitoneal open approach with direct visualization of the aorta followed by interposition grafting at proximal and distal aortic tissues not affected by aneurysmal degeneration. Through research that began in the 1970s, endovascular aortic repair (EVAR) was developed as a minimally invasive approach, first successfully performed as a treatment for AAA in 1990 by Dr. Juan C. Parodi. Today, there are many EVAR stent grafts featuring different technical qualities that a surgeon can select from to suit the individual anatomic needs of each patient. These different features vary in many ways including sizes offered, graft material (No covering-multilayer flow modulator stent, expanded polytetrofluoroetylene or polyester), stent material (stainless steel, nitinol, or cobalt-chromium), proximal fixation (suprarenal stent fixation, polymer ring), deployment method, stent positioning inside or outside the graft, fenestrations (absent, standard "off-the-shelf," customized, or physician-modified), branching, and sac-sealing technology. With every device, attention should be paid to the instructions for use (IFU), and the best practice is to operate within manufacturer guidelines. Despite the variety of options available, there are complications which can occur during the course of EVAR that are independent of which configuration is utilized. Knowledge of what these complications are and how to manage them is critical to the successful treatment of infrarenal AAA.[1]

ACCESS

Correct access technique is essential to EVAR as it is the portal for all subsequent endovascular surgical equipment in the procedure. While open groin cutdown technique has been utilized, percutaneous access is increasing in prevalence with the advent of the large arteriotomy (≥ 14 F) vascular closure devices and development of the "preclose" technique.[2,10] Avoiding open cutdown significantly reduces the complications of wound infection (1% vs 2%),[7] nerve injury (3.4%),[13] and lymphocele (4.8–11.9%).[14] However, without direct visualization, hematoma (17.3%), pseudoaneurysm (5.7%), subintimal wire entry (17.3%), and vessel dissection (3.8%) are just some of the possible complications of percutaneous access.[8,9] A preoperative pulse exam to establish baseline distal perfusion should be routine and used for postoperative comparison. Ultrasound guidance is commonly used to assist with visualization as modified Seldinger technique is applied for atraumatic, anterior, single-entry at the common femoral arteries.[3] Selection of location for percutaneous access is also important and can be anticipated with imaging, either during access or from CTA imaging. Visualized calcifications within the artery should be avoided to prevent vascular dissection, traumatic plaque embolization, or closure device failure.

Once access has been obtained, intraluminal confirmation should be made with angiography before proceeding. Initial access with a 21 G needle (versus 18 G) and 0.018″ wire allows for increased safety in case the first attempt is unsuccessful, in which case, manual pressure can be held for 2 minutes and access reattempted. Angiography may reveal significant atherosclerotic calcifications or tortuosity within the iliac vessels which may warrant pre-dilation, stenting, or stiffer wire placement to facilitate successful sheath and device advancement. Prior to large sheath placement, heparinization (70–90 units/kg) should be utilized to prevent thrombus formation as some sheaths may be occlusive in patients with small-caliber vasculature or preexisting stenotic disease. In the event that vascular occlusion occurs, this may warrant open cutdown at the groin and open thrombectomy. If in the course of access significant vascular dissection occurs, this may be treated by initially attempting prolonged balloon angioplasty or local stenting if the flap continues to be flow-limiting.

At the conclusion of the procedure, cases of incomplete or unsuccessful deployment of closure devices may be assisted toward hemostasis with protamine heparin reversal and application of nonocclusive hemostatic pressure (20+ minutes) to prevent hematoma formation. If this is unsuccessful, or in the event of complete device failure, open cutdown should be performed with direct arterial repair. If wire access is maintained, proximal balloon occlusion can allow for hemorrhagic control during open cutdown and can serve as a directional guide to expedite exposure. Pseudoaneurysm formation is a possible short-term to late complication that can be treated with compression alone or with thrombin injection and compression if the pseudoaneurysm neck is sufficiently narrow and short, short; if this is not successful, it may require direct arterial repair as well.

GRAFT MALDEPLOYMENT

Accurate positioning of the stent grafts ensures proper landing zone length and undisturbed perfusion to aortic branch vessels. Preoperative planning and imaging may predict optimal fluoroscopic visualization angles utilized to eliminate parallax when performing deployment. Aortogram with the device in place, just prior to deployment is important to perform due to the fact that the additional rigidity of the device on the wires may alter aortic alignment. Depending on the device selected, there are features that may allow for adjustments depending on the issue encountered. Some devices allow for unidirectional repositioning after partial deployment or proximal recapturing which can allow for level and orientation adjustments.[4] Once fully deployed, graft repositioning may not be possible due to the radial forces of the stents and/or proximal fixation struts keeping the stent graft fixed in place. If migration occurrs or deployment is too low (preventing optimal proximal fixation), a proximal cuff can be placed for graft extension. If side branches off of the aorta are at risk for malperfusion due to partial or full coverage, adjunctive techniques may need to be considered. In the case of proximal vessels (e.g., renal artery, superior mesenteric artery, celiac artery) being partially or fully covered, brachial access should be obtained to assist with cannulation of the vessels at risk so that either stenting or snorkeling with proximal extension may be performed using either bare metal or covered stents, if needed. Distally, use of a marker catheter for limb measurement is important for accuracy in tortuous anatomy. If partial or complete internal iliac artery coverage occurs, ipsilateral wire access into the internal iliac artery may allow for distal limb extension and internal iliac artery stenting that extends into the external iliac artery to permit retrograde pelvic perfusion via snorkel technique.

After main body deployment for most grafts, the subsequent procedure is to cannulate the contralateral gate; however, this is a challenge if the gate orientation prevents wire access or if the gate does not open completely. In the case of difficult cannulation, brachial access can provide the directional advantage to allow for a snare to capture the wire through the gate. Additionally, if the gate does not open, brachial access may allow for a wire to pass through the contralateral gate from the superior direction, which can be subsequently opened with a noncompliant balloon in the event of external compression.

EMBOLISM

Preoperative imaging should be reviewed for aortic wall thrombus burden as wire manipulation and stent graft positioning during procedure may result in distal embolization. Flexible tip wires, gentle manipulation, and careful catheter exchanges can help to prevent this complication. If embolization is seen during angiography, catheter suction thrombectomy techniques may be applied, however there is risk of further embolization of smaller emboli distally. If a lesion does not respond to suction thrombectomy, exclusion using a covered stent may be attempted, or open cutdown and open thrombectomy when appropriate.

ENDOLEAK

TYPE Ia/Ib

Endoleaks at the proximal and distal portions of stent grafts can have many causes. Appropriate over-sizing (as recommended by manufacturer IFUs) and positioning as part of preoperative planning is important to prevent gaps either due to fabric infolding, inadequate seal zone length, or external compression from aortic wall thrombus or calcifications. With the advent of polymer-based proximal seal zones (e.g., Ovation, Nellix, Alto), this may compensate for neck irregularities by creating a more conformable seal not dependent on a circular seal.[12] Additionally, if snorkel technique is planned to be utilized at the proximal seal zone, consideration of a stent graft where the graft fabric material lies outside rather than within the stent wirecage could allow for a reduction in endoleak potential.[11] When a Ia/Ib endoleak is seen on angiography, initially, local balloon angioplasty may allow for better conformation of the proximal seal to eliminate the endoleak. If snorkeling, it is important to simultaneously inflate a balloon within the snorkel to prevent stent collapse during this procedure. If this does not yield success, it can be an option to see if the endoleak channel is able to be directly accessed to allow for placement of embolization coils, glue, or dimethyl sulfoxideethylene vinyl alcohol (DMSO-EVOH) solution. This can also be performed after the initial EVAR via translumbar approach (Figure 8.1). Endostaples are another option if the issue is severe neck angulation leading to "bird-beaking" to allow for better wall apposition.[5] Stenting at the proximal neck is another option, either with a proximal covered cuff (if there is room below a branching vessel, Figure 8.2) or a Palmaz stent if a branch is within too close of proximity where a covered cuff would potentially lead to branch exclusion. A technique that would maximize proximal extension while safely ensuring a branch is not covered proximally would be to access the branch and simultaneously inflate a balloon within it while deploying a proximal cuff while applying gentle proximal pressure so that the cuff accurately abuts the balloon without overriding the ostium.[6] Distally, if there is not enough distance to allow for adequate seal zone or potentially internal iliac artery calcifications preventing good apposition, utilization of an iliac branch device may be an option or the chimney technique from the common into both the internal and external iliac arteries.

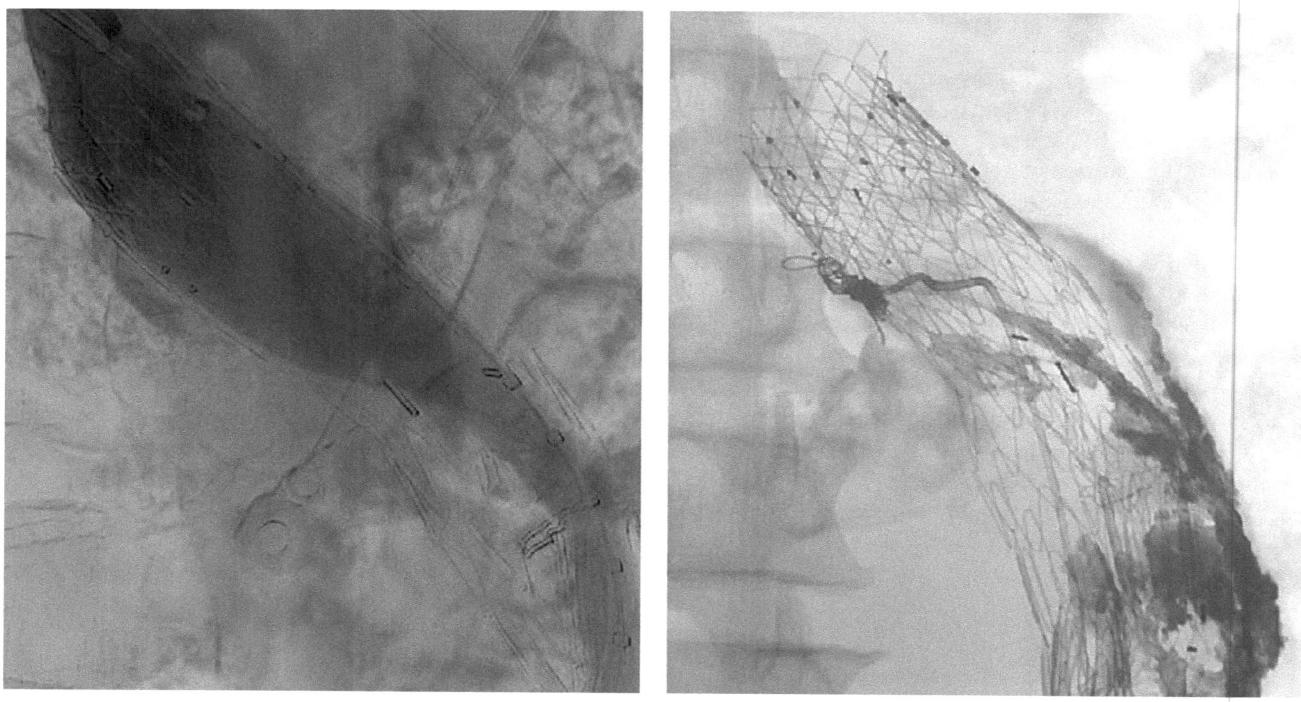

Figure 8.1 61-year-old male with type Ia endoleak repaired with coils and Onyx liquid embolic agent. Left image is an angiogram with lateral oblique angulation demonstrating the endoleak. Right image is from his translumbar embolization.

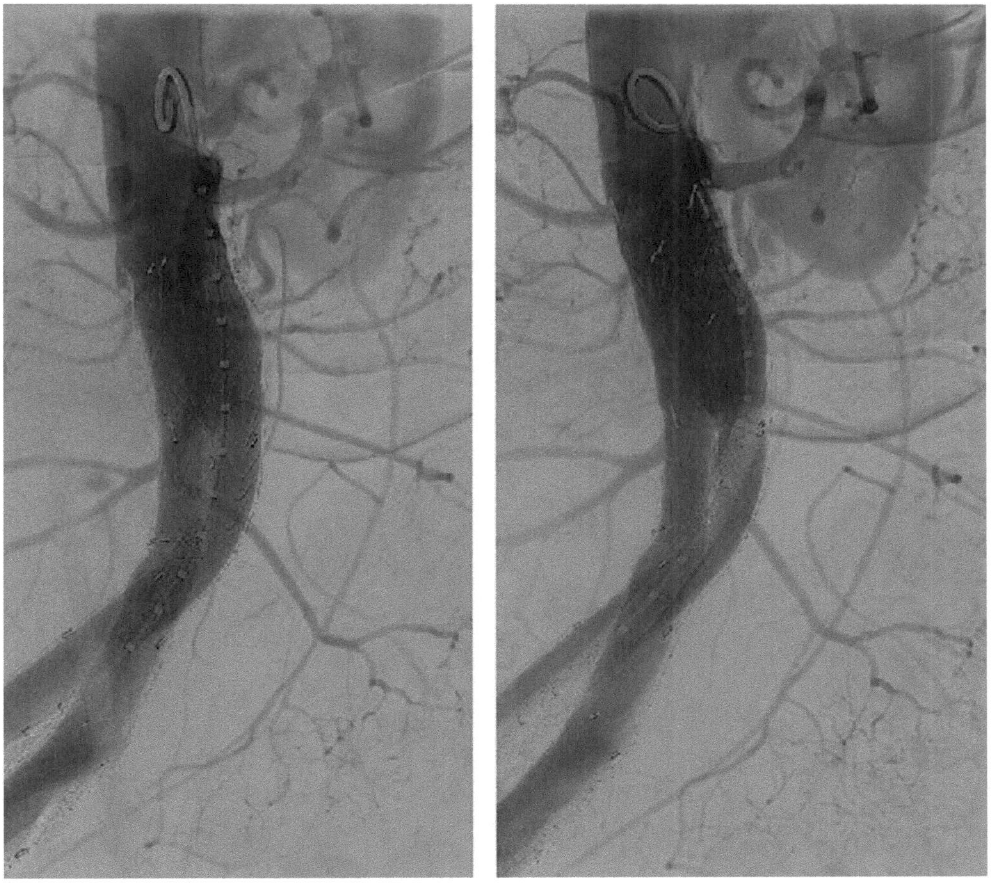

Figure 8.2 79-year-old male with type Ia endoleak repaired with proximal stent graft extension. Images are intraoperative angiography before (left) and after (right) proximal extension stent graft placement.

TYPE II

This endoleak type can often be observed with routine surveillance as it can spontaneously resolve over time with sac thrombosis. However, if it is believed that the collateral flow from either lumbar arteries or the inferior mesenteric artery (IMA) is too significant to resolve, one technique could be to maintain wire access between the stent graft and the aortic wall to allow for direct vessel cannulation and embolization with coils, glue, or DMSO-EVOH solution. Should cannulation prove difficult, having a second wire within the aortic sac to inflate a balloon may create enough space to allow for wire manipulation and vessel access.[6] Additionally, it may be possible to access the IMA via collateral vessels such as the superior mesenteric artery via the marginal artery of Drummond or Arc of Riolan or the lumbar arteries through iliolumbar branches.

TYPE III

In this type of endoleak, maintaining wire access across the two components is highly important in case of complete component separation. Most often, this type of endoleak can be prevented with adequate component overlap during deployment and proper sizing. If the cause is fabric infolding or angulation leading to strut "bird-beaking," the initial approach may be to see if balloon angioplasty is enough to generate proper apposition to resolve the endoleak. If this is not successful, lining the overlap with another stent, either bare-metal or covered, for reinforcement and/or extended overlap coverage should be the next step (Figure 8.3). In the event that neither of these maneuvers is successful, particularly at the limb-main body junction point, complete embolization of the limb proximally from within the main body and distally from the involved iliac in combination with open femoral-femoral bypass may be required as a salvage technique. When this is found as a short-term or late complication of EVAR, re-accessing the luminal portion of the endograft is a key initial step. While most configurations of EVAR grafts have the wirecage component external to the graft fabric material, there are those with the wirecage within, which can complicate repair. Confirmation of the wire passing within the lumen of the wirecage and not behind a strut wire can be

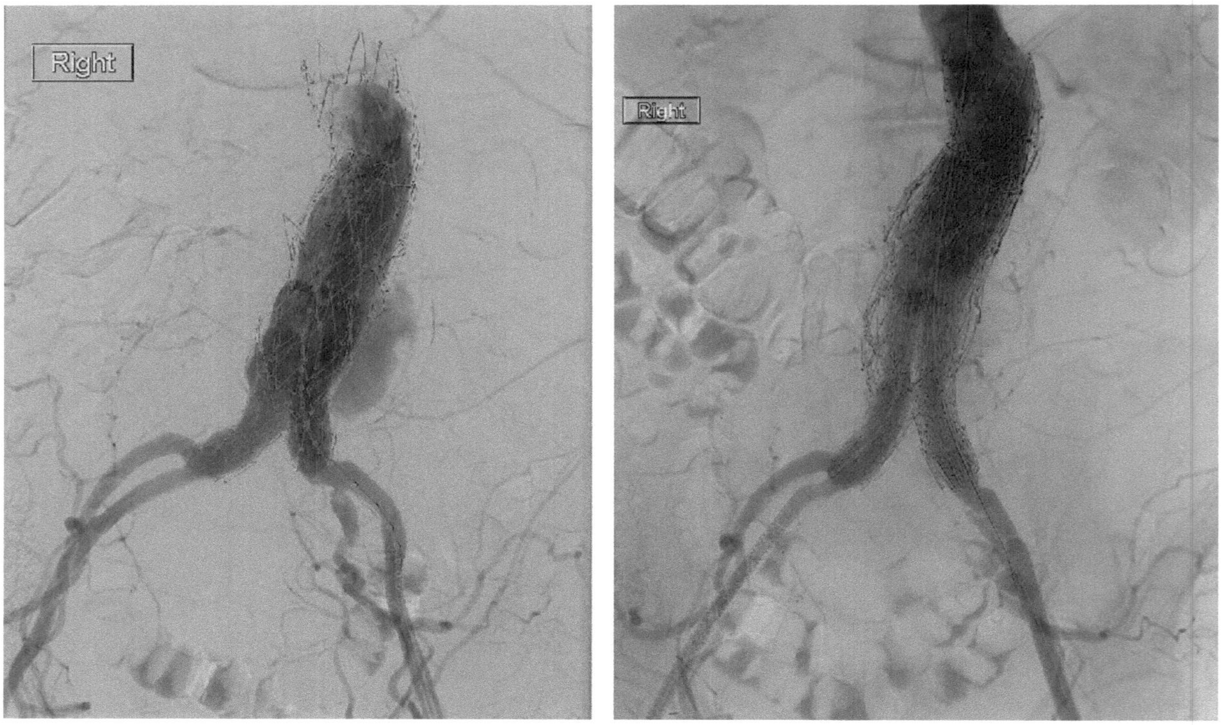

Figure 8.3 75-year-old female with type III endoleak repaired with a re-lining EVAR stent graft. Images are intraoperative angiography before (left) and after (right) relining stent graft placement.

achieved with greater likelihood by advancing a pigtail catheter (partially formed with a small length of wire protruding) up the endograft past the proximal extent and then followed by exchanging the catheter for a large noncompliant balloon that is retracted over the wire through the entire endograft past the wirecage proximally to distally (Figure 8.4).

LIMB OR COMPLETE ENDOGRAFT OCCLUSION

Another short, or long-term complication of EVAR can be limb/endograft occlusion; this rarely occurs during initial EVAR with appropriate systemic heparinization. Occlusion may be due to issues not directly related to technical failure of initial deployment such as proximal-origin embolization or distal thrombosis due to peripheral vascular disease which proximally extends into the iliac EVAR limbs or even the body. This can be endovascularly treated with re-lining of the endografts with covered stents via proximal (brachial) and/or distal (femoral) wire access. Open treatment options can include aorto-bifemoral, axillobifemoral, or femoral-femoral bypass (Figure 8.5).

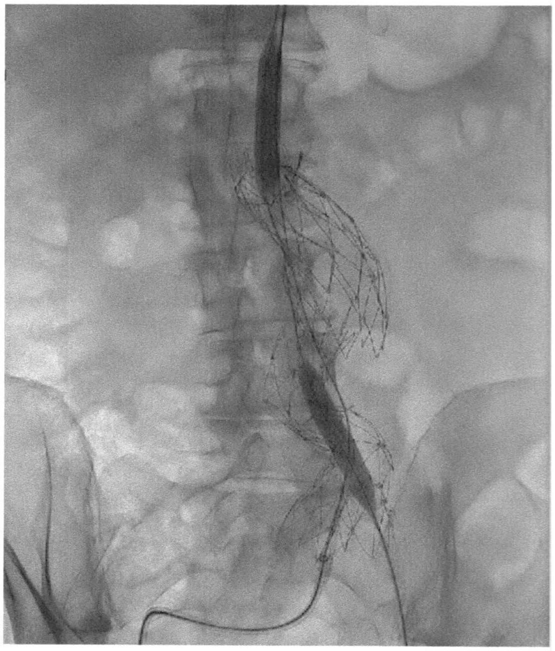

Figure 8.4 67-year-old male with type III endoleak of an EVAR stent graft and proximal extension cuff configured with the graft fabric material external to the stent wirecage. This composite angiogram image demonstrates the technique of using a 12 mm balloon advanced within the stent graft to confirm placement of the working wire as internal to the stent prior to stent graft deployment rejoining the separated components.

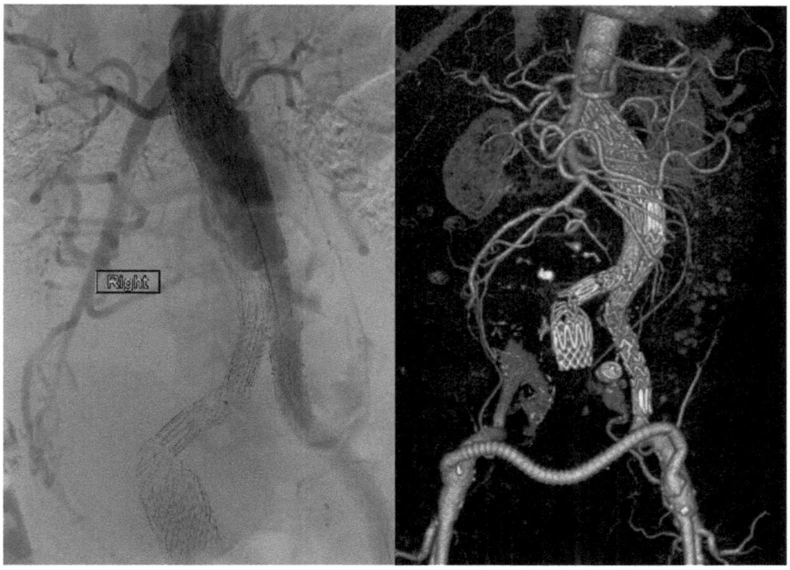

Figure 8.5 61-year-old male with occlusion of his right EVAR limb. This was treated with open left-to-right femoral-femoral bypass. Left image is an angiogram demonstrating the occlusion, and the right image is a 3D reconstruction of the patient's vascular anatomy after open repair.

REFERENCES

1. Cronenwett JL, Rutherford RB. Rutherfords Vascular Surgery. Philadelphia: Saunders/Elsevier; 2014.
2. Schwartz B, Burstein S, Economides C, et al. "Review of Vascular Closure Devices." Cath Lab Digest. https://www.cathlabdigest.com/articles/Review-Vascular-Closure-Devices. Accessed 2018.
3. Bensley RP, Hurks R, Huang Z, et al. Ultrasound-guided percutaneous endovascular aneurysm repair success is predicted by access vessel diameter. Journal of Vascular Surgery. 2012;55(6): 1554–1561. doi:10.1016/j.jvs.2011.12.042.
4. Katsargyris A, Botos B, Oikonomou K, Leistl MPD, Ritter W, Verhoeven E. The New C3 Gore Excluder Stent-graft: Single-center Experience with 100 Patients. European Journal of Vascular and Endovascular Surgery. 2014;47(4): 342–348. doi:10.1016/j.ejvs.2013.12.015.
5. Guimaraes M, Yamada R, and Schonholz C. "Endoleak and the Role of Embolization." Endovascular Today. https://evtoday.com/articles/2015-apr/endoleak-and-the-role of embolization. Accessed 2018.
6. Oderich GS. Endovascular Aortic Repair: Current Techniques with Fenestrated, Branched and Parallel Stent-Grafts. Cham: Springer; 2017.
7. Buck DB, Karthaus EG, Soden PA, et al. Percutaneous versus femoral cutdown access for endovascular aneurysm repair. Journal of Vascular Surgery. 2015; 62(1): 16–21. doi:10.1016/j.jvs.2015.01.058.
8. Samson RH, Sprayregen S, Veith FJ, Scher LA, Gupta SK, Ascer E. Management of angioplasty complications, unsuccessful procedures and early and late failures. Ann Surg. 1984;199(2): 234–240.
9. Dwivedi K, Regi JM, Cleveland TJ, et al. Long-Term Evaluation of Percutaneous Groin Access for EVAR. CardioVascular and Interventional Radiology. October 2018. doi:10.1007/s00270-018-2072-3.
10. Lee WA, Brown MP, Nelson PR, and Huber, TS. Total Percutaneous Access for Endovascular Aortic Aneurysm Repair ("Preclose" Technique). Journal of Vascular Surgery. 45(6): 1095–101. doi:10.1016/j.jvs.2007.01.050.
11. Helo N., Chang AC., Hyun C., Bianchi C., Teruya TH., Yi AC, & Chon, KS. (2017). Retrospective Review of Billowing Phenomenon—A Mimic of Endoleak Following Placement of Endologix Covered Stent for the Treatment of Abdominal Aortic Aneurysm. Annals of Vascular Surgery. 45: 239–246. doi:10.1016/j.avsg.2017.06.127.
12. Greaves NS, Moore A, Seriki D, & Ghosh, J. (2018). Outcomes of Endovascular Aneurysm Repair using the Ovation Stent Graft System in Adverse Anatomy. European Journal of Vascular and Endovascular Surgery. 2018;55(4): 512–517. doi:10.1016/j.ejvs.2017.11.023.
13. Dougherty MJ, & Calligaro KD. How to avoid and manage nerve injuries associated with aortic surgery: Ischemic neuropathy, traction injuries, and sexual derangements. Seminars in Vascular Surgery. 2001;14(4): 275–281. doi:10.1053/svas.2001.27886.
14. Obara A., Dziekiewicz M. A., Maruszynski M., Witkowski A., Dąbrowski M., & Chmielak Z. Lymphatic complications after vascular interventions. Videosurgery and Other Miniinvasive Techniques. 2014;3: 420–426. doi:10.5114/wiitm.2014.43021.

9

Complications of endovascular repair of juxtarenal aortic aneurysms

JORDAN R. STERN AND JASON T. LEE

Endovascular repair of abdominal aortic aneurysms (EVAR) was initially limited to the infrarenal aorta by the requirement of an adequate proximal seal zone below the renal arteries. The introduction and widespread adoption of techniques such as chimney/snorkel parallel grafting (ChEVAR), and custom fenestrated endografts (FEVAR), now allow for total endovascular repair of aneurysms with short or no infrarenal neck (Figure 9.1). Endovascular repair of these "juxtarenal" aortic aneurysms is more technically complex than standard EVAR and carries its own set of unique potential complications. This chapter will review some of the systemic, procedural, and long-term complications related to these procedures.

MEDICAL COMPLICATIONS

Endovascular juxtarenal aortic aneurysm repair generally requires general anesthesia and incurs longer operative times and higher doses of radiation and intravenous contrast than standard EVAR.[1,2] This predictably leads to somewhat higher rates of various perioperative complications including renal, pulmonary, and cardiovascular events when compared to EVAR.[1,3,4] However, when compared to open repair of anatomically similar aneurysms, the morbidity profile is still favorable.[4,5]

A meta-analysis of juxtarenal aneurysm repair by Katsargyris et al.[6] summarized the relevant literature regarding perioperative complications for both FEVAR (10 studies, 931 patients) and ChEVAR (5 studies, 94 patients). For FEVAR, cardiac complications (acute myocardial infarction and arrythmia) occurred in 3.7% of patients, pulmonary complications (pneumonia, ARDS, prolonged ventilation) in 2.3%, sepsis in 0.6%, and ischemic stroke in 0.3%. For ChEVAR, cardiac complications occurred in 7.4%, pulmonary in 3.2%, and ischemic stroke in 3.2%. Only ischemic stroke was significantly different between the two procedures and higher in the ChEVAR group, likely due to upper extremity access issues. This will be specifically discussed later in this chapter.

PERIOPERATIVE AND LATE MORTALITY

Perioperative mortality from endovascular repair of juxtarenal aneurysms has been reported as anywhere from 0–10% in the literature, similar to EVAR and also consistently lower than that of open repair.[1,4,6–9] Long-term mortality appears to be more dependent on cardiac, oncologic, and other factors and is similar for endovascular and open approaches.[5,10,11]

RENAL DYSFUNCTION

Because of the manipulation and stenting of the renal arteries, postoperative renal impairment is one of the primary concerns with endovascular juxtarenal aneurysm repair and deserves some particular attention, especially since acute kidney injury is correlated with increased risk of mortality in these patients.[12,13] The rate of transient renal insufficiency is higher than that seen with standard EVAR, and has been estimated to be around 15–35% following these procedures.[11,14–17] There does not appear to be a major difference in renal complications between FEVAR and ChEVAR.[6]

Longer-term renal outcomes are primarily determined by patency of the branch stents,[18] though even with patent branches there is some evidence for decreasing renal function over time.[11,15] Fortunately, the majority of patients in all of these studies did not require permanent hemodialysis, and this remains a rare event.[15,17] In order to mitigate the risk of postoperative renal failure, volume status should be optimized in the perioperative period, contrast use should be judicious, and renal manipulation should be minimized to only the necessary amount.

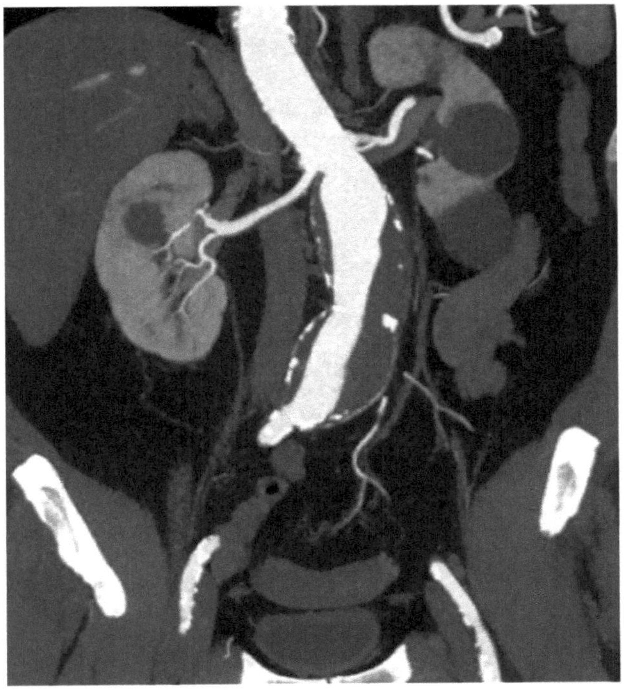

Figure 9.1 Juxtarenal abdominal aortic aneurysm.

ACCESS SITE COMPLICATIONS

FEMORAL ACCESS

The common femoral artery (CFA) remains the primary access site for endovascular aortic aneurysm repair. The CFA is easily accessible either surgically or percutaneously and can accommodate the large sheaths—often 20 Fr or greater—required to deliver the endografts. Although open surgical exposure remains the gold standard, percutaneous, large-bore femoral access has become increasingly common and totally percutaneous endovascular aortic aneurysm repair (PEVAR) is now the preferred approach of many practitioners due to shorter procedure times and lower complication rates.[19–22] Complications related to percutaneous femoral access are well described, and can generally be divided into hemorrhagic concerns such as hematoma and pseudoaneurysm formation, and thrombotic complications involving the access vessels.[23,24] Careful planning is of paramount importance in avoiding complications, and percutaneous access should not be attempted in very small vessels and those with heavy calcific disease, particularly on the anterior surface. The use of ultrasound guidance has been shown to reduce complications as well, and should be considered standard of care for all percutaneous cases.[25,26] Special attention should be paid to safe access during FEVAR, as the larger sheaths required for this procedure have been correlated with a higher incidence of all access site complications, particularly pseudoaneurysm formation.[27,28]

Management of hemorrhagic complications from the puncture site is dependent on the level at which access was obtained. When the common femoral artery is accessed in the correct location, manual pressure can be held against the underlying femoral head even for larger arteriotomies. For punctures above or through the inguinal ligament, direct surgical exposure via a retroperitoneal incision may be required to achieve control. Alternatively, temporary tamponade can be achieved with an angioplasty balloon from a contralateral approach, followed by placement of a self-expanding covered stent in the external iliac artery to seal the arteriotomy.

For heavily calcified aortoiliac segments, there is also a risk of arterial rupture from tracking of sheaths and devices (Figure 9.2).[29,30] When recognized quickly, these potentially life-threatening injuries can also be managed by temporary balloon tamponade and placement of a covered stent. Perhaps the most dreaded access vessel complication occurs when the sheath is withdrawn and the iliac artery is completely avulsed, everted, and pulled out with it—the so-called "iliac on a stick." In these cases, if wire access is still maintained, the avulsed segment can be

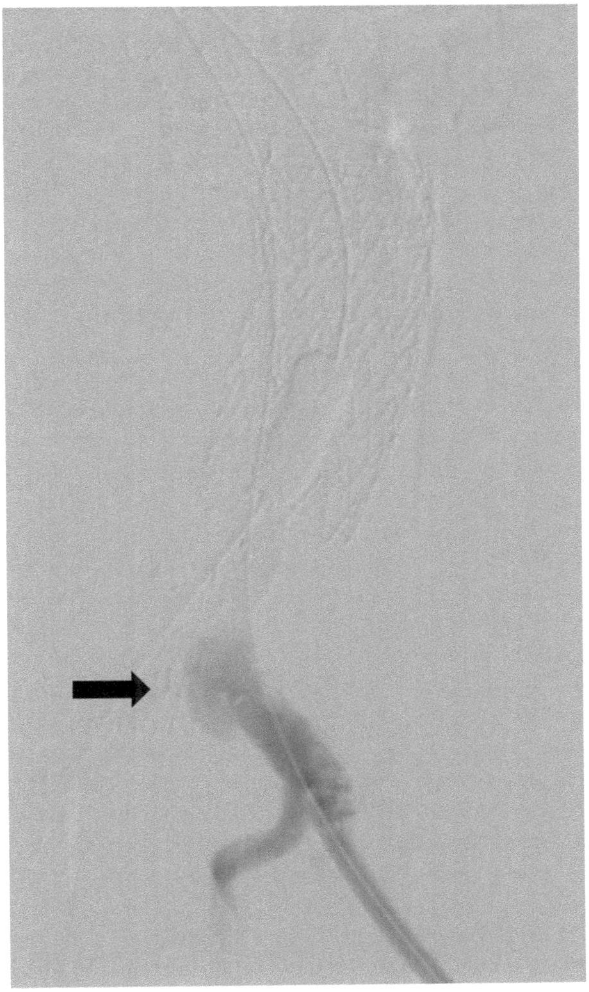

Figure 9.2 Iliac artery rupture.

traversed with a covered stent as well.[31,32] However, if wire access has been lost, then emergent surgical control and open repair is the only option.

Thrombotic complications of femoral access are primarily related to failure of vascular closure devices.[33] A "pre-close" technique using two Proglide Perclose devices (Abbott Vascular, Santa Clara, CA) is the most commonly employed technique for large-bore percutaneous access and has been shown to be safe and effective.[34] However, incorrect deployment can lead to arterial dissection and/or occlusion by lifting of posterior plaque with the footplate.[35] This is generally recognized by a lack of distal pulses or Doppler signals after the sheath is removed and the sutures are tightened. Although some percutaneous methods have been described to address this, open surgical repair with or without endarterectomy and patch angioplasty is the treatment of choice. Once again, early recognition in addition to proper preoperative planning is the key to achieving favorable outcomes.

UPPER EXTREMITY ACCESS

For more complex aortic interventions, upper extremity arterial access may be required. This is particularly true for placement of parallel snorkel or chimney grafts, as these require deployment from above.[36] Use of the upper extremity carries risk of several unique complications, including a 3–10% risk of stroke from wire-catheter manipulation within the aortic arch.[37] The left arm is generally preferred as this obviates the need for crossing the head vessels, though the risk of stroke does not appear to be significantly related to laterality.[38] Whichever side is chosen, manipulation within the arch should be minimized and only performed after systemic heparinization.

Arm access has traditionally been achieved via by either open or percutaneous access of the brachial artery.[39] Sheaths up to 8Fr can be used from this location in most individuals, which is sufficient for the majority of endovascular procedures. Percutaneous brachial access carries a higher risk of complications than open surgical exposure, especially for sheaths larger than 5 Fr.[40] Of particular importance is the risk of brachial sheath hematoma, which can lead to permanent neurologic injury from compression of the median nerve.[40] This risk is alleviated with open access, as the brachial sheath is left open on closure. As such, we advocate for open access whenever possible. When a percutaneous approach is chosen, the safest area to access is several centimeters above the antecubital fossa where manual compression can be held against the distal humerus. The use of vascular closure devices is typically not recommended for the brachial artery.

When larger sheaths are required, the axillary artery may be exposed through a small supra- or infraclavicular incision and accessed either by use of a surgical conduit or via direct puncture. This approach has been shown to be safe, with a low rate of complications primarily related to injury of adjacent structures such as the axillary vein and brachial plexus.[41,42] The presence of pacemakers or tunneled catheters may make exposure difficult and increase the risk of complications, as does a morbidly obese body habitus or previous surgical dissection.

The radial artery can also be used for procedures where a 6Fr sheath is sufficient, and percutaneous radial access can be performed with a low rate of complications such as hematoma (< 1%) and pseudoaneurysm (< 0.1%) by experienced practitioners.[43,44] Preoperative assessment of the collateral flow through the ulnar artery is essential, as with an intact palmar arch even thrombotic occlusion of the radial artery will likely be clinically silent and not lead to overt hand ischemia.[43]

TECHNICAL MISADVENTURES

COMPLICATIONS RELATED TO BRANCH CANNULATION

Several issues can arise when cannulating target vessels and deploying branch stents, whether in a snorkel position or through a fenestration. If the target vessel cannot be accessed then, by definition, no bridging stent component can be deployed. Anatomic factors affecting the ability to cannulate can include heavy calcification at the vessel ostium, tortuosity, and angulation.[45] Careful assessment of preoperative cross-sectional imaging should identify the majority of these issues ahead of time, and any additional materials such as steerable sheaths, angled catheters, and multiple wires can be made available for the case. Pre-wiring of any difficult targets prior to deploying the main body endograft as well as the use of fusion-type imaging systems may also help ensure success. If the failure to cannulate in FEVAR is due to poor device design and malalignment of the fenestration with the target, this may not be a recoverable situation. This is covered below under the topic "shuttering."

Once the target has been cannulated, there is risk of injury to the artery itself or the end-organ it supplies. This tends to occur most frequently in the renal arteries.[46] Perforation of the kidney from an errant wire can be self-limited, but can also lead to significant hemorrhage or fistula formation (Figure 9.3).[45] In rare cases this may necessitate embolization or even emergent operative exploration, so careful attention should be paid to keeping the wire tip in the visual field at all times. Use of softer-tipped or more favorable shapes of stiff wires should be considered, particularly with challenging angles or short renal landing zones.

Dissection of the target vessel can occur from wire manipulation or during placement of the bridging stent.[47] When this occurs and is recognized intraoperatively, the focus should be on maintaining perfusion to the end-organ. If the dissection is small and non-flow-limiting,

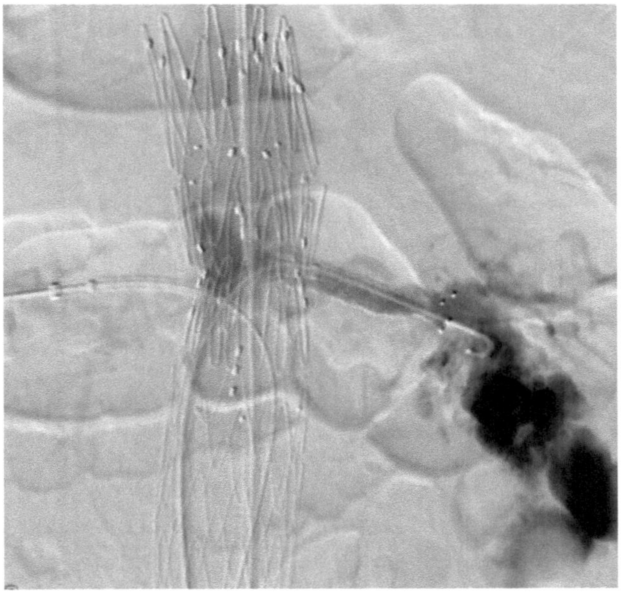

Figure 9.3 Wire perforation of the left kidney during fenestrated aortic aneurysm repair. Significant extravasation of contrast is seen, and ultimately the renal artery was embolized and sacrificed for hemorrhage control.

it can potentially be observed. In more severe cases, an additional self-expanding bare metal stent can be deployed to tack down the flap distally. Intravascular ultrasound (IVUS) can be extremely helpful for more complicated dissections where the true and false lumens are not immediately distinguishable, and to assist with sizing of the additional stent.

SHUTTERING

The success of fenestrated aortic aneurysm repair (FEVAR) is highly dependent on preoperative planning. Fenestrations need to be accurately positioned in order to line up properly with the appropriate target vessel and allow cannulation and/or bridge stenting. Malalignment of the fenestration and target results in a phenomenon called "shuttering," where a portion of the lumen is obstructed. In severe cases, this may even lead to the total inability to cannulate the vessel and loss of the intended visceral target branch (Figure 9.4). The most common configuration for the Zenith Fenestrated device (Cook Medical, Bloomington, IN) involves small fenestrations for the renal arteries, which are then bridged with a covered stent-graft.[48] The stent serves to correct and eliminate any minor shuttering issues and preserve renal blood flow.

Shuttering is much more common with the superior mesenteric artery (SMA), where there is generally a large fenestration or scallop that is not stented.[48–50] Although some degree of shuttering occurs frequently, the clinical consequences are variable. In a study from our group, shuttering with anywhere from 12–40% luminal reduction occurred in 50% of patients, without any consequent clinical events.[49] We generally have not stented large fenestrations during FEVAR. In contrast, Lala et al. found that 43% of unstented SMA fenestrations were significantly shuttered, and this resulted in several SMA stenoses and even one occlusion.[50] The authors therefore advocated for routine stenting of scallops and large fenestrations whenever feasible.

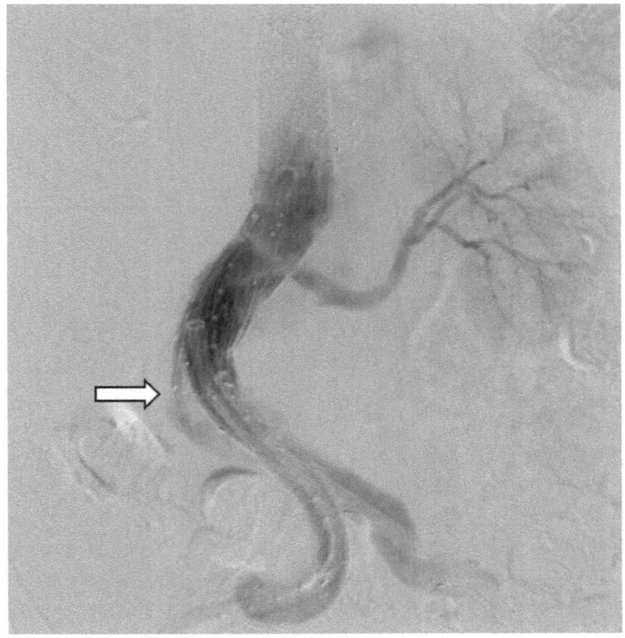

Figure 9.4 Malalignment of renal fenestration. The right renal fenestration was unable to be cannulated due to severe malalignment. Flush aortogram demonstrates good filling of the left renal stent with left nephrogram, but no filling of the right. An endoleak is seen due to contrast extravasation through the open fenestration (white arrow).

The decision to stent to prevent shuttering should be taken on a case-by-case basis. Pre-wiring of the SMA can give some clue as to the alignment of the fenestration once the device is fully deployed. When there is concern for compromised mesenteric blood flow on completion angiogram, the degree of shuttering can be investigated further by a balloon inflation test or intravascular ultrasound (IVUS). Considering the potentially fatal outcome of an acutely occluded SMA, it would be prudent to err on the side of caution and place a bridging stent whenever the suspicion for mesenteric compromise is high.

ENDOLEAKS

There is a risk of endoleak following any endovascular aortic intervention. However, there are some endoleaks specific to juxtarenal aneurysm repair which deserve special attention, primarily related to the proximal seal and branch vessels. This includes gutter leaks for parallel grafting (type 1a), and junctional (type 3) or distal branch (type 1c) leaks for fenestrated repair.

GUTTER LEAKS

When employing a parallel grafting technique in a snorkel or chimney configuration, there is a risk of proximal type 1a endoleak between the parallel components due to the circular shape of the grafts, commonly referred to as a "gutter leak" (Figure 9.5).[36,51] As the number of gutters increases with the number of parallel stents, so does the risk of gutter leak.[52,53] In the PERICLES registry of over 500 patients undergoing snorkel repair, the rate of intraoperative gutter leak was 7.9%.[54] However, this decreased to 2.9% after adjunctive measures such as repeat kissing balloon angioplasty and placement of additional aortic cuffs as indicated. On follow-up, CT imaging demonstrated resolution of all but two of these, though both of these patients eventually required graft explantation. While gutter leaks do affect the proximal seal, there is evidence to suggest that they have a more benign natural history than traditional type 1a endoleaks. In one single-institution study, a 30% gutter leak rate was noted on first postoperative imaging study. At 18 months of follow-up, 88.4% of these had spontaneously resolved and no difference was seen in aneurysm sac diameter between those with gutter leaks and those without.[55]

One novel strategy to mitigate the risk of gutter leak is the so-called "eye of the tiger" technique.[56] Here, an oversized balloon expandable stent is placed for the chimney, and a self-expanding stent is placed inside but not initially deployed. The proximal seal of the main body endograft is then ballooned, effectively crushing and flattening the chimney stent. Finally, the inner self-expanding stent is deployed, creating an "eye" shape that fills the gutter space.

For persistent gutter leaks that lead to continued aneurysm sac expansion, multiple adjunctive procedures are possible. Embolization of the gutter space with coils or other materials has been described,[57] as has the use of EndoAnchors (Medtronic, Minneapolis, MN).[58] In rare cases, this may even require endograft explantation and formal open thoracoabdominal repair.

BRANCH STENT LEAKS

There are several leak points related to the bridging stents that are unique to fenestrated and branch type aortic repairs (B/FEVAR). This primarily includes type III leaks from the graft-branch interface and type 1c leaks from the branch-target vessel interface. Fortunately, with appropriate sizing and planning, these are relatively uncommon. In a series of 650 patients undergoing B/FEVAR with 1679 total branches, Mastracci et al. showed rates of branch-related endoleak requiring intervention of only 2.5% for renal, 3.9% for SMA, and 2.8% for celiac branches.[18] Accurate diagnosis of these leaks is made difficult by the proximal location of the branches within the main body graft, as they occur early and simultaneously with type Ia endoleaks on both angiography and CT.[59]

Junctional, type III leaks at the connection point between the fenestration and main body represent a potential source of continued sac pressurization. In order

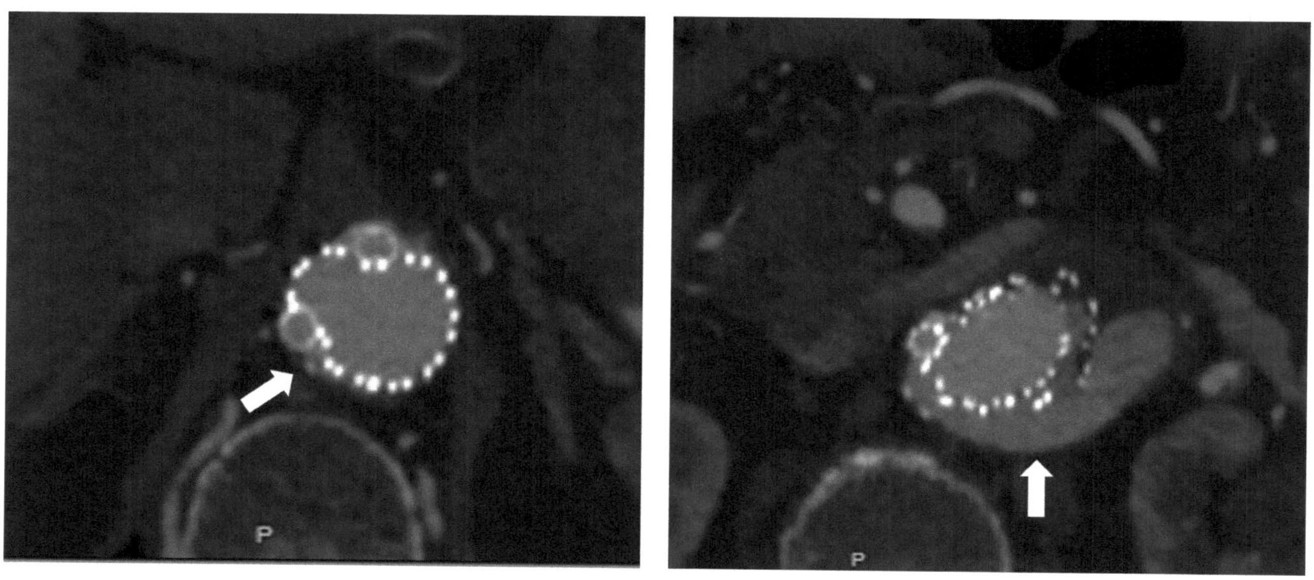

Figure 9.5 Gutter leak during chimney EVAR. There is a small gutter seen posteriorly between the main body and the right renal chimney (left panel, white arrow). This is associated with a significant endoleak on early-phase computed tomography angiogram (right panel, white arrow).

to prevent these from occurring, the bridging stents need to be appropriately sized to the fenestration, and positioned with adequate overlap and protrusion into the main body. While a number of different bridging stents can be used,[60] we recommend using a balloon-expandable, covered stent graft such as the Gore VBX (W.L. Gore, Flagstaff, AZ) or iCast (Atrium Medical, Hudson, NH). These stents can be post-dilated and flared at the proximal end using an angioplasty balloon several millimeters larger than the fenestration. For a standard 6 × 6 mm or 6 × 8 mm fenestration, a 9–10 mm angioplasty balloon provides an excellent flare and helps seal the overlap. When there is inadequate seal, repeat balloon flaring and even placement of additional overlapping stent grafts can be considered. However, even if there is still a small, persistent leak on intraoperative completion angiogram following these maneuvers, the majority of these can be safely observed and will spontaneously resolve without need for intervention.[59]

Type 1c endoleaks at the interface of the branch stent and the target vessel are also quite uncommon,[18] but deserve some special mention. When these occur, it is likely to have been a failure of either the sizing or positioning of the branch stent itself. If the stent is undersized, then gentle post-dilation of the distal seal may resolve the leak. If this fails, or if the stent is malpositioned at a kink or bend in the target artery, then extension with a self-expanding bare metal stent can be considered as well. Extension with covered stents or even a more flexible self-expanding bare metal stent is also possible, but care needs to be taken to avoid covering major branches as this could lead to end-organ ischemia.

Finally, infrequent issues can occur with the branch stents themselves, including fracture and/or fabric tear, component separation (when there are multiple bridging stents), and stent disassociation with from the target vessel. These are generally easily managed with placement of additional stent grafts to maximize overlap and seal.

BRANCH PATENCY AND ASSOCIATED REINTERVENTIONS

Below the visceral segment, these juxtarenal endovascular repairs are subject to the same failure modes as any other EVAR. The unique long-term success (or failure) of these repairs is therefore largely dependent on the patency of the visceral branches, and the associated need for re-intervention.[18] These longer-term complications are certainly significant, but the data suggest that occlusion of branch stents can actually be a salvageable situation in the majority of cases and rarely leads to clinical sequelae such as need for permanent renal replacement therapy in the case of renal stent occlusion.[61] Endovascular rescue may include simple balloon angioplasty and injection of tissue plasminogen activator (tPA), or more complex techniques such as pharmacomechanical thrombectomy with various devices (Figure 9.6).

CHIMNEY/SNORKEL STENTS

The overall patency of parallel chimney stents has been quite good throughout the literature. Short-term (6–12 month) patency of greater than 90% has been consistently reported in multiple series.[36,62–65] The largest series comes from the multicenter PERICLES registry, which has reported outcomes of nearly 900 chimney grafts at a median follow-up of 17 months. Primary patency was 94%, with secondary patency of 95.3%.[54] Other, smaller series have echoed these findings as well. Lachat et al. reported an overall patency of 98% at a mean follow-up of 25 months,[66] and Lee et al. reported a primary patency of 95% at 2 years.[67] Long-term studies of branch patency from parallel graft series are forthcoming and will be important to establish ChEVAR as a reasonable strategy.

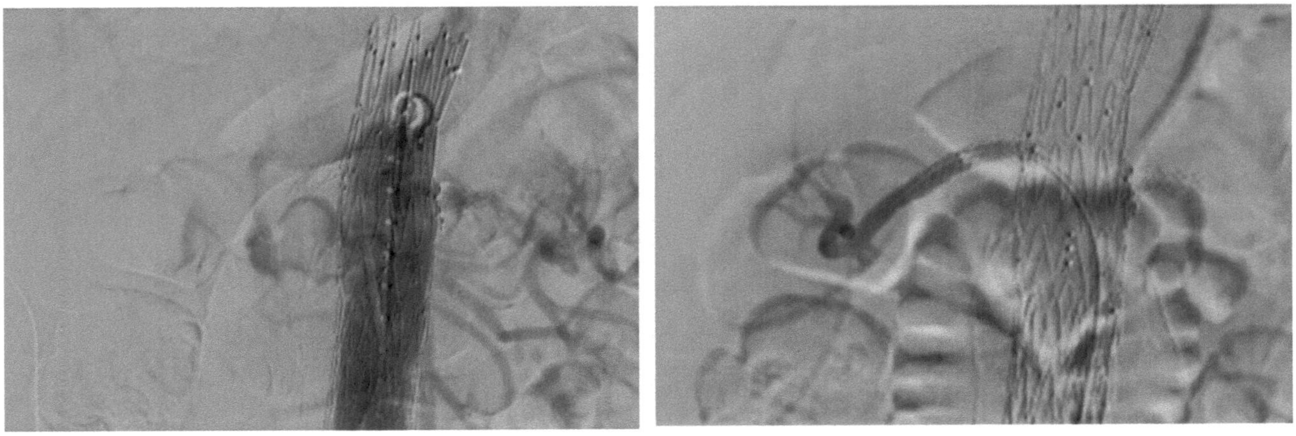

Figure 9.6 Endovascular salvage of occluded renal stent. Initial aortogram demonstrated filling of the left renal stent, but not the right (left panel). After cannulation, injection of tPA, and balloon angioplasty the right renal stent is now widely patent (right panel).

Endovascular rescue of occluded chimney grafts is possible, especially when found acutely. In the PERICLES registry the overall secondary intervention rate was 6.6%, with greater than half of these being performed for branch occlusions.[54] These procedures were successful in 8/13 cases (62%), suggesting that it may at least be worth an attempt at reopening these when occlusion is noted. Overall, reintervention rates have been reported as 4–15% in additional studies, confirming the durability of the ChEVAR strategy.[67,68]

FENESTRATED STENTS

The long-term durability of FEVAR is similarly dependent on patency of the branch stents. In the United States, the only commercially available device is the Zenith Fenestrated graft (ZFEN, Cook Medical, Bloomington, IN), which has demonstrated excellent results in both clinical trial and real-world settings. The pivotal trial for ZFEN reported a secondary reintervention rate of 22% at 33 months average follow-up, 73% of which were performed for branch stent occlusion.[69] Fortunately, the majority of these occluded branches were able to be salvaged, leading to primary and secondary patency rates of 81% and 97%, respectively.

The GLOBALSTAR registry reported real-world outcomes of over 300 patients undergoing FEVAR in the United Kingdom, again with favorable long-term patency results. Freedom from target vessel loss in this series was 93%, 91%, and 85%, and freedom from late secondary intervention was 90%, 86%, and 70% at 1, 2, and 3, years respectively.[70] The high rate of target vessel patency even after occlusion again reinforces the salvageability of this situation. The most robust single-center experiences corroborate these results as well, with long-term patency ranging from 85–92% at 4–5 years of follow-up.[18,71]

CONCLUSION

Endovascular repair of juxtarenal aneurysms is complex, and carries with it a range of potential complications. However, results are overall quite favorable for both the ChEVAR and FEVAR approach. Understanding the unique potential pitfalls for each strategy and planning for them ahead of time will help ensure success and provide the best long-term outcomes for these patients.

REFERENCES

1. Locham S, Faateh M, Dhaliwal J, Nejim B, Dakour-Aridi H, Malas MB. Outcomes and cost of fenestrated versus standard endovascular repair of intact abdominal aortic aneurysm in the United States. J Vasc Surg. 2019 Apr 1;69(4): 1036–1044.e1.
2. Westin GG, Rockman CB, Sadek M, Ramkhelawon B, Cambria MR, Silvestro M, et al. Increased ischemic complications in fenestrated and branched endovascular abdominal aortic repair compared with standard endovascular aortic repair. J Vasc Surg [Internet]. 2020 Feb 17 [cited 2020 Apr 25]; Available from: http://www.sciencedirect.com/science/article/pii/S0741521419325364
3. Glebova NO, Selvarajah S, Orion KC, Black JH, Malas MB, Perler BA, et al. Fenestrated endovascular repair of abdominal aortic aneurysms is associated with increased morbidity but comparable mortality with infrarenal endovascular aneurysm repair. J Vasc Surg. 2015 Mar 1; 61(3): 604–10.
4. Ultee KHJ, Zettervall SL, Soden PA, Darling J, Verhagen HJM, Schermerhorn ML. Perioperative outcome of endovascular repair for complex abdominal aortic aneurysms. J Vasc Surg. 2017;65(6): 1567–75.
5. Doonan RJ, Girsowicz E, Dubois L, Gill HL. A systematic review and meta-analysis of endovascular juxtarenal aortic aneurysm repair demonstrates lower perioperative mortality compared with open repair. J Vasc Surg. 2019 Dec; 70(6): 2054–2064.e3.
6. Katsargyris A, Oikonomou K, Klonaris C, Töpel I, Verhoeven ELG. Comparison of outcomes with open, fenestrated, and chimney graft repair of juxtarenal aneurysms: Are we ready for a paradigm shift? J Endovasc Ther. 2013 Apr 1;20(2): 159–69.
7. Varkevisser RRB, O'Donnell TFX, Swerdlow NJ, Liang P, Li C, Ultee KHJ, et al. Fenestrated endovascular aneurysm repair is associated with lower perioperative morbidity and mortality compared with open repair for complex abdominal aortic aneurysms. J Vasc Surg. 2018 Dec 12.
8. Starnes BW, Heneghan RE, Tatum B. Midterm results from a physician-sponsored investigational device exemption clinical trial evaluating physician-modified endovascular grafts for the treatment of juxtarenal aortic aneurysms. J Vasc Surg. 2017 Feb; 65(2): 294–302.
9. O'Donnell TFX, Boitano LT, Deery SE, Schermerhorn ML, Schanzer A, Beck AW, et al. Open Versus Fenestrated Endovascular Repair of Complex Abdominal Aortic Aneurysms: Ann Surg. 2020 May; 271(5): 969–77.
10. Mastracci TM, Eagleton MJ, Kuramochi Y, Bathurst S, Wolski K. 12-year results of fenestrated endografts for juxtarenal and group IV thoracoabdominal aneurysms. J Vasc Surg. 2015 Feb; 61(2): 355–64.
11. Kristmundsson T, Sonesson B, Dias N, Törnqvist P, Malina M, Resch T. Outcomes of fenestrated endovascular repair of juxtarenal aortic aneurysm. J Vasc Surg. 2014 Jan 1;59(1): 115–20.

12. Boyle JR. Acute kidney injury predicts mortality after endovascular aortic repair. Eur J Vasc Endovasc Surg. 2015 Oct 1;50(4): 431.
13. Black SA, Brooks MJ, Naidoo MN, Wolfe JHN. Assessing the Impact of Renal Impairment on Outcome after Arterial Intervention: A Prospective Review of 1559 Patients. Eur J Vasc Endovasc Surg. 2006 Sep 1;32(3): 300–4.
14. Nordon IM, Hinchliffe RJ, Holt PJ, Loftus IM, Thompson MM. Modern Treatment of Juxtarenal Abdominal Aortic Aneurysms with Fenestrated Endografting and Open Repair – A Systematic Review. Eur J Vasc Endovasc Surg. 2009 Jul 1;38(1): 35–41.
15. Martin-Gonzalez T, Pinçon C, Maurel B, Hertault A, Sobocinski J, Spear R, et al. Renal Outcomes Following Fenestrated and Branched Endografting. Eur J Vasc Endovasc Surg. 2015 Oct 1;50(4): 420–30.
16. Marzelle J, Presles E, Becquemin J. Results and Factors Affecting Early Outcome of Fenestrated and/or Branched Stent Grafts for Aortic Aneurysms: A Multicenter Prospective Study. Ann Surg. 2015 Jan; 261(1): 197–206.
17. Tran K, Fajardo A, Ullery BW, Goltz C, Lee JT. Renal function changes after fenestrated endovascular aneurysm repair. J Vasc Surg. 2016 Aug; 64(2): 273–80.
18. Mastracci TM, Greenberg RK, Eagleton MJ, Hernandez AV. Durability of branches in branched and fenestrated endografts. J Vasc Surg. 2013 Apr 1;57(4): 926–33.
19. Timaran DE, Soto M, Knowles M, Modrall JG, Rectenwald JE, Timaran CH. Safety and effectiveness of total percutaneous access for fenestrated endovascular aortic aneurysm repair. J Vasc Surg. 2016; 64(4): 896–901.
20. Cao Z, Wu W, Zhao K, Zhao J, Yang Y, Jiang C, et al. Safety and Efficacy of Totally Percutaneous Access Compared with Open Femoral Exposure for Endovascular Aneurysm Repair: A Meta-analysis. J Endovasc Ther. 2017 Apr 1;24(2): 246–53.
21. Agrusa CJ, Meltzer AJ, Schneider DB, Connolly PH. Safety and Effectiveness of a "Percutaneous-First" Approach to Endovascular Aortic Aneurysm Repair. Ann Vasc Surg. 2017 Aug; 43: 79–84.
22. Souza LR de, Oderich GS, Banga PV, Hofer JM, Wigham JR, Cha S, et al. Outcomes of total percutaneous endovascular aortic repair for thoracic, fenestrated, and branched endografts. J Vasc Surg. 2015 Dec 1;62(6): 1442–1449.e3.
23. Buck DB, Karthaus EG, Soden PA, Ultee KHJ, van Herwaarden JA, Moll FL, et al. Percutaneous versus femoral cutdown access for endovascular aneurysm repair. J Vasc Surg. 2015 Jul; 62(1): 16–21.
24. Hajibandeh S, Hajibandeh S, Antoniou SA, Child E, Torella F, Antoniou GA. Percutaneous access for endovascular aortic aneurysm repair: A systematic review and meta-analysis. Vascular. 2016 Dec; 24(6): 638–48.
25. Inagaki E, Farber A, Siracuse JJ, Mell MW, Rybin DV, Doros G, et al. Routine use of ultrasound guidance in femoral arterial access for peripheral vascular intervention decreases groin hematoma rates in high-volume surgeons. Ann Vasc Surg. 2018 Aug; 51: 1–7.
26. Kalish J, Eslami M, Gillespie D, Schermerhorn M, Rybin D, Doros G, et al. Routine use of ultrasound guidance in femoral arterial access for peripheral vascular intervention decreases groin hematoma rates. J Vasc Surg. 2015 May; 61(5): 1231–8.
27. Naddaf A, Williams S, Hasanadka R, Hood DB, Hodgson KJ. Predictors of Groin Access Pseudoaneurysm Complication: A 10-Year Institutional Experience. Vasc Endovascular Surg. 2020 Jan; 54(1): 42–6.
28. Levin SR, Farber A, Bertges DJ, Ferris M, Cheng TW, Arinze N, et al. Larger Sheath Size for Infrainguinal Endovascular Intervention Is Associated With Minor but Not Major Morbidity or Mortality. Ann Vasc Surg. 2019 Oct; 60: 327–334.e2.
29. Shah SK, Parodi FE, Eagleton MJ, Bena JF, Clair DG. Iliac injury during abdominal and thoracic aortic endovascular intervention. J Vasc Surg. 2016; 64(3): 726–30.
30. Dahdouh Z, Roule V, Grollier G. Life-threatening iliac artery rupture during transcatheter aortic valve implantation (TAVI): diagnosis and management. Heart Br Card Soc. 2013 Aug; 99(16): 1217–8.
31. Obon-Dent M, Reul RM, Mortazavi A. Endovascular iliac rescue technique for complete arterial avulsion after transcatheter aortic valve replacement. Catheter Cardiovasc Interv Off J Soc Card Angiogr Interv. 2014 Aug 1;84(2): 306–10.
32. Brinster DR. Minimally invasive technique for iliac revascularization after large-bore sheath traumatic avulsion. Innov Phila Pa. 2009 Jan; 4(1): 43–5.
33. Noori VJ, Eldrup-Jørgensen J. A systematic review of vascular closure devices for femoral artery puncture sites. J Vasc Surg. 2018; 68(3): 887–99.
34. Dosluoglu HH, Cherr GS, Harris LM, Dryjski ML. Total percutaneous endovascular repair of abdominal aortic aneurysms using Perclose ProGlide closure devices. J Endovasc Ther Off J Int Soc Endovasc Spec. 2007 Apr; 14(2): 184–8.
35. Bechara CF, Annambhotla S, Lin PH. Access site management with vascular closure devices for percutaneous transarterial procedures. J Vasc Surg. 2010 Dec; 52(6): 1682–96.

36. Lee JT, Greenberg JI, Dalman RL. Early experience with the snorkel technique for juxtarenal aneurysms. J Vasc Surg. 2012 Apr; 55(4): 935–46; discussion 945–46.
37. Lavingia KS, Dua A, Stern JR. Upper extremity access options for complex endovascular aortic interventions. J Cardiovasc Surg (Torino). 2018 Jun;59(3):360–7.
38. Plotkin A, Ding L, Han SM, Oderich GS, Starnes BW, Lee JT, et al. Association of upper extremity and neck access with stroke in endovascular aortic repair. J Vasc Surg. 2020 Nov;72(5):1602–9.
39. Alvarez-Tostado JA, Moise MA, Bena JF, Pavkov ML, Greenberg RK, Clair DG, et al. The brachial artery: a critical access for endovascular procedures. J Vasc Surg. 2009 Feb; 49(2): 378–85; discussion 385.
40. Kret MR, Dalman RL, Kalish J, Mell M. Arterial cutdown reduces complications after brachial access for peripheral vascular intervention. J Vasc Surg. 2016 Jul; 64(1): 149–54.
41. Stern JR, Ellozy SH, Connolly PH, Meltzer AJ, Schneider DB. Utility and safety of axillary conduits during endovascular repair of thoracoabdominal aneurysms. J Vasc Surg. 2017; 66(3): 705–10.
42. Wooster M, Powell A, Back M, Illig K, Shames M. Axillary Artery Access as an Adjunct for Complex Endovascular Aortic Repair. Ann Vasc Surg. 2015 Nov; 29(8): 1543–7.
43. Cortese B, Rigattieri S, Aranzulla TC, Russo F, Latib A, Burzotta F, et al. Transradial versus transfemoral ancillary approach in complex structural, coronary, and peripheral interventions. Results from the multicenter ancillary registry: A study of the Italian Radial Club. Catheter Cardiovasc Interv. 2018 Jan;91(1): 97–102.
44. Stern JR, Elmously A, Smith MC, Connolly PH, Meltzer AJ, Schneider DB, et al. Transradial interventions in contemporary vascular surgery practice. Vascular. 2019 Feb;27(1):110–16.
45. Huang IKH, Renani SA, Morgan RA. Complications and Reinterventions After Fenestrated and Branched EVAR in Patients with Paravisceral and Thoracoabdominal Aneurysms. Cardiovasc Intervent Radiol. 2018 Jul 1;41(7): 985–97.
46. Verhoeven ELG, Vourliotakis G, Bos WTGJ, Tielliu IFJ, Zeebregts CJ, Prins TR, et al. Fenestrated stent grafting for short-necked and juxtarenal abdominal aortic aneurysm: an 8-year single-centre experience. Eur J Vasc Endovasc Surg. 2010 May; 39(5): 529–36.
47. Watanabe Y, Aramoto H, Asano R, Furuichi S, Sumiyoshi T, Takanashi S. Iatrogenic renal artery dissection uncommon complication during aortic endovascular repair. JACC Cardiovasc Interv. 2010 Sep; 3(9): 986–7.
48. Simons JP, Shue B, Flahive JM, Aiello FA, Steppacher RC, Eaton EA, et al. Trends in use of the only Food and Drug Administration-approved commercially available fenestrated endovascular aneurysm repair device in the United States. J Vasc Surg. 2017;65(5): 1260–9.
49. Ullery BW, Lee GK, Lee JT. Shuttering of the superior mesenteric artery during fenestrated endovascular aneurysm repair. J Vasc Surg. 2014 Oct; 60(4): 900–7.
50. Lala S, Knowles M, Timaran D, Baig MS, Valentine J, Timaran C. Superior mesenteric artery outcomes after fenestrated endovascular aortic aneurysm repair. J Vasc Surg. 2016 Sep; 64(3): 692–7.
51. Ullery BW, Lee JT, Dalman RL. Snorkel/chimney and fenestrated endografts for complex abdominal aortic aneurysms. J Cardiovasc Surg (Torino). 2015 Oct; 56(5): 707–17.
52. Donas KP, Pecoraro F, Torsello G, Lachat M, Austermann M, Mayer D, et al. Use of covered chimney stents for pararenal aortic pathologies is safe and feasible with excellent patency and low incidence of endoleaks. J Vasc Surg. 2012 Mar 1;55(3): 659–65.
53. Taneva GT, Criado FJ, Torsello G, Veith F, Scali ST, Kubilis P, et al. Results of chimney endovascular aneurysm repair as used in the PERICLES Registry to treat patients with suprarenal aortic pathologies. J Vasc Surg. 2020 May 1;71(5): 1521–27.e1.
54. Donas KP, Lee JT, Lachat M, Torsello G, Veith FJ, PERICLES investigators. Collected world experience about the performance of the snorkel/chimney endovascular technique in the treatment of complex aortic pathologies: the PERICLES registry. Ann Surg. 2015 Sep; 262(3): 546–53; discussion 552–3.
55. Ullery BW, Tran K, Itoga NK, Dalman RL, Lee JT. Natural history of gutter-related type Ia endoleaks after snorkel/chimney endovascular aneurysm repair. J Vasc Surg. 2017 Apr; 65(4): 981–90.
56. Minion D. Molded Parallel Endografts for Branch Vessel Preservation during Endovascular Aneurysm Repair in Challenging Anatomy. Int J Angiol Off Publ Int Coll Angiol Inc. 2012 Jun; 21(2): 81–4.
57. Ikoma A, Nakai M, Sato M, Nishimura Y, Okamura Y. Embolization of a perigraft gutter leak with coils and N-butyl cyanoacrylate through the pseudolumen using a triple coaxial catheter system after endovascular aortic repair with a chimney graft. J Vasc Interv Radiol. 2014 Oct; 25(10): 1648–50.
58. Donselaar EJ, van der Vijver-Coppen RJ, van den Ham LH, Lardenoye JWHP, Reijnen MMPJ. EndoAnchors to Resolve Persistent Type Ia Endoleak Secondary to Proximal Cuff With Parallel Graft Placement. J Endovasc Ther. 2016 Feb; 23(1): 225–8.

59. Swerdlow NJ, McCallum JC, Liang P, Li C, O'Donnell TFX, Varkevisser RRB, et al. Select type I and type III endoleaks at the completion of fenestrated endovascular aneurysm repair resolve spontaneously. J Vasc Surg. 2019 Aug 1;70(2): 381–90.
60. Torsello GF, Beropoulis E, Munaò R, Trimarchi S, Torsello GB, Austermann M. Outcomes of bridging stent grafts in fenestrated and branched endovascular aortic repair. J Vasc Surg [Internet]. 2020 Jan 19 [cited 2020 Apr 25]; Available from: http://www.sciencedirect.com/science/article/pii/S0741521419326436
61. Heidemann F, Kölbel T, Debus ES, Diener H, Carpenter SW, Rohlffs F, et al. Renal Function Salvage After Delayed Endovascular Revascularization of Acute Renal Artery Occlusion in Patients With Fenestrated-Branched Endovascular Aneurysm Repair or Visceral Debranching. J Endovasc Ther. 2018 Aug 1;25(4): 466–73.
62. Donas KP, Eisenack M, Panuccio G, Austermann M, Osada N, Torsello G. The role of open and endovascular treatment with fenestrated and chimney endografts for patients with juxtarenal aortic aneurysms. J Vasc Surg. 2012 Aug; 56(2): 285–90.
63. Tolenaar JL, Zandvoort HJA, Moll FL, van Herwaarden JA. Technical considerations and results of chimney grafts for the treatment of juxtarenal aneursyms. J Vasc Surg. 2013 Sep; 58(3): 607–15.
64. Igari K, Kudo T, Uchiyama H, Toyofuku T, Inoue Y. Early Experience with the Endowedge Technique and Snorkel Technique for Endovascular Aneurysm Repair with Challenging Neck Anatomy. Ann Vasc Dis. 2014; 7(1): 46–51.
65. Donas KP, Torsello GB, Piccoli G, Pitoulias GA, Torsello GF, Bisdas T, et al. The PROTAGORAS study to evaluate the performance of the Endurant stent graft for patients with pararenal pathologic processes treated by the chimney/snorkel endovascular technique. J Vasc Surg. 2016 Jan 1;63(1): 1–7.
66. Lachat M, Veith FJ, Pfammatter T, Glenck M, Bettex D, Mayer D, et al. Chimney and Periscope Grafts Observed Over 2 Years After Their Use to Revascularize 169 Renovisceral Branches in 77 Patients With Complex Aortic Aneurysms. J Endovasc Ther. 2013 Oct 1;20(5): 597–605.
67. Lee JT, Varu VN, Tran K, Dalman RL. Renal function changes after snorkel/chimney repair of juxtarenal aneurysms. J Vasc Surg. 2014 Sep; 60(3): 563–70.
68. Suominen V, Pimenoff G, Salenius J. Fenestrated and Chimney Endografts for Juxtarenal Aneurysms: Early and Midterm Results. Scand J Surg. 2013 Sep 1;102(3): 182–8.
69. Oderich GS, Greenberg RK, Farber M, Lyden S, Sanchez L, Fairman R, et al. Results of the United States multicenter prospective study evaluating the Zenith fenestrated endovascular graft for treatment of juxtarenal abdominal aortic aneurysms. J Vasc Surg. 2014 Dec; 60(6): 1420–1428.e1-5.
70. British Society for Endovascular Therapy and the Global Collaborators on Advanced Stent-Graft Techniques for Aneurysm Repair (GLOBALSTAR) Registry. Early results of fenestrated endovascular repair of juxtarenal aortic aneurysms in the United Kingdom. Circulation. 2012 Jun 5;125(22): 2707–15.
71. Grimme FAB, Zeebregts CJ, Verhoeven ELG, Bekkema F, Reijnen MMJP, Tielliu IFJ. Visceral stent patency in fenestrated stent grafting for abdominal aortic aneurysm repair. J Vasc Surg. 2014 Feb; 59(2): 298–306.

SUGGESTED READINGS

Oderich GS, Greenberg RK, Farber M, Lyden S, Sanchez L, Fairman R, et al. Results of the United States multicenter prospective study evaluating the Zenith fenestrated endovascular graft for treatment of juxtarenal abdominal aortic aneurysms. J Vasc Surg. 2014 Dec;60(6):1420–1428.e1-5.

Donas KP, Lee JT, Lachat M, Torsello G, Veith FJ, PERICLES investigators. Collected world experience about the performance of the snorkel/chimney endovascular technique in the treatment of complex aortic pathologies: the PERICLES registry. Ann Surg. 2015 Sep;262(3):546–53; discussion 552-553.

10

Complications of endovascular repair of thoracic aortic aneurysms/dissections

HAZEL L. MARECKI AND JESSICA P. SIMONS

Soon after endovascular repair of abdominal aortic aneurysms was described, surgeons and innovators considered application of this strategy to thoracic aortic pathology. First reported by Dake et al. in 1994,[1] thoracic endovascular aortic repair (TEVAR) to treat thoracic aortic aneurysms provided a safe alternative to open repair. The first available TEVAR endograft, the Gore Thoracic Aortic Graft (W. L. Gore & Associates, Flagstaff, AZ) endoprosthesis, was introduced in the United States in 2005. Since that time, several other devices have been marketed, with iterative advances in design including smaller delivery sheath size, enhanced conformability, and an expanded range of diameters and lengths (Figure 10.1).

While first-generation devices were only FDA-approved for treatment of thoracic aortic aneurysms (specifically, aortic diameter > 6 cm, saccular aneurysm > 2 cm, or symptomatic aneurysms),[2] their use for a wide range of aortic pathology is now endorsed by consensus guidelines from both the United States and Europe.[3–5] This includes pseudoaneurysm and traumatic aortic injury, penetrating aortic ulcer (> 20 mm in diameter and 10 mm neck), intramural hematoma, and complicated Type B aortic dissection, as well as thoracic aortic aneurysms > 5.5 cm. The role of TEVAR for uncomplicated Type B aortic dissection has been studied[6,7] but remains controversial at the time of this publication. Relatively few strict contraindications to TEVAR exist, limited mostly to anatomic considerations: inadequate proximal/distal seal zones or inadequate access vessels. Both connective tissue disorders[8] and contaminated fields[9] have been described as relative contraindications, although several reports of TEVAR in both scenarios have been published.[10,11]

In contrast to endovascular repair of abdominal aortic aneurysms, direct comparisons of outcomes of TEVAR versus open thoracic aortic repair have been conspicuously absent, with the majority of information derived from device-specific prospective trials, contrasted with historical controls.)[12] While this relates, in part, to lower disease frequency, it perhaps also reflects the dominant belief that TEVAR has dramatically transformed the morbidity of thoracic aortic repair.[13–16] Historically, open thoracic aortic repair, in the elective setting, was associated with mortality and paraplegia rates of 4.8% and 4.6%, respectively.[17] In the setting of rupture, the surgical mortality increases to over 25% even at centers of excellence.[9]

A retrospective review of patients who underwent TEVAR versus open repair in the United States in 2006–2007 for isolated descending thoracic aortic aneurysms, showed shorter hospital length of stay by 1.3 days and 60% fewer complications in the TEVAR group, despite being used on patients over a decade older overall than patients who underwent open repair.[18] A systematic review and meta-analysis showed a reduction in 30-day all-cause mortality and paraplegia for TEVAR compared with open surgery.[8] When comparing TEVAR for ruptured descending thoracic aortic aneurysm, TEVAR showed an improved 30-day mortality (19% vs 33%) with decreased 30-day rates of myocardial infarction, stroke and paraplegia when compared with open repair.

With such compelling outcomes, particularly when compared to historical controls of open thoracic aortic repair, it is important to note that TEVAR is not free from risk of complications. These will be described herein. For the purposes of clarity, they are organized according to timeframe and potential root cause, although in many cases there may be overlap and/or co-existence. In the tradition of surgical morbidity and mortality conferences, perioperative complications are described as related to planning (judgment) or to execution (technique). The etiologies of mid- and long-term complications after TEVAR may be less clear, may be multifactorial, or may reflect the natural history of the disease. In this chapter, the most prevalent and/or clinically significant complications of thoracic endovascular aortic repair are covered, from perioperative to long term.

Table 1 U.S. Food and Drug Administration (FDA) - Approved Devices for Thoracic Endovascular Aortic Repair

Device System	Manufacturer	FDA Approval	Indications	Stent Material	Graft Material	Fixation	Minimum Non-Aneurismal Aortic Seal Zone Length (mm) Prox. and Dist.	Sheath Outer Diameter (French) for 34 mm diameter graft size	Overall Delivery Sheath Profile (French)	Graft Diameter Range (mm)	Aortic Vessel Diameter Range (mm)
RelayPlus	Bolton Medical	2012	TAA, PAU	Nitinol	Polyester Woven	Uncovered stent wire	15-25	23	22-26	22-46	19-42
Zenith	Cook	2015	TAA, PAU	Nitinol	Polyester Woven	Barbs, uncovered stent wire	20	18	16-20	24-46	20-42
cTAG	Gore	2011	TAA, BTAI, Type B dissection	Nitinol	ePTFE	Partially covered stent wire	20	25*	20-24	21-45	16-42
Valiant	Medtronic	2011	TAA, BTAI, Type B dissection	Nitinol	Polyester Woven	Uncovered stent wire	20	24	22-25	22-46	18-44

ePTFE - Polytetrafluoroethylene; Nitinol - nickel-titanium; TAA - descending thoracic aortic aneurysm; PAU - penetrating atherosclerotic ulcer; BTAI - blunt traumatic aortic injury
*Requires separate 22 fr dryseal sheath; outer diameter measures 8.2mm, which is equivalent to 25 fr

Figure 10.1 FDA-approved thoracic endografts, as of September 2018. (Bodell B et al. Thoracic Endovascular Aortic Repair: Review of Current Devices and Treatment Options. *Techniques in Vascular and Interventional Radiology* 2018; Vol 21: 137–145.)

PERIOPERATIVE COMPLICATIONS

The overall perioperative complication rate associated with TEVAR remains very low, but an awareness of some specific risks is necessary to ensure favorable outcomes. For the purposes of organizing and understanding these complications, we present them according to root cause (errors in planning or errors in execution). However, it is important to note that there can be overlap between these categories; conversely, even in the best of situations, most complications will have a non-zero incidence.

In this chapter, perioperative complications are defined as those occurring within the first 30 days post-operatively and related to the device itself; discussion of general medical complications will not be covered.

RELATED TO ERRORS IN PLANNING

SPINAL CORD ISCHEMIA

Spinal cord ischemia (SCI) is perhaps one of the most dreaded complications of thoracic aortic surgery, occurring in up to 10% of TEVAR cases.[14–16] Several factors are recognized to contribute to the risk of development of SCI, including:

1. Length of aortic coverage
2. Prior aortic surgery (both endovascular and open)
3. Occluded collaterals such as internal iliac or vertebral arteries
4. Intraoperative hypotension
5. Perioperative anemia

Each of these risk factors must, therefore, be carefully considered to prevent SCI.[19] First, a thorough history and physical exam should be performed to document surgical history and a baseline neurologic exam. Next, careful review of imaging should be performed. Again, this should focus on identifying any prior aortic repair as well as the patency of collateral circulation (Figure 10.2).

Preoperative planning should also carefully consider the necessary length of coverage. A balance must be struck between ensuring adequate seal proximally and distally, while not covering unnecessary aortic length, particularly at the level most commonly associated with the origin of the anterior spinal artery (artery of Adamkiewicz, T9-T12). A proximal seal of at least 20 mm of healthy, parallel-walled aorta is appropriate; if coverage of the left subclavian is necessitated to achieve this, revascularization (either staged or at the same time as the TEVAR) is advisable, to preserve the collateral flow via the left vertebral artery). Distally, a 20 mm seal is also desirable; high-quality computed tomography angiographic (CTA)

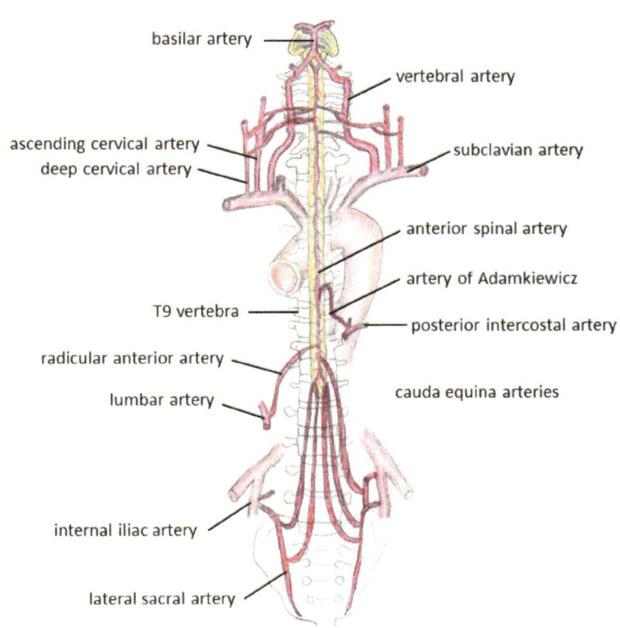

Figure 10.2 Anatomy of spinal cord perfusion and collateral pathways.

imaging can often reveal any particularly robust intercostals that can be spared, if possible, while still achieving adequate seal.[20]

Intraoperative hypotension and anemia should be avoided. With TEVAR, access artery injury is one of the most common precipitators of such a state. Efforts to mitigate this are discussed below.

Once a careful risk assessment has been conducted, cerebrospinal fluid (CSF) drainage can be considered as an adjunct to prevent/manage SCI. For coverage lengths of 200 mm or greater, or other high-risk settings, CSF drainage catheters can be placed preoperatively.[21] Intraoperatively, once the device is deployed, CSF drainage can be initiated, while simultaneously increasing the mean arterial pressure to > 90 mmHg. Drainage can be performed (up to 10–20 cc per hour) to maintain an intracranial pressure of 10 mmHg or less.[22]

RETROGRADE TYPE A AORTIC DISSECTION

Retrograde Type A aortic dissection (RTAD) is a rare complication of TEVAR, but highly morbid; a meta-analysis of nearly 9000 patients calculated an incidence of 2.5%, with associated mortality of 37%.[23] While several mechanisms have been proposed, the low incidence does not lend itself to statistical methods. In general, risk of RTAD may be increased when TEVAR is used:

1. Among patients with Marfan syndrome
2. For acute/chronic dissection (as compared with aneurysm pathology)
3. With more proximal landing zones (zone 0–2)
4. When proximal diameter is oversized greater than 15%
5. When aggressive wire manipulation or balloon molding is performed

Concerns have also been raised regarding graft configurations with proximal bare metal stents; however, the literature has yielded conflicting results.[23,24] Given the lack of robust evidence, all of the factors listed above should be considered for any individual patient.

POSTERIOR CIRCULATION STROKE

Another rare but devastating complication of TEVAR is posterior circulation stroke, occurring in ~3.1% of patients.[25] It typically occurs in the context of coverage of the left subclavian artery. In more than 20% of aneurysms and dissections, it is necessary to cover the left subclavian artery to achieve adequate proximal seal.[26] The left subclavian artery perfuses the brain via the left vertebral artery, which is dominant in over 60% of patients. While most perioperative strokes are believed to be embolic (discussed below), a subset are posterior circulation strokes, in watershed regions secondary to loss of left vertebral artery perfusion. While coverage of the left subclavian is generally well tolerated with respect to arm perfusion, coverage of the left subclavian without revascularization, dramatically increases the risk for stroke (and posterior circulation stroke, in particular) to > 5% as compared to < 2% with preoperative revascularization.[27] When left subclavian coverage is planned, if there is a compelling reason to try to avoid revascularization, preoperative imaging is necessary to first demonstrate a patent right vertebral artery in continuity with a patent Circle of Willis. Anatomic factors that increase the risk of posterior circulation stroke include:

1. Dominant left vertebral artery in the setting of intended left subclavian coverage
2. Aberrant/hypoplastic/absent right subclavian artery
3. Left vertebral terminating in posterior inferior cerebellar artery
4. Anomalous origin of the left vertebral from the aortic arch

Revascularization of the vertebrals should be carefully considered in those circumstances.

ACCESS ARTERY INJURY

Access artery injuries include iliac artery dissection, rupture, and thrombosis. In fact, transfemoral access is considered feasible in only 70% of cases.[28] One large series reported an incidence of nearly 20%, despite the use of iliac conduits in > 20% of patients.[29] Thrombosis most commonly occurs in the setting of inadequate intraoperative anticoagulation and an occlusive or near-occlusive sheath; an activated clotting time (ACT) goal of > 250 seconds is advised. Factors associated with access artery dissection and rupture include:

1. Inadequate iliac artery diameter
2. High-grade and/or long-segment stenoses
3. High degree of calcification
4. Tortuosity

Specifically, iliac diameter must be 7 mm or greater. While precise definitions for tortuosity that correspond with risk of iliac injury do not exist, careful review of preoperative imaging, with consideration for how the vector of force of an advancing device may interact with iliac tortuosity (leading to shear stress at fixed points, such as the internal iliac origin) can be helpful. Similarly, heavy calcification and stenoses can lead to additional friction as the device is advanced.

When these concerns are identified preoperatively, it is advisable to consider adjunctive measures to mitigate the risk of access artery injury. Specifically, small iliac diameter may be overcome with the use of serial hydrophilic dilators, as long as there is not concomitant heavy calcification. Open or endovascular conduits should also be considered. Open conduits may make use of either an aortic or a common iliac proximal anastomosis, exposed via a retroperitoneal approach. Endovascular conduits typically span the common iliac to distal external iliac segment, or even the common femoral; a 12 mm diameter graft should be chosen due to the additional friction they impart, compared with native iliac vessel.

TYPE Ia OR Ib ENDOLEAK

In the case of TEVAR for thoracic aortic aneurysm, Type Ia or Ib endoleaks can occur and should be treated intraoperatively. In a large international registry, the incidence was < 1%.[30] In general, they result from inadequate over-sizing or implantation of the device in an unintended segment where the aortic diameter is larger than expected. Careful preoperative planning based on high-quality axial imaging, with attention to device-specific instructions for use should largely prevent this. Some authors have advocated adjunctive measures to enhance the precision of deployment such as rapid ventricular pacing or use of adenosine to temporarily halt the aortic impulse.[50]

In cases where a Type Ia or Ib endoleak is identified intraoperatively, it should be addressed. Options include either balloon molding of the seal zone, or extension of coverage with an additional device. Balloon molding of the proximal seal should be carefully considered due to the possibility of RTAD (see above) and avoided in cases of TEVAR for aortic dissection.

RELATED TO ERRORS IN EXECUTION

STROKE

Perioperative stroke is a dreaded complication of TEVAR, occurring in 3–5% of cases, with an associated in-hospital mortality of 16–20%.[31,32] Most strokes are related to embolic events that occur inadvertently throughout endovascular manipulation in the arch and thoracic aorta. While the instance of clinically significant stroke is low, postoperative diffusion-weighted MRIs show small "silent" embolic strokes in as many as 60% of TEVAR patients. This section will briefly review nonmodifiable risk factors but will focus on modifiable factors associated with perioperative stroke during TEVAR.

i. *Comorbidities*
   One of the strongest associations of perioperative stroke is a personal history of stroke, associated with at least a five-fold higher odds of stroke.[33] Perioperative stroke is also associated with a history of ischemic coronary disease, renal failure, and female sex.
ii. *Intraoperative considerations*
   Given that embolic phenomena are largely responsible for intraoperative stroke, certain pharmacologic maneuvers can help mitigate this risk. Intravenous heparinization should occur with the introduction of large sheaths. Although guidelines do vary in terms of goals for activated clotting time (ACT), 250–300 seconds is generally desired for work in the aortic arch. Longer operative time is also associated with higher stroke risk,[25] likely related to technical difficulty resulting in excess wire manipulation with more resulting inadvertent strokes.

   Perioperative hypotension and anemia also contribute to stroke risk by reducing intracranial perfusion.[27] Intraoperative blood loss greater than 800 cc has been correlated with increased stroke risk.[33] While precise thresholds for goal hemoglobin levels and goal blood pressure ranges have not been defined, these principles can be considered on a case-by-case basis.
iii. *Wire manipulation*
   While endovascular interventions are considered minimally invasive, it is important to consider the potential trauma that wires, catheters, and devices may cause to the intima. Preoperative imaging should be carefully evaluated for the presence of thrombus and atherosclerotic disease (Figure 10.3). Analysis of the EUROSTAR registry found that a "shaggy aorta" was associated with a thirty-fold increase in the odds of perioperative stroke.[25] Other predictors of perioperative stroke related to wire manipulation include the use of a through-and-through wire,[25] presence of a penetrating aortic ulcer, and Grade V atheroma of the aortic arch.[31,32] While many of these factors may not be modifiable, strictly speaking, their presence should impact the assessment of risk/benefit ratio and preoperative patient counseling.
iv. *Extent of proximal coverage*
   In order to achieve technical success in TEVAR, with adequate proximal seal, it is sometimes necessary to extend coverage across the left subclavian (Zone 2) or across the left common carotid artery (Zone 1), both of which are associated with increased risk of perioperative stroke. One or both of these could also be inadvertently covered if the endograft is deployed too proximally. Coverage of these great vessels can lead to stroke by either malperfusion (if revascularization is not performed) or embolization from arch disease or thrombus that forms on the endograft itself.[31,32] Subclavian artery revascularization has been shown to decrease the incidence of perioperative stroke from 6.4% to 2.3%, and specifically posterior circulation stroke rates from 5.5% to

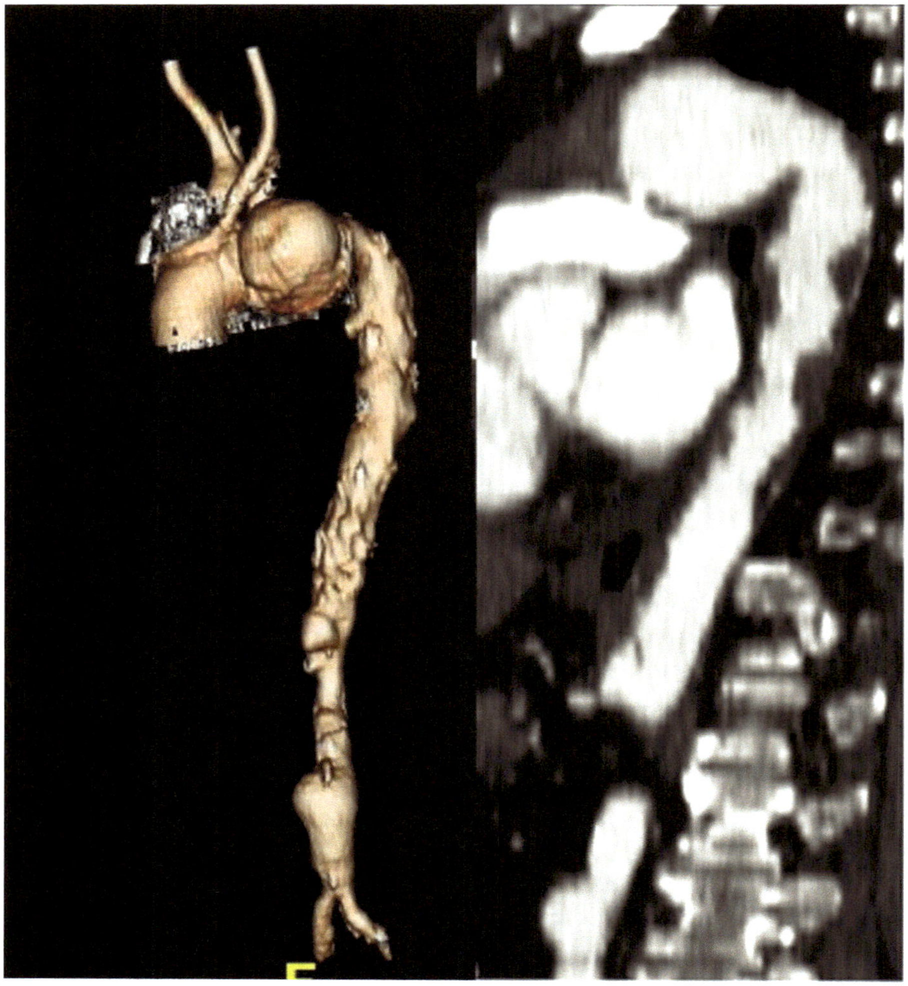

Figure 10.3 Computed tomography angiography demonstrating a "shaggy" thoracic aorta.

1.2%. Since left common carotid artery revascularization is always advised in cases where it will be covered, the reduction in stroke risk associated with this is not known.

Efforts to mitigate this risk include performing an arch aortagram with the device introduced, and advanced to the anticipated level of deployment. The optimal obliquity for identifying their origins can be anticipated by careful review of preoperative imaging (Figure 10.4).

MESENTERIC ISCHEMIA

Intentional coverage of the celiac artery with the distal extent of the endograft has been described, with one large series reporting coverage in 4% of cases in order to achieve a distal seal.[34] Estimates of clinically evident foregut ischemia have ranged from 0–12%.[35–37] Manifestations are variable, including ischemic pancreatitis, perforated gastric ulcer, splenic infarction, acalculous cholecystitis, and shock liver; multiorgan failure and death have also been reported. In addition to the obvious consideration that coverage results in inadequate collateral circulation via the superior mesenteric artery, partial coverage of the celiac has also been associated with mesenteric ischemia.[38] The mechanism for this may be microembolization; for that reason, complete coverage, rather than partial, is advocated.[36] Adequate evaluation of mesenteric collateral circulation is imperative prior to intentional celiac coverage. CTA is typically adequate, with selective angiography, with or without balloon occlusion of the celiac, only when the CTA is unclear.[39]

A related consideration is the adequacy of distal seal in cases where celiac coverage is performed to achieve seal in an ectatic visceral segment (see above section on Type 1b endoleak). In these cases, postoperative mesenteric ischemia may result from distal migration of the endograft and inadvertent coverage of the superior mesenteric artery.[36] In these cases where the distal seal is tenuous due to ectasia, alternative strategies such as fenestrated/branched endovascular aneurysm repair may be better options to avoid these complications.

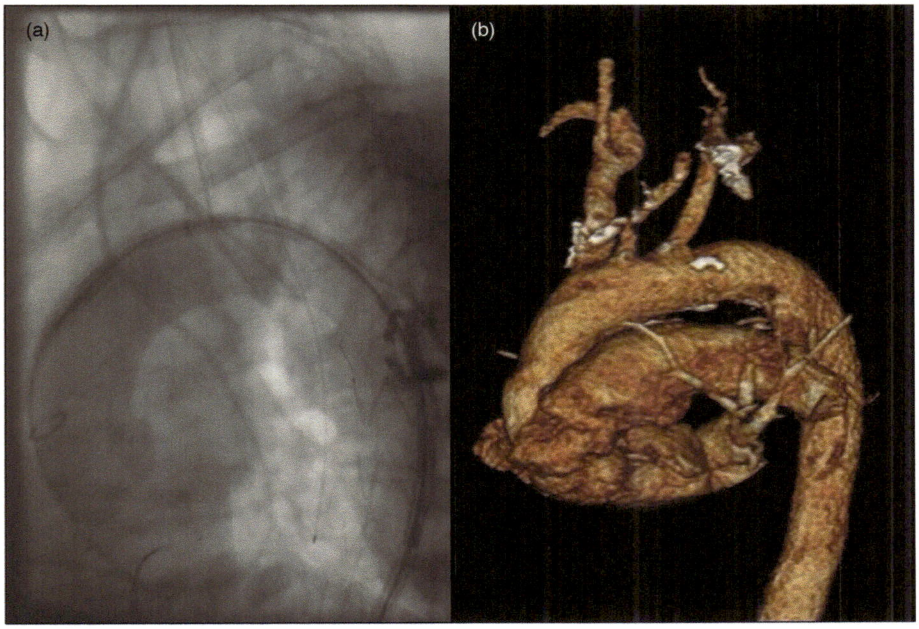

Figure 10.4 Patient treated for acute complicated Type B aortic dissection. (a) Intraoperative arch angiogram at 60° left anterior oblique and 9° cranial to visualize origin of left subclavian artery. (b) Preoperative 3D reconstruction used for determining necessary gantry angles (60° left anterior oblique and 9° cranial) to optimize visualization of origin of left subclavian.

MALDEPLOYMENT IN THE FALSE LUMEN OF ACUTE TYPE B AORTIC DISSECTION

In cases of complicated acute Type B aortic dissection (TBAD), TEVAR is indicated to manage the site of entry tear in the descending thoracic aorta. While there are some case reports of intentional deployment in the false lumen for chronic TBAD,[40,41] in acute TBAD, great care should be taken to ensure deployment in the true lumen. The true incidence of maldeployment in the false lumen is unknown and likely under-reported, but it is important to consider given the potentially catastrophic consequences, namely malperfusion of critical branch vessels and death.[42] This complication likely occurs in settings where the dissection is extensive, with multiple fenestrations throughout the aorta. Prevention requires multiple efforts to ensure there is definitive identification of the true lumen intraoperatively prior to deployment. First, careful study of the preoperative CTA is imperative; this includes careful identification of true and false lumen, with note made of which branches are perfused via the true lumen. Second, even with open exposure of femoral access vessels, it may be difficult to identify true and false lumen on inspection. Given that multiple fenestrations exist, even if the true lumen is definitely accessed in the groin, this does not ensure that the wire will remain in the true lumen as it is advanced retrograde. Instead, adjuncts such as intravascular ultrasound should be employed to help confirm the true lumen where the endograft will be deployed.

Third, digital subtraction angiography should be performed to verify true lumen access. This can be achieved with an imaging catheter placed via the right brachial artery (which is perfused via the true lumen, by definition, in TBAD). It can also be accomplished with the use of a long, 14 Fr sheath from the femoral artery, through which angiography can be performed via the side-arm at the level of each branch vessel, without loss of wire access. Again, it is imperative to study the preoperative CTA to understand branch vessel perfusion, and correlate it with intraoperative angiography.

MID- AND LONG-TERM COMPLICATIONS

In the case of mid- and long-term complications, the etiology is often multifactorial, unclear, unavoidable, or a combination of all of these. This underscores the importance of lifelong surveillance of the repair to identify and treat complications before they have clinical implications.

GRAFT INFECTION

The true incidence of TEVAR graft infection is unknown. However, the incidence of endograft infection of either EVAR or TEVAR is reported as < 1%.[43] In a large systematic review of EVAR and TEVAR infections, the mean time to presentation ranged widely (115–991 days).[10] Diagnosis is often confirmed by the presence of perigraft inflammation or air (Figure 10.5). While in many cases the exact mechanism may remain unknown, potential

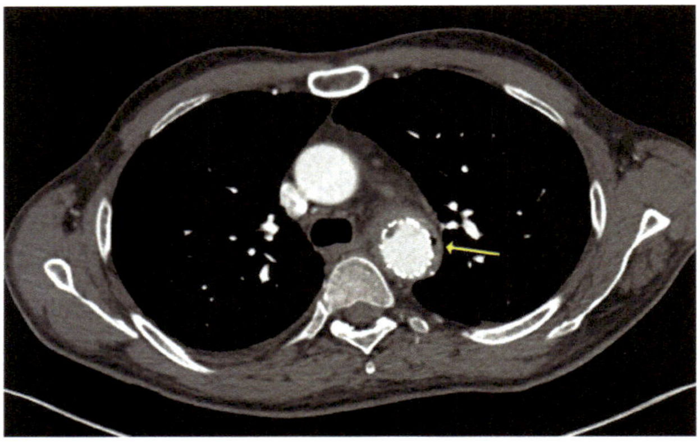

Figure 10.5 Patient presenting with failure to thrive 8 years after TEVAR for traumatic aortic injury; periaortic inflammation and perigraft air (yellow arrow) seen on axial imaging, diagnostic for graft infection.

mechanisms are the same as those common to all vascular graft infections: seeding from blood stream infection, contamination from an infection in an adjacent structure, or break in sterile technique at the time of implantation. The incidence may rise in the future, as TEVAR is increasingly reported as a management strategy for mycotic aneurysms, and aortoesophageal and aortobronchial fistulae.[11,44,45] In these cases, it is prudent to collaborate with infectious disease specialists for consideration of long-term treatment with antibiotics and/or antifungals.[46]

GRAFT MIGRATION/COMPONENT SEPARATION

Thoracic endografts are subject to a relatively more forceful aortic impulse than infrarenal endografts. Over the long term this may lead to device migration (typically defined as > 10 mm) or component separation (Figure 10.6), and resultant Type Ia or Type III endoleak. Incidence of migration has been reported as 7% in a series of 123 patients over a median follow up of 3 years; the associated incidence of Type I or III endoleak was 44%.[47] Risk factors for graft migration and/or component separation include:

1. Neck angulation > 60 degrees
2. Neck length < 15 mm
3. Inadequate overlap between components (< 5 cm)
4. High degree of tortuosity in the thoracic segment

Careful attention to these factors preoperatively may potentially reduce these complications. However, it is important to note that, in cases of dissection and aneurysm, the aortic wall may be diseased over a long segment, subject to progressive degeneration over time. This degeneration can manifest as either dilation or elongation of the aorta that, in turn, can cause loss of proximal/distal seal, device migration, or both.

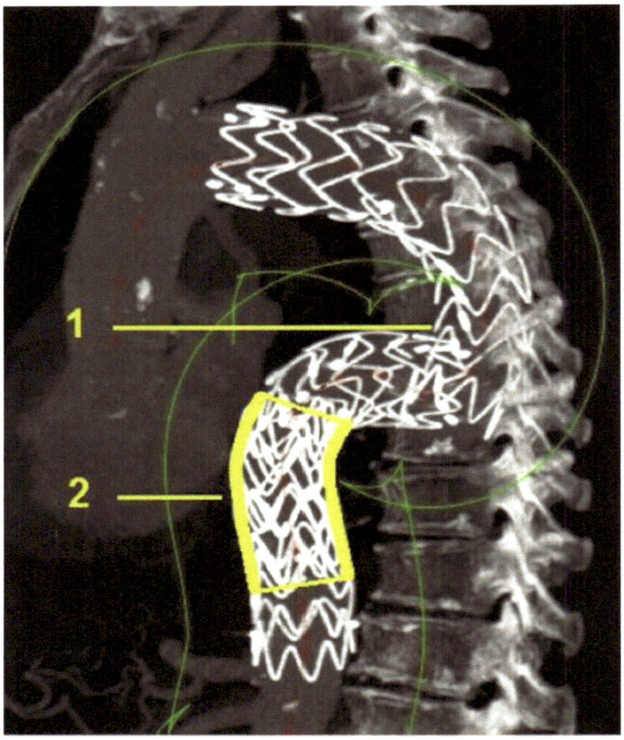

Figure 10.6 Device migration resulting in component separation at 54 months. (Geisbusch P, et al. Endograft Migration after Thoracic Endovascular Aortic Repair. J Vasc Surg 2018 Dec 12. pii: S0741-5214(18)32141-4.)

With respect to device type and configuration, no specific endograft has been shown to be significantly associated with migration. However, bird-beaking (lack of apposition to the aortic wall along the lesser curvature) has been associated with device migration. Bird-beaking, in turn, has been associated with lack of a proximal bare stent.[48]

ENDOLEAKS

Reported incidence of endoleak and/or residual aneurysm sac expansion after TEVAR for aneurysm has ranged from 7–12% at 1 year, and up to 38% overall[14–16] (Figure 10.7). Type 1 endoleaks are the most common type after TEVAR, likely reflecting the complexity of achieving a durable seal in the setting of chronic aortic pulsation pressure, arch tortuosity, and potential aortic radial degeneration and elongation over time. As for any endovascular aneurysm repair, the likelihood of endoleak relates both to the appropriateness of seal zones chosen preoperatively as well as the natural history of aneurysmal degeneration. A 2 cm seal length is recommended, as well as careful adherence to instructions for use with respect to oversizing the device diameter.[49] Ultimately, the importance of preoperative patient education and counseling around the need for rigorous long-term surveillance of the repair cannot be understated.

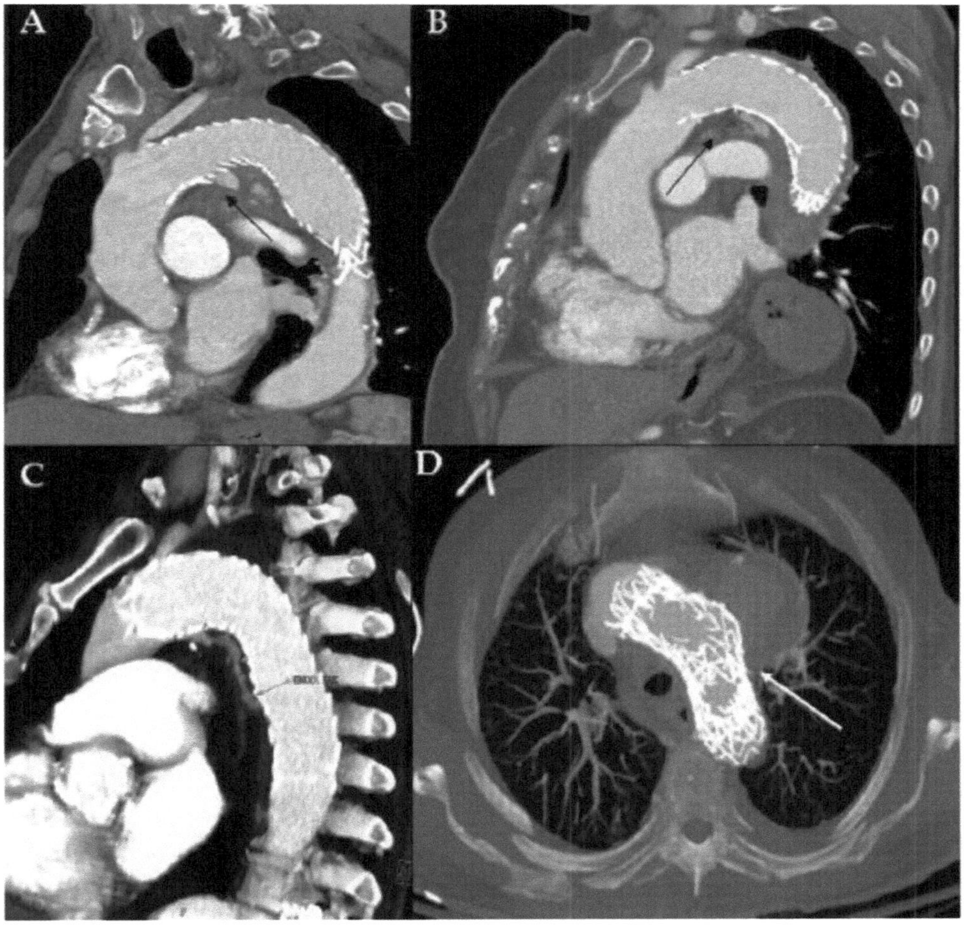

Figure 10.7 Classification of endoleak after thoracic aortic endograft repair. (Ricotta JJ. Endoleak management and postoperative surveillance following endovascular repair of thoracic aortic aneurysms. J Vasc Surg. 2010;52(4 Suppl): 91S-9S. doi: 10.1016/j.jvs.2010.06.149.)

REFERENCES

1. Dake MD, Miller DC, Semba CP, Mitchell RS, Walker PJ, Liddell RP. Transluminal placement of endovascular stent-grafts for the treatment of descending thoracic aortic aneurysms. N Engl J Med. 1994;331(26): 1729–1734. doi: 10.1056/NEJM199412293312601. PubMed PMID: 7984192.
2. Nation DA, Wang GJ. TEVAR: Endovascular Repair of the Thoracic Aorta. Semin Intervent Radiol. 2015;32(3): 265–271. doi: 10.1055/s-0035-1558824. PubMed PMID: 26327745; PubMed Central PMCID: PMCPMC4540616.
3. Hiratzka LF, Bakris GL, Beckman JA, Bersin RM, Carr VF, Casey DE, et al. 2010 ACCF/AHA/AATS/ACR/ASA/SCA/SCAI/SIR/STS/SVM guidelines for the diagnosis and management of patients with Thoracic Aortic Disease: a report of the American College of Cardiology Foundation/American Heart Association Task Force on Practice Guidelines, American Association for Thoracic Surgery, American College of Radiology, American Stroke Association, Society of Cardiovascular Anesthesiologists, Society for Cardiovascular Angiography and Interventions, Society of Interventional Radiology, Society of Thoracic Surgeons, and Society for Vascular Medicine. Circulation. 2010;121(13): e266–369. doi: 10.1161/CIR.0b013e3181d4739e. PubMed PMID: 20233780.
4. Erbel R, Aboyans V, Boileau C, Bossone E, Bartolomeo RD, Eggebrecht H, et al. 2014 ESC Guidelines on the diagnosis and treatment of aortic diseases: Document covering acute and chronic aortic diseases of the thoracic and abdominal aorta of the adult. The Task Force for the Diagnosis and Treatment of Aortic Diseases of the European Society of Cardiology (ESC). Eur Heart J. 2014;35(41): 2873–2926. doi: 10.1093/eurheartj/ehu281. PubMed PMID: 25173340.
5. Grabenwöger M, Alfonso F, Bachet J, Bonser R, Czerny M, Eggebrecht H, et al. Thoracic Endovascular Aortic Repair (TEVAR) for the treatment of aortic diseases: a position statement from the European Association for Cardio-Thoracic

Surgery (EACTS) and the European Society of Cardiology (ESC), in collaboration with the European Association of Percutaneous Cardiovascular Interventions (EAPCI). Eur J Cardiothorac Surg. 2012;42(1): 17–24. doi: 10.1093/ejcts/ezs107. PubMed PMID: 22561652.

6. Nienaber CA, Kische S, Zeller T, Rehders TC, Schneider H, Lorenzen B, et al. Provisional extension to induce complete attachment after stent-graft placement in type B aortic dissection: the PETTICOAT concept. J Endovasc Ther. 2006;13(6): 738–746. doi: 10.1583/06-1923.1. PubMed PMID: 17154712.
7. Nienaber CA, Rousseau H, Eggebrecht H, Kische S, Fattori R, Rehders TC, et al. Randomized comparison of strategies for type B aortic dissection: the INvestigation of STEnt Grafts in Aortic Dissection (INSTEAD) trial. Circulation. 2009;120(25): 2519–2528. doi: 10.1161/CIRCULATIONAHA.109.886408. PubMed PMID: 19996018.
8. Cheng D, Martin J, Shennib H, Dunning J, Muneretto C, Schueler S, et al. Endovascular aortic repair versus open surgical repair for descending thoracic aortic disease a systematic review and meta-analysis of comparative studies. J Am Coll Cardiol. 2010;55(10): 986–1001. doi: 10.1016/j.jacc.2009.11.047. PubMed PMID: 20137879.
9. Crawford ES, Hess KR, Cohen ES, Coselli JS, Safi HJ. Ruptured aneurysm of the descending thoracic and thoracoabdominal aorta. Analysis according to size and treatment. Ann Surg. 1991;213(5): 417–425; discussion 25-6. PubMed PMID: 2025061; PubMed Central PMCID: PMCPMC1358463.
10. Li HL, Chan YC, Cheng SW. Current Evidence on Management of Aortic Stent-graft Infection: A Systematic Review and Meta-Analysis. Ann Vasc Surg. 2018;51: 306–313. doi: 10.1016/j.avsg.2018.02.038. PubMed PMID: 29772328.
11. Tigkiropoulos K, Stavridis K, Lazaridis I, Saratzis N. Endovascular Repair of Aortobronchial Fistula due to Saccular Aneurysm of Thoracic Aorta. Case Rep Vasc Med. 2017;2017: 3158693. doi: 10.1155/2017/3158693. PubMed PMID: 29279784; PubMed Central PMCID: PMCPMC5723941.
12. Wang GJ, Jackson BM, Foley PJ, Damrauer SM, Goodney PP, Kelz RR, et al. National trends in admissions, repair, and mortality for thoracic aortic aneurysm and type B dissection in the National Inpatient Sample. J Vasc Surg. 2018;67(6): 1649–1658. Epub 2018/03/02. doi: 10.1016/j.jvs.2017.09.050. PubMed PMID: 29506945.
13. Demetriades D, Velmahos GC, Scalea TM, Jurkovich GJ, Karmy-Jones R, Teixeira PG, et al. Operative repair or endovascular stent graft in blunt traumatic thoracic aortic injuries: results of an American Association for the Surgery of Trauma Multicenter Study. J Trauma. 2008;64(3): 561–570; discussion 70-1. doi: 10.1097/TA.0b013e3181641bb3. PubMed PMID: 18332794.
14. Makaroun MS, Dillavou ED, Wheatley GH, Cambria RP, Investigators GT. 5-year results of endovascular treatment with the Gore TAG device compared with open repair of thoracic aortic aneurysms. J Vasc Surg. 2008;47(5): 912–918. doi: 10.1016/j.jvs.2007.12.006. PubMed PMID: 18353605.
15. Fairman RM, Criado F, Farber M, Kwolek C, Mehta M, White R, et al. Pivotal results of the Medtronic Vascular Talent Thoracic Stent Graft System: the VALOR trial. J Vasc Surg. 2008;48(3): 546–554. doi: 10.1016/j.jvs.2008.03.061. PubMed PMID: 18572352.
16. Matsumura JS, Cambria RP, Dake MD, Moore RD, Svensson LG, Snyder S, et al. International controlled clinical trial of thoracic endovascular aneurysm repair with the Zenith TX2 endovascular graft: 1-year results. J Vasc Surg. 2008;47(2): 247–257; discussion 57. doi: 10.1016/j.jvs.2007.10.032. PubMed PMID: 18241743.
17. Svensson LG, Kouchoukos NT, Miller DC, Bavaria JE, Coselli JS, Curi MA, et al. Expert consensus document on the treatment of descending thoracic aortic disease using endovascular stent-grafts. Ann Thorac Surg. 2008;85(1 Suppl): S1–41. doi: 10.1016/j.athoracsur.2007.10.099. PubMed PMID: 18083364.
18. Gopaldas RR, Huh J, Dao TK, LeMaire SA, Chu D, Bakaeen FG, et al. Superior nationwide outcomes of endovascular versus open repair for isolated descending thoracic aortic aneurysm in 11,669 patients. J Thorac Cardiovasc Surg. 2010;140(5):1001–1010. doi: 10.1016/j.jtcvs.2010.08.007. PubMed PMID: 20951252.
19. Khoynezhad A, Donayre CE, Bui H, Kopchok GE, Walot I, White RA. Risk factors of neurologic deficit after thoracic aortic endografting. Ann Thorac Surg. 2007;83(2): S882–9; discussion S90-2. doi: 10.1016/j.athoracsur.2006.10.090. PubMed PMID: 17257946.
20. Ullery BW, Cheung AT, Fairman RM, Jackson BM, Woo EY, Bavaria J, et al. Risk factors, outcomes, and clinical manifestations of spinal cord ischemia following thoracic endovascular aortic repair. J Vasc Surg. 2011;54(3): 677–684. doi: 10.1016/j.jvs.2011.03.259. PubMed PMID: 21571494.
21. Hnath JC, Mehta M, Taggert JB, Sternbach Y, Roddy SP, Kreienberg PB, et al. Strategies to improve spinal cord ischemia in endovascular thoracic aortic repair: Outcomes of a prospective cerebrospinal fluid drainage protocol. J Vasc Surg. 2008;48(4): 836–840. doi: 10.1016/j.jvs.2008.05.073. PubMed PMID: 18723308.

22. Fedorow CA, Moon MC, Mutch WA, Grocott HP. Lumbar cerebrospinal fluid drainage for thoracoabdominal aortic surgery: rationale and practical considerations for management. Anesth Analg. 2010;111(1): 46–58. doi: 10.1213/ANE.0b013e3181ddddd6. PubMed PMID: 20522706.
23. Chen Y, Zhang S, Liu L, Lu Q, Zhang T, Jing Z. Retrograde Type A Aortic Dissection After Thoracic Endovascular Aortic Repair: A Systematic Review and Meta-Analysis. J Am Heart Assoc. 2017;6(9). doi: 10.1161/JAHA.116.004649. PubMed PMID: 28939705; PubMed Central PMCID: PMCPMC5634245.
24. Canaud L, Ozdemir BA, Patterson BO, Holt PJ, Loftus IM, Thompson MM. Retrograde aortic dissection after thoracic endovascular aortic repair. Ann Surg. 2014;260(2): 389–395. doi: 10.1097/SLA.0000000000000585. PubMed PMID: 24441822.
25. Buth J, Harris PL, Hobo R, van Eps R, Cuypers P, Duijm L, et al. Neurologic complications associated with endovascular repair of thoracic aortic pathology: Incidence and risk factors. a study from the European Collaborators on Stent/Graft Techniques for Aortic Aneurysm Repair (EUROSTAR) registry. J Vasc Surg. 2007;46(6): 1103–1110; discussion 10-1. doi: 10.1016/j.jvs.2007.08.020. PubMed PMID: 18154984.
26. Biglioli P, Roberto M, Cannata A, Parolari A, Fumero A, Grillo F, et al. Upper and lower spinal cord blood supply: the continuity of the anterior spinal artery and the relevance of the lumbar arteries. J Thorac Cardiovasc Surg. 2004;127(4): 1188–1192. doi: 10.1016/j.jtcvs.2003.11.038. PubMed PMID: 15052221.
27. Feezor RJ, Martin TD, Hess PJ, Klodell CT, Beaver TM, Huber TS, et al. Risk factors for perioperative stroke during thoracic endovascular aortic repairs (TEVAR). J Endovasc Ther. 2007;14(4): 568–573. doi: 10.1177/152660280701400420. PubMed PMID: 17696634.
28. Henretta JP, Karch LA, Hodgson KJ, Mattos MA, Ramsey DE, McLafferty R, et al. Special iliac artery considerations during aneurysm endografting. Am J Surg. 1999;178(3): 212–218. PubMed PMID: 10527442.
29. Jackson BM, Woo EY, Bavaria JE, Fairman RM. Gender analysis of the pivotal results of the Medtronic Talent Thoracic Stent Graft System (VALOR) trial. J Vasc Surg. 2011;54(2): 358–363, 63.e1. doi: 10.1016/j.jvs.2010.12.064. PubMed PMID: 21397440.
30. Tsilimparis N, Debus S, Chen M, Zhou Q, Seale MM, Kölbel T. Results from the Study to Assess Outcomes After Endovascular Repair for Multiple Thoracic Aortic Diseases (SUMMIT). J Vasc Surg. 2018;68(5): 1324–1334. doi: 10.1016/j.jvs.2018.02.027. PubMed PMID: 29748101.
31. Ullery BW, McGarvey M, Cheung AT, Fairman RM, Jackson BM, Woo EY, et al. Vascular distribution of stroke and its relationship to perioperative mortality and neurologic outcome after thoracic endovascular aortic repair. J Vasc Surg. 2012;56(6): 1510–7. doi: 10.1016/j.jvs.2012.05.086. PubMed PMID: 22841287.
32. Kotelis D, Bischoff MS, Jobst B, von Tengg-Kobligk H, Hinz U, Geisbüsch P, et al. Morphological risk factors of stroke during thoracic endovascular aortic repair. Langenbecks Arch Surg. 2012;397(8): 1267–1273. doi: 10.1007/s00423-012-0997-6. PubMed PMID: 22956054.
33. Kanaoka Y, Ohki T, Maeda K, Baba T, Fujita T. Multivariate Analysis of Risk Factors of Cerebral Infarction in 439 Patients Undergoing Thoracic Endovascular Aneurysm Repair. Medicine (Baltimore). 2016;95(15): e3335. doi: 10.1097/MD.0000000000003335. PubMed PMID: 27082585; PubMed Central PMCID: PMCPMC4839829.
34. Leon LR, Mills JL, Jordan W, Morasch MM, Kovacs M, Becker GJ, et al. The risks of celiac artery coverage during endoluminal repair of thoracic and thoracoabdominal aortic aneurysms. Vasc Endovascular Surg. 2009;43(1): 51–60. doi: 10.1177/1538574408322655. PubMed PMID: 18996912.
35. Jim J, Caputo FJ, Sanchez LA. Intentional coverage of the celiac artery during thoracic endovascular aortic repair. J Vasc Surg. 2013;58(1): 270–275. doi: 10.1016/j.jvs.2013.04.003. PubMed PMID: 23711693.
36. Rose MK, Pearce BJ, Matthews TC, Patterson MA, Passman MA, Jordan WD. Outcomes after celiac artery coverage during thoracic endovascular aortic aneurysm repair. J Vasc Surg. 2015;62(1): 36–42. doi: 10.1016/j.jvs.2015.02.026. PubMed PMID: 25937603.
37. Kawatani Y, Kurobe H, Nakamura Y, Suda Y, Okuma Y, Sato S, et al. Acute pancreatitis caused by pancreatic ischemia after TEVAR combined with intentional celiac artery coverage and embolization of the branches of the celiac artery. J Surg Case Rep. 2017;2017 (2): rjx029. doi: 10.1093/jscr/rjx029. PubMed PMID: 28458836; PubMed Central PMCID: PMCPMC5400475.
38. Ayad M, Senders ZJ, Ryan S, Abai B, DiMuzio P, Salvatore DM. Chronic mesenteric ischemia after partial coverage of the celiac artery during TEVAR, case report, and review of the literature. Ann Vasc Surg. 2014;28(8): 1935.e1–6. doi: 10.1016/j.avsg.2014.08.001. PubMed PMID: 25108090.

39. Mehta M, Darling RC, Taggert JB, Roddy SP, Sternbach Y, Ozsvath KJ, et al. Outcomes of planned celiac artery coverage during TEVAR. J Vasc Surg. 2010;52(5): 1153–1158. doi: 10.1016/j.jvs.2010.06.105. PubMed PMID: 20709480.
40. Simring D, Raja J, Morgan-Rowe L, Hague J, Harris PL, Ivancev K. Placement of a branched stent graft into the false lumen of a chronic type B aortic dissection. J Vasc Surg. 2011;54(6): 1784–1787. doi: 10.1016/j.jvs.2011.05.053. PubMed PMID: 21784607.
41. Kamman AV, Williams DM, Patel HJ. Thoracic Endovascular Aortic Repair into the False Lumen in Chronic Aortic Dissection. Ann Vasc Surg. 2017;42: 303.e11–e14. doi: 10.1016/j.avsg.2016.11.027. PubMed PMID: 28390917.
42. Han SM, Gasper WJ, Chuter TA. Endovascular rescue after inadvertent false lumen stent graft implantation. J Vasc Surg. 2016;63(2): 518–522. doi: 10.1016/j.jvs.2014.11.072. PubMed PMID: 25595403.
43. Hobbs SD, Kumar S, Gilling-Smith GL. Epidemiology and diagnosis of endograft infection. J Cardiovasc Surg (Torino). 2010;51(1): 5–14. PubMed PMID: 20081758.
44. Kan CD, Lee HL, Yang YJ. Role of Endovascular Aortic Repair in the Treatment of Infected Aortic Aneurysms Complicated by Aortoenteric or Aortobronchial Fistulae. Thorac Cardiovasc Surg. 2018;66(3): 240–247. doi: 10.1055/s-0037-1608834. PubMed PMID: 29207434.
45. Jonker FH, Schlösser FJ, Moll FL, van Herwaarden JA, Indes JE, Verhagen HJ, et al. Outcomes of thoracic endovascular aortic repair for aortobronchial and aortoesophageal fistulas. J Endovasc Ther. 2009;16(4): 428–440. doi: 10.1583/09-2741R.1. PubMed PMID: 19702348.
46. Sörelius K, Wanhainen A, Wahlgren CM, Langenskiöld M, Roos H, Resch T, et al. Nationwide Study on Treatment of Mycotic Thoracic Aortic Aneurysms. Eur J Vasc Endovasc Surg. 2018. doi: 10.1016/j.ejvs.2018.08.052. PubMed PMID: 30340857.
47. Geisbüsch P, Skrypnik D, Ante M, Trojan M, Bruckner T, Rengier F, et al. Endograft migration after thoracic endovascular aortic repair. J Vasc Surg. 2018. doi: 10.1016/j.jvs.2018.07.073. PubMed PMID: 30553729.
48. Banno H, Akita N, Fujii T, Tsuruoka T, Takahashi N, Sugimoto M, et al. Proximal Bare Stent May Reduce Bird-Beak Configuration, Which is Associated with Distal Migration of Stent Graft in the Aortic Arch. Ann Vasc Surg. 2018. doi: 10.1016/j.avsg.2018.08.081. PubMed PMID: 30342207.
49. Ricotta JJ. Endoleak management and post-operative surveillance following endovascular repair of thoracic aortic aneurysms. J Vasc Surg. 2010;52 (4 Suppl): 91S–9S. doi: 10.1016/j.jvs.2010.06.149. PubMed PMID: 20724097.
50. Bokoch MP, Hiramoto JS, Lobo EP, Shalabi A. Rapid Ventricular Pacing for Landing Zone Precision During Thoracic Endovascular Aortic Arch Repair: A Case Series. J Cardiothorac Vasc Anesth. 2017;31(6): 2141–2146. doi: 10.1053/j.jvca.2017.03.034. PubMed PMID: 28764987.

SUGGESTED READINGS

Nienaber CA, Rousseau H, Eggebrecht H, Kische S, Fattori R, Rehders TC, et al. Randomized comparison of strategies for type B aortic dissection: the INvestigation of STEnt Grafts in Aortic Dissection (INSTEAD) trial. Circulation. 2009;120(25):2519–28. doi: 10.1161/CIRCULATIONAHA.109.886408. PubMed PMID: 19996018.

Hiratzka LF, Bakris GL, Beckman JA, Bersin RM, Carr VF, Casey DE, et al. 2010 ACCF/AHA/AATS/ACR/ASA/SCA/SCAI/SIR/STS/SVM guidelines for the diagnosis and management of patients with Thoracic Aortic Disease: a report of the American College of Cardiology Foundation/American Heart Association Task Force on Practice Guidelines, American Association for Thoracic Surgery, American College of Radiology, American Stroke Association, Society of Cardiovascular Anesthesiologists, Society for Cardiovascular Angiography and Interventions, Society of Interventional Radiology, Society of Thoracic Surgeons, and Society for Vascular Medicine. Circulation. 2010;121(13):e266-369. doi: 10.1161/CIR.0b013e3181d4739e. PubMed PMID: 20233780.

11

Complications of stent grafts for popliteal aneurysms

NATHAN J. ARANSON AND TRUC M. TA

Although a rare entity with a prevalence of 7.39/100,000, popliteal artery aneurysms (PAA) are the most common peripheral artery aneurysm encompassing 70% of all those diagnosed.[1,2] Ranging from 0.5 to 1.1 cm, a normal popliteal artery is a continuation of the superficial femoral artery in the thigh, extending from the adductor magnus (Hunter's) canal to the origin of the anterior tibial artery below the knee. Most popliteal artery aneurysms occur in the proximal part or midportion of the artery and are considered to be present if the diameter is 50% greater than the diameter of a normal adjacent segment of artery.[3] These aneurysms are most frequently found in men (95%), and are often bilateral (39–54%), and a synchronous aneurysm is found in up to 60% of patients.[1,4–7] Unlike abdominal aortic aneurysms, PAAs rarely rupture (1.4%) and rather manifest with limb ischemia due to aneurysm thrombosis or distal embolization.[8] Although most patients present without symptoms, more than two thirds of patients will develop some degree of limb ischemia during a 5 year surveillance.[5,9,10] Due to the prevalence of symptomatic complications leading to a heightened risk of limb loss (40%), an escalating approach to surgical management has been recommended.[11,12]

The typical threshold for surgical candidacy is any asymptomatic popliteal artery aneurysm greater than 2 cm diameter or those with mural thrombus of any size. Symptomatic aneurysms (compression, embolization, thrombosis, rupture) should be treated regardless of their diameter.[9,12,13] Historically, the inflow artery was either surgically ligated or occluded with compression.[14–16]

Since 1969, open surgical repair with autologous saphenous vein bypass and aneurysm exclusion has been regarded as the gold standard, although a posterior approach with aneurysmorrhaphy and interposition bypass has been popularized by some.[17,18] The first endovascular treatment of a PAA was described in 1994 by Marin et al. and a multitude of literature since that time has shown improved results that rival open repair.[19–22] As a testament to improved results and increased documentation of primary and secondary patency the overall utilization of endovascular popliteal artery aneurysm repair (EPAR) is on the rise being used in over 45% of patients in some centers.[23–25]

BRIEF TECHNICAL SUMMARY

With the documented benefits of endovascular repair for the treatment of abdominal aortic aneurysms, there has been much interest in developing a successful technique resulting in a durable repair of popliteal artery aneurysms. Many studies have shown benefits of this endovascular treatment option with documented reduction in operative time, wound complications, and length of hospital stay.[6,7,22,23,26–31] Initially, the benefit of this approach was paradoxically outweighed by an increased perioperative graft occlusion rate leading to an increase in 30 day re-interventions.[6,24–27,31,32] Subsequent studies have adjusted patient selection criteria and operative technique to obtain primary and secondary patency rates which are comparable to the success and durability of open repair.[29,33]

Much of the contemporary literature on the endovascular treatment of popliteal artery aneurysm centers around the use of the Gore Viabahn endoprosthesis (W.L. Gore & Associates, Flagstaff, AZ). The progeny of the Gore Hemobahn graft, used until 2003, this is a Nitinol stent with an ultrathin (100 μm) inner lining of heparin bonded expanded PTFE.[34] Advantages of the Viabahn endoprosthesis are that it is flexible (which allows it to tolerate bending at the knee joint), its inner lining is PTFE instead of irregular stent material, and the present construct has a contoured proximal edge designed to minimize endpoint inflammation which can lead to stenosis. Alternate stents and grafts have been used and documented in the literature but with less frequency.[21,35]

The patient can be treated with minimal anesthetic, utilizing intravenous sedation and injectable local anesthetic. The patient is placed supine, and an external radiopaque ruler is placed adjacent to the knee. When anatomically acceptable, antegrade access into the common femoral artery can be utilized with planned use of a percutaneous closure device. The patient should have an infrageniculate popliteal artery which is >= 4.5 mm and has at least 20 mm of normal artery proximal to the anterior tibial artery ostium. In this disease process, the artery elongates as it enlarges in diameter, which can create a tortuous transition zone between the stented and the non-stented segments.[5] As this morphologic change can lead to kinking, less tortuous anatomy is preferable. Due to the embolic potential of PAAs, the tibial outflow can be compromised, but for best long-term results, at least one vessel runoff is recommended to enhance durability.[33] The Viabahn endoprosthesis should not be oversized more than 15% of the normal artery diameter (or 1 mm) and best results are seen with 10–20 mm seal within a non-diseased artery. When overlapping grafts, 20 mm over overlap should be sought and the grafts should not differ in diameter by more than 1–2 mm to minimize the risk of infolding, which can lead to early thrombosis. Additional completion imaging should be obtained with the knee flexed to ensure there is no graft kinking.[28–30,33,36] Postoperative medical optimization with dual antiplatelet therapy is recommended and has been shown to improve primary patency rates.[37,38]

COMPLICATIONS

The majority of studies on the topic of endovascular repair of popliteal artery aneurysms quote 100% technical success as defined by complete aneurysm exclusion without evidence of endoleak and with preservation of the preoperative infrageniculate runoff.[26,27,31,36,38,39] Unfortunately, the durability of the procedural outcome has been called into question as the repetitive biomechanical forces at the knee flexion joint can lead to endoprosthesis migration, and endoleak or fracture, infolding, and thrombosis.[36] Even though much literature has suggested that the perioperative thrombosis rate is higher, there has been no proof of an increased rate of amputation and a general acceptance of lower complication rates.[6,21,23–27,31]

ACCESS SITE COMPLICATIONS

In order to treat a PAA with a Viabahn endoprosthesis, a 7Fr–12Fr delivery sheath must be placed into the femoral artery. This requires eventual closure of a 3–4 mm arteriotomy which can be accomplished via primary repair, endovascular closure device, or manual pressure. Most procedures are still performed with surgical exposure of the femoral artery access site.[26,28] However, due to the myriad benefits of minimally invasive endovascular therapy, an increasing number of endovascular procedures for popliteal artery aneurysms are being performed via percutaneous access rather than open surgical exposure.[32,36] More contemporary literature uses the well documented "preclosure" technique with Proglide sutures similarly used with large-caliber arterial access sites in percutaneous endovascular repair of abdominal aortic aneurysms (PEVAR).[40]

Likely secondary to the discrepancy between the open and endovascular procedures with respect to incisional burden, it is not surprising that wound complications are five-fold higher in open treatment.[22] Documented wound complications in EPAR range from 0–7% with bleeding complications being more frequent than wound complications.[6,7,33] Bleeding complications ranged from hematoma and pseudoaneurysm to retroperitoneal hemorrhage, with hematoma being the most common (3–6%).[7,33] Only one study described a patient with a retroperitoneal bleed.[5] Three studies each described one patient with an access site bleeding complication requiring intervention.[9,28,31] Overall access site complications are quite rare.

In order to prevent access site complications, standard endovascular practices should be upheld. Ultrasound should be used for percutaneous access to confirm common femoral artery anterior wall entry in a non-diseased segment. Similar techniques and exclusionary criteria should be employed as are utilized in PEVAR. In addition, there are certain patient populations who have increased risk of percutaneous access site complications, including those with atherosclerotic femoral arteries, small-caliber vessels, and morbidly obese patients.[40] Generally, these patients will benefit from an open surgical exposure for arterial access.

THROMBOSIS

Description and incidence

As is true with all peripheral interventions, the longevity of patency allows for comparison of success. When comparing open versus endovascular treatment of PAA, most studies compare primary, primary assisted, and secondary patency in a longitudinal fashion. The timeline for calculation is typically perioperative (immediate), within 30 days (short-term), or anything at or beyond 1 year (long term). The historical gold standard with respect to the treatment of PAA is aneurysm exclusion with saphenous vein graft bypass, which has a documented long-term primary and secondary patency of 80–95%.[23,25] The largest and most recent meta-analysis of over 4500 patients did find a significantly lower 1 year primary patency rate (88.3% vs 81.2%; $p = 0.01$) in the endovascular treatment but no clinical adverse sequelae was elucidated ($p = 0.79$).[22] An Italian multicenter study of endovascular repair of popliteal artery aneurysms in 2018 aimed to assess the effectiveness of endovascular treatment of PAA at short- and long-term follow-up treated a total of 48 aneurysms,

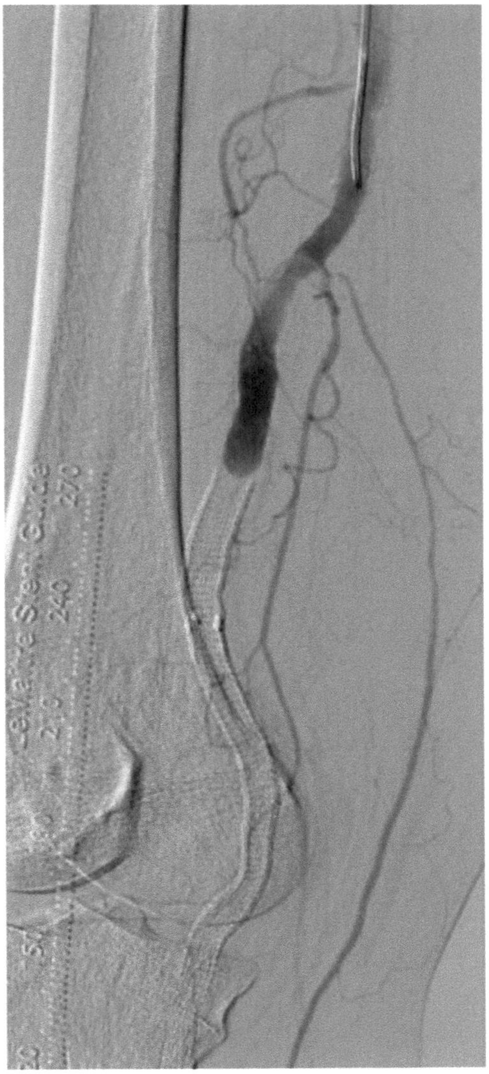

Figure 11.1 Angiogram of thrombosis of popliteal artery stent graft.

deploying a total of 79 endoprostheses.[41] They found that, at a mean follow-up of 24.5 months, a total of 12 grafts thrombosed (25%), requiring thrombolytic treatment followed by angioplasty. They did not observe any type II endoleak at either short- or long-term follow-up. They also found that there was a slight tendency of higher stent graft thrombosis and reduced patency after re-intervention in the long term in patients with longer lesions and with fewer runoff vessels. An example of graft thrombosis visualized on angiogram is shown in Figure 11.1.

Prevention/avoidance

In order to prevent thrombotic complications, the operative surgeon is encouraged to choose the diameter and length of the stent graft carefully. This should be chosen with the assistance of centerline imaging through the preoperative CT angiography or utilization of intravascular ultrasound (IVUS) through the treatment zone. Once the inner diameter of the target vessel is elucidated for the proximal and distal seal, an appropriately sized stent graft should be used based on the instructions for use (IFU) of the endoprosthesis (https://www.goremedical.com/products/viabahn—ifu/instructions). Data suggest that the use of longer stents or multiple stents is an independent predictor of stent graft thrombosis.[42] The surgeon is encouraged to optimize endoprosthesis length, diameter, and overlap in order to prevent thrombosis.

Long-term implications/outcomes

Although technical success in most studies approaches 100%, the largest concern is related to the durability of this form of treatment. Multiple studies have looked at the long-term outcome of placing an endoprosthesis into the femoropopliteal arterial system, with greatest concern crossing the knee flexion joint. Most studies found insignificant differences between open and endovascular repair at 1 year with primary patency over 80%. Despite this initial success, long-term follow-up out to 3 years yielded a primary patency of less than 70%.[20] This was found to be significantly lower than the long-term success of open repair.[21,23,30] Figure 11.2 shows a Forest plot from a meta-analysis comparing open versus endovascular treatment of PAAs. Despite this, the endovascular treatment patients had a higher rate of secondary patency, and most studies found that the endovascular treatment patients had less invasive secondary interventions after thrombosis with most patients undergoing catheter-directed thrombolysis with eventual angioplasty or stent extension.[22] In order to prevent stent thrombosis, most studies recommend dual antiplatelet agents use or even anticoagulants.[37,38]

MIGRATION/ENDOLEAK

Description and incidence

At the completion of endovascular treatment for popliteal artery aneurysm, nearly all patients had reported success. This was defined as exclusion of aneurysm, absence of endoleak, and preservation of distal run-off. On follow-up imaging some patients were found to have re-perfusion of the aneurysm sac. As popliteal artery aneurysm is not as commonly found to exert mass effect and rupture as it is to thrombose or embolize, this has been deemed less of an issue with respect to guiding subsequent treatments. Endoleak types mirror those as described with endovascular repair of abdominal aortic aneurysm (EVAR).[43] Most studies suggest absence of definable endoleak upon completion imaging.[36,37,39] Despite this initial success, 5–10% of these patients were found to have evidence of endoleak on follow-up imaging modalities.[5,9,29] One study suggested that upward of 15% (8/57) of interventions were complicated long term by stent graft migration leading to Type I or III endoleak.[37] See Figures 11.3 and 11.4.

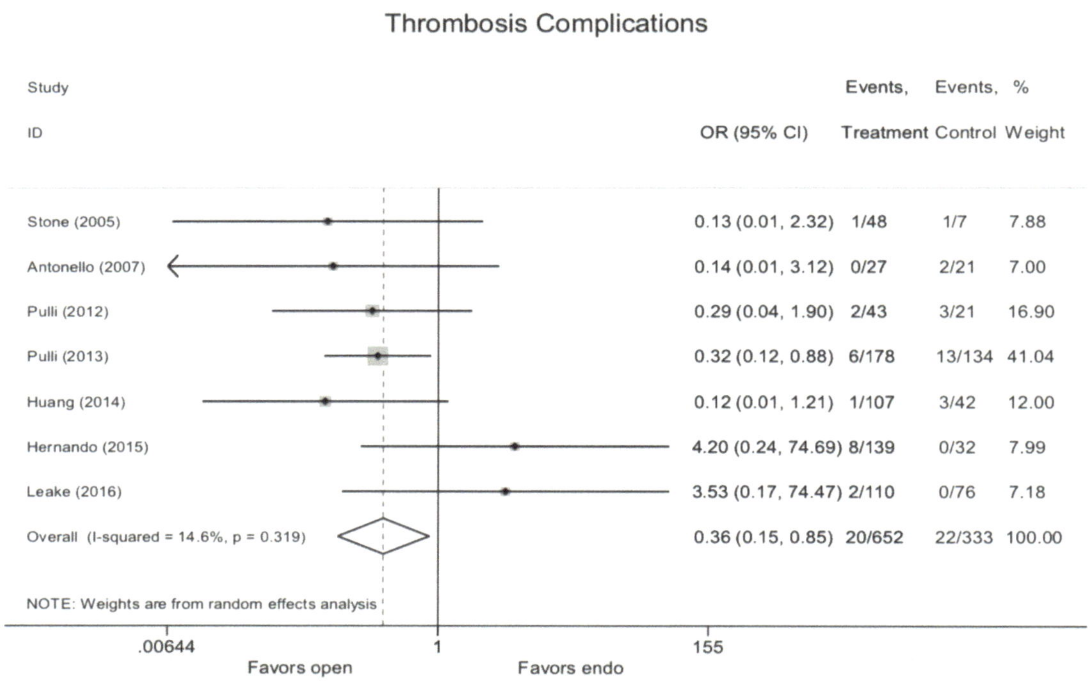

Figure 11.2 Meta-analysis of open and endovascular repair of PAAs: Forest plot.[22]

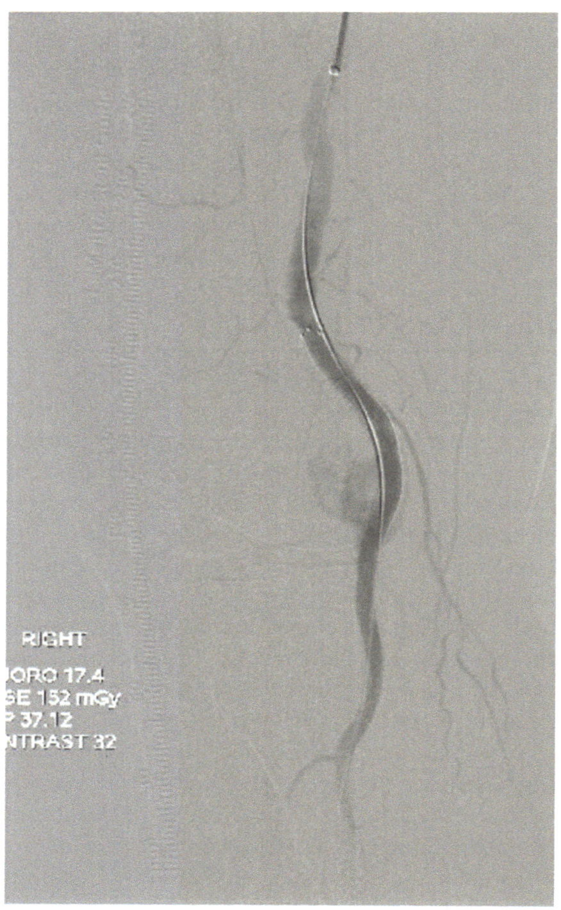

Figure 11.3 Endoleak seen on completion angiogram after stent graft deployment.

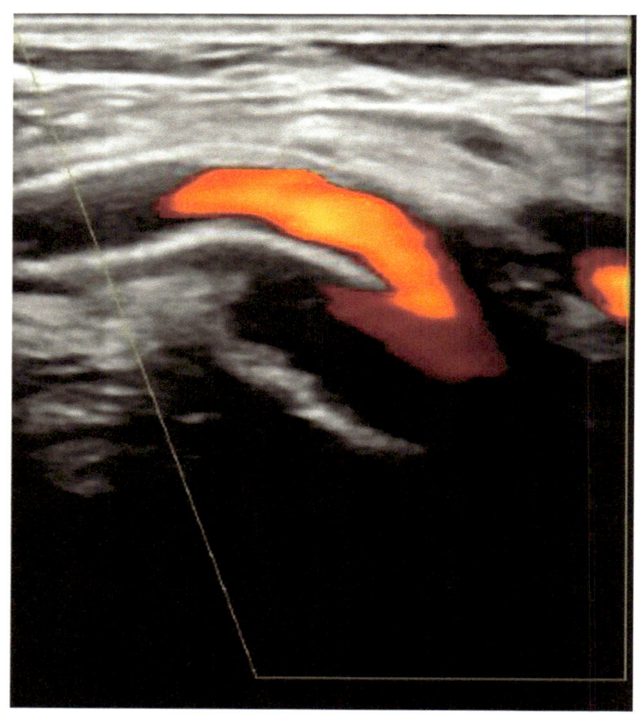

Figure 11.4 Type I endoleak seen on follow-up duplex ultrasound.

Prevention/avoidance

From a technical standpoint, it is thought that insufficient overlap with normal artery in the proximal or distal seal zone, under-sizing of the stent, or the forces incurred by repetitive knee flexion are some of the reasons why stent migration and endoleak are seen.[5] Much of the technical literature on the topic recommends use of centerline imaging to determine the true diameter of the target vessel as well as use of IVUS to guide diameter measurements along with identification of normal uniform vessel. The instructions for use for the Viabahn endoprosthesis suggest a 5–20% diameter oversizing along with a 10 mm graft-to-vessel overlap and a 10 mm graft-to-graft overlap without a > 1 mm difference between stent graft diameters. It is also recommended that all patients be imaged with the knee extended and flexed to 90 degrees. Many operators will recommend against voluntary knee flexion past 90-degrees in the postoperative period to avoid graft-to-graft separation or graft kinking, which can lead to occlusion.

Long-term implications/outcomes

A recent systematic review of endovascular popliteal aneurysm repair using Hemobahn/Viabahn stent graft found that a common indication for re-intervention following popliteal aneurysm repair was type I or III endoleaks.[20] The study found the incidence of endoleaks to be 0–20% between mean follow-up periods of 14–54 months. All type I or III endoleaks were treated by re-lining, and all type II endoleaks were managed conservatively. This is in comparison to open repair where persistent enlargement was seen in over 30% of patients.[44]

FRACTURE/INFOLDING

Description and incidence

The Gore Viabahn stent graft is the most common endoprosthesis used to treat PAAs. Although they are hailed for their flexibility and resistance to fracture and infolding, when these issues occur, they can lead to thrombosis. In a meta-analysis of 14 total studies detailing endovascular PAA repair, 5 of them (total of 514 popliteal artery aneurysms) examined the incidence of stent-graft fracture. Three studies revealed no fractures during follow-up, and the overall reported incidence ranged from 0–27.3% in studies with mean follow-up between 21.3 and 50 months. All studies reported the routine use of > 1 stent graft to achieve successful exclusion of the aneurysm, with acceptable targeted overlap. To this regard, one group reported a 16.7% incidence of stent fractures after endovascular repair, but fewer than 40% of these patients experienced thrombosis.[37] Comparatively, graft infolding is less commonly seen but more often leads to graft thrombosis. One study revealed rates upward of 10%, yet all of the patients who developed graft infolding also had stent graft thrombosis.[5]

Prevention/avoidance

Prevention of stent fracture begins with patient and stent selection. There is a documented higher incidence with the use of overlapping stents and in younger patients.[45] When possible, the treatment length should be minimized and the overlapping lengths optimized between 1–2 cm to avoid rigid stent-to-stent forces. The construct of the Viabahn endoprosthesis has a flexible self-expanding stent on the exterior mounted to thin-walled PTFE. Due to this, if the stent is oversized too much with respect to the artery, the inner PTFE can infold, leading to occlusion and thrombosis. Preventing this from happening relies on the proper sizing of the graft with respect to the artery it lines. In addition, when overlapping stents, the inner stent should be no larger than 1 mm in diameter compared with the outer stent.[5] These are the two highest-yield methods to avoid stent fracture and infolding. In addition, most studies advocate for completion angiogram with knee extended and flexed to ensure on-table patency and no graft infolding with the forced curvature of the graft.[33]

Long-term implications/outcomes

The long-term data on stent fractures is sparse, but in one study by Golchehr et al. patients were followed on average more than 5 years. They reported stent fractures in over 25% of the patients at 5 years, but most of these were seen in patients treated with Hemobahn stent grafts. Of the patients with stent fractures, the majority were asymptomatic, but one-third had claudication symptoms and one patient had limb-threatening ischemia. Three-quarters of the fractures were circumferential, but fewer than half of the patients with stent fractures had multiple fractures.[7] Comparing patients with and without fractures found 38.5% of graft occlusions in the stent fracture group versus 24.6% in the group without any stent fracture. However, their analysis did not show any statistical difference between the two groups in terms of long patency rate. They did note that multiple stent grafts and younger patient age were independent predictors of stent graft fracture.[45]

With regard to graft-related complications, one study revealed almost 10% incidence of graft infolding, and interestingly all cases had graft occlusion at long-term follow-up. Conversely, despite this finding with respect to graft infolding, the same was not true for those patients with graft dislocation or stent fracture.[5]

REFERENCES

1. Dent, TL, et al. Multiple Arteriosclerotic Arterial Aneurysms. JAMA Archives of Surgery. 1972;105: 338–344.
2. Lawrence PF, Lorenzo-Riviero S, Lyon JL. The incidence of iliac, femoral, and popliteal artery aneurysms in hospitalized patients. Journal of Vascular Surgery. 1995 Oct;22(4): 409–416.
3. Callum KG, Gaunt JI, Thomas ML, Browse NL. Physiological studies in arteriomegaly. Cardiovascular Research. 1974 May;8(3): 373–383.
4. Ravn H, Pansell-Fawcett K, Bjorck M. Popliteal Artery Aneurysm in Women. Eur J Vasc Endovasc Surg. 2017;54: 738–743.
5. Maraglino, Cosimo, et al. Endovascular Treatment of Popliteal Artery Aneurysms: A Word of Caution after Long-Term Follow-up. Annals of Vascular Surgery. 2017 May;41: 62–68.
6. Shahin Y, Barakat H, Shrivastava V. Endovascular Versus Open Repair of Asymptomatic Popliteal Artery Aneurysms: A Systematic Review and Meta-Analysis. JVIR. 2016 May;27(5): 715–722.
7. Golchehr B, et al. Long-term outcome of endovascular popliteal artery aneurysm repair. Journal of Vascular Surgery. 2018 Jun;67(6): 1797–1804.
8. Brown SL, Lewis M, Morrow, DB. Endovascular Repair of Ruptured Popliteal Artery Aneurysms: A Case Report and Review of the Literature. European Journal of Vascular and Endovascular Surgery. 2016;32: 24–28.
9. Golchehr B, et al. Clinical Outcome of Isolated Popliteal Artery Aneurysms Treated with a Heparin-bonded Stent Graft. Eur J Vasc Endovasc Surg. 2016;52: 99–104.
10. Dawson I, et al. Asymptomatic popliteal aneurysm: elective operation versus conservative follow-up. British Journal of Surgery. 1994 Octr;81(10): 1504–1507.
11. Ascher E, Markevich N, Schutzer RW, Kallakuri S, Jacob T, Hingorani AP. Small popliteal artery aneurysms: Are they clinically significant? Journal of Vascular Surgery. 2003 Apr;37(4): 755–760.
12. Ravn H, Wanhainen A, Bjorck M. Surgical technique and long-term results after popliteal artery aneurysm repair: Results from 717 legs. Journal of Vascular Surgery. 2007 Aug;46(2): 236–243.
13. Szilagyi DE, Schwartz RL, Reddy DJ. Popliteal Arterial Aneurysms: Their Natural History and Management. JAMA Archives of Surgery. 1981 May;116: 724–728.
14. Galland RB. History of the Management of Popliteal Artery Aneurysms. Eur J Vasc Endovasc Surg. 2008;35: 466–472.
15. Perry MO. John Hunter - Triumph and Tragedy. Journal of Vascular Surgery. 1993;17: 7–14.
16. Clark A. Clinical Lecture on Aneurysm of the Popliteal Artery. British Medical Journal. 1895 Nov;(28): 1557–1558.
17. Edwards WS. Exclusion and saphenous vein bypass of popliteal aneurysms. Surg Gyneco Obstet. 1969;128: 829–830.
18. Beseth BD, Moore WS. The posterior approach for repair of popliteal artery aneurysms. Journal of Vascular Surgery. 2006 May;43(5): 940–945.
19. Marin ML, et al. Transfemoral endoluminal stented graft repair of a popliteal artery aneurysm. Journal of Vascular Surgery. 1994 Apr;19(4): 754–757.
20. Patel SR, et al. A Systematic Review and Meta-analysis of Endovascular Popliteal Aneurysm Repair Using the Hemobahn/Viabahn Stent-Graft. Journal of Endovascular Therapy. 201;22(3): 330–337.
21. Cina CS. Endovascular Repair of Popliteal Artery Aneurysms. Journal of Vascular Surgery. 2010 Apr;51(4): 1056–1060.
22. Leake AE, et al. Meta-analysis of open and endovascular repair of popliteal artery aneurysms. Journal of Vascular Surgery. 2017 Jan;65(1): 246–256.
23. Eslami MH, et al. Open repair of asymptomatic popliteal artery aneurysm is associated with better outcomes than endovascular repair. Journal of Vascular Surgery. 2015 Mar;61(3): 663–669.
24. Bjorck M, et al. Editor's Choice: Contemporary Treatment of Popliteal Artery Aneurysm in Eight Countries: A Report from the Vascunet Collaboration of Registries. European Journal of Vascular and Endovascular Surgery. 2014 Feb;47(2): 164–171.
25. Cervin A, et al. Treatment of Popliteal Aneurysm by Open and Endovascular Surgery: A Contemporary Study of 592 Procedures in Sweden. Eur J Vasc Endovasc Surg. 2015;50: 342–350.
26. Antonello M, et al. Open repair versus endovascular treatment for asymptomatic popliteal artery aneurysm: Results of a prospective randomized study. Journal of Vascular Surgery. 2005 Aug 42(2): 185–193.
27. Huang Y, et al. Outcomes of endovascular and contemporary open surgical repairs of popliteal artery aneurysm. Journal of Vascular Surgery. 2014 Sep;60(3): 631–638.
28. Curi MA, et al. Mid-term outcomes of endovascular popliteal artery aneurysm repair. Journal of Vascular Surgery. 2007 Ma;45(3): 505–510.
29. Leake AE, et al. Contemporary outcomes of open and endovascular popliteal artery aneurysm repair. Journal of Vascular Surgery. 2016 Jan;63(1): 70–76.
30. Dorigo, Walter, et al. A matched case-control study on open and endovascular treatment of popliteal artery aneurysms. Scandanavian Journal of Surgery. 2018;107(3): 236–243.

31. Pulli R, et al. Comparison of Early and Midterm Results of Open and Endovascular Treatment of Popliteal Artery Aneurysms. Annals of Vascular Surgery. 2012 Aug;26(6): 809–818.
32. Stone, Patrick A, et al. The value of duplex surveillance after open and endovascular popliteal aneurysm repair. Journal of Vascular Surgery. 2005 Jun;41(6): 936–941.
33. Del Tatto B, et al. Open and Endovascular Repair of Popliteal Artery Aneurysms. Annals of Vascular Surgery. 2018;50: 119–127.
34. Mollenhoff, C, Katsargyris, A, Steinbauer, M. Current status of Hemobahn/Viabahn endografts for treatment of popliteal aneurysms. Journal of Cardiovascular Surgery (Torino). 2013;54: 785–791.
35. Argenteri A, Bianchi G. Use of a Multilayer Flow Modulator in the Treatment of Aneurysms. s.l.: Minerva Medica, 2012.
36. Rajasinghe HA, et al. Endovascular Exclusion of Popliteal Artery Aneurysms With Expanded Polytetrafluoroethylene Stent-Grafts: Early Results. Vascular and Endovascular Surgery. 2007;40(6): 460–466.
37. Tielliu IFJ, et al. Endovascular treatment of popliteal artery aneurysms: Results of a prospective cohort study. Journal of Vascular Surgery. 2005 Apr;41(4): 561–566.
38. Speziale F, et al. Ten Years' Experience in Endovascular Repair of Popliteal Artery Aneurysm Using the Viabahn Endoprosthesis: A Report from Two Italian Vascular Centers. Annals of Vascular Surgery. 2015;29: 941–949.
39. Wissgott C, Lüdtke CW, Vieweg H, Scheer F, Lichtenberg M, Schlöricke E, Andresen R. Endovascular Treatment of Aneurysms of the Popliteal Artery By a Covered Endoprosthesis. Clin Med Insights Cardiol. 2014;8(Suppl 2): 15–21.
40. Aranson N, Watkins M. Percutaneous Interventions in Aortic Disease. Circulation. 2015 Apr;131; 1291–1299.
41. Guzzardi G, Natrella M, Del Sette B, Petullà M, Fanelli G, Porta C, Carriero A, Laganà D. Endovascular repair of popliteal artery aneurysms: an Italian multicenter study. Radiol Med. 2019 Jan;124(1): 79–85.
42. Garg K, Rockman CB, Kim BJ, Jacobowitz GR, Maldonado TS, Adelman MA, Veith FJ, Cayne NS. Outcome of endovascular repair of popliteal artery aneurysm using the Viabahn endoprosthesis. J Vasc Surg. 2012 Jun;55(6): 1647–1653.
43. Eliason JL, Upchurch GR. Endovascular Abdominal Aortic Aneurysm Repair. Circulation. 2008;117: 1738–1744.
44. Mehta M, Champagne B, Darling RC, Roddy SR, Kreienberg PB, Ozsvath KJ, Paty PSK, Chang BB, Shah DM. Outcome of popliteal artery aneurysms after exclusion and bypass: Significance of residual patent branches mimicking type II endoleaks. Journal of Vascular Surgery. 2004 Nov;40(5): 886–890.
45. Tielliu IF, Zeebregts CJ, Vourliotakis G, Bekkema F, van den Dungen JJ, Prins TR, Verhoeven EL. Stent fractures in the Hemobahn/Viabahn stent graft after endovascular popliteal aneurysm repair. J Vasc Surg. 2010 Jun;51(6): 1413–1418.

SUGGESTED READINGS

Shahin Y, Barakat H, and Shrivastava, V. Endovascular Versus Open Repair of Asymptomatic Popliteal Artery Aneurysms: A Systematic Review and Meta-Analysis. JVIR, 2016 May;27(5): 715–722.

Szilagyi DE, Schwartz RL, and Reddy DJ. Popliteal Arterial Aneurysms: Their Natural History and Management. JAMA Arch Surg 1981 May;116: 724–728.

12

Complications of inferior vena cava filters

MATTHEW T. MAJOR, PAUL G. BOVE, AND GRAHAM W. LONG

Venous thromboembolic disease (VTE) is relatively common, 70–113 cases/100,000/year,[1] and carries a 15% mortality rate from pulmonary embolism (PE).[2] First-line treatment is systemic anticoagulation. However, a subset of patients develop bleeding complications or sustain a PE while on therapeutic anticoagulation. These patients, and others with relative indications, may benefit from inferior vena cava (IVC) filter placement. The placement rate for IVC filters increased from 1994 to 2008, from 65 to 202 per 100,000, during the period after retrievable filters were introduced into the market. However, placement rates decreased after 2008 to 129 per 100,000 beneficiaries, possibly due to changing views regarding long-term safety and efficacy. Despite the advent of these retrievable filters, the vast majority are never removed with only 18% recovered in 2015.[3,4] Complications related to IVC filters vary depending on filter type, with the majority attributable to retrievable filters.[5–8] This chapter will characterize complications from IVC filter placement, such as access issues and filter malposition; late complications, such as filter fracture, migration, perforation and thrombosis; and those related to filter retrieval.

VASCULAR ACCESS COMPLICATIONS

Vascular access complications for IVC filter insertion vary from 4–11%, similar to those for central venous catheter insertion. The authors routinely perform ultrasound-guided sheath placement, which may decrease access site complications. Bleeding and thrombosis are most common, with bleeding in 6–15% and thrombosis in 2–35%. Significant bleeding requiring transfusion is rare. Pneumothorax and air embolism are other rare complications. Arteriovenous fistula is also uncommon (0.02%) and presents with localized pain, distal ischemia, and palpable thrill.[9] Small fistulas can be observed and often resolve spontaneously; larger, symptomatic fistulas require open repair if they involve the common or profunda femoral arteries, or endovascular repair with a covered stent if they involve the external iliac or superficial femoral arteries.

FILTER MALPOSITION

Filter tilt is defined as greater than 15 degrees angulation of the filter from the long axis of the vena cava (Figure 12.1). This is encountered with all filter designs, except the Bird's Nest Filter (Cook Medical, Bloomington, IN) due to its inherent design. Increased tilt angle may increase the risk of PE, but it does not increase the risk of thrombosis. Most manufacturers recommend against attempting to adjust the filter position to correct the tilt. A few advocate for the placement of a second filter in this circumstance, although this is not supported in the literature.[9]

Ideal positioning of an IVC filter is with the apex just inferior to the renal veins and the base superior to the caval bifurcation. Misplacement or migration of the device above the level of the renal veins may lead to renal vein thrombosis, while positioning in a unilateral iliac vein leaves the contralateral side unprotected. Inadvertent lack of identification of aberrant anatomy such as a duplicated vena cava could also result in leaving one side unprotected (Figure 12.2). One method to avoid this complication would be routine left femoral vein access and venography. Reviewing prior computed tomographic (CT) imaging preoperatively assists with detecting caval anomalies and determining appropriate caval sizing. Placement into the gonadal or lumbar veins has also been described.[9] There have been rare cases of inadvertent placement into the infra-renal aorta, one of which remained asymptomatic for 16 years and was discovered incidentally on abdominal CT scan.[10] Inadvertent filter placement into the spinal canal at the level of L2-L3 as a result of wire/sheath perforation into the retroperitoneum has also been encountered.[11] Incorrect filter orientation may also occur for systems utilizing an asymmetric design, such as using a femoral delivery system on an internal jugular approach

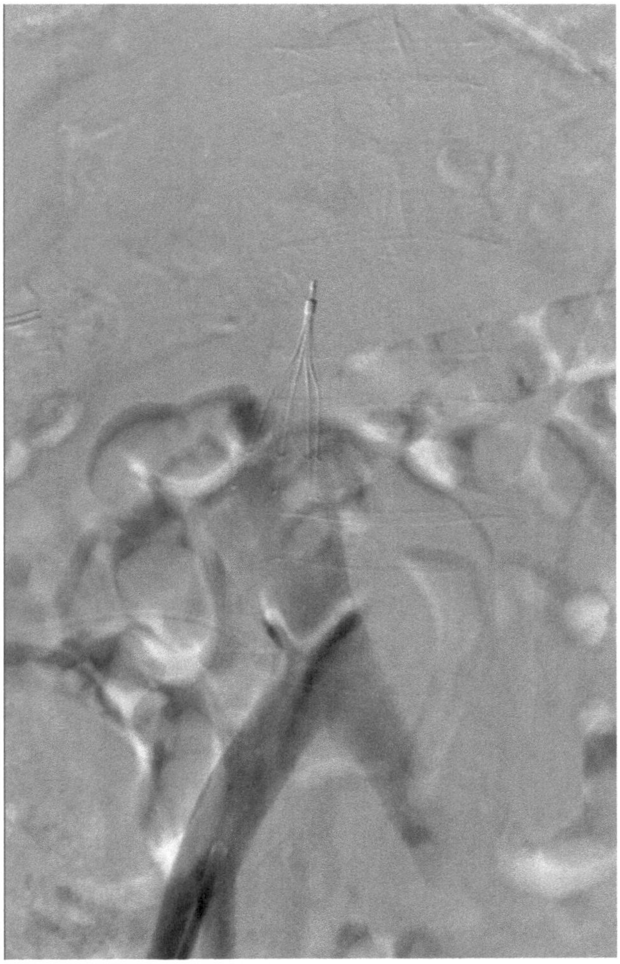

Figure 12.1 Post-deployment venogram demonstrating filter tilt.

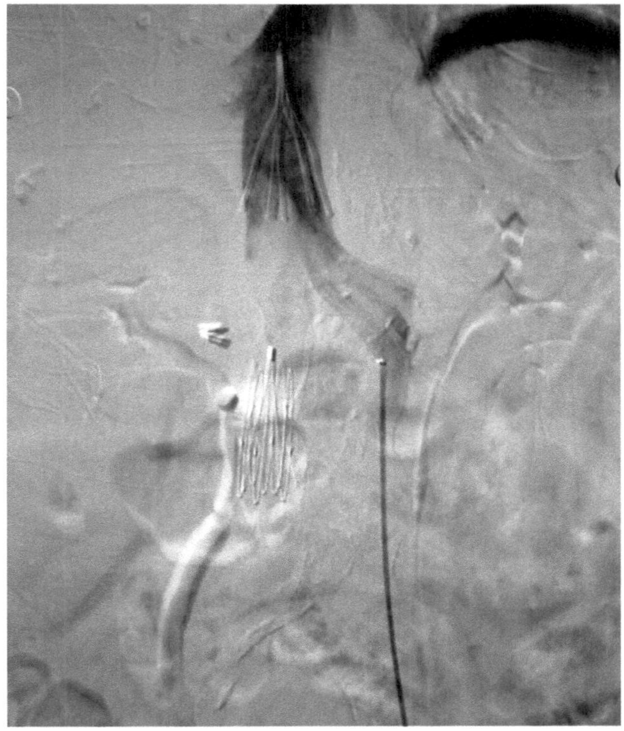

Figure 12.2 Completion cavagram in patient with a duplicated IVC. The second, superior filter is placed above the confluence of the left-sided IVC and left renal vein with the right-sided IVC. The inferior filter was placed in the right-sided IVC. Note the left renal pelvis at the level of the left-sided IVC and left renal vein confluence.

and vice versa.[9] Immediate retrieval followed by replacement with a correctly oriented filter should be performed if possible. In the case of permanent filters, consideration should be made for insertion of an additional, properly oriented filter to provide adequate protection from PE.

FILTER FRACTURE

In a review of the FDA Manufacturer and User Facility Device Experience (MAUDE) database from 2014, the most common late complication after IVC filter placement was fracture, accounting for 5.9–27.1% of all complications.[12] Filter fracture can occur when there is structural integrity failure of the material, most commonly seen 1 year following placement, and may lead to fragment embolization. Fracture is more often seen in the retrievable filter design and is uncommonly seen with permanent filters. This can result in alterations in flow dynamics within the IVC, which may place these patients at higher risk for thrombosis and decrease the effectiveness of PE prevention as well. Fragment embolization has been reported within the pulmonary vasculature, renal veins, and heart.[9] Filter and fragment retrieval is recommended for patients upon discovery of fracture.[8]

A prospective single-institution study evaluated 82 consecutive patients who presented with IVC filter fracture as an outpatient. All underwent catheter-based main filter retrieval after diagnosis; removal of fragments was attempted if they were deemed to be intravascular and accessible on imaging. There were 185 fragments were identified, most commonly within the IVC (81), followed by the retroperitoneum (51), pulmonary artery (33), heart (16), hepatic vein (2), renal vein (1), and aorta (1). Of these, 47% were deemed eligible for endovascular retrieval, and 89.7% were successfully retrieved. Minor complications were seen in 6.9% and one major complication (cardiac tamponade) was seen. There were 19 cases of retained cardiopulmonary fragments, 81% of which remained asymptomatic over a mean follow-up period of 845 days. Two patients pursued surgical removal (2 cardiac fragments and 1 pulmonary fragment) due to persistent pain and anxiety regarding the fragments.[13]

FILTER EMBOLIZATION

Filter embolization is defined as post deployment movement of the filter to a distant anatomic site. This should be distinguished from filter migration, which is defined as a > 2 cm change in filter position compared to that at the time of deployment.[8] Intracardiac or intrapulmonary embolization is a rare life-threatening event (Figure 12.3). In a 2009 review,[14] 98 such cases were identified in the literature over a 30-year period. The majority (77%) presented with one or more symptoms of chest pain, shortness of breath, cardiac arrhythmia, or hypotension; 30% demonstrated evidence of myocardial wall injury, damage to the chordae tendineae, or tricuspid valve. Embolization occurred most often during filter deployment (33%); an additional 14% were seen in the acute period (within 24 hours of deployment), 17% in the subacute period (between 24 hours and 1 week), and 30% in the delayed period (more than 1 week after deployment). Average time to presentation for delayed cases was 2.9 months. The most common cause reported in this study was operator error during initial placement, such as premature or inadvertent deployment or difficulty passing a guide wire during filter delivery. In 12 cases, authors reported a large embolus had dislodged the filter from the vena cava and carried it into the heart via a "sail" effect. Other common causes include a mega cava (> 28 mm), wire entrapment during central venous catheter placement, during transfemoral cannula placement for cardiopulmonary bypass, and cannula removal after extracorporeal membrane oxygenation (ECMO) (Figure 12.4). While some are asymptomatic, the long-term consequences of intracardiac or intrapulmonary filter components are unknown. Retrieval by either endovascular or open surgical technique is recommended whenever feasible.[14]

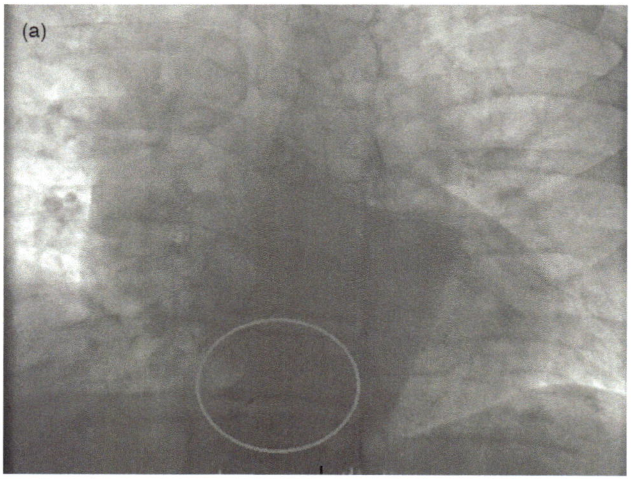

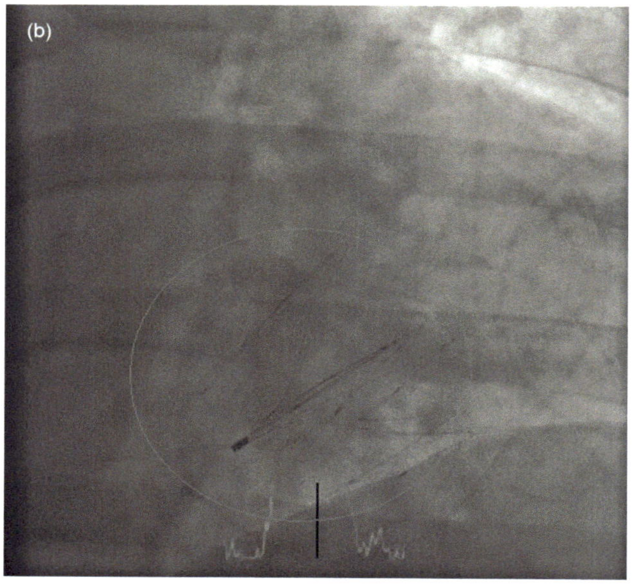

Figure 12.3 Fluoroscopic images showing filter embolization to the right ventricle (a) and magnified views of the same filter (b). This patient required surgical removal through a sternotomy and cardiopulmonary bypass.

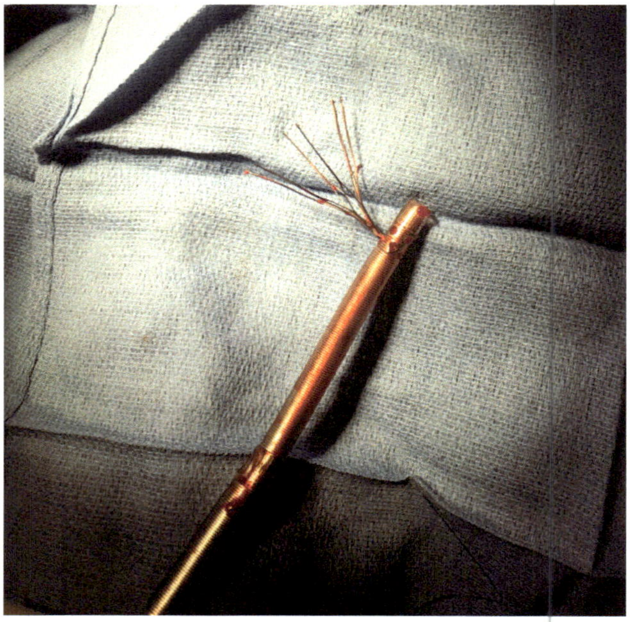

Figure 12.4 IVC filter embedded in veno-venous ECMO cannula, removed simultaneously during bedside de-cannulation.

IVC PERFORATION

IVC perforation is defined as a filter strut or anchor extending > 3 mm outside the vessel wall and entering the retroperitoneum or surrounding anatomic structures (Figures 12.5–12.7). The majority are asymptomatic, and some suggest filter perforation may be more common than previously estimated. In a literature review of IVC

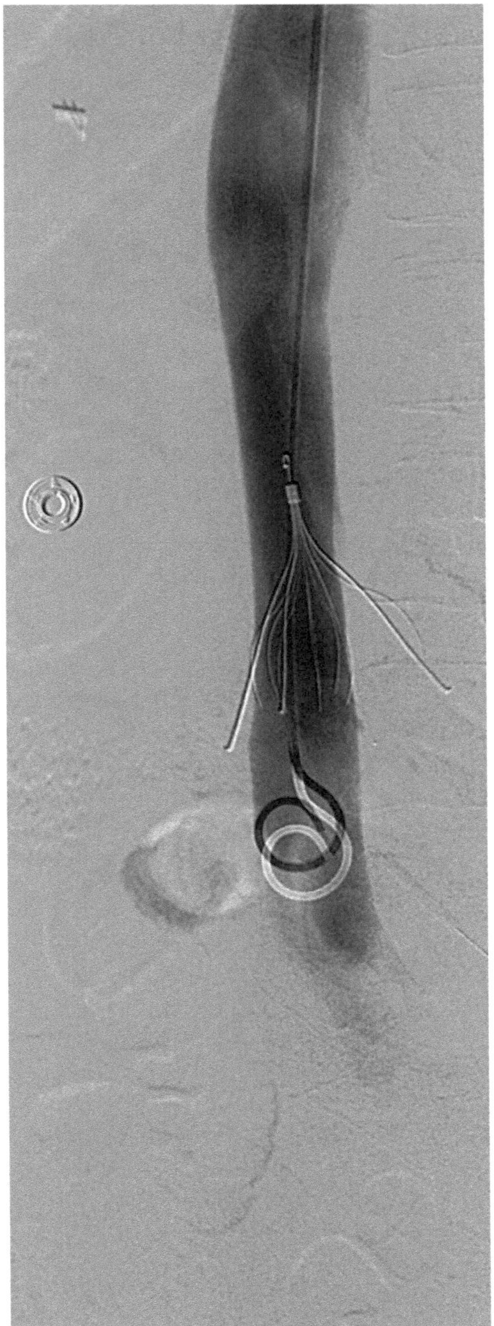

Figure 12.5 Cavagram demonstrating transmural filter strut penetration at the time of retrieval, approximately 2 months after placement.

filters, caval perforation was reported in 19% of 9002 reviewed cases. Among the cases of filter perforation, 8% were symptomatic. For symptomatic patients, pain was most commonly reported (77%); 5% had major complications requiring unplanned intervention, which included surgical removal of the IVC filter (63), endovascular stent graft placement for aortic pseudoaneurysm (8), endovascular retrieval of permanent filter (4), arterial embolization for bleeding (2), endovascular stent graft with

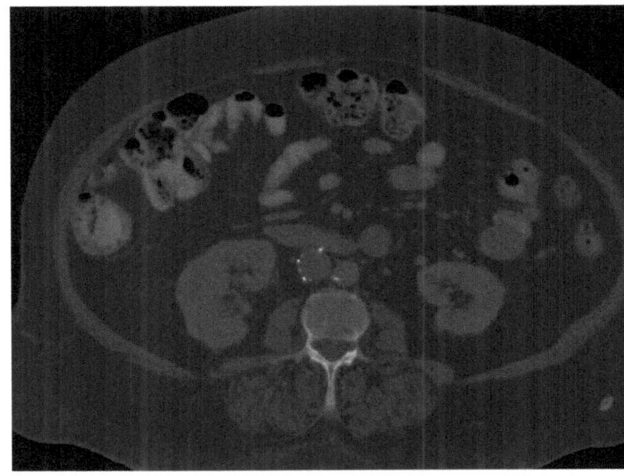

Figure 12.6 Axial CT image showing filter strut penetration of the aorta. This patient was asymptomatic and treated conservatively.

embolization (1), percutaneous nephrostomy (1), ureteral stent placement (1), and percutaneous nephrostomy with ureteral stent (1). Perforated struts involved other organs or anatomic structures 19% of the time, with the duodenum, lumbar vertebra, and aorta being the most commonly affected. Less common presentations reported in the literature include pancreatitis, ureteral injury, retroperitoneal hematoma, and chronic pain syndrome.[15]

The mechanism of IVC penetration is not well understood, but some data suggest that conically shaped filters with free struts have a higher frequency of penetration compared to those without free struts. While these filters without free struts may decrease the rate of perforation, they may increase the risk of caval thrombosis. Other proposed mechanisms of caval penetration include an increase in filter span, sharpness of the barbs, decreased strength of the native caval wall, significant filter tilt (> 15 degrees), and smaller caliber IVC. Caval motion with the cardiorespiratory cycle, postural changes, abdominal trauma and physical pressure may also contribute.[16]

Treatment of patients with asymptomatic filter perforation is debatable, but should be considered for cases involving adjacent organs or structures. For patients with symptomatic filter perforation, retrieval should be considered. Endovascular removal is often feasible with a high success rate; however, this is related to operator experience and familiarity with advanced retrieval techniques. Of note, iatrogenic fracture of a strut outside the cava has been reported. Retroperitoneal hemorrhage from IVC filters is typically self-limiting and can be managed with supportive care, although some patients may require arterial embolization or open surgery for hemorrhage control. A literature review regarding symptomatic duodenal perforation from IVC filters identified 21 case reports. Diagnosis for these patients often required multiple imaging modalities or esophagogastroduodenoscopy, but the authors suggest a high level of clinical suspicion for patients presenting with a history of IVC filter placement,

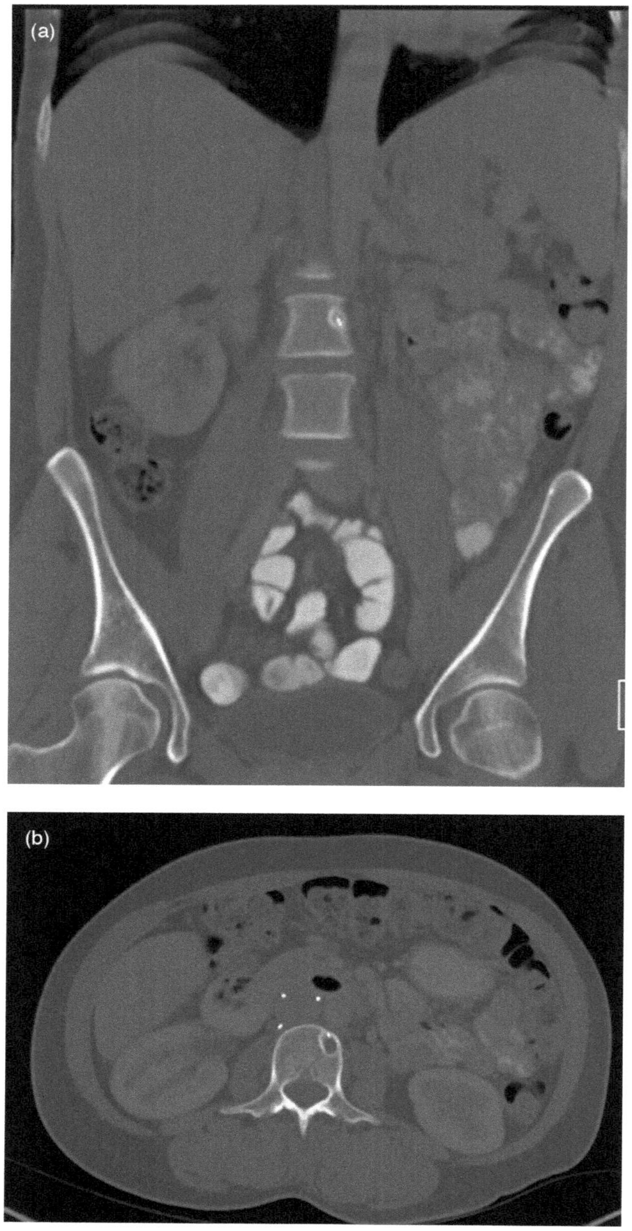

Figure 12.7 Filter strut penetration into the L3 vertebral body on coronal (a) and axial (b) CT. This patient was asymptomatic and managed conservatively.

and persistent abdominal pain or an episode of gastrointestinal bleeding. Regarding management, only 1 of these patients was successfully treated with endovascular retrieval, and the majority were treated with laparotomy. Those who had surgical exploration often demonstrated intense inflammatory reaction around the vena cava, precluding removal in 19% of patients. The cava was explored and the filter successfully removed in 48%. All patients who underwent caval exploration were closed using patch angioplasty, except for one which was closed primarily. For patients whose filters were unable to be removed, the offending struts were often trimmed with wire cutters. Complications following abdominal exploration were reported in one patient who had IVC and bilateral iliac vein thrombosis after trimming of the struts without caval exploration. No surgical deaths or incidents of pulmonary embolism were reported.[15,17]

IVC THROMBOSIS

Inferior vena cava thrombosis after IVC filter placement is reported in 2–30% of patients. Symptoms include bilateral lower extremity pain and edema; renal failure may occur if thrombus extends above the level of the renal veins. The risk of PE is also increased if the thrombus extends above the filter with recurrent pulmonary embolism occurring in 1–7%. The cause of filter thrombosis may be related to the patient's initial risk factors for thrombosis or the presence of foreign material within the body with progressive accumulation of thrombus on the struts. There is also the possibility of an entrapped, mobile thrombus within the filter rather the formation of new thrombus caused by the filter. There is no statistical difference in IVC thrombosis between patients with and without malignancy, although patients with metastatic disease may be at increased risk of recurrent PE despite filter placement. Rates of recurrent PE for patients with metastatic disease are reported at 10.4%, compared to 2.3% in those with non-metastatic malignancy. Tumor subtype (carcinoma vs sarcoma) does not appear to influence the likelihood of thrombotic complications.[5]

Once caval thrombosis is discovered, current practice includes systemic anticoagulation, with the majority managed without additional intervention. Acutely symptomatic patients may be managed with catheter-directed thrombolysis; however, the thrombus may be more subacute or chronic, and therefore refractory to thrombolytic therapy. In these patients, endovascular stent placement through the occluded filter has been described. Of note, prophylactic anticoagulation with an indwelling filter does not seem to improve the rate of IVC thrombosis.[9,18]

Another strategy for management includes pharmacomechanical thrombolysis. One device used for iliocaval thrombosis is the AngioJet device (Boston Scientific, Marlborough, MA), whose treatment mechanism uses the Venturi-Bernoulli principle. It uses high-pressure pulsatile jets with tissue plasminogen activator (tPA) solution to create low-pressure zones for thrombus maceration and aspiration. This reduces the duration and dose of thrombolytic therapy. AngioJet efficacy may be limited in large-diameter vessels such as the IVC, since the thrombectomy effect may not reach the vessel wall as it creates a channel through the clot (Figure 12.8).[19] Another example is the AngioVac system (AngioDynamics, Latham, NY) which removes large thrombi from the IVC. It uses an extracorporeal venovenous bypass system consisting of a 22F cannula with an expandable tip to create a suction vortex allowing for removal of large thrombi while maintaining flow with an extracorporeal centrifugal pump. This technique avoids the need for thrombolytic medication. There are several case reports in the literature describing successful use of the AngioVac for iliocaval thrombosis with an indwelling IVC filter.[20] A third device used for large vessel venous thrombosis is the ClotTriever system (Inari Medical, Irvine, CA) which also does not use thrombolytic medication. It is an over-the-wire device that uses a nitinol coring element and braided collection bag for mechanical thrombectomy. Reports in the literature describe its successful use for acute iliocaval thrombosis.[27]

RECURRENT PE AND DVT

The reported incidence of recurrent PE after IVC filter placement is between 0.5%–6%, although estimating the true incidence is difficult due to the number of unreported or unrecognized events. The PREPIC study randomized 400 patients with DVT at high risk for PE to either filter or nonfilter groups, and then further randomized them to receive low molecular weight heparin or unfractionated heparin. The 8 year follow-up results demonstrated a PE rate of 6.2% in the filter group compared to 15.1% in the non-filter group, but there was significant increase in the rate of DVT in those with IVC filter (35.7% vs 27.5%).[21] Current recommendations for IVC filter patients with recurrent PE are that systemic anticoagulation be used unless contraindicated. The presence of a filter should not alter the duration or intensity of anticoagulation.[8]

DVT is a common late complication of an indwelling IVC filter with an incidence as high as 43%. In the PREPIC study, filter recipients treated with anticoagulation were more likely to develop DVT compared to those on anticoagulation alone.[22] At 2 years, the risk of DVT in patients with an IVC filter was double those without. The etiology is thought to be from alterations in venous blood flow and the underlying coagulopathy of patients requiring an IVC filter. This risk may be mitigated by a retrievable filter, but only if they are removed. The incidence of DVT for indwelling retrievable filters is comparable to permanent filters (11.3% vs 12.6%).[9,23]

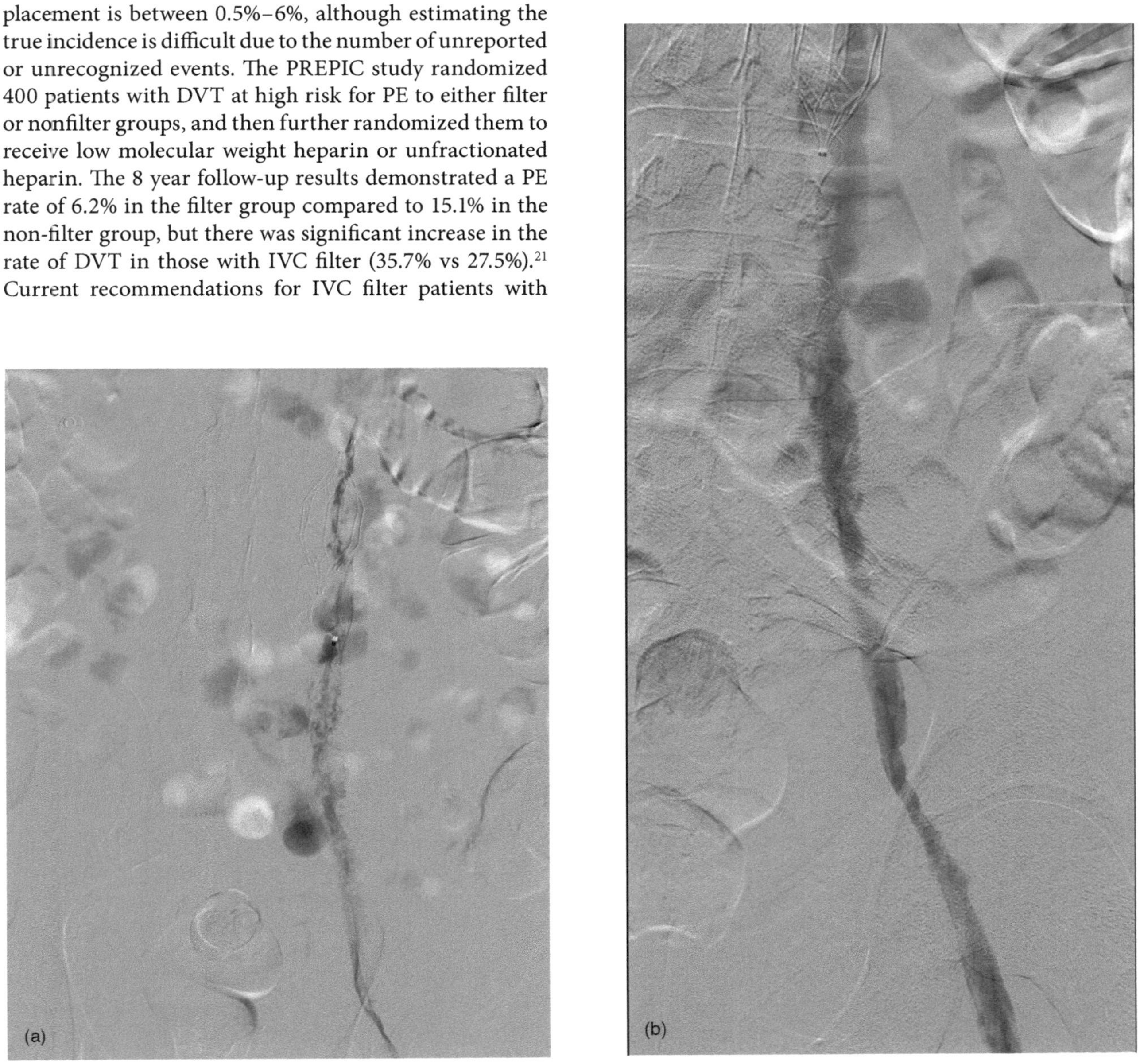

Figure 12.8 (a) Venogram showing iliocaval thrombosis in association with an existing filter, (b) treated with pharmacomechanical thrombolysis.

RETRIEVAL COMPLICATIONS

In 2010, the FDA published a warning regarding 146 cases of filter migration and 56 fractures that may have been associated with long-term placement of retrievable filters, and ended with the recommendation that "implanting physicians and clinicians responsible for the ongoing care of patients with retrievable IVC filters consider removing the filter as soon as protection from PE is no longer needed."[16] Retrieval rates for retrievable IVC filters have historically been as low as 5.2%, despite relatively high success and low complication rates associated with the procedure. In a retrospective review of 605 patients with retrievable IVC filters, a retrieval rate of 23% was demonstrated with an overall technical success rate of 93%. The most common reason for technical failure was large thrombus burden within the filter. Average indwelling filter time for this study was 111 days. Predictive risk factors for non-retrieval included age > 80 years, acute bleed, current malignancy, post-filter anticoagulation, and history of VTE.[24]

Complications associated with filter retrieval include device fracture, caval intussusception, dissection, and hemorrhage. Several factors increase the rate of complications during retrieval, including: longer indwelling times, increased tilt angle, and hook embedment. Complications for retrieval performed within 30 days of filter placement are rare, and there are increasing numbers of reports demonstrating safe retrieval with increasing dwell times.[9] An extreme example of this is a report of a Gunther-Tulip filter (Cook Medical, Inc.) removal 4753 days after placement. The apex of this filter was embedded into the caval wall and a Hangman technique was utilized. This uses a subapical guidewire loop to dissect the tissue and allows for release of the embedded filter. Once released, the apex was snared and a 16Fr sheath was advanced in an attempt to collapse the filter struts. This was unsuccessful despite significant traction force. To improve force on the struts, the CloverSnare (Cook Medical, Inc.) kit was used, consisting of a 10Fr outer and 8Fr inner sheath which were inserted through the 16Fr sheath with gradual telescopic advance of the sheaths over the struts to allow them to release from the fibrous tissue. This allowed for collapse of the struts and retrieval. This particular retrieval was performed in conjunction with stent reconstruction for post-thrombotic iliocaval obstruction using a combination of Wallstent (Boston Scientific, Natick, MA) in the distal IVC and two Protégé GPS stents (EV3 Endovascular, Inc., Plymouth, MN) at the bilateral iliocaval junction overlapping the IVC stent. The patient tolerated this well without complication.[25] An emerging strategy to facilitate retrieval of longstanding embedded filters is photothermal tissue ablation with an excimer laser. This technique is frequently used as an adjunct for removal of adherent venous pacemaker leads. In 2017, a 5-year prospective study of 251 consecutive patients undergoing laser-assisted IVC filter retrieval with the excimer sheath system was published. Mean dwell time was 979 days. The laser-assisted technique was employed after three failed attempts using standard retrieval force (measured digitally). The laser-assisted retrieval was successful in 99.2% of patients with a complication rate of 1.6%. The average force needed for retrieval was significantly less than during the failed attempts (6.7 vs 3.8 lbs).[26] These latter techniques should be considered as aggressive approaches to filter retrieval and require advanced catheter skills with appropriate patient selection.

FOLLOW-UP FOLLOWING FILTER INSERTION

Lack of follow-up and overall low removal rate for retrievable IVC filters has led some centers to develop dedicated IVC filter or thrombosis clinics to mitigate this issue. These measures increase retrieval rates and physician awareness of filter-related complications. Dedicated clerical staff arrange follow-up appointments and maintain patient databases, which were effective in improving follow-up and facilitating filter retrieval.[28,29] Other measures shown to improve retrieval rates include development of an institutional surveillance protocol identifying patients with filters on rounds, education of trauma providers, electronic tracking of filter patients, and automated email reminders for admitting physicians. Inadequate documentation of filter placement in patient charts and discharge instructions is likely another cause for low retrieval rates. In a multicenter retrospective review of retrievable IVC filters at tertiary care institutions over a 12-year period, filter insertion was documented in 342 of 810 cases (42%) and discharge instructions for filter removal or follow-up were seen in only 129 (16.3%). This group noted that if only the filter placement was mentioned in the discharge note, retrieval rates were not changed. However, if specific discharge instruction, for filter management were given, a statistically higher likelihood of filter removal was seen.[28]

CONCLUSION

Inferior vena caval filters offer a strategy for protecting patients against life-threatening PE in those who cannot tolerate systemic anticoagulation or in whom anticoagulation is not effective. Increasing numbers and types of IVC filters with longer dwell times result in a variety of complications at the time of placement and, more importantly, in the long term. Redoubling efforts to remove all filters in a timely fashion may mitigate the incidence of these complications. Likewise, awareness of these long-term risks relative to the natural history of a given thrombus may bring into question placement of a filter at all.

REFERENCES

1. White, RH. The Epidemiology of Venous Thromboembolism. Circulation. 2003. 107(23_suppl_1): p. I4-I8.
2. Horlander, KT, Mannino DM, and Leeper KV. Pulmonary embolism mortality in the United States, 1979-1998: an analysis using multiple-cause mortality data. Arch Intern Med, 2003;163(14): p. 1711–1717.
3. Duszak, R, Jr., et al. Placement and removal of inferior vena cava filters: national trends in the medicare population. J Am Coll Radiol. 2011,8(7): p. 483–489.
4. Morris E., et al. National Trends in Inferior Vena Cava Filter Placement and Retrieval Procedures in the Medicare Population Over Two Decades. J Am Coll Radiol. 2018;15(8): p. 1080–1086.
5. Abtahian, F., et al., Inferior vena cava filter usage, complications, and retrieval rate in cancer patients. Am J Med. 2014;127(11): p. 1111–1117.
6. Desai, TR, et al., Complications of indwelling retrievable versus permanent inferior vena cava filters. J Vasc Surg Venous Lymphat Disord. 2014;2(2): p. 166–173.
7. Wassef, A, Lim, W, and Wu, C. Indications, complications and outcomes of inferior vena cava filters: A retrospective study. Thromb Res. 2017;153: p. 123–128.
8. Sella, DM and Oldenburg, WA. Complications of inferior vena cava filters. Semin Vasc Surg. 2013;26(1): p. 23–28.
9. Grewal, S, Chamarthy, MR, and Kalva, SP. Complications of inferior vena cava filters. Cardiovasc Diagn Ther. 2016;6(6): p. 632–641.
10. Nguyen, NT, et al. Natural history of an intra-aortic permanent inferior vena cava filter. J Vasc Surg. 2014;60(3): p. 784.
11. Cuadra, SA, et al. Misplacement of a vena cava filter into the spinal canal. J Vasc Surg. 2009;50(5): p. 1170–1172.
12. Andreoli, JM, et al. Comparison of complication rates associated with permanent and retrievable inferior vena cava filters: a review of the MAUDE database. J Vasc Interv Radiol. 2014;25(8): p. 1181–1815.
13. Kesselman, AJ, et al. Endovascular Removal of Fractured Inferior Vena Cava Filter Fragments: 5-Year Registry Data with Prospective Outcomes on Retained Fragments. J Vasc Interv Radiol. 2018;29(6): p. 758–764.
14. Owens, CA, et al. Intracardiac migration of inferior vena cava filters: review of published data. Chest. 2009;136(3): p. 877–887.
15. Jia, Z, et al. Caval Penetration by Inferior Vena Cava Filters. Circulation. 2015;132(10): p. 944–952.
16. Ayad, MT and Gillespie, DL. Long-term complications of inferior vena cava filters. J Vasc Surg Venous Lymphat Disord. 2019;7(1): p. 139–144.
17. Malgor, RD. and Labropoulos, N. A systematic review of symptomatic duodenal perforation by inferior vena cava filters. J Vasc Surg. 2012;55(3): p. 856–861.e3.
18. Desai, KR, et al. Retrievable IVC Filters: Comprehensive Review of Device-related Complications and Advanced Retrieval Techniques. Radiographics. 2017;37(4): p. 1236–1245.
19. Golowa, Y, et al. Catheter directed interventions for inferior vena cava thrombosis. Cardiovasc Diagn Ther. 2016;6(6): p. 612–622.
20. Smith, SJ, et al. Vacuum-assisted thrombectomy device (AngioVac) in the management of symptomatic iliocaval thrombosis. J Vasc Interv Radiol. 2014;25(3): p. 425–430.
21. Decousus, H, et al. 8-year follow-up of patients with permanent vena cava filters in the prevention of pulmonary embolism: the PREPIC (Prevention du Risque d'Embolie Pulmonaire par Interruption Cave) randomized study. Circulation. 2005;112(3): p. 416–422.
22. Decousus, H, et al. A clinical trial of vena caval filters in the prevention of pulmonary embolism in patients with proximal deep-vein thrombosis. Prevention du Risque d'Embolie Pulmonaire par Interruption Cave Study Group. N Engl J Med. 1998;338(7): p. 409-415.
23. Kim, HS, et al. A comparison of clinical outcomes with retrievable and permanent inferior vena cava filters. J Vasc Interv Radiol. 2008;19(3): p. 393–399.
24. Siracuse, JJ, et al. Risk factors of nonretrieval of retrievable inferior vena cava filters. Ann Vasc Surg. 2015;29(2): p. 318–321.
25. Doshi, MH. and Narayanan, G. Late endovascular removal of Gunther-Tulip inferior vena cava filter and stent reconstruction of chronic post-thrombotic iliocaval obstruction after 4753 days of filter dwell time: a case report with review of literature. Radiol Case Rep. 2016;11(4): p. 348–353.
26. Kuo, WT, et al. Laser-Assisted Removal of Embedded Vena Cava Filters: A 5-Year First-in-Human Study. Chest. 2017;151(2): p. 417–424.
27. Crowner, JR, and Marston, WA. Percutaneous Thrombectomy Using a Novel Single-Session Device for Acute Iliocaval Deep Venous Thrombosis. J Vasc Surg Venous Lympat Disord. 2018;6: 300–301.
28. Tao, MJ, et al. Temporary inferior vena cava filter indications, retrieval rates, and follow-up management at a multicenter tertiary care institution. J Vasc Surg. 2016;64(2): 430–437.
29. Minocha, J et al. Improving Inferior Vena Cava Filter Retrieval Rates: Impact of a Dedicated Inferior Vena Cava Filter Clinic. J Vasc Interv Radiol. 2010;21: 1847–1851.

13

Complications of carotid endarterectomy

LAURA T. BOITANO AND MARK F. CONRAD

DESCRIPTION OF CAROTID ENDARTERECTOMY

INDICATIONS

Virtually all available practice guidelines recommend the use of degree of stenosis as the most important factor in determining the appropriateness of intervention in patients with carotid disease. Current indications for carotid endarterectomy (CEA) in the United States are the following: Asymptomatic patients with 70–99% stenosis on duplex ultrasound or axial imaging with a 3- to 5 year life expectancy and institutional combined perioperative stroke/death rates of ≤ 3%.[1] Although the Asymptomatic Carotid Atherosclerosis Study (ACAS) and the Asymptomatic Carotid Surgery Trial (ACST-1) demonstrated an advantage of CEA over best medical therapy in the prevention of stroke for patients with a 60% or greater stenosis, most surgeons reserve intervention for asymptomatic plaques to 70–99% stenosis.[2–4] In symptomatic patients, indications for CEA include ≥ 50% stenosis.

PROCEDURE

Carotid endarterectomy can be performed under local, regional, or general anesthesia. The type of anesthesia used is determined by patient risk factors, surgeon preference, and institutional familiarity with each approach. CEA should be performed with attention to the neurologic status of the patient while the internal carotid artery is clamped. Depending on the anesthetic chosen, different neuromonitoring strategies can be employed to reduce the risk of perioperative stroke due to lack of collateral flow. This will be discussed later in the chapter. There are no randomized trial data suggesting superiority of one anesthetic technique over another.[5] However, for access to a high bifurcation (above C2), maneuvers to assist with exposure including nasotracheal intubation and subluxation of the mandible must be performed under general anesthesia.[1]

The patient is positioned on the table with the neck turned toward the contralateral side, and a rolled towel or thyroid bag is placed under the shoulders in order to hyperextend the neck, thus facilitating access to the carotid bifurcation. It is important to ensure that the head does not float above the table and the head is held in position with 1-inch cloth tape. The incision is made along the anterior border of the sternocleidomastoid muscle (Figure 13.1). A pitfall at this point in the operation would be making the incision too medial so the larynx becomes an obstacle or too lateral, which can injure the spinal accessory or greater auricular nerves. The incision is carried towards the ear and should stop 1–2 cm below the mandible to reduce injury to the marginal mandibular branch of the facial nerve. The platysma is divided and the deep cervical fascia is incised anterior to the sternocleidomastoid muscle, which is retracted laterally. The carotid sheath is incised to then expose the internal jugular vein, which is exposed along its medial border. The common facial vein is divided to further allow lateral mobilization of the internal jugular vein. It is important to skeletonize the facial vein to avoid inadvertent ligation of the hypoglossal nerve, which can lie posterior to the vein in patients with a high bifurcation. The jugular vein is retracted laterally, and the common carotid artery is exposed. Heparin should be given at this time as a bolus, usually 100 units/kg.

The vagus nerve usually lies posterior to the common carotid artery but can be anterior in 15% of patients so it is important to identify its location prior to ligating any structures anterior to the common carotid. The ansa hypoglossi nerve also runs anterior to the common carotid artery and may be divided after the vagus nerve

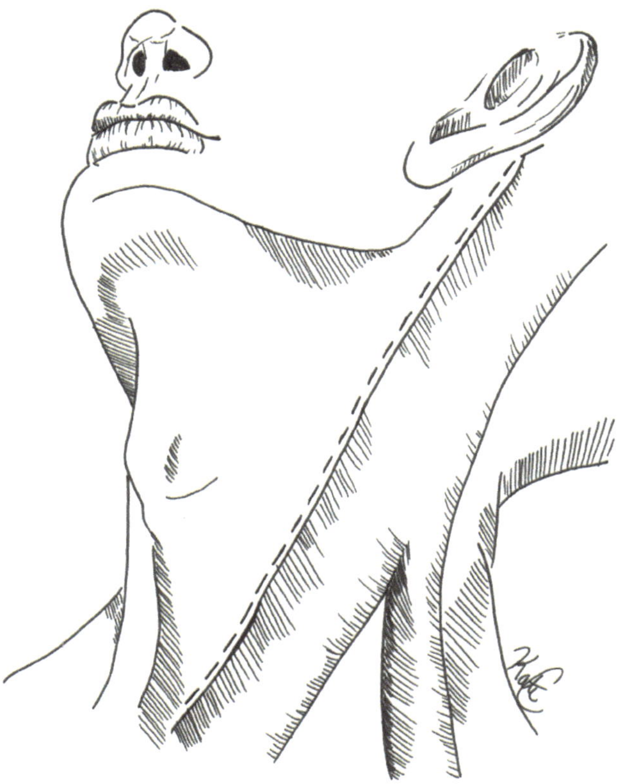

Figure 13.1 With the neck flexed and the head rotated away from the lesion, the incision is made along the anterior border of the sternocleidomastoid muscle.

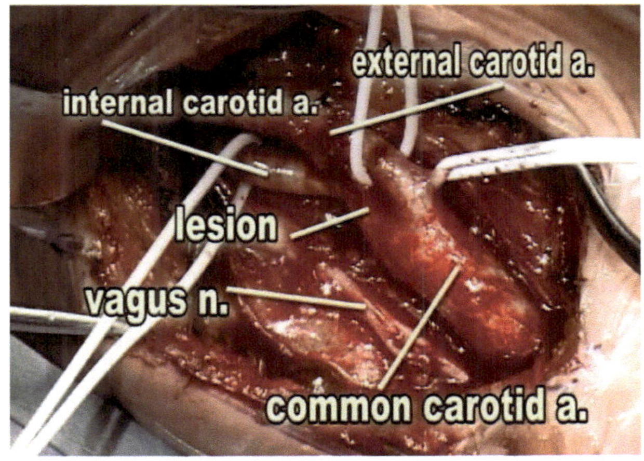

Figure 13.2 Dissected carotid artery.

has been identified. The ansa travels cephalad and joins the hypoglossal nerve, and its course should be traced prior to ligation. The common carotid artery is dissected and surrounded with an umbilical tape and tourniquet that can be used for proximal control if a shunt is needed. The carotid is freed from surrounding tissue, taking care not to disturb the bulb. The first branch of the external carotid artery, the superior thyroid artery is identified and circled with a loop. The external carotid artery (ECA) and internal carotid arteries (ICA) are then isolated. The hypoglossal nerve crosses the ICA at a variable distance from the bifurcation; in most cases, manipulation is unnecessary. However, if mobilization is required, there is usually a small arterial or venous branch from the sternocleidomastoid that acts as a sling around the nerve. Ligating this with suture or clips allows mobilization away from the ICA. Once the ICA is mobilized, the distal point should be palpated against a right angle to identify a soft spot above the plaque for clamping. If plaque can be palpated, the dissection must be carried higher (Figure 13.2).

The clamping sequence is as follows: the ICA is clamped distal to the area of disease, then CCA and ECA are clamped. Make sure that the vagus nerve is not clamped with the common carotid artery. An arteriotomy is made on the CCA with an 11-blade and extended to the ICA using Potts scissors. It is important to make big cuts through the plaque to avoid spiraling the arteriotomy posteriorly. The arteriotomy on the ICA is extended beyond the plaque to normal carotid artery. If a shunt is needed, it can be placed at this time into the ICA first, then it is allowed to flow backwards prior to placing it in the CCA to prevent any air from going to the brain. The flow in the shunt can be evaluated with a Doppler. The endarterectomy should be performed by removing the plaque and developing a plane between the media and adventitia of the artery. The distal plaque often feathers nicely but can be transected with a fine scissor if necessary. The proximal endpoint of the plaque usually needs to be excised with a Potts scissors. Plaque is removed from the ECA via an eversion technique. After the plaque is removed, heparinized saline irrigation is used to ensure that all of the plaque is adequately removed and to look for residual fibers that can act as a nidus for platelet plug formation. Following this, the prosthetic or vein patch is tailored to length and sewn onto the carotid artery with prolene suture. If a shunt was placed, it should be removed prior to closing the patch and clamps applied to the ICA and CCA. Before closure, all vessels are flushed to remove any potential emboli; then flow is restored. The appropriate sequence for clamp removal is from the ICA, then the ECA, then occlude the ICA with a Debakey forceps and open the CCA, allowing 5–6 heartbeats to push blood into the ECA. The wound bed is then inspected for hemostasis. Protamine can be administered. Once the wound is dry, the neck is closed in three layers with absorbable sutures to the fascia to the SCM followed by closure of the platysma and then staples on the skin. A subcuticular closure can also be used, but staples allow any bleeding to release before leading to airway compromise, and if removed on postoperative day 5 or 6, will leave a nice cosmetic result.

COMPLICATIONS

STROKE—PREVENTION

Intraoperatively, there are several techniques that can be used to reduce the risk of stroke. There should be minimal manipulation of the carotid bifurcation where the plaque is particularly bulky to reduce the risk of distal embolization during the dissection. Prior to clamping, a heparin bolus is given (100 units/kg) and a full three minutes should pass prior to application of any clamps. The heparin bolus is usually given after ligation of the facial vein and prior to manipulation of the carotid artery to reduce the risk of significant embolic events during dissection. The sequence of clamping is important and should always begin with the ICA to reduce the risk of embolization during application of other clamps, and the placement of this clamp should be on a soft area of the artery, distal to the plaque. The endpoint of the arteriotomy is critical to the success of the operation, and it should sit flush with the arterial wall with no lifting when heparinized saline is applied; tacking sutures may be placed distally if necessary.

Cerebral protection and monitoring during the CEA are critical to prevent stroke due to lack of collateral circulation to the brain. There are three ways to assess blood flow to the brain during carotid cross clamping: electroencephalography (EEG) monitoring, carotid stump pressures, and neurologic changes in an awake patient. The gold standard for neuromonitoring is awake neurologic monitoring, which requires CEA to be performed under regional or local anesthesia. In this situation, neurologic symptoms following arterial clamp placement would mandate shunting. However, it is often difficult for awake patients to lie still for the duration of the operation and many anesthesiologists struggle with regional neck blocks, making availability hospital-dependent. Under general anesthesia there are multiple modalities to monitor cerebral blood flow during carotid clamping. These include: EEG, carotid stump measurements, somatosensory evoked potentials, transcranial Doppler measurement of middle cerebral artery flow, or cerebral oximetry measurements. EEG is the most commonly employed strategy; it is very sensitive, which results in a fairly high false positive rate requiring use of shunting in situations where shunts could be avoided.[6] However, the rate of selective shunting with EEG is around 5% in most series. Shunting is an important aspect of all strategies of neuromonitoring. Indeed, it is imperative that the shunt be placed properly to avoid risk of embolic stroke, air embolus, or dissection. Based on the most recent Society for Vascular Surgery Guidelines for the management of extracranial carotid disease, there is no clear benefit of routine shunting versus selective shunting, and individual practices will vary depending on availability of the various forms of neuromonitoring.[1] Non-shunting, on the other hand, is not advocated. A recent meta-analysis found that stroke rate after routine shunting was 1.4%, whereas after routine non-shunting the stroke rate was 2%, and the stroke rate after selective shunting ranged from 1.1% to 4.8% depending on the neuromonitoring strategy employed.[7]

Timing of carotid endarterectomy following stroke is an area of some controversy as the surgeon must balance the need to remove the embolic risk of atherosclerotic plaque to prevent future stroke and the risk of hemorrhagic conversion or worsening of the ischemic penumbra when performing surgery in the peri-stroke time period.[8] Traditionally, it was recommended that CEA be delayed 6 weeks after a major stroke; however, with newer imaging technology, patients can be stratified into those who are high risk for hemorrhagic conversion with early surgery and those who are not. In the advent of this, several studies have tried to determine the optimal timing of CEA after stroke; initially studies favored treatment within 48 hours of the index stroke,[9] but the updated guidelines from the Society for Vascular Surgery, taking into account all available evidence, suggest that treatment after symptomatic carotid disease should take place within 2 weeks after patients are medically stabilized.[1] Recently, a study by Tanious et. al. suggested that CEA should be delayed for more than 48 hours after the index stroke, and the optimal timing is between 2 and 14 days after the index stroke, as this was shown to be associated with lower odds of postoperative stroke/death and stroke compared with an earlier or later intervention.[8]

STROKE—MANAGEMENT

Following completion of the carotid endarterectomy, all patients should undergo a neurologic examination upon emergence from anesthesia. If new neurologic abnormalities are identified in the operating room before travel to the post-anesthesia care unit, anesthesia should be restarted and the incision should be opened and flow within the ICA should be checked with a Doppler probe. If there is flow within the ICA and it appears normal, further investigation is warranted in terms of duplex ultrasonography or arteriography in the operating room (OR). In this situation, most commonly the etiologies are distal embolization or dissection; however, ischemia during clamping is also a potential etiology. Angiography is the preferred modality in this case as intracranial vessels can be evaluated and potentially treated with neuro-salvage techniques if an embolus is found. This should be done in conjunction with neurosurgical or neuro-interventional colleagues.

If Duplex evaluation shows that there is no flow identified in the ICA, the endarterectomy must be explored. In this scenario, there is a high suspicion for a technical issue with the endarterectomy endpoints or patch closure. In this scenario, it is recommended that distal ICA clamping be avoided. Thrombus may extrude from the arteriotomy without maneuvers due to backpressure; however, if the thrombus persists, balloon embolectomy may be required. In this case, caution should be exercised as over-distention of a balloon in the distal ICA can result in a carotid artery-cavernous fistula. Following thrombectomy, the endarterectomy must be inspected carefully to identify the technical issue and this should be repaired prior to re-patch closure. This often requires extension of the arteriotomy proximally and distally to better visualize the endpoints and look for dissection flaps.

A patient who is neurologically intact initially and develops a neurologic deficit in the post-anesthesia care unit or later in recovery should be managed differently than a patient who awakes in the OR with an immediate deficit. In this case, a stat duplex should be performed at the bedside. If there is evidence for stenosis, intimal flap, occlusion, or other abnormality, the patient should be taken immediately to the operating room for re-exploration. If there are no stat ultrasound capabilities at the hospital or there is no defect found on carotid duplex ultrasound, the patient should undergo a stat non-contrast CT of the head followed by a CTA head and neck. This will identify a hemorrhagic stroke and characterize the carotid system to find the cause of the problem such as a dissection, occlusion, or defect that has embolic potential (Figure 13.3). If there is an embolus, anticoagulation can be initiated, and the patient should be immediately taken to the angiography suite for clot retrieval. However, a hemorrhagic stroke warrants reversal of any anticoagulation and may require discussion with neurosurgery. Strokes are rare after carotid surgery, and early identification with a swift and deliberate response can limit the long-term sequelae of this dreaded complication.

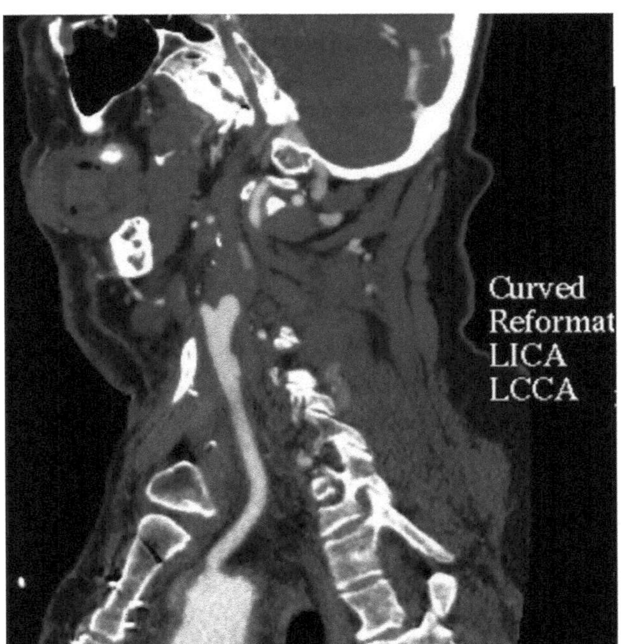

Figure 13.3 3D reconstruction of acutely occluded carotid artery after CEA.

CARDIAC-MI—PREVENTION

Coronary artery disease often accompanies carotid artery disease. Cardiac complications, including myocardial infarction (MI), are associated with significantly higher perioperative mortality, and a recent study found that such complications account for the majority of deaths following CEA.[10] The Carotid Revascularization Endarterectomy Versus Stenting Trial (CREST) found that patients who had an MI with EKG changes or postoperative biomarker elevation were significantly more likely to die in the follow-up period, even after adjusting for other risk-factors for mortality.[11] Fortunately, over time the rate of cardiac complications have decreased due to improved preoperative risk stratification and management as well as improved medication regimens. Indeed, a recent systematic review and meta-analysis found that the rate of MI after CEA was under 1% in contemporary series.[12]

With regard to cardiac risk stratification, CEA is considered an intermediate risk procedure. Patients who have a functional capacity of at least 4.0 METS, which is consistent with moderate activity, do not require further preoperative cardiac testing.[13] Patients who have a history of coronary angiography and/or revascularization within the last 5 years or a normal stress test within 2 years do not need a formal cardiac evaluation prior to CEA unless there has been a change in their exercise capacity and/or new-onset symptoms such as angina or shortness of breath. In patients without such functional capacity or with recent onset of symptoms, cardiac evaluation including a stress test is recommended. In addition to appropriate screening, perioperative optimal medical therapy is essential for successful long-term outcomes. The PeriOperative Ischemic Evaluation (POISE) trial showed a reduction of cardiac events with beta-blocker therapy.[14] The most recent Society for Vascular Surgery guidelines suggest beta-blocker therapy is "nearly universally required in this patient group," given the concomitant nature of carotid and coronary disease.[1] In addition to beta-blocker therapy, aspirin and statin as well as most home medications should be continued through the perioperative period.

CARDIAC-MI—MANAGEMENT

The diagnosis of MI is confirmed with an elevated troponin above the person's baseline in addition to symptoms of ischemia, or electrocardiogram findings consistent with a new MI including: new ST-segment, T wave changes, new left bundle branch block, or pathological Q waves. Once the diagnosis is confirmed, immediate consultation with cardiology is indicated.

CRANIAL NERVE INJURY—PREVENTION

Cranial nerve injury is usually related to stretch, retraction, clamping, and very rarely transection.[15,16] The rate of cranial nerve injury varies in the literature. Some of this variation has to do with the method of assessing for, and the definition of, cranial nerve injury. For instance, in the CREST trial, cranial nerve injury occurred in about 5% of patients undergoing CEA.[17] This was echoed in a recent report of the Vascular Study Group of New England, which reported a rate of 5.6% at discharge.[18] In contrast, a study which utilized an exam by an otolaryngologist reported an incidence of 27%; however, only 7% of injuries were permanent, and none were disabling.[19] Consistent with this, most cranial nerve injury is transient and most studies report permanent cranial nerve injury in less than 1% of patients.[18,20] The most commonly injured nerve is the hypoglossal nerve.[18,20] Conditions that may increase the rate of cranial nerve injury include high-risk anatomic conditions such as history of previous neck radiation, previous neck surgery (i.e., for cancer or previous CEA), and tracheostomy. These conditions can distort tissue planes and make identification of cranial nerves more difficult, so the decision to pursue CEA is based on imaging as well as local skin and neck conditions.[21]

Cranial nerve injury can be minimized by knowledge of anatomy and anticipation of anatomic variations. The first potential encounter with cranial nerve is with the placement of the incision. The marginal mandibular branch of the facial nerve can be injured if the incision is extended to the mandible which is why the distal extent of the incision should be limited to 1–2 cm from the angle of the jaw. If cranial extension of the incision is required, it should be curved posteriorly to reduce the risk of nerve injury. If injured, there is a distortion in the smile expression.[19] The greater auricular nerve, which is a cutaneous sensory nerve, can also be encountered at the superior aspect of the longitudinal CEA incision. Injury manifests as numbness of the earlobe as well as numbness of the angle of the mandible.

The vagus nerve should be immediately identified after ligation and transection of the facial vein. It typically lies posterior to the common carotid artery, however, on occasion it can be found anterior.[15] It is imperative that this nerve not be confused with the ansa cervicalis, which can be divided without consequence. Rarely, the recurrent laryngeal nerve branches from the vagus at the carotid bifurcation, a phenomenon called "nonrecurrent recurrent laryngeal nerve." Injury to the vagus or the non-recurrent laryngeal nerve results in ipsilateral vocal cord paralysis, which manifests as hoarseness and weak cough.[19] The superior laryngeal nerve is a branch of the vagus nerve and courses posterior to the external and internal carotid artery to the larynx. It isn't usually seen in the operative field but may be injured if clamps on the ICA or ECA are not applied appropriately or when dissection of the superior thyroid artery. Injury to this nerve may result in early fatigability of the voice, changes in voice quality, or difficulty swallowing. The hypoglossal nerve crosses a variable distance from the carotid bifurcation and usually behind the posterior belly of the digastric muscle.[15] In cases of a high carotid bifurcation or a long carotid lesion extending well into the ICA, the nerve may be encountered and often requires mobilization. Safe mobilization can be performed by dividing the ansa hypoglossi. Dissection should be continued along the posterior border of this nerve to avoid injury to the hypoglossal. The more mobilization that is required, the higher likelihood of injury. Hypoglossal nerve injury can be an obvious finding on postoperative examination as the tongue will deviate to the affected side (ipsilateral to the CEA) due to tongue weakness. In cases of transection, patients will have difficulty swallowing and with speech articulation. Bilateral nerve injury can result in airway obstruction and, in some cases, may require tracheostomy.[15] The glossopharyngeal nerve is typically more cephalad to the operative field. An important branch is the nerve of Hering, which innervates the carotid sinus; extensive dissection around the carotid bifurcation may injure this nerve, resulting in bradycardia and hypotension.

In addition to knowledge of anatomy, care should be taken during the procedure to avoid nerve injury. This includes sharp dissection on the artery and meticulous use of forceps, retractors, clamps, and cautery.[16]

CN INJURY—MANAGEMENT

If a cranial nerve injury is suspected, immediate consultation with an otolaryngologist is recommended. Nerve injury is most commonly due to edema rather than transection. Steroids and bed elevation are often employed with resolution of the deficit. However, in cases of transection, immediate repair is required.

BLEEDING—PREVENTION

Bleeding after CEA is an important complication to avoid as large neck hematomas can result in airway compromise and death.[22] Luckily, significant bleeding is rare due to meticulous evaluation of the operative field prior to closure. Postoperative bleeding is reported to occur in under 3.0% of cases.[23,24] A valsava maneuver can be given by the anesthesia team to test the anastomosis. In addition, the blood pressure should be artificially raised briefly to simulate a hypertensive episode postoperatively. If significant bleeding is identified during these maneuvers, it should be treated with ligation, suture, or electrocautery. Some surgeons prefer to place a drain prior to closing the incision to monitor bleeding. Furthermore, many surgeons reverse the therapeutic anticoagulation administered intraoperatively with protamine, and there is evidence that this reduces bleeding complications after CEA without increasing the incidence of stroke.[24] In a study of a regional CEA registry, authors found bleeding requiring reoperation was rare but significantly higher in patients who did not receive protamine (1.7% no protamine vs 0.6% protamine). Furthermore, hypertension should be avoided in the perioperative period to reduce the incidence of hematoma (Figure 13.4).

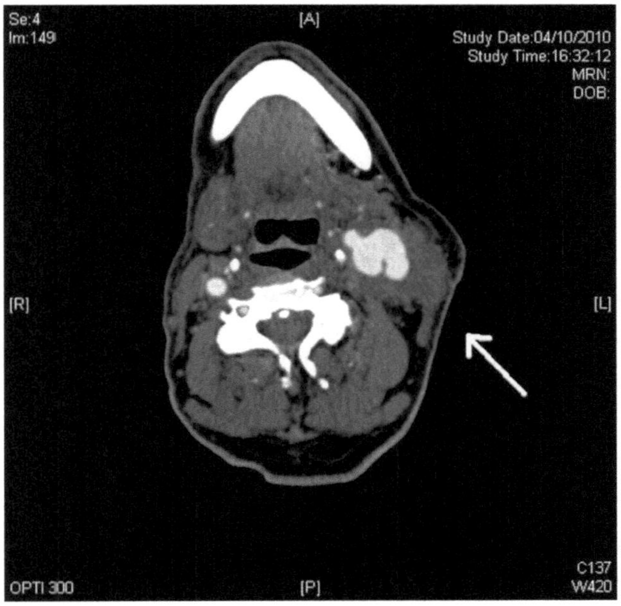

Figure 13.4 Carotid pseudoaneurysm after CEA.

BLEEDING—MANAGEMENT

If a significant cervical hematoma is identified, the patient should be immediately taken back to the operating room for wound exploration and hematoma evacuation. Anticoagulation should be reversed. Most commonly bleeding is from an arterial source, so management at the bedside is not optimal. Furthermore, if bright red blood is pouring into the drain, the patient should be rushed to the operating room. In cases of a small, nonexpanding hematoma, anticoagulation can be reversed and the site can be monitored. However, there should be a low threshold for returning to the operating room should there be evidence for expansion.

HYPERTENSION AND CEREBRAL HYPERPERFUSION SYNDROME—PREVENTION

Cerebral hyperperfusion syndrome results from an "unexpected increase in cerebral blood flow > 100%, potentially leading to cerebral hemorrhage."[25] The mechanism by which this occurs is related to chronic ischemia resulting in maximal dilation of cerebral vessels and lack of autoregulation followed by normal or elevated blood flow after carotid revascularization. This results in cerebral edema and potentially hemorrhage.[25–28] Though a rare complication after CEA (0–3% in the literature), it is associated with high mortality of up to 50%.[26,27] The syndrome typically occurs as a delayed perioperative complication on postoperative day 3 to 6. Clinical manifestations include headache, which is ipsilateral to the CEA, focal neurologic deficits, cerebral edema, brain hemorrhage, and seizures.[26–28] In its early stages, the edema is reversible so early recognition is critical to prevention of catastrophic consequences.

Preoperative or intraoperative risk factors include high-grade carotid artery stenosis, impaired cerebrovascular reserve including contralateral carotid artery stenosis, intraoperative distal carotid pressure < 40 mmHg, intraoperative ischemia, and recent contralateral CEA.[26,27] Timing of CEA has also been shown to play a role in the development of cerebral hyperperfusion; CEA performed in close proximity to an ischemic event, either TIA or stroke, increases the risk of cerebral hyperperfusion. Furthermore, ipsilateral CEA should be performed at least 3 months after contralateral CEA to reduce the risk of cerebral hyperperfusion. The most important risk factor cited by many studies, however, is perioperative hypertension.[25–27] Hypertension has been shown to be the most influential factor in the development of cerebral hyperperfusion, so strict blood pressure control is imperative to preventing this complication.

HYPERTENSION AND CEREBRAL HYPERPERFUSION SYNDROME – MANAGEMENT

The most important management strategy for cerebral hyperperfusion syndrome is prevention. This includes strict blood pressure control with a goal systolic blood pressure of less than 150 mmHg. Intravenous agents such as labetalol, nitroprusside, and nitroglycerin can be utilized to meet this goal. Patients who present with a severe ipsilateral headache should undergo head CT and have strict blood pressure control. Seizures can be treated with standard antiepileptic medication. In severe cases, patients may receive platelet transfusions to ameliorate the antiplatelet effect of aspirin or other antiplatelet medication (Table 13.1).

RESTENOSIS

Restenosis is rare after CEA but can occur up to 5% of the time. This can be minimized by performing either a patch angioplasty technique or eversion endarterectomy. Regarding patch angioplasty, there is no superiority of one patch material over another, but clearly patching is superior to primary closure in terms of perioperative outcomes including stroke and restenosis.[1,29] Indeed, the most recent SVS guidelines recommend these closures as the standard of care over primary repair. Following application and suturing of the patch but before the final knot is tied, the CCA and ICA clamps are released to remove air and potential embolic material from the artery. It should be noted that an alternative to patch angioplasty is an eversion technique which is most effective for tortuous and redundant carotid arteries. The EVEREST study compared eversion to standard CEA in a randomized prospective fashion and found no statistically

Table 13.1 Cerebral hyperperfusion syndrome: Prevention, signs/symptoms, and management

Prevention	Explanation
Blood pressure control	Even patients with normal blood pressure preoperatively may have fluctuations in pressure. Beta-blockers and clonidine are the treatment of choice as they reduce cerebral perfusion and mean arterial pressure without directly affecting cerebral blood flow.
Timing of CEA	For patients with bilateral disease requiring treatment, wait at least 3 months to revascularize the contralateral side
Signs/Symptoms	
Ipsilateral headache, seizures, neurologic symptoms from hyperperfusion-related stroke and intracranial hemorrhage	Headache is usually the first symptom to develop, seizures typically follow, and late (and rare) manifestations include infarct extension and intracerebral hemorrhage
Management	
Blood pressure control	Blood pressure control after recognizing cerebral hyperperfusion is important. Beta-blockers and clonidine should similarly be used.
Anti-epileptic medications	Should be utilized for patients with EEG consistent with seizure or if clinically the patient develops a seizure
Mannitol or hypertonic saline	Cerebral edema treatment with these agents may be effective
Corticosteroids	Unclear benefit

significant differences in outcomes.[30] Furthermore, the use of completion imaging remains an area of unclear benefit according to the most recent Society for Vascular Surgery guidelines, and usage is a personal preference as it is unclear if all detected abnormalities on completion imaging are clinically meaningful.[1] Patients should undergo regular surveillance after CEA to monitor for restenosis.

REFERENCES

1. Ricotta JJ, Aburahma A, Ascher E, Eskandari M, Faries P, Lal BK, et al. Updated Society for Vascular Surgery guidelines for management of extracranial carotid disease: Executive summary. J Vasc Surg. 2011;54(3): 832–836.
2. Endarterectomy for asymptomatic carotid artery stenosis. Executive Committee for the Asymptomatic Carotid Atherosclerosis Study. JAMA. 1995;273(18): 1421–1428.
3. Halliday AW, Thomas DJ, Mansfield AO. The asymptomatic carotid surgery trial (ACST). Int Angiol. 1995;14(1): 18–20.
4. Halliday A, Harrison M, Hayter E, Kong X, Mansfield A, Marro J, et al. 10-year stroke prevention after successful carotid endarterectomy for asymptomatic stenosis (ACST-1): a multicentre randomised trial. Lancet. 2010;376(9746): 1074–1084.
5. Group GTC, Lewis SC, Warlow CP, Bodenham AR, Colam B, Rothwell PM, et al. General anaesthesia versus local anaesthesia for carotid surgery (GALA): A multicentre, randomised controlled trial. Lancet. 2008;372(9656): 2132–2142.
6. Stoughton J, Nath RL, Abbott WM. Comparison of simultaneous electroencephalographic and mental status monitoring during carotid endarterectomy with regional anesthesia. J Vasc Surg. 1998;28(6): 1014–1021; discussion 21-3.
7. Aburahma AF, Mousa AY, Stone PA. Shunting during carotid endarterectomy. J Vasc Surg. 2011;54(5): 1502–1510.
8. Tanious A, Pothof AB, Boitano LT, Pendleton AA, Wang LJ, de Borst GJ, et al. Timing of carotid endarterectomy after stroke: Retrospective review of prospectively collected national database. Ann Surg. 2018;268(3): 449–456.
9. Ferrero E, Ferri M, Viazzo A, Labate C, Berardi G, Pecchio A, et al. A retrospective study on early carotid endarterectomy within 48 hours after transient ischemic attack and stroke in evolution. Ann Vasc Surg. 2014;28(1): 227–238.
10. Musser DJ, Nicholas GG, Reed JF 3rd. Death and adverse cardiac events after carotid endarterectomy. J Vasc Surg. 1994;19(4): 615–622.
11. Blackshear JL, Cutlip DE, Roubin GS, Hill MD, Leimgruber PP, Begg RJ, et al. Myocardial infarction after carotid stenting and endarterectomy: results from the carotid revascularization endarterectomy versus stenting trial. Circulation. 2011;123(22): 2571–2578.
12. Boulanger M, Cameliere L, Felgueiras R, Berger L, Rerkasem K, Rothwell PM, et al. Periprocedural myocardial infarction after carotid endarterectomy and stenting: Systematic review and meta-analysis. Stroke. 2015;46(10): 2843–2848.
13. Fleisher LA, Fleischmann KE, Auerbach AD, Barnason SA, Beckman JA, Bozkurt B, et al. 2014 ACC/AHA guideline on perioperative

cardiovascular evaluation and management of patients undergoing noncardiac surgery: A report of the American College of Cardiology/American Heart Association Task Force on Practice Guidelines. Circulation. 2014;130(24): e278–333.

14. Group PS, Devereaux PJ, Yang H, Yusuf S, Guyatt G, Leslie K, et al. Effects of extended-release metoprolol succinate in patients undergoing non-cardiac surgery (POISE trial): A randomised controlled trial. Lancet. 2008;371(9627): 1839–1847.
15. Schauber MD, Fontenelle LJ, Solomon JW, Hanson TL. Cranial/cervical nerve dysfunction after carotid endarterectomy. J Vasc Surg. 1997;25(3): 481–487.
16. Kakisis JD, Antonopoulos CN, Mantas G, Moulakakis KG, Sfyroeras G, Geroulakos G. Cranial nerve injury after carotid endarterectomy: Incidence, risk factors, and time trends. Eur J Vasc Endovasc Surg. 2017;53(3): 320–335.
17. Brott TG, Hobson RW 2nd, Howard G, Roubin GS, Clark WM, Brooks W, et al. Stenting versus endarterectomy for treatment of carotid-artery stenosis. N Engl J Med. 2010;363(1): 11–23.
18. Fokkema M, de Borst GJ, Nolan BW, Indes J, Buck DB, Lo RC, et al. Clinical relevance of cranial nerve injury following carotid endarterectomy. Eur J Vasc Endovasc Surg. 2014;47(1): 2–7.
19. Zannetti S, Parente B, De Rango P, Giordano G, Serafini G, Rossetti M, et al. Role of surgical techniques and operative findings in cranial and cervical nerve injuries during carotid endarterectomy. Eur J Vasc Endovasc Surg. 1998;15(6): 528–531.
20. Cunningham EJ, Bond R, Mayberg MR, Warlow CP, Rothwell PM. Risk of persistent cranial nerve injury after carotid endarterectomy. J Neurosurg. 2004;101(3): 445–448.
21. Tsantilas P, Kuehnl A, Brenner E, Eckstein HH. Anatomic criteria determining high-risk carotid surgery patients. J Cardiovasc Surg (Torino). 2017;58(2): 152–160.
22. Greenstein AJ, Chassin MR, Wang J, Rockman CB, Riles TS, Tuhrim S, et al. Association between minor and major surgical complications after carotid endarterectomy: Results of the New York Carotid Artery Surgery study. J Vasc Surg. 2007;46(6): 1138–1144; discussion 45-6.
23. Nunn DB. Carotid endarterectomy: an analysis of 234 operative cases. Ann Surg. 1975;182(6): 733–738.
24. Stone DH, Nolan BW, Schanzer A, Goodney PP, Cambria RA, Likosky DS, et al. Protamine reduces bleeding complications associated with carotid endarterectomy without increasing the risk of stroke. J Vasc Surg. 2010;51(3): 559–564, 64e1.
25. De Rango P. Cerebral hyperperfusion syndrome: the dark side of carotid endarterectomy. Eur J Vasc Endovasc Surg. 2012;43(4):377.
26. Wang GJ, Beck AW, DeMartino RR, Goodney PP, Rockman CB, Fairman RM. Insight into the cerebral hyperperfusion syndrome following carotid endarterectomy from the national Vascular Quality Initiative. J Vasc Surg. 2017;65(2): 381–389e2.
27. Farooq MU, Goshgarian C, Min J, Gorelick PB. Pathophysiology and management of reperfusion injury and hyperperfusion syndrome after carotid endarterectomy and carotid artery stenting. Exp Transl Stroke Med. 2016;8(1): 7.
28. Sundt TM Jr., Sharbrough FW, Piepgras DG, Kearns TP, Messick JM Jr., O'Fallon WM. Correlation of cerebral blood flow and electroencephalographic changes during carotid endarterectomy: With results of surgery and hemodynamics of cerebral ischemia. Mayo Clin Proc. 1981;56(9): 533–543.
29. Rockman CB, Halm EA, Wang JJ, Chassin MR, Tuhrim S, Formisano P, et al. Primary closure of the carotid artery is associated with poorer outcomes during carotid endarterectomy. J Vasc Surg. 2005;42(5): 870–877.
30. Cao P, Giordano G, De Rango P, Zannetti S, Chiesa R, Coppi G, et al. A randomized study on eversion versus standard carotid endarterectomy: study design and preliminary results: The Everest Trial. J Vasc Surg. 1998;27(4): 595–605.

SUGGESTED READINGS

Halliday A, Harrison M, Hayter E, Kong X, Mansfield A, Marro J, et al. 10-year stroke prevention after successful carotid endarterectomy for asymptomatic stenosis (ACST-1): a multicentre randomised trial. Lancet. 2010;376(9746):1074–84.

Boulanger M, Cameliere L, Felgueiras R, Berger L, Rerkasem K, Rothwell PM, et al. Periprocedural Myocardial Infarction After Carotid Endarterectomy and Stenting: Systematic Review and Meta-Analysis. Stroke. 2015;46(10):2843–8.

14

Complications of extracranial carotid aneurysm repair and resection of carotid body tumor

SACHINDER SINGH HANS AND MARY LEE

CAROTID ANEURYSM REPAIR

Extracranial carotid aneurysms are uncommon and are often the result of atherosclerotic degenerative disease, fibromuscular dysplasia, or trauma.[1,2] Because of the risk of cerebral embolization with resultant stroke and occasional risk of rupture, repair of the carotid aneurysm is recommended in most patients.[1,2] In addition, patients with large extracranial carotid aneurysm may develop local compression symptoms. In contemporary practice, aneurysm resection with interposition grafting, patch angioplasty, or simple end-to-end anastomosis following resection of the aneurysm can be performed because of the associated redundancy of the internal carotid artery (ICA). Operative repair often presents a clinical challenge to the surgeon due to associated inflammation, small diameter thin wall ICA, and in patients in whom the carotid aneurysm is located 2–3 cm above the carotid bifurcation extending toward the base of the skull (Figure 14.1). Recent reports have advocated the use of covered stents in high-risk patients with suitable anatomy. In patients with distal location of the aneurysm, mandibular subluxation may become necessary in order to gain distal exposure. Surgical repair is effective but has a combined mortality/major stroke rate of 4–9%.[1] In patients with distal ICA aneurysm, the incidence of postoperative cranial nerve dysfunction can be as high as 44%.[2]

COMPLICATIONS

The most common postoperative complication of carotid aneurysm repair is carotid nerve injury in the range of 3–17%.[2] The stroke rate of untreated carotid aneurysm can be as high as 50%, and the postoperative stroke-free rate is excellent with 80–87% of patients remaining symptom free.[2] Zhou et al. reported 42 cases of carotid aneurysm and divided them into two groups: group one (1985–1994) had 22 patients, and group two (1995–2004) had 20 patients.[2] In group one all patients underwent open repair, while in group two 14 patients underwent endovascular interventions, 5 interposition grafting following resection, and 1 carotid ligation. Most aneurysms in their series were atherosclerotic but 36% were pseudoaneurysms.[2] The incidence for cranial nerve palsy was 14% in group one and 5% in group two. The 30-day mortality/major stroke was 14% in group one and 5% in group two ($p < .04$).[2]

CAROTID BODY TUMOR RESECTION

Carotid body tumor (cervical paraganglioma) are the most common head and neck paragangliomas.[3,4] These tumors arise from the paraganglia cells that migrate from the neural crest near the sympathetic ganglia.[3,4] These tumors may go undetected as they are benign and indolent. Large tumors, especially if they are larger than 3 cm in size, are palpable on physical examination as a neck mass anterior to sternomastoid and overlying the carotid bifurcation.[3,4] The carotid body tumors are mobile in a medial-to-lateral plane. A recent review of carotid body tumors revealed a mean age of 55 years (18–94 years) at time of diagnosis with male-to-female ratio of 1:1.9.[3,4] Most tumors were on the right side (57%) with 25% on the left and 17% bilateral. These tumors are usually sporadic but are familial in 10–20% of patients.[3,4] These tumors can have malignant potential (4.3%); spread to

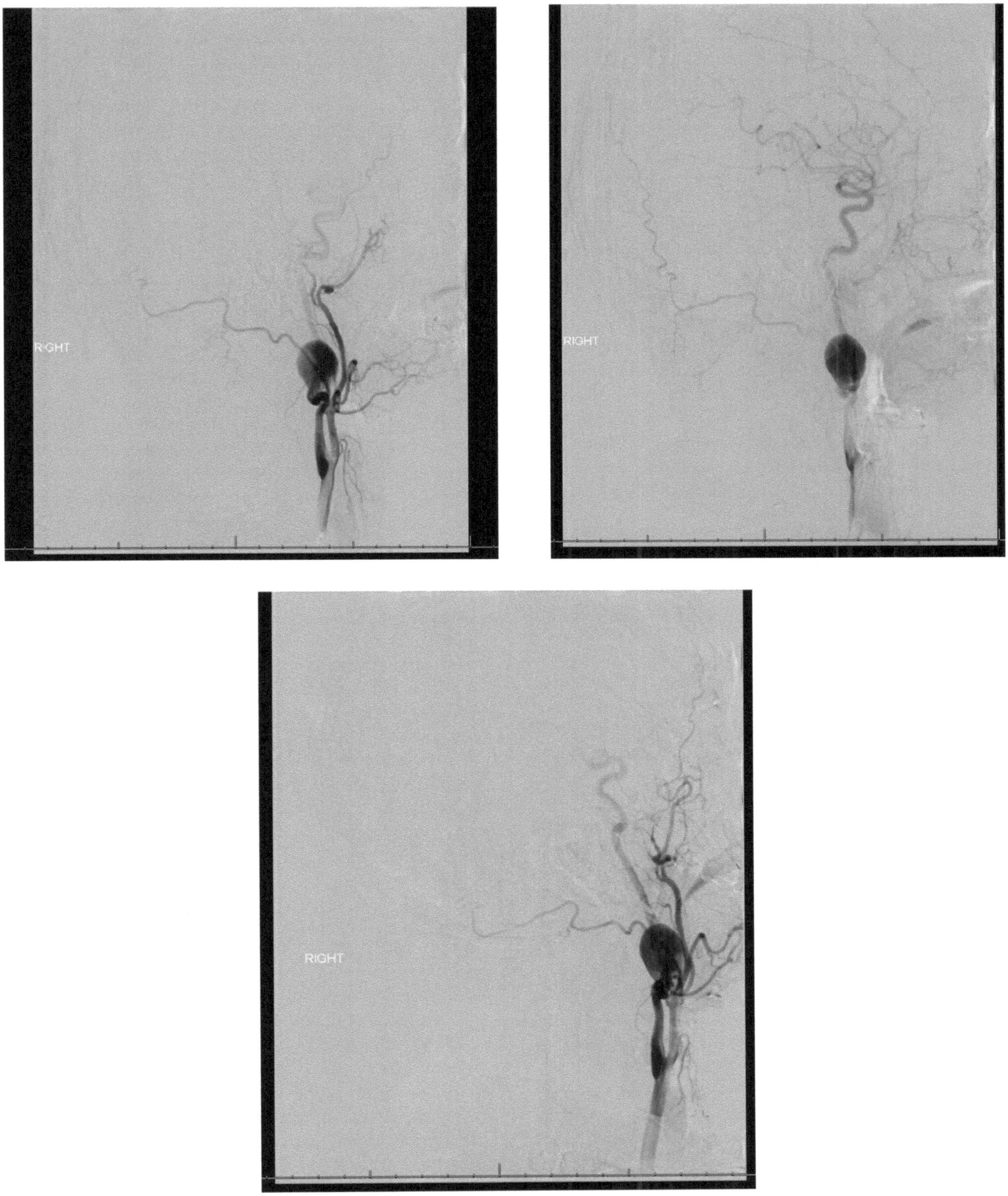

Figure 14.1 Selective right carotid arteriogram showing high internal carotid aneurysm. (Distal right ICA aneurysm.)

the local (cervical) lymph nodes is the most common, and spread to liver, lung, and bone occurs in less than 5% of cases.[3,4] Preoperative embolization should typically be reserved, tumors greater than 5 cm in transverse diameter.[3,4] When embolization is performed, surgical resection is recommended within 24–48 hours to avoid post embolization inflammation.[3,4] If the need for exposure for distal ICA for tumors extending toward the base of the skull by preoperative imaging, nasotracheal intubation, and/or mandibular subluxation should be considered.[5] In our institution, both ENT and oral-maxillofacial surgeons perform this procedure.[5] Due to forward displacement of the mandible, a narrow triangular field becomes a rectangular field, increasing the width of distal exposure. There is associated local distortion of the local anatomy with displacement of posterior belly of digastric and hypoglossal nerve anteriorly and superiorly, and the carotid bifurcation and right ICA are rotated medially following mandibular subluxation.[5] Intraoperative cerebral monitoring with electroencephalography and median nerve evoked potentials should be considered in patients undergoing resection of large carotid body tumors. As a first step, the common carotid artery is exposed at the base of the neck with early identification of the vagus nerve. The dissection plane is carried out in subadventitial base with the aid of bipolar cautery. This avascular space was first described by Gordon-Taylor as the "white line." Distal exposure can be facilitated with division of the posterior belly of digastric muscle and stylohyoid, avoiding injury to the glossopharyngeal nerve. Ligation and division of the occipital artery facilitates high exposure. If further exposure is required, division of stylohyoid process by the Rongeur and tip of the mastoid process may become necessary, but this can increase risk of glossopharyngeal nerve injury.

An internal-to-external artery dissection technique by beginning the dissection from the ICA and then dissecting the tumor from the ICA with external carotid artery to be the last to be dissected has been advocated by some authors. In Shamblin III tumors, where the arteries are completely encased by the tumor, resection of the involved artery with the tumor should be carried out. The typical blood supply in patients with carotid body tumors arises from the external carotid artery, and there are multiple feeding arteries which are ligated and divided. For larger tumors, the external carotid artery is ligated and divided to assist with mobilization and resection of the tumor. In a minority of cases, lateral arteriorrhaphy, patch angioplasty, or even a bypass may become necessary if there is associated injury of the ICA. Greater saphenous vein (GSV) from the groin and thigh is the preferred method of interposition grafting in patients where removal of the tumor and the artery is required.

AVOIDING NERVE INJURY

The most common cranial nerves injured are the vagus and hypoglossal. As there are multiple cranial nerves along the lateral border of the distal ICA (7th, 9th, 10th, and 12th) dissection in this area should be carefully performed.[3,4] Routine exposure of hypoglossal and vagus nerve should be carried out, and 11th spinal accessory nerve should be undertaken if the tumor is extending towards the accessory nerve.[4] Deep retraction near the mandible may result in injury to the marginal mandibular branch of the facial nerve.[3,4]

COMPLICATIONS

Barorecetor failure is a very rare but an important complication following bilateral carotid body tumor resection. It should be suspected in patients with tachycardia and labile hypertension 24–72 hours following tumor removal.[4] Other symptoms include headache, emotional lability, and anxiety. Prompt diagnosis of this syndrome is imperative as patients can develop hypertensive encephalopathy with stroke.[4] The baroreflex failure has not been described following unilateral carotid body tumor resection, suggesting that contralateral preservation of baroreceptor is adequate to maintain normal physiology.[4] Interruption of the baroreceptors results in unopposed sympathetic signals from the brain stem leads to tachycardia and labile hypertension with BP increasing to very high values. An incidence of 20% of baroreflex failure following bilateral common carotid body tumor resection has been reported.[4] Treatment is largely empiric. Antihypertensive complications with quick onset of action and short half-life such as labetalol, phentolamine, hydrolozine, and nitroprusside are recommended. For long-term management, clonidine is a preferred therapy. Clonidine treats both hypertension and tachycardia associated with this syndrome by stimulating alpha-2 receptors in the brain stem and stimulating parasympathetic outflow.[4]

STROKE, PSEUDOANEURYSM, AND MORTALITY

In a series of over 500 contemporary cases, stroke rate following carotid body tumor resection is reported to be about 4%.[4] A mortality rate as high as 8.8% has been reported in complex cases requiring arterial resection.[3,4] Cranial nerve injury is the most common complication, and incidence of cranial nerve dysfunction can be as high as 40%. Permanent cranial nerve injury occurs in about 20% of patients (8–39%).[3,4] Pseudoaneurysm is an extremely uncommon complication of resection of carotid body tumor.[4] Complete resection of carotid body tumor can be performed in most patients, and the survival of the patients following complete resection is similar to general population. Recurrence can occasionally occur. Patients with malignant carotid body tumor (exceedingly rare) require post-radiation therapy and late metastatic disease has been reported.[5]

Case Example 1

A 52-year-old male with history of hypertension presented to emergency room with vague neurological symptoms. CTA of the head and neck showed a large right carotid body tumor with upper extent of the tumor extending to the junction of C1-C2 vertebral body. Patient underwent catheter-based carotid and cerebral angiography, which showed a very large vascular carotid body tumor extending towards the base of the skull (Figure 14.2). The tumor was 5.3 cm in length and 4.8 cm in transverse diameter (Figure 14.2). Under nasotracheal intubation, mandibular subluxation was performed by the maxillofacial surgeon. Electoencephalographic monitoring (EEG) and SSEPs (somatosensory evoked potentials) were performed. Following a curved hockey stick incision, extending behind the lobule of the ear, carotid sheath was opened and vagus nerve was exposed and preserved. Cephalad end of the dissection was carried out after exposure of the posterior belly of the digastric and hypoglossal nerve was exposed. Dissection was performed along the lateral wall of the ICA as well as along the external carotid artery. Tumor was completely mobilized in the subadventitial plane. There was a small tear in the ICA in the anterolateral wall, which was repaired with a transverse 7-0 cardiovascular polypropylene. As the dissection was proceeding, cephalad ischemic changes in the EEG were observed, and there was no pulse in the ICA. Patient was given 10,000 units of heparin. Common carotid artery was clamped, and an incision was made in the common and ICA; a grayish white platelet thrombus was removed with brisk backbleeding. After removal of the thromboembolus, a bovine pericardial patch was applied, and a completion arteriogram was performed, which showed minor irregularities at the site of patch grafting (Figure 14.3). There was satisfactory filling of the anterior cerebral artery and superior branch of the middle cerebral artery but poor filling of the inferior branch of middle cerebral artery (Figures 14.4, 14.5). In the recovery room, patient was found to have weakness of the left upper extremity; he was kept on ventilatory support and nasogastric tube feeding and subsequently underwent tracheostomy and peg tube placement. MRI of the brain showed infarct in the distribution of inferior branch of the middle cerebral artery. Patient underwent IVC filter placement for deep venous thrombosis of right lower extremity. He continued to improve from the stroke effecting his left upper extremity and was subsequently discharged to an extended care facility. At 1 year follow-up, patient has grade 4/5 motor function of the left upper extremity, although he has limited shoulder movement due to "frozen shoulder."

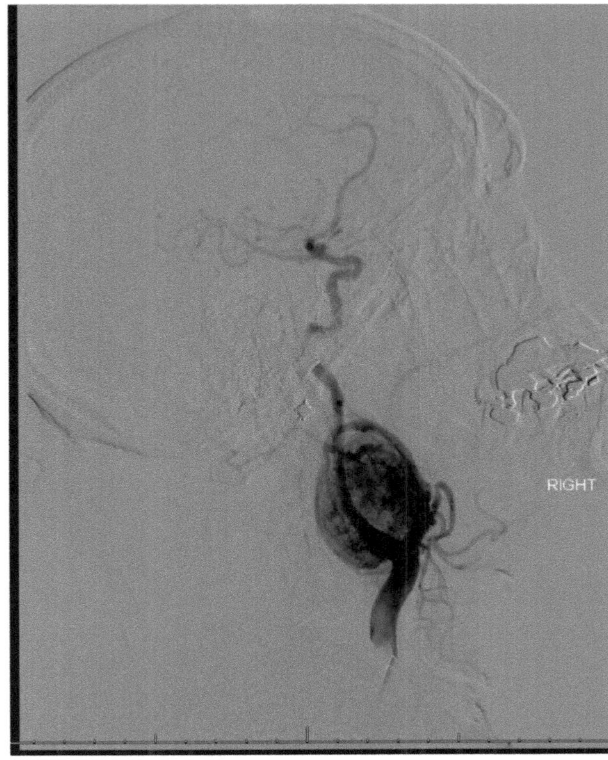

Figure 14.2 Selective right carotid arteriogram showing large carotid body tumor.

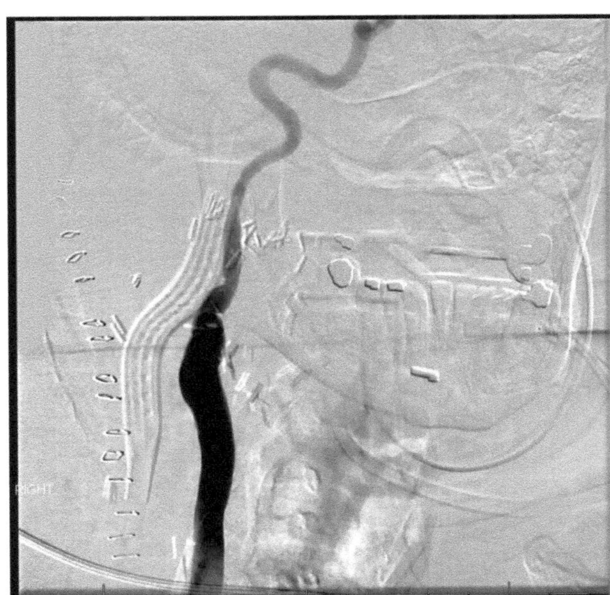

Figure 14.3 Operative arteriogram following removal of the tumor with minor irregularities at the site of patch graft.

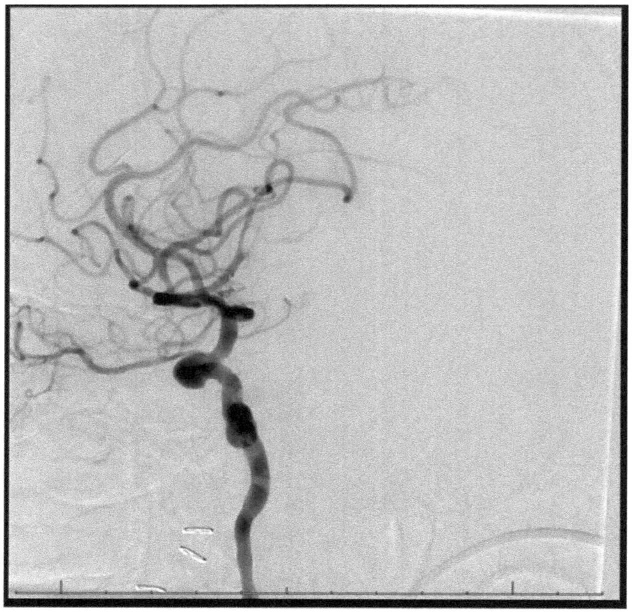

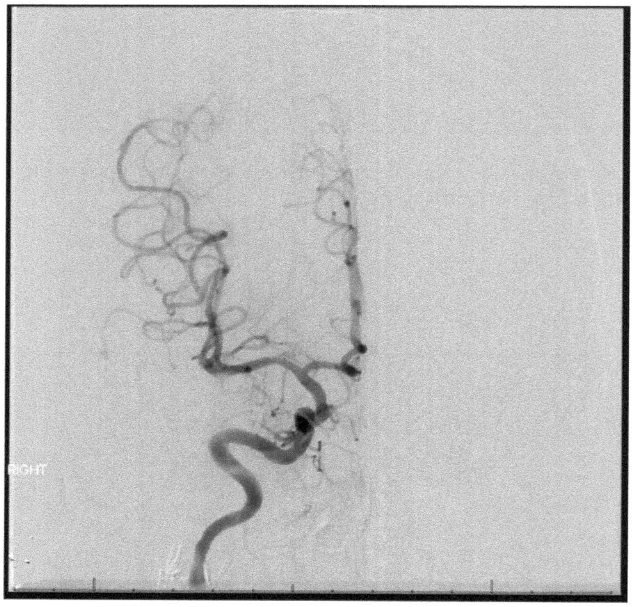

Figure 14.4, 14.5 Intracerebral view (Lateral and AP) showing absent filling of inferior branches of middle cerebral artery.

REFERENCES

1. Hans SS. Extracranial carotid and vertebral artery aneurysms in Extracranial carotid and vertebral artery disease. Edited by Hans SS. Springer International 2018; 261–266.
2. Zhou W, Lin PH, Bush RL, Peden E, et al. Carotid artery aneurysm: evolution of management of over two decades. J Vasc Surg. 2006;43: 493–6.
3. Weaver MR, Reddy DJ. Resection of carotid body tumor in endovascular and open vascular reconstruction. Edited by Hans SS, Shepard AD, Weaver MR, Bove PG, Long GW. CRC Press. Boca Raton, FL 2017. 167–172.
4. Davis FM, Obi A, Osborne N. Carotid body tumors in open vascular and endovascular reconstructions. Extracranial carotid and vertebral artery disease. Edited by Hans SS. Springer International 2018; 253–260.
5. Hans SS. Resection of a malignant carotid body tumor with carotid artery resection, in Challenging arterial reconstructions: 100 clinical cases. Springer International 2020.

SUGGESTED READINGS

Surgical and medical management of extracranial carotid artery aneurysms Grant T. Fankhauser, MD,a William M. Stone, MD,a Richard J. Fowl, MD,a Mark E. O'Donnell, MD,a Thomas C. Bower, MD,b Fredric B. Meyer, MD,b et.al

Current surgical management of carotid body tumors Victor J. Davila, MD,a James M. Chang, MD,a William M. Stone, MD,a Richard J. Fowl, MD,a Thomas C. Bower, MD,b Michael L. Hinni, MD,c et.al

15

Complications of open reconstruction for aneurysmal and occlusive diseases of aortic arch vessels

SRIHARI LELLA AND SAMUEL SCHWARTZ

The great vessels, also known as the vessels of the aortic arch (innominate, left common carotid, and subclavian arteries), supply blood flow to the head, neck, and upper extremities. A number of disease processes can affect these vessels, including atherosclerosis causing stenosis, aneurysmal disease, dissections, and a host of genetic and inflammatory conditions. Repair options include endarterectomy with patch angioplasty, transposition of vessels to adjacent great vessels, resection with interposition graft placement, or various forms of transthoracic bypass. Open repair holds particular challenges due to the angulation of the aortic arch; the dynamic nature of this vessel also places it at risk for damage during the operation. Additionally, clamping the aorta at this location, at close proximity to the heart, has its own set of potential complications. Many of the complications associated with these procedures could be devastating with resultant high morbidity and mortality.

Special mention must be made of Takayasu's arteritis (TA). TA is a large-vessel arteritis that tends to involve the aorta and/or its branch vessels. In the acute stage, the arterial walls can get disrupted with degeneration of the media and subsequent aneurysm formation. With more chronic inflammation, the arterial walls become thickened and fibrosed, leading to stenosis with thrombosis.[1] Generally steroid/immunosuppressive therapy is provided during the acute inflammatory phase. Surgery is predominantly performed during a state of quiescence.

AORTIC CLAMPING

Open repair of the great vessel branches invariably requires clamping of the aorta, generally with a side-biting clamp. While the effects of side-biting clamping may not cause as profound changes on the hemodynamic physiology as complete cross-clamping of the aorta, it may still cause significant hemodynamic responses.

CARDIAC EFFECTS

When the aorta is clamped, there is a significant rise in afterload due to the impedance of blood flow. This in turn results in increased left ventricular end-systolic wall stress with left ventricular dilation. There is also an increase in myocardial oxygen demand. Autoregulation of the coronary blood flow generally allows for the oxygen demand to be met, resulting in a positive inotropic response thereby relieving the myocardial wall stress.

However, the majority of patients undergoing these surgeries have some form of coronary artery disease (CAD). As such, some of them may not have enough reserve for such autoregulation that puts them at risk for myocardial impairment. Additionally, in patients with CAD, the rise in afterload and preload can result in elevated filling pressures with left ventricular decompensation. Rarely, in patients with advanced preexisting disease, acute heart failure or an acute coronary event are a possibility.[2]

DISSECTION

Iatrogenic dissection is a rare complication but can cause devastating consequences depending on the location. These can occur from both the aortic clamp site as well as at the anastomoses. The consequences of a dissection in the aortic arch vessels can range from no symptoms to ischemic symptoms to the upper extremities or stroke. The vast majority of these are caused from technical aspects of the surgery.

Aortic dissection from clamp injury can result in both Type A and B dissections. Early intraoperative recognition and management is key to improved patient outcomes. Occasionally, it may cause a blue purple discoloration to the aorta that may be visible. There can also be dilation with progression intraoperatively to more distal aortic segments. Type A dissections can result in significant aortic regurgitation as well as cardiac tamponade. They should be promptly repaired with the assistance of cardiac surgery. Type B dissections may be managed with an endovascular stent or conservative therapy.[3]

STROKE

Stroke warrants its own discussion as it can be caused by the above-mentioned factors, but it is more likely to be caused by emboli. This can be due to the atherosclerotic debris or thrombus along the vessel wall that is manipulated during vessel exposure or clamping. The more diseased the arch vessels are, the more likely they are to cause emboli to the brain. Nevertheless, the severity of the stroke can be variable. The stroke rates after transthoracic bypass or endarterectomy of the brachiocephalic artery have been between 2.9 to 8%.[4–7]

Generally, when operating on the right brachiocephalic and left common carotid artery, it is important to perform a neurologic exam at the end of the procedure once the patient is off sedating anesthetics. If there is a major lateralizing deficit and there is concern from a technical standpoint, it is essential to re-explore the surgical site. A cerebral angiogram by Interventional Neuroradiology should also be considered if there is concern for an embolus; mechanical thrombectomy can be performed without additional anticoagulation. Should the patient develop signs concerning for a stroke postoperatively, emergent head imaging should be obtained with a plan for management with either reoperation, angiography, or conservative therapy based on the association with the initial procedure.

STERNAL WOUND INFECTION

In addition to the superficial surgical site infections, deep sternal wound infection (DSWI, also referred to as mediastinitis) is a serious concern. While studies looking at such infections after aortic arch vessel surgery are lacking, the incidence for patients undergoing cardiac surgery has been shown to be between 1% and 5%.[8] Risk factors for the development of DSWI include obesity, chronic obstructive pulmonary disease, tobacco use, diabetes, osteoporosis, and reoperation.[8] DSWI carries with it a high morbidity and may often lead to fatal outcomes with reported mortality rates between 10% and 47%.[8–9]

Pairolero et al. divided DSWI into three types.[10] Type I has the earliest presentation occurring within several days after sternotomy. These patients may present with wound separation, drainage (usually not suppurative), and with or without sternal instability; Type I is without extensive cellulitis, osteomyelitis, or costochronditis. They are generally treated with antibiotics and operative debridement. Type II usually occurs between the first and fourth weeks after sternotomy and is the most common type of presentation. There is generally cellulitis with purulent drainage and underlying mediastinal suppuration. Osteomyelitis is common in this type of infection, but costochondritis is rare. Exploration and debridement of all necrotic tissue should be excised. Exposed healthy cartilage should also be resected back to bone. All foreign material also should be removed. The wound should be closed with muscle transposition if there is dead space, with the pectoralis major muscle being the most commonly used muscle. Other flaps that have been described include omental and rectus flaps. Finally, Type III infections are chronic infections on the order of months to years with chronically draining sinus tracts into the sternum or costochondral arches. While osteomyelitis and costochondritis are commonly seen, mediastinitis is rare in this type. These wounds are generally packed and may need chronic debridements. If the wound is deemed to be clean, closure with muscle transpositions similar to those used in Type II can be utilized.[10–11]

The most common types of bacteria isolated from surgical wound cultures of DSWI are coagulase-negative Staphylococcus, which often leads to Type I DSWI, and *Staphylococcus aureus*, which is usually the cause of Type II infections. Other less commonly found pathogens include *Enterobacter cloacae*, *Klebsiella oxytoca*, *Klebsiella pneumoniae*, *Propionibacterium acnes*, *Escherichia coli*, and *Bacteroides fragilis*.[12–13] These less common organisms are often the cause of Type III chronic infections.

REFERENCES

1. Johnston SL, Lock RJ, Gompels MM. Takayasu arteritis: a review. Journal of Clinical Pathology. 55(7): 481–486. doi:10.1136/jcp.55.7.481.
2. Gelman S. The Pathophysiology of Aortic Cross-clamping and Unclamping. Anesthesiology. 1995;82(4): 1026–1057. doi:10.1097/00000542-199504000-00027.
3. Singh A, Mehta Y. Intraoperative aortic dissection. Annals of Cardiac Anaesthesia. 2015;18(4): 537. doi:10.4103/0971-9784.166463.
4. Berguer R, Morasch MD, Kline RA. Transthoracic repair of innominate and common carotid artery disease: Immediate and long-term outcome for

100 consecutive surgical reconstructions. Journal of Vascular Surgery. 1998;27(1): 34–42. doi:10.1016/s0741-5214(98)70289-7.
5. Crawford ES, Stowe CL, Powers RW. Occlusion of the innominate, common carotid, and subclavian arteries: long-term results of surgical treatment. Surgery. 1983;94(5): 781–791.
6. Kieffer E, Sabatier J, Koskas F, Bahnini A. Atherosclerotic innominate artery occlusive disease: Early and long-term results of surgical reconstruction. Journal of Vascular Surgery. 1995;21(2): 326–337. doi:10.1016/s0741-5214(95)70273-3.
7. Rhodes JM, Cherry KJ, Clark RC, et al. Aortic-origin reconstruction of the great vessels: Risk factors of early and late complications. Journal of Vascular Surgery. 2000;31(2): 260–269. doi:10.1016/s0741-5214(00)90157-5.
8. Gummert JF, Barten MJ, Hans C, et al. Mediastinitis and Cardiac Surgery - an Updated Risk Factor Analysis in 10,373 Consecutive Adult Patients. The Thoracic and Cardiovascular Surgeon. 2002;50(2): 87–91. doi:10.1055/s-2002-26691.
9. Losanoff J. Disruption and infection of median sternotomy: a comprehensive review. European Journal of Cardio-Thoracic Surgery. 2002;21(5): 831–839. doi:10.1016/s1010-7940(02)00124-0.
10. Pairolero PC, Arnold PG. Management of Infected Median Sternotomy Wounds. The Annals of Thoracic Surgery. 1986;42(1): 1–2. doi:10.1016/s0003-4975(10)61822-x.
11. Singh K, Anderson E, Harper JG. Overview and Management of Sternal Wound Infection. Seminars in Plastic Surgery. 2011;25(01): 025–033. doi:10.1055/s-0031-1275168.
12. Ståhle E. Sternal wound complications—incidence, microbiology and risk factors. European Journal of Cardio-Thoracic Surgery. 1997;11(6): 1146–1153. doi:10.1016/s1010-7940(97)01210-4.
13. Sjögren J, Malmsjö M, Gustafsson R, Ingemansson R. Poststernotomy mediastinitis: a review of conventional surgical treatments, vacuum-assisted closure therapy and presentation of the Lund University Hospital mediastinitis algorithm. European Journal of Cardio-Thoracic Surgery. 2006;30(6): 898–905. doi:10.1016/j.ejcts.2006.09.020.

SUGGESTED READINGS

Charlton-Ouw KM, Pratt WB, Safi HJ. Brachiocephalic Artery Disease and its Surgical Treatment, in Rutherford's Vascular Surgery and Endovascular Therapy, 9th Edited by Sidawy AN, Perler BA. Philadelphia: Elsevier; 2019: 1291–1303.

16

Complications of upper extremity bypass grafting for occlusive and aneurysmal disease

ADAM TANIOUS AND MARK F. CONRAD

Upper extremity occlusive and atherosclerotic disease is rare when compared to other peripheral arterial beds and accounts for less than 3% of extremity bypass cases.[1] The refinement of minimally invasive tools and techniques has led many operators to take an endovascular-first approach to upper extremity disease. This has made open surgery less common despite the fact that historical outcomes are well documented to be favorable. This chapter will cover the workup and treatment of upper extremity disease with open surgery. It will outline the morbidity and mortality associated with these procedures, suggest ways to avoid negative outcomes, and detail a management approach that addresses each complication in a systematic fashion.

INCIDENCE OF UPPER EXTREMITY DISEASE

ATHEROSCLEROTIC LESIONS

Arterial occlusive disease of the upper extremity occurs rarely when compared to other peripheral arterial beds.[2,3] A Dutch study found that upper arm pulse differences occurred in 2% of patients, while lower extremity disease was identified in 20–30% of the same population.[3] However, occlusive disease is the most commonly encountered arterial pathology of the upper extremity. In a report of 20 years of experience with innominate lesions, Brewster et al. reported that 52% were due to atherosclerosis followed by aneurysms, dissections, infection, and trauma.[4] The most common sites of upper extremity atherosclerosis are the innominate and subclavian arteries. Indeed, atherosclerosis is extremely rare distal to the subclavian artery. Most arm lesions are asymptomatic, and disease of vessels proximal to the wrist account for only about 10% of symptomatic cases. The most common symptoms encountered are arm claudication (usually with movements above the head), hand or finger pain (usually do to embolus), ulcerations, or gangrene, and the most common cause of upper extremity ischemia is palmar or digital artery occlusion.

ANEURYSMAL DISEASE

Aneurysms of the upper extremity are rare as well and comprise around 0.4–4% of all aneurysms encountered.[4] The pathology is most commonly degenerative, and this accounts for approximately 60% of patients presenting with upper extremity aneurysms, while the remaining causes are related to iatrogenic injury or trauma.[3,5] Cury et al. looked at 74 supra-aortic aneurysms and found that the subclavian artery is most commonly involved, making up 50% of the cohort while only 3% were in the innominate artery. Almost 70% were asymptomatic upon presentation, but when symptoms did occur, embolization, not rupture, was the most common presenting symptom and was the source in 68% of symptomatic patients.[5]

INDICATION FOR BYPASS

The most common cause of acute arm ischemia is embolic disease, which is usually treated with an open embolectomy with a high rate of successful restoration of blood flow. Patients who have asymptomatic atherosclerotic disease should be managed with risk factor modification including smoking cessation, blood pressure control, addition of lipid-lowering and antiplatelet agents, and control of diabetes. Patients with claudication should be similarly managed conservatively with the addition of an upper extremity exercise regimen. Patients with severe symptoms of chronic upper extremity ischemia should undergo intervention, and although many will opt for an endovascular option, there is a paucity of data regarding the initial success and long-term durability of these procedures. To wit, open repair remains the gold standard for treatment. Hughes et al. described a single-institutional experience with upper extremity bypass over 13 years and reported that lifestyle-limiting arm claudication was the most common indication (55%), followed by tissue loss (30%) and rest pain (15%).[6]

Aneurysms of the upper extremity pose the same risks as those of other vascular beds including: rupture, thrombosis, and local symptoms secondary to compression. When a patient presents with symptoms, the decision to intervene is clear, and historically up to 50% of patients with upper extremity aneurysms were symptomatic. However, with the improvement of axial imaging, the incidental finding of aneurysmal degeneration of the upper extremity is increasing and, in contemporary practice, up to 70% of upper extremity aneurysms are asymptomatic when discovered.[5] There are no guidelines that provide a size threshold for repair in asymptomatic patients. The larger series report a mean aneurysm size of 3.0–3.5 cm with a range of 2.2–4.5 cm, and it appears that, for most, the presence of an aneurysm is an indication for repair.[5,7]

OPEN SURGICAL REPAIR

Open repair of arteries at the level of the aortic arch are covered in Chapter 15, and the operative focus of this chapter will be bypasses in the upper extremity and dissection of possible inflow and outflow vessels.

EXPOSURE OF THE SUBCLAVIAN ARTERY

The subclavian artery can be approached from above or below the clavicle (Figure 16.1). The supraclavicular approach provides excellent exposure to the subclavian artery and vein and the vertebral artery. The patient is positioned with the head turned away from the incision, and a scapular roll or thyroid bag is used to extend the neck and the supraclavicular fossa. The incision is made 1 finger breadth (1–2 cm) above the clavicle and parallel to it. It should begin at the sternal head of the sternocleidomastoid muscle (SCM) and extend laterally. The platysma, omohyoid muscle, and the clavicular head of the SCM are all divided to widen the exposure. At this level, the internal jugular vein is identified and retracted medially. The vagus nerve is usually located posteriorly between the internal jugular vein and the common carotid artery, but it can be anterior and should be avoided. Another structure to identify at this point is the thoracic duct, which is located on the left side near the point where the internal jugular vein drains into the left subclavian vein.

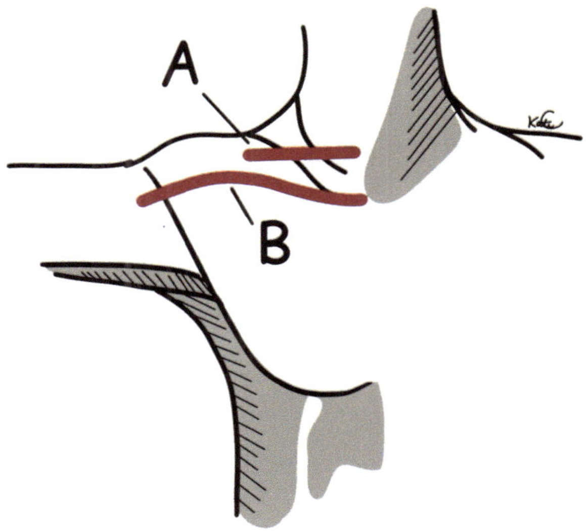

Figure 16.1 Incisions for exposure of the subclavian artery. (A) The supraclavicular approach. (B) The infraclavicular approach.

Some authors recommend routine ligation of the thoracic duct to avoid injury with a chylous fistula or chylothorax. Continuing the dissection, the scalene fat pad is mobilized and reflected laterally to expose the anterior scalene muscle (ASM). The phrenic nerve should be identified on and freed from the anterior surface of the ASM and is unique because it is the only nerve that courses from a lateral to a medial position. The ASM attachment to the first rib is divided carefully to avoid injury to the subclavian vein; once the ASM is divided, the subclavian artery can be isolated (Figure 16.2).

EXPOSURE OF THE AXILLARY ARTERY

The axillary artery can be exposed for bypass from the infraclavicular or delta-pectoral approaches. For the infraclavicular approach, the patient is positioned with the arm extended, and a shoulder roll is placed to help

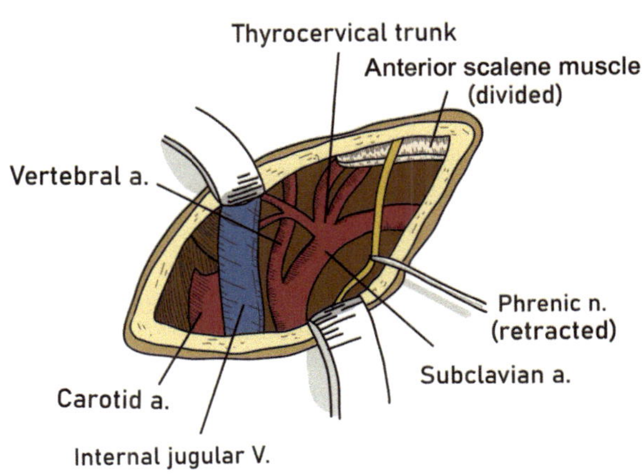

Figure 16.2 Supraclavicular exposure of the subclavian artery.

with exposure. The incision is made a finger breadth (1–2 cm) below the middle third of clavicle, and the pectoral fascia is divided. The pectoralis major muscle fibers are separated in the direction of the incision. This exposes the clavipectoral fascia, which is divided to reveal the axillary neurovascular bundle. The pectoralis minor is retracted laterally to improve exposure. The vascular structures encountered will be the axillary vein first as it is anterior to the artery, which is posterior and superior to the vein. Overlying vein branches are ligated and the vein is retracted inferiorly to expose the artery. The brachial plexus usually lies deep to the axillary artery and should be identified to avoid an inadvertent clamp injury. At this juncture, the artery can be dissected free. The lateral pectoral nerve can cross the axillary artery and should be identified to avoid injury.

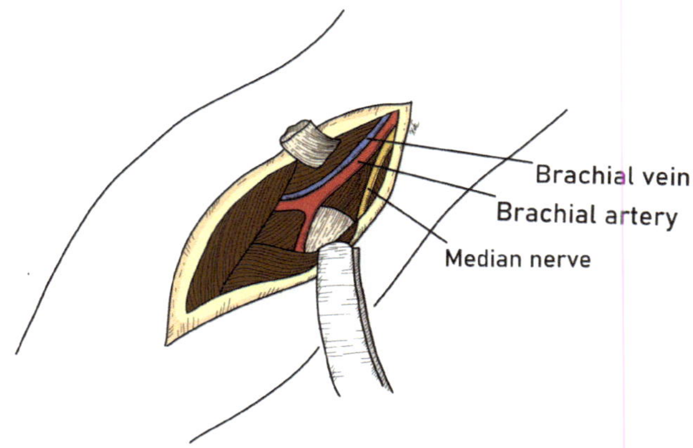

Figure 16.3 Exposure of the brachial artery.

EXPOSURE OF THE BRACHIAL ARTERY

Exposure of the brachial artery in the antecubital fossa is not complicated. The patient is positioned with the arm abducted to 90 degrees at the shoulder and the hand supinated. Overextension of the shoulder should be avoided to prevent traction injury to the brachial plexus. The arm should be circumferentially prepped to allow for flexibility in positioning and access to the radial pulse during the procedure. The incision is made along the medial bicipital groove, which is the longitudinal plane between the biceps and triceps muscle. The basilic vein is located in this area and should be identified and retracted inferiorly as the dissection continues. The neurovascular bundle is located below the deep fascia of the medial border of the biceps muscle; once this is incised, the biceps muscle is retracted superiorly. The most superficial structure encountered is usually the median nerve, which needs to be mobilized and retracted without traction. The brachial artery is deep to the median nerve and is flanked by paired brachial veins. The ulnar nerve runs posterior to the brachial artery. Crossing vein branches are ligated and the artery is controlled, taking care not to include the ulnar nerve. If two arteries are encountered at this location, it represents a high bifurcation of the brachial artery and these arteries will become the radial and ulnar arteries in the forearm (Figure 16.3).

EXPOSURE OF THE RADIAL ARTERY

The radial artery can be exposed at the mid-forearm or at the wrist. For both exposures, the arm is prepped circumferentially for intraoperative manipulation and is positioned with shoulder abducted to 90 degrees and the hand in the supinated position. The radial artery in the forearm follows a path along the medial edge of the brachioradialis muscle, and the incision should be made along this line. It can be useful to first identify the artery with ultrasound and mark the incision on the skin, especially when an abundance of adipose tissue obscures the surface anatomy of the arm. The antebrachial fascia is thick, and division will expose the radial artery in the proximal two-thirds of the forearm between the brachioradialis and pronator teres muscles. The radial artery is again flanked by paired veins and crossing veins must be ligated to fully expose the artery. In the middle third of the forearm, the superficial radial nerve runs in close proximity to the radial artery and should be identified and avoided.

Exposure of the radial artery in the wrist again begins with the hand and forearm circumferentially prepped and the shoulder abducted to 90 degrees with the hand supinated. The radial artery runs lateral to the flexor carpi radialis tendon in the wrist. For direct arterial exposure, a longitudinal incision is made just next to the tendon; however, for fistula creation, the incision is moved more laterally to position between the radial artery and the cephalic vein; this is usually along the lateral border of the radius. The antebrachial fascia is excised and the artery runs deep to this with paired veins. The superficial radial nerve is superficial to the fascia in the wrist and runs laterally between the radial artery and the cephalic vein.

EXPOSURE OF THE ULNAR ARTERY

The ulnar artery can be exposed at the mid-forearm or at the wrist. For both exposures, the arm is prepped circumferentially for intraoperative manipulation and is positioned with shoulder abducted to 90 degrees and the hand in the supinated position. The ulnar artery in the proximal forearm crosses under the superficial flexor muscles, so exposure is easier in the mid-forearm. The incision is made along an imaginary line drawn from the medial epicondyle of the humerus to the pisiform in the wrist. However, it is useful to first identify the artery with ultrasound and mark the incision on the skin. The antebrachial fascia is divided, and the flexor carpi ulnaris and flexor digitorum superficialis are separated to expose the ulnar artery. The ulnar artery is flanked by paired veins and crossing veins must be ligated to fully expose the artery. In the middle third of the forearm, the ulnar nerve runs along the medial boarder of the ulnar artery and should be identified and avoided.

Exposure of the ulnar artery in the wrist again begins with the hand and forearm circumferentially prepped and the shoulder abducted to 90 degrees with the hand supinated. The ulnar artery runs medial to the flexor carpi ulnaris tendon in the wrist. For direct arterial exposure, a longitudinal incision is made next to the tendon. The antebrachial fascia is excised and the artery runs deep to this with paired veins. The palmar branch of the ulnar nerve is superficial to the fascia in the wrist and should be avoided.

TUNNELING THE BYPASS

As in the leg, the autogenous vein is the best conduit for upper extremity bypass, and both the great saphenous and cephalic veins have been used with good success. The vein can be reversed or non-reversed depending on the size of the vein and proposed inflow and outflow targets. Prosthetic conduits can be used but have been shown to have inferior results, especially when they cross at least one joint.[8] When the bypass originates from the subclavian or axillary artery, it is best to tunnel anatomically to avoid distortion with shoulder movement. If placed superficially, the bypass will be more prone to injury during extended abduction of the shoulder; this can be minimized by leaving a small amount of redundancy. If the bypass originates from the brachial artery, it is usually tunneled subcutaneously to avoid injury to the nerves in the forearm. In addition, when the arm veins are of good quality, in situ bypasses have been used with good success.

COMPLETION IMAGING

Early graft failure is predictive of long-term adverse outcomes such as limb loss and death and can often be attributed to technical issues, low flow, or high peripheral resistance.[9]

These are issues that can be identified with completion imaging once the bypass is open. While the majority of data regarding completion imaging comes from the lower extremity bypass literature, they also apply to the upper extremity. Arteriography remains the gold standard for technical evaluation postprocedure, but Duplex scanning has become popular because it is readily available and has the ability to not only detect structural issues but have also hemodynamic parameters which may suggest a problem with an otherwise technically adequate bypass.[10] However, although it is recommended for all upper extremity bypass, a review of the VQI database showed that completion imaging did not affect long-term graft patency.[11]

COMPLICATIONS

ARTERIAL AND VENOUS INJURY

The vessels of the upper extremity can be fragile and prone to injury, especially the subclavian and axillary arteries. Common injuries include: arterial occlusion, tear, transection, thermal injury from electrocautery, or distal embolization.[12] Once an injury is recognized, the artery should be completely mobilized and exposed to allow for safe control of the vessel and repair under direct vision. Blindly throwing stitches into a bleeding field in an attempt to control hemorrhage leads to further injury, and young surgeons should resist this urge. The most difficult injuries to repair are in the proximal subclavian artery because it is prone to retract into the chest, so it is important to obtain proximal control without making the injury worse. The exact method of repair will depend upon the injury identified. For transections and tears, the margins should be cleaned and the injury can be closed primarily. This will often require a doubly pledgeted suture in a friable artery to prevent further injury. If the ends of the artery cannot be re-approximated without tension, then an interposition bypass may be required. These are often short, and prosthetic conduits have been shown to have similar outcomes to autogenous vein.

Venous injuries can be more difficult to identify and control than arterial injuries because the blood appears to well up in the wound without an obvious direct source. However, in the trauma literature, venous injury is associated with lower risk of morbidity and mortality compared to arterial injury.[13] It is again important to fully expose the vein and identify the injury prior to any attempts at repair. If the injured vein is friable or fragile, it can typically be ligated with minimal morbidity.

THORACIC DUCT INJURY

The thoracic duct is the largest lymphatic structure in the body. It begins at the level of the second lumbar vertebra when lumbar and intestinal lymphatic trunks converge. It then travels up the left side of the spine and eventually drains into the left subclavian vein around the 7th cervical vertebra. If the duct is injured, it will release a milky fluid called chyle that contains fat droplets and lymph. Chyle leaks from thoracic duct injuries during neck dissections have been reported in up to 8% of cases, and a quarter of these are caused by right neck surgery.[14] Often, the injury is identified at surgery when chyle is seen in the operative field and in this situation all attempts should be made to identify and ligate the source. Postoperatively, the patient may present with neck edema, erythema, fluid in the chest, or increased drainage after resumption of a regular diet. The drainage is not always milky, and a triglyceride level of greater than 100 mg/dL in the fluid collection will confirm the diagnosis.[15] If the leak is identified in the early postoperative period, the wound should be re-explored, the leak identified, and after repair, it should be covered with a muscle flap to promote healing. A low-output leak (< 500 mL/day) can often be treated conservatively with bed rest, a low-fat or medium-chain fatty acid diet, and wound care.[16] In addition, subcutaneous octreotide dosed at 100–200 ug every 8–12 hours has been shown to be helpful in getting chyle leaks to resolve with low-volume leaks stopping in 2–4 days and high-volume leaks in 2 weeks.[17] Late surgical exploration may be required if the leak does not resolve, but it is best if done within the first week. Newer endovascular techniques for duct occlusion have been described but remain anecdotal.[18]

NERVE INJURY

Peripheral nerve injury can occur during exposure of the arteries of the upper extremity and will differ based upon the location of the dissection. In order to identify and treat these injuries in a timely manner, it is important to have a keen understanding of the neurovascular anatomy of the dissection area and the subsequent deficits that will be encountered if an issue is to occur. Although a traumatic division or ligation of surrounding nerves during dissection is often identified at the time of the injury, other peripheral nerve trauma such as thermal injury, compressive injury, or traction injury is more likely to be diagnosed postoperatively when the patient has a deficit on postoperative neurologic exam.

Dissection of the subclavian artery can lead to injury of the vagus and phrenic nerves. If the vagus nerve is injured near the common carotid artery, the patient will experience paralysis of the ipsilateral vocal cord from the recurrent laryngeal nerve. This can cause life-threatening airway issues, and any persistent hoarseness after surgery should prompt an evaluation of the cords. Injury to the phrenic nerve will lead to paralysis of the diaphragm. Unilateral diaphragmatic paralysis results in loss of lung volume on chest x-ray. Many patients are asymptomatic at rest but will experience shortness of breath with exertion. For traction injuries, this may be transient, but in some cases, the patient's condition never improves.

The brachial plexus runs along the course of the subclavian and axillary arteries and can be encountered with exposure of either of these vessels. The posterior and medial cords of the brachial plexus run inferior to the subclavian artery, which splits these as it passes below the clavicle. The superior, middle, and inferior trunks of the brachial plexus surround the axillary artery on 3 of its 4 sides. Occasionally, one of the trunks can run anterior to the axillary artery, and no cord-like structures should be divided during the dissection. Injuries to the brachial plexus are clinically divided into branches of the upper plexus and the lower plexus. Injuries to the upper plexus can manifest as the "waiter's tip" position with the arm abducted, the shoulder internally rotated the elbow extended and the forearm pronated.[19] Injuries of the lower plexus can affect the thoracodorsal nerve leading to inability to adduct the shoulder or portions of the radial, median, and ulnar nerves.

As the axillary artery becomes the brachial artery, the median and ulnar nerve are the most adjacent neurologic structures. The median nerve changes its relative location to the brachial artery, switching from a lateral position in the upper arm to a medial position as both pass through the bicipital aponeurosis. In the forearm, the surgeon must be cognizant of the ulnar nerve as it becomes more intimately associated with the ulnar artery. Injuries to the ulnar nerve are divided into low and high categories. If the nerve is injured distal to the motor branch of the flexor carpi ulnaris muscle, it is considered a low injury and the patient loses sensation in the ulnar portion of the palm. If the injury is high, there is loss in the function of the intrinsic muscles of the hand that results in the "claw" hand where the fourth and fifth fingers have hyperextension at the metacarpal joints and flexion at the intraphalangial joints.[20] The median nerve innervates the pronator teres, palmaris longus and flexors carpi radialis and digitorum superficialis, so injury leads to an inability to oppose the thumb and a weak grip. The patient may also experience numbness of the forearm, palm, thumb, digits 2, 3 and half of 4. Finally, a radial nerve injury will manifest as wrist weakness and loss of finger extension.

There are a variety of tests that can be used to quantify the degree of nerve injury. Electrophysiological assessment with electroneuromyography (EMG) is considered the gold standard for verification of the diagnosis, and the results can be used to plan treatments in nerve injury patients.[21] Prior to EMG, initial evaluation included a peripheral ultrasound to determine if the nerve is in continuity.[22] If the nerve is found to be transected, then the treatment algorithm is simple and the patient should undergo expedient intervention to re-approximate the nerve. If the nerve is in continuity, then it is up to the consulting provider to move forward with EMG in the inpatient setting or give time for possible traction and thermal injuries to resolve.[22] EMG can be used measure all of the following values: sensorial nerve axon potential peak amplitude, transmission speed of sensorial nerve fibrils, motor nerve axon potential peak amplitude, distal motor latency, and speed of motor nerve fibrils. Indeed, EMG is a critical tool in the identification of peripheral nerve injury; a study of approximately 2500 patients with suspected upper extremity neuropathy showed that EMG confirmed nerve damage in 55% and showed normal nerve activity in the rest of patients.[21]

GRAFT FAILURE/LONG-TERM PATENCY

Bypass patency is affected by factors such as the patency of the inflow and outflow vessels and the quality of conduit used. It is accepted that a single vein should be the conduit of choice if available as this leads to better long-term patency, but Jain et al. showed that excellent results can be achieved with PTFE as they reported a 3 year patency of 88%.[23,24]

In addition to the usual factors, the patency of an upper extremity bypass can be negatively affected by the number of joints it traverses.[23]

The data regarding upper extremity bypass are sparse in comparison to the lower extremity literature because they are rare. Indeed, in a 15-year experience from Northwestern, Mesh et al. described 31 upper extremity bypasses.[24] Open bypass for upper extremity critical limb ischemia is generally successful with a reported secondary patency of 91% and limb salvage rates of 100%.[25] In a 10 year study with a mean follow up of 34 months, Spinelli et al. found a graft thrombosis rate of 17%.[25] More recently, Cheun et al. reported on distal upper extremity bypass in 21 patients using saphenous vein to radial or ulnar targets. After 2 years of follow-up, the primary-assisted and secondary patency rate was 90% with a 5-year secondary patency of 67% despite having a high prevalence of diabetic and chronic renal failure patients in the cohort.[26]

While it is clear that patients who undergo bypass for occlusive disease and have a history of diabetes have a higher risk for long-term bypass complications, both aneurysmal and occlusive disease patients warrant follow up of their repair. Noninvasive testing proves useful in these patients, particularly duplex ultrasound with measurement of flow velocities and waveform analysis. While currently there are no set criteria for upper extremity bypass velocity targets, general duplex criteria should guide the surgeon regarding the status of a bypass and alert to pending issues: spectral broadening, blunted upstroke, or monophasic signals waveform analysis; reduced peak systolic velocities from pre-procedure or immediate postprocedure assessment; and differences noted when compared to the contralateral extremity.[27] Particular attention should be paid to patients with a known incomplete palmar arch as this, combined with poor digital run-off, have been shown to predict amputation after upper extremity bypass.[26]

Once a significant stenosis is identified, further imaging should be obtained to plan for re-intervention for symptom improvement or graft salvage. Angiographic imaging will help determine appropriate sources of inflow and possible targets for repeat bypass or possible endovascular solutions. CTA provides a noninvasive anatomic representation of the vascular tree and can identify structural problems such as kinking and external compression.

GRAFT INFECTION

Graft infection is a rare complication of upper extremity bypass grafting, but it can have devastating consequences. In the available literature regarding upper extremity bypass grafting for both occlusive and aneurysmal disease pathologies, noted infections have been limited to the incision sites, with no graft infections reported.[24–26,28,29] Rhodes et al. describe increased incisional infection rates in patients with radiation arteritis and atherosclerosis obliterans.[29] One explanation for the paucity of infections in upper extremity bypasses could be that the vast majority of patients are treated with autologous conduits, which can be infection resistant.[25–26]

Diagnosis of a bypass infection is usually straightforward. Systemic signs of illness such as fever, chills, or mental status changes should alert the surgeon to the possibility of a graft-related issue, particularly in patients with prosthetic bypass grafts. All incisions should be inspected to identify any cellulitis or a draining sinus tract. In addition, palpation over the bypass tunnel may reveal fluctuance or edema. The workup of the patient includes obtaining blood cultures and imaging. Contrast-enhanced computed tomography is the preferred initial imaging technique as it can identify subtle loss of normal tissue planes (fat density), fluid or gas collections surrounding the graft, and the presence of pseudoaneurysms. Gas collections adjacent to a prosthetic bypass are expected to dissipate within the first month of surgery; therefore, their presence in late follow-up is a very specific marker of graft infection even if the patient is otherwise asymptomatic.[30] CTA can also be used for planning of future intervention with regard to anatomy at clamp sites, determination of inflow and outflow vessels, and planning of clean bypass tunneling tracts.

Bypass infection requires removal of the graft material and a plan to re-establish arterial flow outside of the infected field. The standard teaching is that all infected material should be removed, and it is rare that portions of an infected graft can be salvaged. These are extensive operations and it can seem prudent to try to avoid re-operative areas, but it is rare to get away with this approach, especially if a prosthetic conduit was used. This is especially true if either anastomosis is involved as these patients will experience exsanguinating hemorrhage if surgery is delayed.[31] Because there are little data specific to the treatment of upper extremity bypass infections, these recommendations are extrapolations of graft infections from other arterial beds.

REFERENCES

1. McCarthy WJ, Flinn WR, Yao JST, Williams LR, Bergan JJ. Result of bypass grafting for upper limb ischemia J Vasc Surg. 1986; 3(5): 741–746.
2. Dent TL, Lindenauer SM, Ernst CB, Fry WJ. Multiple arteriosclerotic arterial aneurysms. Arch Surg. 1972;105(2):338–344.
3. Mackaay AJ, Beks PJ, Dur AH, et al. The distribution of peripheral vascular disease in a Dutch Caucasian population: Comparison of type II diabetic and non-diabetic subjects. European Journal of Vascular & Endovascular Surgery. 1995;9(2):170–175.
4. Brewster DC, Moncure AC, Darling RC, Ambrosino JJ, Abbott WM. Innominate artery lesions: Problems encountered and lessons learned. J Vasc Surg. 1985; 2:99–112.

5. Cury M, Greenberg RK, Morales JP, Mohabbat W, Hernandez AV. Supra-aortic vessels aneurysms: diagnosis and prompt intervention. J Vasc Surg. 2009;49(1):4–10.
6. Hughes K, Hamdan A, Schermerhorn M, Giordano A, Scovell S, Pomposelli F. Bypass for chronic ischemia of the upper extremity: Results in 20 patients. J Vasc Surg. 2007; 46: 303–307.
7. Pairolero PC, Walls JT, Payne WS, Hollier LH, Fairbairn JF. Subclavian-axillary artery aneurysms. Surgery. 1981; 90(4): 757–763.
8. Roddy SP, Darling RC, Chang BB, Keienberg PB, Paty PSK, Lloyd WE, Shah DM. Brachial artery reconstruction for occlusive disease: A 12-year experience. J Vasc Surg. 2001; 33(4). 802–805.
9. Johnson BL, Bandyk DF, Back MR, Avino AJ, Roth SM. Intraoperative duplex monitoring of infrainguinal vein bypass procedures. J Vasc Surg. 2000;31: 679–690.
10. Scali ST, Beck AW, Nolan BW, et al. Completion duplex ultrasound predicts early graft thrombosis after crural bypass in patients with critical limb ischemia. J Vasc Surg. 2011;54(4): 1006–1010.
11. Woo K, Palmer OP, Weaver FA, Rowe VL. Society for Vascular Surgery Vascular Quality Initiative. Outcomes of completion imaging for lower extremity bypass in the Vascular Quality Initiative. J Vasc Surg. 2015;62(2): 412–416.
12. Cormier B, Nezhat F, Sternchos J, Sonoda Y, Leitao MM. Electrocautery-associated vascular injury during robotic-assisted surgery. Obstet Gynecol. 2012;120(2 Pt 2): 491–493.
13. Giannakopoulos TG, Avgerinos ED. Management of Peripheral and Truncal Venous Injuries. Front Surg. 2017;4: 46–46.
14. Crumley RL, Smith JD. Postoperative chylous fistula prevention and management. The Laryngoscope. 1976;86(6): 804–813
15. Polistena A, Monacelli M, Lucchini R, Triola R, Conti C, Avenia S, Barillaro I, Sanguinetti A, Avenia N. Surgical morbidity of cervical lymphadenectomy for thyroid cancer: A retrospective cohort study over 25 years. Int J Surg. 2015; 21: 128–134.
16. Campisi CC, Boccardo F, Piazza C, Campisi C. Evolution of chylous fistula management after neck dissection. Current Opinion in Otolaryngology and head and Neck Surgery. 2013; 21(2): 150–156.
17. Jain A, Singh SN, Singhal P, Sharma MP, Grover M. A prospective study on the role of Octreotide in management of chyle fistula neck. Laryngoscope. 2015; 125(7): 1624–1627.
18. Higgins M, Park AW, Angle JF. Chylothorax: Percutaneous embolization of the thoracic duct. Operative Techniques in Thoracic and Cardiovasc Surg. 2015;20(4): 402–412.
19. Cunningham J, Hoskins W, Ferris S. Upper trunk brachial plexus palsy following chiropractic manipulation. Front Neurol. 2016;7: 211.
20. Woo A, Bakri K, Moran SL. Management of ulnar nerve injuries. J Hand Surg Am. 2015; 40(1): 173–181.
21. Cirakli A, Ulusoy EK, Ekinci Y. The role of electrophysiological examination in the diagnosis of carpal tunnel syndrome: Analysis of 2516 patients. Niger J Clin Pract. 2018;21(6): 731–734.
22. Houdek MT, Shin AY. Management and complications of traumatic peripheral nerve injuries. Hand Clinics. 2015;31(2): 151–163.
23. Jain KM, Simoni EJ, Munn JS, Madson DL. Long-term follow-up of bypasses to the brachial artery across the shoulder joint. AJS. 1996;172(2): 127–129.
24. Mesh CL, McCarthy WJ, Pearce WH, Flinn WR, Shireman PK, Yao JS. Upper extremity bypass grafting. A 15-year experience. Arch Surg. 1993;128(7): 795–802.
25. Spinelli F, Benedetto F, Passari G, et al. Bypass surgery for the treatment of upper limb chronic ischaemia. Eur J Vasc Endovasc Surg. 2010;39(2): 165–170.
26. Cheun TJ, Jayakumar L, Sheehan MK, Sideman MJ, Pounds LL, Davies MG. Outcomes of upper extremity interventions for chronic critical ischemia. J Vasc Surg. 2019;69(1): 120–128.
27. Brumberg RS, Back MR, Armstrong PA, et al. The relative importance of graft surveillance and warfarin therapy in infrainguinal prosthetic bypass failure. J Vasc Surg. 2007;46(6): 1160–1166.
28. Whitehouse WM, Zelenock GB, Wakefield TW, Graham LM, Lindenauer SM, Stanley JC. Arterial bypass grafts for upper extremity ischemia. J Vasc Surg. 1986;3(3): 569–573.
29. Rhodes JM, Cherry KJ, Clark RC, et al. Aortic-origin reconstruction of the great vessels: Risk factors of early and late complications. J Vasc Surg. 2000;31(2): 260–269.
30. Kilic A, Amaoutakis DJ, Reifsnyder T, Black JH, Abularrage CJ, Perler BA, Lum YW. Management of infected vascular grafts. Vascular Medicine. 2016;21(1): 53–60.
31. Bandyk DF, Novotney ML, Back MR, Johnson BL, Schmacht DC. Expanded application of in situ replacement for prosthetic graft infection. J Vasc Surg. 2001;34(3): 411–9 discussion 419–20.

SUGGESTED READING

Roddy SP, Darling RC, Chang BB, Keienberg PB, Paty PSK, Lloyd WE, Shah DM. Brachial artery reconstruction for occlusive disease: A 12-year experience. *J Vasc Surg* 2001; 33(4): 802–805.

17

Complications of open repair of unruptured abdominal aortic aneurysm

SACHINDER SINGH HANS

INDICATION

Small fusiform aneurysms (less than 4 cm in maximum AP/transverse diameter) are at a low risk of rupture, and therefore can be safely observed. The threshold for repair of an abdominal aortic aneurysm (AAA) is 5 cm in women and 5–5.5 cm in men. These diameters for repair are general guidelines.[1] However, patient's age, medical comorbidities, and life expectancy should be considered before recommending open repair of AAA. In general, the indication for repair in saccular aneurysm is 4.5 cm in anterior-posterior (AP)/transverse diameter.[1] An important consideration is the diameter of the aorta at or just below the renal arteries in relation to the largest transverse/AP diameter of the AAA. In women, AAA repair should be considered if the transverse/AP diameter of the AAA is twice the diameter of the aorta at the aortic neck. For example, if the aorta at the level of the renal arteries measures only 20–22 mm, it is appropriate to recommend repair in a patient with a 4.5 cm AAA provided the patient's general medical condition is satisfactory. Similarly, in men with a large diameter aortic neck, 30–32 mm repair can be deferred until the aneurysm reaches 6 cm in transverse/AP diameter, particularly in high risk patients. Open repair of infrarenal AAA is infrequently performed as the preferred method of treatment of infrarenal AAA is endovascular repair in patients with suitable anatomy. However, in patients with complex anatomy, open repair should be considered despite the availability of fenestrated grafts or branched endografts. These grafts at the present time should preferably be considered in high-risk patients only. The surgeon should be familiar with various open techniques as each has its distinct advantages and disadvantages.[2]

Transperitoneal approach is the most common method for exposing the infrarenal aorta, using either a midline or a transverse incision. A left flank retroperitoneal approach is exceedingly useful in patients with complex aortic neck anatomy and significant chronic obstructive pulmonary disease. The entire abdominal aorta from diaphragmatic hiatus to its bifurcation can be approached by a left flank approach. The main limitation of this exposure is the lack of good visualization of the right common iliac artery bifurcation and mid to distal right renal artery. In patients with associated horseshoe kidney, large or inflammatory AAA, multiple prior intra-abdominal operations, and prior ileostomy or colostomy, this approach is highly recommended.[2]

PREOPERATIVE PREPARATION

Preoperative computed tomographic angiography (CTA) is extremely useful to determine the site of aortic and iliac clamping and help in planning the type of aortic reconstruction. In addition, the CT scan should be reviewed for the presence of venous anomalies such as a retroaortic left renal vein, posterior collar renal vein, and the presence of arterial occlusive disease or aneurysmal disease in the celiac, superior mesenteric, and inferior mesenteric arteries. It is important to identify any other unexpected intra-abdominal pathology or structural anomalies, including a presence of a horseshoe or pelvic kidney, in order to appropriately plan the aortic repair.

TRANSPERITONEAL REPAIR

The abdomen is opened through a long xiphoid-to-suprapubic midline incision. The stomach, greater omentum, and transverse colon are retracted cephalad, and the small bowel is packed by warm saline soaked towels to the right. A self-retaining retractor such as a Bookwalter (Codman and Shurtleff Incorporated. Raynham, MA) or Omni (Integra) or Omni-Tract (Integra Life Sciences

Corporation, Plains Borough, NJ), Thompson retractor (Thompson Surgical Instruments, Traverse City, MI) is applied.[2] Ligament of Treitz is divided in a relatively avascular plane. The third and fourth portions of the duodenum are mobilized to the right periaortic lymphatics, and connective tissue containing small blood vessels are ligated and divided using 2-0 silk ties.[2] Inferior mesenteric vein can usually be preserved unless the aneurysm involves the pararenal aorta. Left renal vein is mobilized and a Silastic vessel loop is passed around it. The dissection in the posterior peritoneum is carried caudally to the right of the midline to protect inferior mesenteric artery (IMA) and avoid injury to the sympathetic nerve plexus. The accessory renal arteries if present and gonadal arteries should be carefully dissected.[2] Gonadal arteries are ligated and divided, but significant size accessory renal artery or abnormal origin of the main renal artery should be preserved with aortic cuff following the division of the anterior wall of the aorta and should be reimplanted into prosthetic graft as a Carrel patch.

PARARENAL AORTA

In the era of endovascular repair, most patients who required open repair have either juxtarenal or pararenal aortic aneurysms. In order to obtain optimal exposure of the pararenal aorta, the left renal vein may have to be divided and ligated, which is performed close to the inferior vena cava preserving collateral flow via adrenal and gonadal vein. Each adrenal artery just above the renal arteries needs to be ligated with 5-0 cardiovascular polypropylene suture (Ethicon, Somerville, NJ) and a silver clip is applied distally prior to its division.

Aortic bifurcation is carefully identified and both common iliac arteries are carefully mobilized in patients needing aortobi-iliac reconstruction. Anterior, medial, and lateral walls of the common iliac arteries are mobilized, but author does not completely dissect the posterior wall to prevent injury to the confluence of common iliac veins. On the left side, sigmoid colon may need to be mobilized along the white line of Toldt in patients with aneurysmal common iliac arteries. In patients with heavily calcified or diseased aorta at the aortic neck, supraceliac clamping is often safer than attempting to clamp a significantly diseased artery. Distal anastomosis to femoral arteries should be avoided unless the patient has concomitant iliac artery occlusive disease. Anastomosis to femoral arteries is associated with increased risk of surgical site infection in the groin and late development of an anastomotic aneurysm. Inferior mesenteric artery is looped with double looped Silastic tape. Prior to aortic clamping, heparin is administered intravenously (100 international units/per kg to maintain ACT of 250–300s). Standard repair is accomplished using intraluminal technique. In patients with mycotic aneurysms, the entire aneurysm sac should be removed. Knitted Dacron graft for aortic and aortoiliac reconstruction is preferred. After removal of mural laminated thrombus bleeding from lumbar arteries is controlled with 2-0 GI silk suture. In patients with heavily calcified posterior wall of the aorta, local endarterectomy of the ostia of the lumbar arteries is performed to secure a transfixation suture. Reconstructions performed with a tube or a bifurcated graft. The aortic neck is prepared for proximal anastomosis by "T-ing" of the aortotomy between the normal and the aneurysmal aorta. With a continuous "3-0" or "4-0" polypropylene suture is used for anastomosis.[2] In patients with friable aorta, author prefers interrupted horizontal mattress sutures tied on pledgets and reinforced with a second layer of continuous suture. Before checking the integrity of proximal anastomosis, BioGlue (CryoLife, Kennesaw, GA) is applied in patients with friable aortic neck. Distal anastomosis to the aortic bifurcation or to the common iliac artery is performed with continuous suture.

SUPRACELIAC AORTA

The left lobe of the liver is retracted towards the right following division of the left triangular ligament. Dissection is done after opening of the gastrohepatic omentum. The esophagus is encircled and retracted to the left with a penrose drain with palpation of the nasogastric tube as guide. Deep blades of the surgical retractor system are inserted to expose the right crus of the diaphragm, and the muscular fibers of the right crus are separated with the help of Metzenbaum scissors and about 5 cm opening is made in the right crus. The fascia surrounding the aorta is divided. The index and middle fingers of the right hand are placed over the lateral wall of the aorta to guide the application of a vascular clamp with the left hand.

IMA RECONSTRUCTION

If backbleeding from IMA is poor and the patient has a large IMA with arc of Riolan, reimplantation of IMA into the graft is necessary as a Carrel patch. After a small disk of Dacron graft is excised, a 5-0 or 6-0 cardiovascular polypropylene suture is used for anastomosis.

MAINTENANCE OF PELVIC CIRCULATION

Inadequate antegrade flow to at least one hypogastric artery (HA) may lead to sexual dysfunction, gluteal claudication, and sigmoid or spinal cord ischemia. Therefore, in patients in whom antegrade flow to at least one HA cannot be established, a separate bypass to the HA with a 6 mm or 8 mm Dacron graft should be performed.[2]

RETROPERITONEAL APPROACH

The proper positioning of the patient is important for retroperitoneal exposure. The patient is placed in a modified right lateral decubitus position with the shoulder positioned 60–70 degrees to the table and the hips rotated as far posteriorly as possible. A beanbag is helpful in making the alignment.[2] We usually have a break in the table above the iliac crest. The table is jackknifed to open the left flank. For infrarenal aortic procedure, the standard flank incision extending from the lateral margin of the left rectus sheath midway between the symphysis pubis and the umbilicus laterally into the 11th intercostal space for 10–12 cm is made.[2] For exposure of the pararenal aorta, a 10th intercostal incision is more appropriate.[2] The abdominal wall and the intercostal musculature are divided in the line of the incision and extraperitoneal space is entered at the tip of the 12th rib. The peritoneum and overlying transversalis fascia are stripped away from the abdominal wall musculature anteriorly as far as the lateral border of the rectus sheath. The psoas muscle is exposed posterolaterally behind the left kidney. The abdominal aorta and the left common iliac artery are exposed. An attempt is made to identify the left renal artery. The posterolateral wall of the aorta is then exposed. The neck of the aneurysm is exposed, and the dissection planes anterior and posterior to the aorta for application of proximal aortic clamping are carefully exposed and mobilized. A circumferential dissection of the aortic neck is not necessary if the distal end of the clamp extends beyond the wall of the aortic neck. For suprarenal control of the aorta, dissection is continued cephalad along the lateral wall of the aorta toward the left crus. The fibers of the crus are divided 2–3 cm along the axis of the aorta.[2] A pair of lumbar arteries and adrenal arteries should be carefully avoided. Author prefers 5-0 cardiovascular Prolene suture proximally at the origin of these vessels and silver clips distally before division. As the dissection proceeds cephalad, supraceliac aorta is exposed and clamped as the most optimal site of proximal clamping as determined by preop CTA.[2]

During anterior mobilization of peritoneal sac, the ureter should be carefully protected from excessive stretching by careful retraction and keeping the dissection close to the wall of the aneurysm. Injury to the ureter is extremely uncommon and tends to occur in the distal one-third if precautions are not taken. Once diagnosed, ureteral stent with or without nephrostomy may become necessary at the recommendation of a urologist.

The peritoneal sac is stripped off the left iliac fossa to expose the iliac arteries. Left ureter is mobilized anteromedially with the peritoneal envelope.[2] Proximal portions of the right common iliac artery are exposed, and endoluminal control may be necessary to avoid injury to the iliac vein. More distal right common iliac artery exposure is aided by continuing the flank incision all the way to the linea alba. When more distal exposure is required, a small right lower quadrant incision, a few centimeters above the inguinal ligament with rotation of the operating table to the left, may become necessary complications.

VASCULAR STUDY GROUP OF NEW ENGLAND

Lifeline registry of patients who underwent open repair of non-ruptured infrerenal AAA demonstrated 26% serious and 11% major adverse events noted in the perioperative period. Data from the National Surgical Quality Improvement Program [NSQIP] and the Vascular Study Group and New England [VSGNE], as well as data from individual centers, have shown that the rate of complications increase as the procedure complexity increases.[1]

1. **Delirium:** Delirium is common following open AAA repair in patients above 65 years old. Delirium is more common in patients who have preoperative cognitive impairment. Onset of delirium results in increased incidence of adverse events and length of stay. Postoperative use of narcotics, hypoxia, and infection are other precipitating factors.
2. **Postoperative pulmonary failure:** Pulmonary failure occurs in 8–12% of patients undergoing open AAA repair. The need for ventilator support is quite common following repair of complex AAA. In most patients, tracheostomy is not necessary. Postoperative pulmonary complications have been associated with reduced long-term survival. Predictors of respiratory complications include preoperative chronic obstructive pulmonary disease, congestive heart failure, intraoperative blood transfusion, and preoperative renal dysfunction.[3]
3. **Postoperative renal failure:** Postoperative renal failure occurs in 5–12% of patients undergoing elective open AAA repair.[1] The results from European Vascular Registry revealed postoperative renal failure in 140 (6%) of 2347 patients undergoing open AAA repair. Rates of postoperative renal insufficiency in the Medicare population approach 10% with 0.5% requiring renal replacement therapy. Risk factors for postoperative renal failure include age greater than 75 years, symptomatic AAA, suprarenal or juxtarenal AAA, elevated preoperative serum creatinine, intraoperative blood transfusion, and chronic obstructive pulmonary disease. Patients with postoperative renal failure have a significantly higher 30-day mortality. A meta-analysis of patients undergoing open repair in patients with pararenal aortic aneurysm reported 15–20% incidence of postoperative renal insufficiency with 3.5% patients requiring dialysis support.[1] Close attention to volume status, and adequate

hydration with crystalloids and colloids during the operation and in the postoperative period. Although clinical trials have not demonstrated a reduction in the incidence of renal failure in patients receiving mannitol in aortic cross-clamping, most surgeons empirically infuse 25–50 g of mannitol during the procedure.

4. **Postoperative cardiac complications:** These complications occur in 15% of patients undergoing elective AAA repair. Myocardial injury occurs in 3–8% of adults undergoing major non-cardiac surgery and is associated with significant morbidity with death in 1%–1.6% patients.[5,6] Secondary prevention with cardiovascular drugs (such as aspirin and statins reduces the risk of major cardiac complications and mortality). Myocardial ischemia was reported in 3% of the patient's with death in 1.67% from a large database (10.5 million in hospital surgeries) by reported by Smilowitz et al.[6] In their study, vascular operations were the largest group among patients undergoing noncardiac surgery. According to 2014 ESC/ESA guidelines, preoperative noninvasive testing should be considered in high-risk surgery such as open AAA repair, and patients with more than two clinical risk markers (systolic heart failure, recent MI and poor functional capacity). However, coronary artery revascularization before elective vascular surgery does not significantly alter the long-term outcome. The risk factors for predicting cardiac complications are based on revised cardiac risk index (ESC guidelines 2014):
   A. Type of surgery: Out of all the non-cardiac surgeries, open AAA results in the highest incidence of cardiac complications.
   B. History of ischemic heart disease.
   C. History of heart failure.
   D. A history of cerebrovascular disease.
   E. Preoperative insulin treatment for Type 1 diabetes mellitus.
   F. Creatinine greater than 2 mg/dL.

5. **Postoperative atrial fibrillation:** Peak onset of paroxysmal atrial fibrillation occurs between 0–4 days. It really does not recur if the underlying cause is corrected. Rate control is the treatment strategy of choice in many patients with a goal of ventricular rate between 80–100 per minute. Beta-blockers like metoprolol, calcium channel blockers (diltiazem and amiodarone) are usually administered.[8] Direct current cardioversions are the preferred treatment option in patients with hemodynamic compromise and should be considered in patients associated with chest pain, pulmonary edema, and loss of consciousness.[8] Despite achieving sinus rhythm, there is a significant long-term risk of atrial fibrillation and stroke among the patient with the new onset of paroxysmal atrial fibrillation. Most patients with new onset of paroxysmal atrial fibrillation will convert to normal sinus rhythm 2 months after surgery. When atrial fibrillation persists for longer than 48 hours, antithrombotic therapy should be considered to reduce the risk of stroke and systemic embolism. The risk of bleeding in patients with recent open AAA repair should be considered before starting anticoagulation.
6. **Intestinal ischemia:** The incidence of intestinal ischemia has varied from 0.2% to as high as 10% usually due to differences in diagnostic criteria and diagnostic methods. Clinically, significant colon ischemia occurs in 1–2% of patients following abdominal aortic aneurysm reconstruction resulting in 50–75% mortality. Mortality can reach 90% if the bowel resection is required for infarction.[1] Colon ischemia is far more common than small bowel ischemia.[1] The presence of early postoperative diarrhea, melena, hematochezia mandates definitive diagnostic aids such as fiberoptic sigmoidoscopy. Ligation of a large IMA, particularly in the presence of meandering mesenteric artery (arc of Riolan), SMA and celiac artery occlusive disease, and atheroembolism or retractor blade injury to superior mesenteric artery, prior colon resection, all contribute to intestinal ischemia. In patients with severe SMA stenosis and presence of mesenteric collaterals and a large IMA may need reimplantation of the IMA into the body or a limb of the aorto/aortobiiliac graft using Carrel patch.[2] Once the diagnosis of bowel ischemia is suspected and confirmed by fiberoptic sigmoidoscopy or colonoscopy, the patient should be adequately resuscitated and started on intravenous antibiotics targeted towards intestinal microorganisms. The patients with disease localized to mucosa and muscularis mucosa can be managed expectantly whereas those with full-thickness infarction of the bowel wall will require emergent laparotomy and bowel resection. In patients with ischemia limited to mucosa and muscularis mucosa, late development of bowel stricture may require intervention.
7. **Lower extremity ischemia:** Lower extremity ischemia occurs in 1–4% of patients undergoing elective AAA repairs. Distal perfusion should be checked after distal anastomosis completed. In patients with preoperative palpable posterior tibial and dorsalis pedis pulses, one should be able to palpate the pulses; however, in patients with associated infrainguinal arterial occlusive disease, Doppler flow should be present at least in posterior tibial or dorsalis pedis artery at the ankle/foot.[2] In some patients in whom body

temperature has fallen during the procedure, the feet should be wrapped with warm blankets.[2] Presence of a limb ischemia usually suggests technical anastomotic complications at the distal anastomosis. Clamp injury causing dissection, acute thrombosis or distal embolization or other causes of lower limb ischemia.[2] Spasm of distal arterial bed with loss of Doppler flows is an uncommon cause. Because of the de-clamping shock following opening of the distal anastomosis, aggressive fluid resuscitation by anesthesia is necessary and close communication between the surgeon and the anesthesia team is very important as the distal clamps are gradually released. Besides meticulous technique during sewing atherosclerotic arteries, care should be undertaken in selecting the clamp sites to prevent atheroemboli or vessel injury. Adequate systemic anticoagulation should be maintained during the aortic crossclamping and dose of heparin adjusted to maintain activated clotting time between 250 and 300. Forward and backbleeding should be carried out before the anastomosis is completed.

8. **Spinal cord ischemia:** Spinal cord ischemia following repair of intact AAA is extremely rare (less than 1%), but rates can be higher in patients undergoing repair of type 4 thoracoabdominal aortic aneurysm.[1,2,4] Previous thoracic aortic graft, aortic crossclamping, and prolonged aortic crossclamp time, and failure to establish flow to at least one hypogastric artery, intraoperative and postoperative hypotension are factors leading to spinal cord ischemia. Abnormally low origin of artery of Adamkiewicz (arteria radicularis magna) can also contribute to a spinal cord ischemia. Typically, arteria radicularis magna arises from a left posterior intercostal artery at the level of T9-T12 and supplies the lower two-third of the spinal cord via anterior spinal artery. When damaged, it can result in anterior spinal syndrome with fecal and urinary incontinence with impaired motor function, but intact sensory function in most patients.
9. **Venous thrombosis:** Following AAA infrequent (1%), however, in patients sustaining major venous injury (iliac veins undergoing primary repair), the incidence of venous thrombosis is higher. Some patients develop deep venous thrombosis (DVT) after discharge. DVT following a AAA repair is associated with higher mortality.
10. **Pancreatitis, duodenal obstruction, ileus:** Pancreatitis, duodenal obstruction and ileus are uncommon complication of AAA repair. These complications are slightly more common after open repair due to large retroperitoneal hematoma and trauma to the pancreas by retractors. Most patients improve with nasogastric suction, correction of electrolytes, and intravenous fluids as well as TPN as necessary. Injuries to the ureter, small bowel, and colon are uncommon and should be managed by urologist and general surgeon.

11a. **Graft-related complications:** Limb occlusion graft, graft infection, para-anastomotic aneurysm tends to develop in 5–10% patients undergoing AAA repair. The most common complications are anastomotic pseudoaneurysm, graft thrombosis, graft enteric fistula. Most complications appear late (3–8 years).[9] Graft infections occurs in less than 1% of patient undergoing elective AAA repair. An implanted aortic graft is at risk of infection at the time of implantation or later by hematogenous spread. This will be described in the chapter on ruptured AAA.

11b. **Para-anastomotic aneurysms** following open AAA repair includes pseudoaneurysm, resulting from disruption of the anastomosis and a true aneurysm that develop proximal to the proximal anastomosis or distal to distal anastomosis. Predisposing factors include hypertension, nicotine abuse, and COPD. The incidence of 4–9% at 10 years follow-up has been reported. Indolent graft infection though rare should be suspected in all patients with anastomotic pseudoaneurysms. Large and rapidly expanding para-anastomotic aneurysms often need repair depending upon the general condition and life expectancy of the patient. Endovascular options whenever feasible are preferable.

11c. **Incisional hernia:** Retroperitoneal incisions for aortic aneurysm can lead to injury to the 11th intercostal nerve, which can lead to paresthesia and in about 30% patients, a "bulge" in the lateral abdominal wall with muscle atrophy in 7–15%. Transperitoneal repair is associated with higher incidence of late small-bowel obstruction and approximately 10–15% patients develop incisional hernia within first 6 years following AAA repair.

11. **Early mortality**: Mortality following open AAA repair is affected by age of the patient, urgency of the procedure in symptomatic patients, associated comorbidities and proximal extension of the aneurysm.[4] A 30-day mortality in most contemporary single-center series have reported 1.5–4%.[1,4] However, data from state and National Registries have reported much higher mortality of 4–8%. A 30-day mortality of 3.0–4.7% have been reported from the results of multi-center post-operative randomized trial with the increasing use of endovascular aneurysm repair.[4] The aneurysms requiring open repair in the present era are more complex often requiring suprarenal or supraceliac crossclamping. Mortality of 3.6% was reported from the vascular study group of New England Registry among 443 patients undergoing open AAA repair for complex aneurysms.

IATROGENIC VENOUS INJURIES

Major venous injury during aortic reconstruction (less than 2%) though rare can lead to major morbidity and mortality. Since the introduction of transluminal repair and abandonment of aneurysm resection, incidence of major venous injury has decreased. Factors associated with major venous injury include anomalies of the left renal vein (left renal vein, retroaortic and left renal collar vein), double or left-sided vena cava, venous injury during clamping of iliac arteries, repair of inflammatory aneurysm, and redo aortoiliac repair.

Case Example 1

Repair of Juxtarenal Abdominal Aortic Aneurysm with Aortorenal Bypass

A 68-year-old male presented with a 5 cm aneurysm (AP/Transverse diameter) juxtarenal abdominal aortic aneurysm (JAAA) with associated 2.8 cm bilateral common iliac artery aneurysms, and 2 cm left hypogastric artery aneurysm. Preoperative aortography showed accessory left lower pole renal artery. Medical comorbidities included history of atrial flutter, hypertension, and post-thrombotic syndrome involving both lower extremities.

Procedure: Through midline transperitoneal incision, AAA was exposed. Exposure for proximal control of the aorta, included ligation of the left renal vein which was performed close to the inferior vena cava. The aneurysm arose at the level the left renal artery and was saccular with a bulge to the left. Left crus of the diaphragm were divided by electrocautery. Both common iliac artery aneurysms were mobilized along with mobilization of the origin of the hypogastric and external iliac arteries. Following systemic heparinization, the aorta was clamped above the left renal artery and below the right renal artery. Arterial reconstruction was performed with end to end anastomoses using bifurcated 22 × 11 mm knitted Dacron graft (Meadox-Boston Scientific, Malborough, MA). The proximal anastomosis was performed in two layers with a first layer of interrupted horizontal mattress suture on pledgets with 3-0 cardiovascular polypropylene (Ethicon, Somerville, NJ) and a second layer of continuous suture. As the proximal clamp was released there was excessive bleeding at 7'o clock of the suture line. Re-application of the clamp a few centimeters proximally resulted in a tear of the aorta. A 30 cc balloon was introduced through the left limb of the Dacron graft and inflated supra at the celiac level. Left renal artery was transected at its origin from the aorta. Proximal stump of the renal artery was suture ligated and deep bites into the left lateral wall of the aorta were taken using horizontal mattress sutures of 3-0 cardiovascular Prolene on pledgets. Bio-glue (Cryolife, Kennesaw, GA) was applied to achieve hemostasis. A 6 mm PTFE graft (W L Gore, Newark, DE) was anastomosed to the main body of the Dacron graft on the left side just above the bifurcation of the graft taking out a small disc of Dacron graft using 5-0 CV polypropylene and distally was anastomosed end to end to the divided left renal artery. The left lower pole renal artery was re-implanted into the left limb of the Dacron graft using 5-0 CV polypropylene as well. The left hypogastric aneurysm was excised, and backbleeding was controlled with 4-0- CV polypropylene suture. Because of severe calcific disease in the left external iliac artery, left limb of the graft was anastomosed to the left common femoral artery in an end to side fashion. Left common iliac aneurysm was opened and its wall was partially removed, and proximal left external iliac artery was ligated. On the right side, anastomosis of the right limb of the Dacron graft was performed end to end to the common iliac artery at the bifurcation after removal of the aneurysm. The patient received 600 cc of blood from the cell saver and one unit of PRBCs were given to the patient. Patient's postop course was complicated by respiratory failure which improved with ventilatory support.

The patient was extubated on the third postoperative day. The patient had transient renal dysfunction. Postoperative aortography showed patent aortoiliac and femoral graft and patent left aortorenal bypass (Figures 17.1 and 17.2). Patient did well and underwent repair of 3.5 cm left femoral anastomotic aneurysm 8 years after the original follow up procedure (Figure 17.3). The patient later expired from complications of Alzheimer's dementia 12 years following his AAA repair.

Discussion: Operative repair of juxtarenal AAA is a technically challenging operation. In absence of the need to visualize distal right common iliac artery (as was the case for this patient due to 2.8 cm right iliac aneurysm), a left flank retroperitoneal approach is increasingly used for open repair of proximal complex AAA. In patients with need to explore the aorta proximal to the renal arteries, redo aortic surgery, AAAs

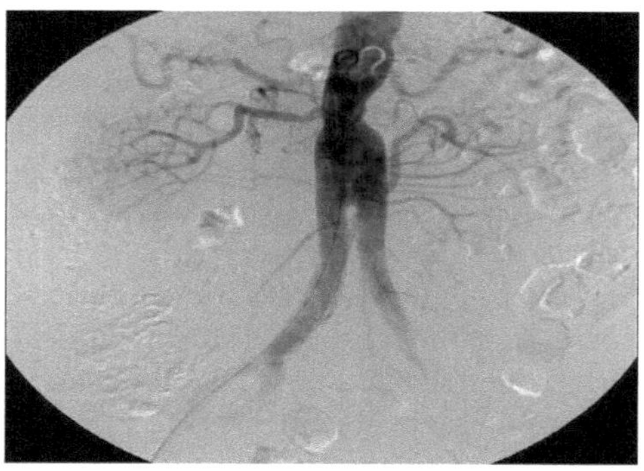

Figure 17.1 Showing aortic reconstruction with aorto-renal bypass.

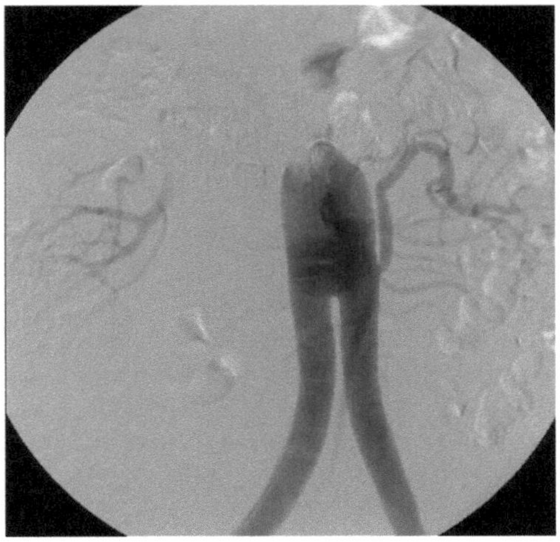

Figure 17.2 Aortography showing aortic bifurcation graft and left aortorenal bypass.

in the presence of a horseshoe kidney, hostile abdomen with prior osteotomies, or inflammatory AAA, concomitant renal artery bypass became necessary as proximal aortic clamp resulted in tear of the aorta above the renal arteries.[1] Because of the improvements in medical management of renovascular hypertension, concomitant renal artery bypass with open AAA is rarely indicated. In order to perform suprarenal dissection via trans peritoneal approach, mobilization of left renal vein or ligation of left renal vein close to the inferior vena cava preserving gonadal and adrenal vein as venous outflow from the kidneys is necessary. Mobilization of the left renal vein without division often requires ligation of adrenal vein and gonadal vein. In addition, left crus of the diaphragm needs to be divided to gain proximal aortic exposure.

Follow-up aortography showed satisfactory proximal anastomosis, patent left aortorenal bypass, occluded lower pole renal artery reimplantation (Figure 17.2), and an anastomotic aneurysm involving the graft and left femoral artery. Though not always possible, either tube graft (aorto-aortic) or aortoiliac anastomosis should be preferred as femoral anastomosis may result in increased incidence of surgical site infection, lymphoceles, and late development of anastomotic aneurysms.[10] Repair of left femoral anastomotic aneurysm was performed by interposition of an 8 mm knitted Dacron graft. A left flank approach through 9th or 10th ICS, 9th ICS for paravisceral extent IV thoracoabdominal aneurysms and 10th ICS for pararenal aortic aneurysms is preferable.[10] Renal, visceral, and occasionally spinal cord ischemia may occur with prolonged proximal clamping.[10] Renal artery reconstruction at the time of open repair of paravisceral aneurysm is associated with increased incidence of acute renal failure and mortality.[11,12] Minimizing renal ischemia time to less than 40 minutes is important in reducing the risk of acute kidney injury. Before aortic

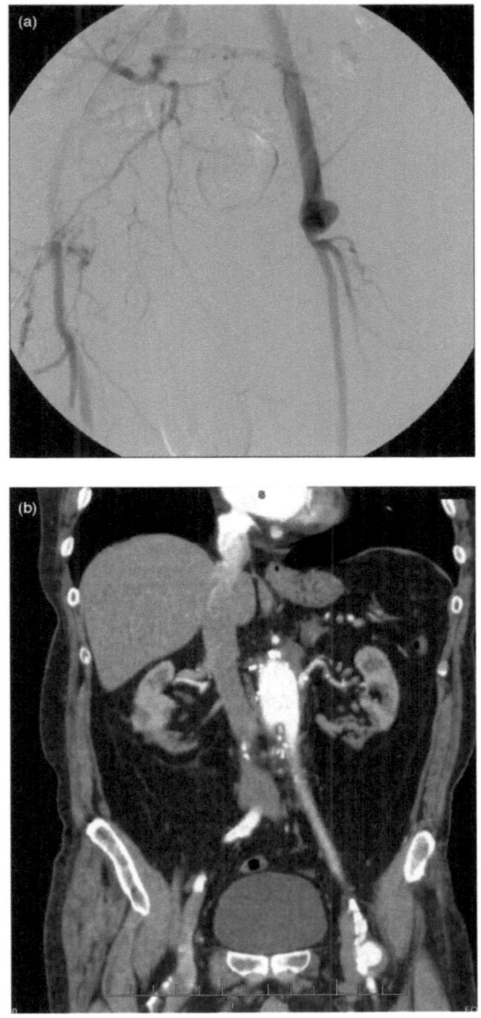

Figure 17.3A and 17.3B Aortogram and CTA showing patent left aortorenal bypass graft and aortic bifurcation graft with left femoral anastomotic aneurysm.

cross clamping above the suprarenal or supraceliac level, hemodynamics needs to be optimized. Mannitol 25 g is administered 30 minutes prior to aortic cross clamping, though its benefit in preventing renal dysfunction has not been proven. Deery et al. reported from vascular surgery group of New England registry for the repair of complex AAA (defined by need of suprarenal or supraceliac clamping) had higher perioperative mortality (3.2% compared to 1.2% standard infrarenal AAA repair).[13] Renal or visceral ischemia independently predicted cardiac, respiratory, and renal complications according to results of their study. [13]

Case Example 2

A 68-year-old female underwent open AAA repair and bilateral common iliac artery aneurysm repair for 4 cm Tr/Ap diameter juxtarenal aneurysm and 4 cm Rt common iliac aneurysm and 2.4 cm left

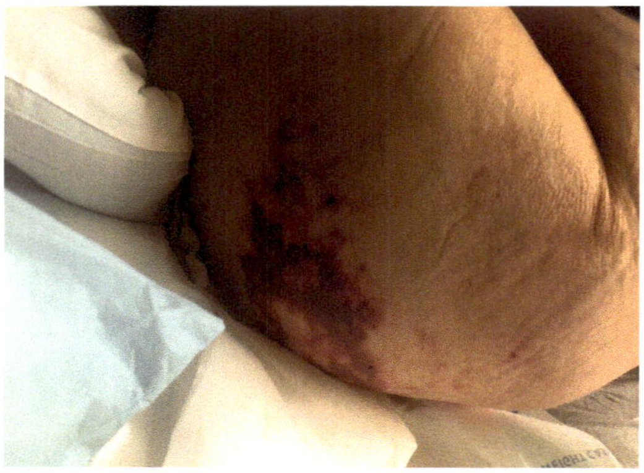

Figure 17.4 Gluteal skin ischemia on the left side due to hypogastric artery malperfusion.

common iliac aneurysm. There was occlusion of right hypogastric artery. There was foreshortening of sigmoid mesocolon with marked adherence to the ureter secondary to remote diverticulitis. Aorto-right external iliac and left common femoral graft with ligation of left common iliac artery above its bifurcation so that left hypogastric artery was established in a retrograde fashion. Postop period was complicated by ATN and ischemic skin over the left gluteal area (Figure 17.4). She did not have any weakness of either lower extremity. Ischemic lesion over the left gluteal area healed in 4 weeks.

Antegrade flow to at least one hypogastric artery should be maintained following open repair of AAA. Failure to do so may result in pelvic ischemia resulting in sigmoid colon ischemia, paraplegia, gluteal muscle and skin necrosis. Because of chronic occlusion of right hypogastric artery with devolpment of pelvic collaterals helped in preventing other manifestations of pelvic ischemia except skin ischemia in this patient.

REFERENCES

1. Chaikof EL, Dalman RL, Eskandari MK, Jackson BM, Lee WA, Mansour MA, et al. The Society for Vascular Surgery practice guidelines on the care of patients with an abdominal aortic aneurysm. J Vasc Surg. 2018;67(1): 2–77.e72. doi:10.1016/j.jvs.2017.10.044
2. Shepard A. Open nonruptured infrarenal aortic aneurysm repair. In Hans S, Shepard A., Weaver M., et al (Ed.), Endovascular and Open Vascular Reconstruction: A Practical Approach. Taylor & Francis Group: Boca Raton, FL, LLC; 2017: (197–204).
3. Zettervall SL, Soden PA, Shean KE, Deery SE, Ultee KH, Alef M, et al. Early extubation reduces respiratory complications and hospital length of stay following repair of abdominal aortic aneurysms. J Vasc Surg. 2017;65(1): 58–64.e51. doi:10.1016/j.jvs.2016.05.095
4. Nathan DP, Brinster CJ, Jackson BM, Wang GJ, Carpenter JP, Fairman RM, Woo EY. Predictors of decreased short- and long-term survival following open abdominal aortic aneurysm repair. J Vasc Surg. 2011;54(5): 1237–1243. doi:10.1016/j.jvs.2011.05.028
5. Khan J, Alonso-Coello P, Devereaux PJ. Myocardial injury after noncardiac surgery. Curr Opin Cardiol. 2014;29(4): 307–311. doi:10.1097/hco.0000000000000069
6. Smilowitz NR, Gupta N, Ramakrishna H, Guo Y, Berger JS, Bangalore S. Perioperative Major Adverse Cardiovascular and Cerebrovascular Events Associated With Noncardiac Surgery. JAMA Cardiol. 2017;2(2): 181–187. doi:10.1001/jamacardio.2016.4792
7. Danelich IM, Lose JM, Wright SS, Asirvatham SJ, Ballinger BA, Larson DW, Lovely JK. Practical management of postoperative atrial fibrillation after noncardiac surgery. J Am Coll Surg. 2014;219(4): 831–841. doi:10.1016/j.jamcollsurg.2014.02.038
8. Davenport DL, Xenos ES. Deep venous thrombosis after repair of nonruptured abdominal aneurysm. J Vasc Surg. 2013;57(3): 678–683.e671. doi:10.1016/j.jvs.2012.09.048
9. Hallett JW Jr, Marshall DM, Petterson TM, Gray DT, Bower TC, Cherry KJ, Jr, et al. Graft-related complications after abdominal aortic aneurysm repair: reassurance from a 36-year population-based experience. J Vasc Surg. 1997;25(2): 277–284; discussion 285–276.
10. Shepard AD. Proximal Abdominal Aortic Aneurysm repair in Endovascular and Open Vascular Reconstruction: A Practical Approach. Hans SS, Weaver MR, Bove PG, Long GW. (Eds.) CRC Press. Boca Raton, FL; 2018: 213–220.
11. Ultee KHJ, Soden PA, Zettervall SL, McCallum JC, Siracuse JJ, Alef MJ, Vascular Study Group of New England. The perioperative effect of concomitant procedures during open infrarenal abdominal aortic aneurysm repair. J. Vasc Surg. 2016;64(4): 934–940.e1. https://doi.org/10.1016/j.jvs.2016.01.048.
12. Wooster M, Back M, Patel S, Tanious A, Armstrong P, Shames M. Outcomes of concomitant renal reconstruction during open paravisceral aortic aneurysm repair. J. Vasc Surg. 2017;66(4): 1149–1156. https://doi.org/10.1016/j.jvs.2017.04.051.
13. Deery SE, Lancaster RT, Baril DT, Indes JE, Bertges DJ, Conrad MF, Patel VI. Contemporary outcomes of open complex abdominal aortic aneurysm repair. J Vasc Surg. 2016;63(5): 1195–1200. doi:10.1016/j.jvs.2015.12.038

SUGGESTED READING

The Society for Vascular Surgery practice guidelines on the care of patients with an abdominal aortic aneurysm. Elliot L. Chaikof, MD, PhD,a Ronald L. Dalman, MD,b Mark K. Eskandari, MD,c Benjamin M. Jackson, MD,d W. Anthony Lee, MD,e M. Ashraf Mansour, MD,f et.al

18

Complications following isolated common iliac artery and hypogastric artery aneurysm repair

MONICA ABDELMASIH, DIPANKAR MUKHERJEE, AND AHMED KAYSSI

Isolated iliac artery aneurysms are uncommon, with autopsy studies estimating a prevalence in the general population of 0.03–0.1%.[1,2] They account for fewer than 2% of all arterial aneurysms.[3–5] Among iliac artery aneurysms, common iliac artery (CIA) aneurysms are the most common.[1,3,4,6–10] Conversely, external iliac artery (EIA) aneurysms are the rarest, which may be explained by the EIA's embryological development from a different cell population than the aorta and other iliac arteries. An aneurysm of the CIA is generally defined as having a diameter greater than 1.5 cm in women and 1.8 cm in men.[1,12] The hypogastric artery, also known as the internal iliac artery (IIA), is generally considered to be aneurysmal when the dimeter is greater than 0.8 cm.[12] While often asymptomatic and diagnosed incidentally, some of these aneurysms can cause abdominal pain, obstructive symptoms involving the gastrointestinal, genitourinary, pelvic venous, or nervous systems, limb ischemia, or fistulization, and; rupture can be associated with significant morbidity and mortality. Hypogastric artery aneurysms in particular have been found to cause symptoms, such as abdominal pain or extremity symptoms, in more than 50% of patients, even in those without free rupture.[13] The expansion rate of CIA aneurysms has been reported as 0.5–1.5 mm/year in those less than 3 cm in diameter compared with 2.5–2.8 mm/year in those measuring greater than 3 cm.[7] The median expansion rate of CIA aneurysms is approximately 2.9 mm/year.[14] Brin et al. reported that 38% of patients with hypogastric artery aneurysms presented with rupture.[15] Another study demonstrated a similarly high hypogastric artery rupture rate of 49%, with hypogastric artery aneurysms rupturing more frequently than CIA aneurysms.[8] The average mortality rate following rupture of an isolated iliac artery aneurysm is approximately 28%, but has been reported to be up to 60%.[5]

INDICATIONS FOR REPAIR

Iliac artery aneurysms should be considered for repair based on size criteria or the presence of patient symptoms. Following a chart review of 50 patients with isolated iliac artery aneurysms, McCready et al. recommended repair of hypogastric artery aneurysms greater than 3 cm.[16] Similarly, Kasirajan et al. recommended that CIA aneurysms greater than 3 cm should also be considered for repair.[17] After a mean follow-up of 57 months, they reported that enlargement was not observed in aneurysms measuring less than 3 cm in diameter. A retrospective analysis of 63 patients, however, found that only 6.3% of hypogastric artery aneurysms ruptured at a size less than 4 cm, which may be a more appropriate threshold for repair.[11] The authors argued that this rupture rate may be similar to that of abdominal aortic aneurysms (AAA) less than 5.5 cm in diameter (8%). This seems to be reflected in practice, as a survey of European vascular surgeons reported that most would treat an asymptomatic CIA aneurysm at a size threshold of 4 cm.[18] The European Society for Vascular Surgery (ESVS) recommends in its 2019 guidelines that elective repair of an iliac artery aneurysm should be considered at a size threshold no smaller than 3.5 cm (class IIb, level C evidence).[12] Regardless of size, however, repair should be considered in patients presenting with new or worsening abdominal pain as this may indicate impending rupture.

OPTIONS FOR REPAIR

Repair of isolated iliac artery aneurysms was traditionally performed with open surgery. However, advances in endovascular technology have allowed for more minimally invasive options, avoiding the challenges of operating deep within the pelvis. Hybrid procedures, including both open and endovascular components, can be used as well. The most appropriate mode of repair should consider the extent and distribution of aneurysmal disease and patient characteristics in order to develop a suitable operative plan (Figure 18.1).[5,11]

A number of studies have compared open and endovascular repair of iliac artery aneurysms and found no significant difference in long-term survival rates.[10] Huang et al. reported a 5-year survival rate of 65% in those who underwent repair for CIA aneurysms. There was no significant difference between open and endovascular repair in terms of 3-year survival, primary patency (open repair 97%, endovascular repair 95%), secondary patency (open repair 99.6%, endovascular repair 100%), or freedom from re-intervention.[14] Patel et al. reported a similar overall primary patency rate of 98% and no significant difference between open and endovascular repair for iliac artery aneurysms (primary patency 100% and 96% in open and endovascular repair, respectively).[6] This pattern of similar survival rates has been reported in open and endovascular repair of isolated hypogastric artery aneurysms as well at 30 days and up to 18 months.[11] Chaer et al. reported that freedom from re-intervention at 1 and 2 years was not significantly different between patients who underwent open and endovascular repair.[19] While Zhorzel et al. also found no significant difference in survival at 1 and 5 years following repair of isolated iliac artery aneurysms, they did find that freedom from re-intervention was significantly greater in open repair compared to endovascular repair (97% compared to 40% at 5 years).[9]

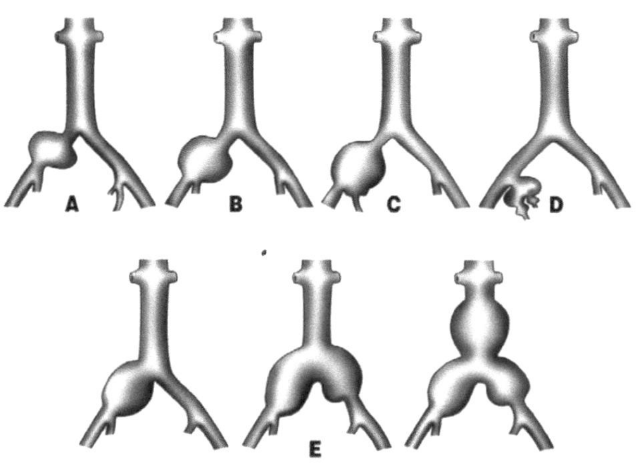

Figure 18.1 Categories of iliac artery aneurysms based on anatomical characteristics. (A) Isolated, unilateral common iliac artery (CIA) aneurysm without involvement of the iliac bifurcation. (B) Isolated, unilateral CIA aneurysm extending to the common iliac bifurcation. (C) Unilateral CIA with involvement of the hypogastric artery. (D) Isolated, unilateral hypogastric artery aneurysm with or without involvement of its distal branches. (E) Unilateral or bilateral CIA aneurysms with involvement of the aortic bifurcation or an abdominal aortic aneurysm. (Sandhu RS, Pipinos II. Isolated iliac artery aneurysms. *Semin Vasc Surg.* 2005;18(4):209–215.)

OPEN REPAIR

Open repair can take place using a trans- or retroperitoneal approach depending on the extent of repair and the presence of bilateral aneurysms. In bilateral disease, a trans-peritoneal approach is more likely to facilitate access. Caution should be maintained around the iliac veins and ureters, which are vulnerable to damage during the dissection. There are a number of options for management depending on the anatomy of aneurysmal disease. In isolated unilateral CIA aneurysms, a straight interposition graft may be placed, allowing for treatment of the aneurysm while maintaining hypogastric artery perfusion. If this is not feasible, then the CIA may be ligated and an extra-anatomic bypass performed. This may be accomplished with a femoral-femoral or femoral-EIA bypass. A bifurcated aortoiliac graft should be used when addressing bilateral CIA aneurysms or combined AAAs and iliac aneurysms. For CIA aneurysms that involve the iliac bifurcation, a bifurcated graft may be used to perfuse both the EIA and hypogastric artery. Alternatively, a straight graft can be anastomosed to the EIA with re-implantation of the hypogastric artery onto the graft, and vice versa. From a technical perspective, placement of the distal anastomosis at the hypogastric artery may be easier as this allows for the more superficial and often more redundant EIA to be re-implanted. This approach can also be used for combined aneurysms of the CIA and hypogastric artery if the distal hypogastric artery or its branches are not involved. A jump graft to the distal hypogastric artery from a CIA to EIA interposition graft is another option. If branches of the hypogastric artery are involved or an isolated hypogastric artery aneurysm without CIA disease is present, the hypogastric artery aneurysm can be excluded with oversewing of its branches from inside the aneurysm sac. There have also been reports of isolated hypogastric artery interposition grafts and aneurysm resection with primary end-to-end anastomosis.[4]

ENDOVASCULAR REPAIR

Endovascular repair may be performed under a general, spinal, or even local anesthetic. Access via the femoral arteries can be obtained with a groin cutdown or percutaneously. In some instances, brachial access may also be required depending on the device used. In general, endovascular repair falls into two categories: exclusion with or without preservation of the hypogastric artery. The complexity of the repair will depend on the aneurysm location, available landing zones, and presence of additional contralateral or ipsilateral iliac aneurysms.

In unilateral isolated CIA aneurysms that do not involve the aortic or iliac bifurcation, a straight covered stent graft can be used. Proximal and distal landing zones of at least 10–15 mm are required to establish an appropriate seal.[20] In the setting of bilateral CIA aneurysms, a bifurcated aortoiliac stent graft should be employed. Alternatively, if required, the CIA aneurysm can be embolized and an aorto-uni-iliac endograft device may be implanted followed by a femoral-femoral bypass graft placement using a hybrid approach.

In cases where the iliac bifurcation or hypogastric artery is aneurysmal, a distal seal may not be achieved with the above approach. Depending on the size of the iliac bifurcation, a bell-bottom graft may be adequate, although the largest currently available size is 28 mm. This would not be suitable for a CIA aneurysm larger than 26 mm, and type Ib endoleaks have been reported in 2.2–4% of patients with this approach.[21] The operator must also decide whether to preserve the hypogastric artery. If the hypogastric artery will not be preserved, then it can be embolized with placement of a covered stent extending from the CIA into the EIA. The embolization of the hypogastric artery is to avoid backbleeding that would prevent aneurysm thrombosis. There are also reports, however, of acceptable outcomes following coverage of the ostium of the hypogastric artery without embolization.[22] If the hypogastric artery is to be preserved, a number of techniques can be used to maintain flow. Bekdache et al. reviewed a number of current devices that can be employed.[21] The trifurcation technique utilizes multiple bifurcated stent graft devices and requires left arm access for cannulation of the hypogastric artery (Figure 18.2). A snorkel technique may also be used whereby two covered stents are placed parallel into the EIA and hypogastric artery then extended into the iliac limb of a bifurcated aortic graft (Figure 18.3).

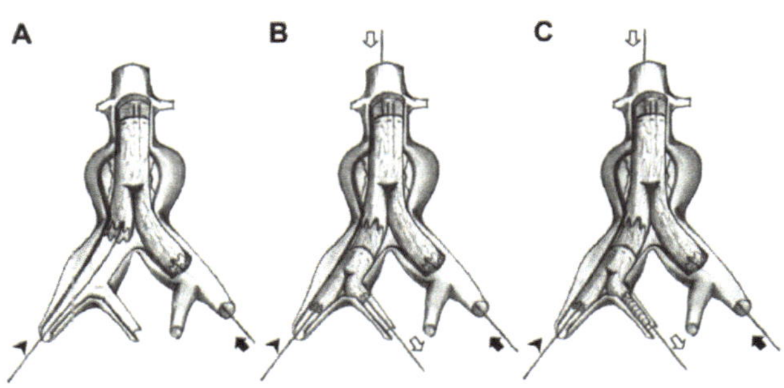

Figure 18.2 Trifurcation technique using multiple bifurcated main body grafts followed by a stent graft into the hypogastric artery. Brachial artery access in additional to femoral artery access is required for the deployment of the stent graft. (Bekdache K, Dietzek AM, Cha A, Neychev V. Endovascular hypogastric artery preservation during endovascular aneurysm repair: a review of current techniques and devices. *Ann Vasc Surg.* 2015;29(2):367–376.)

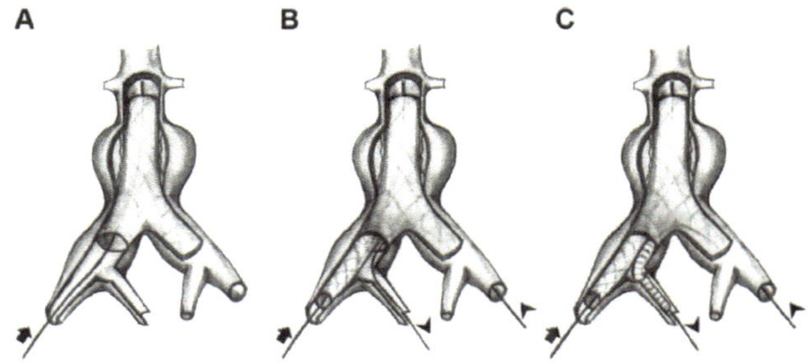

Figure 18.3 Snorkel technique using side-by-side deployment of two individual endografts placed proximally into the iliac limb of a bifurcated main body graft and distally into the external and hypogastric arteries. Only femoral access is required with an up-and-over approach for deployment of the stent graft into the hypogastric artery. (Bekdache K, Dietzek AM, Cha A, Neychev V. Endovascular hypogastric artery preservation during endovascular aneurysm repair: a review of current techniques and devices. *Ann Vasc Surg.* 2015;29(2):367–376.)

Depending on the anatomy, an iliac branched device (IBD) may also be considered. Commercially available IBDs include the Cook Medical Zenith IBD, Gore Excluder Iliac Branched Endoprostheses, and Jotec E-liac IBD.[23] While the Gore and Jotec devices can be used in isolation, the Cook device requires an aortic graft to be placed.[23] In order to utilize these devices, there are a number of anatomical criteria that must be taken into consideration (Figure 18.4). In general, to consider using an IBD, the aortic to iliac bifurcation length must be > 5 cm,

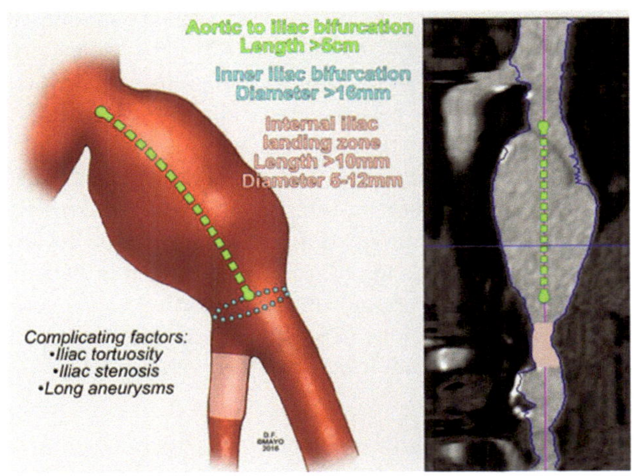

Figure 18.4 Sizing criteria for using an iliac branched device (IBD) for the treatment of a common iliac artery (CIA) aneurysm. Centerline analysis is important for accurate measurement. Factors such as iliac tortuosity or stenosis and long aneurysms can pose challenges for repair. (D'Oria M, Mastrorilli D, DeMartino R, Lepidi S. Current status of endovascular preservation of the internal iliac artery with iliac branch devices (IBD). *Cardiovasc Intervent Radiol.* 2019;42(7):935–948.)

inner iliac bifurcation diameter > 16 mm, and hypogastric artery diameter 5–12 mm with a landing zone > 10 mm.[23] Through-and-through femoral wire access is required regardless of the device type. IBDs have high technical success rates[24,25] and 30-day patency rates between 89–98.8%.[23] Outcomes 5 years after IBD placement have been reported with reasonable durability. Overall survival has been reported as 70.4% with a patency rate of 91.4%, freedom from re-intervention rate of 78.2–81.3%, and freedom from persistent endoleak rate of 100% at 5 years.[24,25] Freedom from IBD occlusion is reported as 83–86% at 5 years.[25]

In the case of isolated hypogastric artery aneurysm, embolization of the aneurysm with placement of a covered stent extending from the CIA to the EIA can be performed. It is recommended, however, to maintain perfusion to at least one hypogastric artery if possible. In cases of bilateral hypogastric artery aneurysms, an effort should be made to preserve flow to at least one of the hypogastric arteries. Domoto et al. reported a case series of 6 patients with isolated hypogastric artery aneurysms in whom a covered stent extending into the superior gluteal artery with embolization of other branches was performed.[26] At 6–12 months, they achieved 100% patency with no migration, endoleaks, or need for re-intervention.

There is some debate regarding whether embolization of the hypogastric artery is necessary when a covered stent graft extends from the CIA to the EIA.[27] A number of retrospective studies have demonstrated that coverage of the orifice of the hypogastric artery without embolization is associated with significantly lower rates of buttock claudication and no significant difference in type II endoleaks.[28,29] Other studies found no significant difference in buttock claudication between groups but still reported no difference in endoleaks.[30,31] A retrospective cohort study of 137 patients by Papazogglou et al. showed that although 6% of patients who did not undergo embolization had a type II endoleak, none of those patients required re-intervention, resulting in no significant difference in the need for re-intervention between coverage with or without embolization.[32] In a systematic review, major complications were significantly higher in patients who underwent coverage with embolization (29%) compared to coverage alone (6%) while there was no significant difference in endoleaks or re-intervention rate.[22]

MANAGEMENT OF POTENTIAL COMPLICATIONS

INTRAOPERATIVE BLEEDING AND INJURIES

Operating deep within the pelvis can be challenging, and the potential for significant bleeding must be anticipated preoperatively. Caution must be taken during dissection around the iliac vessels, as iliac veins lie posterior and medial to the iliac arteries. Blood conservation adjuncts such as a cell saver can be beneficial, if available. Balloon occlusion catheters can also be helpful in controlling backbleeding from pelvic branches that can otherwise be difficult to control. In the case of arteriovenous fistula between the iliac artery aneurysm and adjacent vein, control of the fistula is best obtained from within the iliac artery aneurysm sac, thereby allowing for adequate visualization and control of the defect. To assist in avoiding injury to the ureters, which in some cases may be distorted or adherent secondary to inflammation, ureteral stents can be considered. These can be placed prior to repair and may be used to facilitate identification of the ureters intraoperatively.

PELVIC ISCHEMIA

Occlusion of the hypogastric artery is often performed when repairing a CIA or hypogastric artery aneurysm. Generally, this is thought to be safe as there is often adequate collateral blood supply from the contralateral hypogastric artery in addition to other sources such as the femoral and iliac circumflex vessels. Furthermore, occlusion of both hypogastric arteries can sometimes be performed, either simultaneously or in a staged fashion.

However, occlusion of the hypogastric artery is not completely benign and may lead to pelvic ischemia that can result in buttock claudication, erectile dysfunction, ischemic colitis, and, in severe cases, pelvic necrosis or spinal cord ischemia. Rates of buttock claudication range between 1.6–56% with an incidence of 29.2% in the first 30 days following repair.[21,33] Symptoms are more frequent following bilateral compared to unilateral occlusion, and persist in up to 15–20% of patients.[33,34] However, Patel et al. found that although buttock claudication occurred in 22% of patients who underwent endovascular repair with coil embolization of the hypogastric artery, all resolved within 6 months.[6] Other studies have reported resolution within 3 months to 1 year in all cases of buttock claudication.[35] Similarly, Machado et al. found that despite bilateral hypogastric artery aneurysm embolization in 44% of cases, only one patient experienced buttock claudication and none suffered serious acute pelvic ischemia.[36] Rates of erectile dysfunction and colonic ischemia following aneurysm repair are between 10–45% and 0–9%, respectively, and severe complications such as buttock necrosis, scrotal skin ulceration, and sciatic nerve ischemia occur in fewer than 1% of patients.[21] Regardless of the approach used for repair of an iliac artery aneurysm, pelvic ischemic events occur in over 30% of patients with hypogastric artery interruption compared to fewer than 4% of those with preservation.[33]

Special consideration should be given to patients with contralateral iliac atherosclerotic disease, patients with previous aortic repair, and those with previous colon resection. In these patients, there may be a pre-existent compromise of blood supply to pelvic structures, spinal cord, and bowels. During open repair involving the aorta, re-implantation of the IMA should be considered. Spinal cord protection should also be taken into consideration in high-risk patients. In addition, buttock claudication may be significantly debilitating in a younger patient who is more active.

The risk of pelvic ischemia can be mitigated in a number of ways. Overall, if possible, preservation of the hypogastric artery during repair is preferred. If bilateral embolization is required, performing this in a staged fashion may allow for collateralization. It is recommended to embolize the hypogastric artery proximally rather than distally in order to preserve branches for collateral pelvic blood flow.[12,21] Coverage of the hypogastric artery without embolization may also be considered and has been shown in a number of studies to be associated with less buttock claudication and major complications as previously discussed. During open repair, re-implantation of the IMA, bypass from the femoral artery or EIA to the hypogastric artery, and femoral-femoral crossover are options to maximize collateral or retrograde flow to the pelvis. If technically feasible, bypass to the anterior or posterior branches of the hypogastric artery can be attempted as well.

ENDOLEAK AND MIGRATION

While endovascular repair has allowed for minimally invasive options, surveillance is required to detect stent graft migration or endoleaks that may develop postoperatively (Table 18.1). Endoleaks have been reported in 20–32% of patients who underwent endovascular repair for iliac artery aneurysms.[9,14] Serial Doppler ultrasound or computed tomography angiogram (CTA) studies are typically used for postoperative surveillance, although the utility of Doppler ultrasound studies can be limited in visualizing deep pelvic structures and in patients with a larger body habitus. If there are inadequate landing zones or a bell-bottom graft is used, a type I endoleak may occur requiring re-intervention. Similarly, patients with multi-component repairs such as snorkels or IBDs also need to be assessed for type III endoleaks. Management may include extension of the landing zones with additional stents or further embolization and close monitoring.

Table 18.1 Categories of endoleaks that may be identified at the time of repair or on subsequent follow-up imaging

TABLE 18.1 TYPES OF ENDOLEAK	
Type	**Definition**
Type I	Persistent filling of the aneurysm sac due to incomplete seal or ineffective seal at the proximal (type IA) or distal (type IB) end of the stent graft
Type II	Persistent filling of the aneurysm sac due to retrograde branch flow from collateral vessels
Type III	Blood flow into the aneurysm sac due to inadequate or ineffective sealing of overlapping graft joints or rupture of the graft fabric
Type IV	Blood flow into the aneurysm sac due to the porosity of the graft fabric, causing blood to pass through from the graft and into the aneurysm sac
Type V	Aneurysm sac expansion without clear evidence of endoleak origin

Source: Guimaraes M, Yamada R, Schonholz C. Endoleak and the role of embolization. *Endovascular Today.* 2015: 68–74.

LIMB THROMBOSIS

Limb thrombosis resulting in lower limb ischemia or pelvic ischemia is uncommon but can occur with both open and endovascular repair.[19] A number of factors, such as tortuous iliac vessels, iliac occlusive disease or poor runoff vessels, and technical approaches can make a repair prone to graft kinking or thrombosis (Figure 18.5). Buckley et al. reported only 1 limb occlusion at 54 months following different endovascular techniques, including straight endografts with or without embolization and bell-bottom grafts.[20] Fargion et al. found that IBD occlusion and isolated hypogastric artery or EIA occlusion with a patent IBD occurred in 5.6% and 3.5% of cases respectively during follow-up.[25] Patients with thrombosed grafts may present with symptoms of lower extremity or pelvic ischemia, depending on the region of thrombosis. Expedited CTA imaging should be obtained. Options for management include thrombolysis or thrombectomy with stenting or extra-anatomic bypass with a femoral-femoral crossover graft.

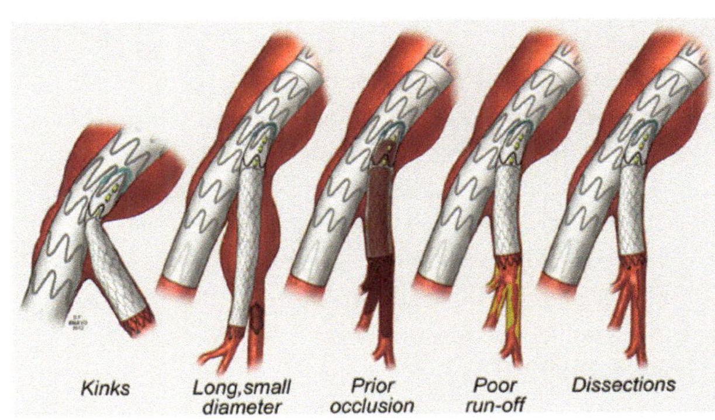

Figure 18.5 Common causes of hypogastric artery stent graft thrombosis during or following hypogastric artery aneurysm repair. (D'Oria M, Mastrorilli D, DeMartino R, Lepidi S. Current status of endovascular preservation of the internal iliac artery with iliac branch devices (IBD). *Cardiovasc Intervent Radiol.* 2019;42(7):935–948.)

REFERENCES

1. Brunkwall J, Hauksson H, Bengtsson H, Bergqvist D, Takolander R, Bergentz SE. Solitary aneurysms of the iliac arterial system: an estimate of their frequency of occurrence. J Vasc Surg. 1989;10(4): 381–384.
2. Kunz R. Aneurysmata bei 35380 autopsien. Schweiz Med Wochenschr. 1980;110: 142–148.
3. Matsumoto K, Matsubara K, Watada S, et al. Surgical and endovascular procedures for treating isolated iliac artery aneurysms: 10-year experience. World J Surg. 2004;28(8): 797–800.
4. Dorigo W, Pulli R, Troisi N, et al. The treatment of isolated iliac artery aneurysm in patients with non-aneurysmal aorta. Eur J Vasc Endovasc Surg. 2008;35(5): 585–589.
5. Sandhu RS, Pipinos, II. Isolated iliac artery aneurysms. Semin Vasc Surg. 2005;18(4): 209–215.
6. Patel NV, Long GW, Cheema ZF, Rimar K, Brown OW, Shanley CJ. Open vs. endovascular repair of isolated iliac artery aneurysms: a 12-year experience. J Vasc Surg. 2009;49(5): 1147–1153.
7. Santilli SM, Wernsing SE, Lee ES. Expansion rates and outcomes for iliac artery aneurysms. J Vasc Surg. 2000;31(1): 114–121.
8. Hiromatsu S, Hosokawa Y, Egawa N, Yokokura H, Akaiwa K, Aoyagi S. Strategy for isolated iliac artery aneurysms. Asian Cardiovasc Thorac Ann. 2007;15(4): 280–284.
9. Zhorzel S, Busch A, Trenner M, et al. Open Versus Endovascular Repair of Isolated Iliac Artery Aneurysms. Vasc Endovascular Surg. 2019;53(1): 12–20.
10. Garbaisz D, Boros A, Legeza P, Szeberin Z. Open and endovascular repair of iliac artery aneurysms. Orv Hetil. 2018;159(13): 520–525.
11. Laine MT, Bjorck M, Beiles CB, et al. Few internal iliac artery aneurysms rupture under 4 cm. J Vasc Surg. 2017;65(1): 76–81.
12. Wanhainen A, Verzini F, Van Herzeele I, et al. Editor's Choice - European Society for Vascular Surgery (ESVS) 2019 Clinical Practice Guidelines on the Management of Abdominal Aorto-iliac Artery Aneurysms. Eur J Vasc Endovasc Surg. 2019;57(1): 8–93.
13. Wilhelm BJ, Sakharpe A, Ibrahim G, Baccaro LM, Fisher J. The 100-year evolution of the isolated internal iliac artery aneurysm. Ann Vasc Surg. 2014;28(4): 1070–1077.
14. Huang Y, Gloviczki P, Duncan AA, et al. Common iliac artery aneurysm: Expansion rate and results of open surgical and endovascular repair. J Vasc Surg. 2008;47(6): 1203–1211.e1202.
15. Brin BJ, Busuttil RW. Isolated hypogastric artery aneurysms. Arch Surg. 1982;117: 1329–1333.
16. McCready RA, Pairolero PC, Gilmore JC, Kazmier FJ, Cherry KJ, Hollier LH. Isolated iliac artery aneurysms. Surgery. 1983;93(5): 688–693.
17. Kasirajan V, Hertzer NR, Beven EG, O'Hara PJ, Krajewski LP, Sullivan TM. Management of isolated common iliac artery aneurysms. Cardiovasc Surg. 1998;6(2): 171–177.
18. Williams SK, Campbell WB, Earnshaw JJ. Survey of management of common iliac artery aneurysms by members of the Vascular Society of Great Britain and Ireland. Ann R Coll Surg Engl. 2014;96(2): 116–120.
19. Chaer RA, Barbato JE, Lin SC, Zenati M, Kent KC, McKinsey JF. Isolated iliac artery aneurysms: a contemporary comparison of endovascular and open repair. J Vasc Surg. 2008;47(4): 708–713.
20. Buckley CJ, Buckley SD. Technical tips for endovascular repair of common iliac artery aneurysms. Semin Vasc Surg. 2008;21(1): 31–34.
21. Bekdache K, Dietzek AM, Cha A, Neychev V. Endovascular hypogastric artery preservation during endovascular aneurysm repair: a review of current techniques and devices. Ann Vasc Surg. 2015;29(2): 367–376.
22. Kontopodis N, Tavlas E, Papadopoulos G, Galanakis N, Tsetis D, Ioannou CV. Embolization or Simple Coverage to Exclude the Internal Iliac Artery During Endovascular Repair of Aortoiliac Aneurysms? Systematic Review and Meta-analysis of Comparative Studies. J Endovasc Ther. 2017;24(1): 47–56.
23. D'Oria M, Mastrorilli D, DeMartino R, Lepidi S. Current Status of Endovascular Preservation of the Internal Iliac Artery with Iliac Branch Devices (IBD). Cardiovasc Intervent Radiol. 2019;42(7): 935–948.
24. Parlani G, Verzini F, De Rango P, et al. Long-term results of iliac aneurysm repair with iliac branched endograft: a 5-year experience on 100 consecutive cases. Eur J Vasc Endovasc Surg. 2012;43(3): 287–292.
25. Fargion AT, Masciello F, Pratesi C, et al. Results of the multicenter pELVIS Registry for isolated common iliac aneurysms treated by the iliac branch device. J Vasc Surg. 2018;68(5): 1367–1373. e1361.
26. Domoto S, Azuma T, Yokoi Y, Isomura S, Takahashi K, Niinami H. Minimally invasive treatment for isolated internal iliac artery aneurysms preserving superior gluteal artery flow. Gen Thorac Cardiovasc Surg. 2019;67(10): 835–840.
27. Kouvelos GN, Koutsoumpelis A, Peroulis M, Matsagkas M. In endovascular aneurysm repair cases, when should you consider internal iliac artery embolization when extending a stent into the external iliac artery? Interact Cardiovasc Thorac Surg. 2014;18(6): 821–824.

28. Tefera G, Turnipseed WD, Carr SC, Pulfer KA, Hoch JR, Acher CW. Is coil embolization of hypogastric artery necessary during endovascular treatment of aortoiliac aneurysms? Ann Vasc Surg. 2004;18(2): 143–146.
29. Farahmand P, Becquemin JP, Desgranges P, Allaire E, Marzelle J, Roudot-Thoraval F. Is hypogastric artery embolization during endovascular aortoiliac aneurysm repair (EVAR) innocuous and useful? Eur J Vasc Endovasc Surg. 2008;35(4): 429–435.
30. Wyers MC, Schermerhorn ML, Fillinger MF, et al. Internal iliac occlusion without coil embolization during endovascular abdominal aortic aneurysm repair. J Vasc Surg. 2002;36(6): 1138–1145.
31. Bharwani N, Raja J, Choke E, et al. Is internal iliac artery embolization essential prior to endovascular repair of aortoiliac aneurysms? Cardiovasc Intervent Radiol. 2008;31(3): 504–508.
32. Papazoglou KO, Sfyroeras GS, Zambas N, Konstantinidis K, Kakkos SK, Mitka M. Outcomes of endovascular aneurysm repair with selective internal iliac artery coverage without coil embolization. J Vasc Surg. 2012;56(2): 298–303.
33. Kouvelos GN, Katsargyris A, Antoniou GA, Oikonomou K, Verhoeven EL. Outcome after Interruption or Preservation of Internal Iliac Artery Flow During Endovascular Repair of Abdominal Aorto-iliac Aneurysms. Eur J Vasc Endovasc Surg. 2016;52(5): 621–634.
34. Lin PH, Chen AY, Vij A. Hypogastric artery preservation during endovascular aortic aneurysm repair: is it important? Semin Vasc Surg. 2009;22(3): 193–200.
35. Igari K, Kudo T, Toyofuku T, Jibiki M, Inoue Y. Comparison between endovascular repair and open surgery for isolated iliac artery aneurysms. Surg Today. 2015;45(3): 290–296.
36. Machado RM, Rego DN, de Oliveira P, de Almeida R. Endovascular Treatment of Internal Iliac Artery Aneurysms: Single Center Experience. Braz J Cardiovasc Surg. 2016;31(2): 127–131.

19

Complications of open repair of ruptured abdominal aortic aneurysm

SACHINDER SINGH HANS

Most patients with ruptured abdominal aortic aneurysm (AAA) with sudden-onset back or flank pain and associated diaphoresis. The patients may or may not be hypotensive at the time of presentation. In some instances, blood pressure may be elevated secondary to pain. Patients presenting to ER with ruptured AAA are not aware of the presence of aneurysm in most instances. The site of rupture is usually posterolaterally with blood extravasation from the rupture initially contained in the retroperitoneum. This contained hematoma may allow the patient to may remain hemodynamically stable for an uncertain amount of time.[1,2] Anterior rupture (free) results in severe shock secondary to massive blood loss.[2] Rarely, an AAA may present as "chronic contained rupture" as the linear split in the posterior wall of the aneurysm is sealed by anterior spinal ligament. Such patients are hemodynamically stable and present often with low back pain.[2] There is no associated retroperitoneal hematoma in the patient with chronic contained rupture.

Early transportation to the emergency department and prompt diagnosis by CTA and judicious resuscitation with blood products, allowing permissive hypotension with a goal of keeping the blood pressure close to 90 mm systolic, are necessary in the acute management of a patient with ruptured AAA.[1] While ultrasound is useful in making an expeditious diagnosis of the presence of an AAA, it is not beneficial in treatment planning be that open or endovascular repair. Therefore, CTA of the abdomen and pelvis with thin cuts is necessary in most patients who are hemodynamically stable. Patient's with extreme hypotension should be taken to the operating room (preferably a hybrid operating room) immediately where, under ultrasound guidance, the femoral artery is punctured and a 12-French sheath is placed to advance a balloon occlusion catheter in the suprarenal segment of the aorta.[2] Following this, arteriography with an Omniflush marker catheter will help in deciding between open and endovascular repair.

OPERATIVE TECHNIQUE

One of the most important factors determining the outcome of the patient's ruptured AAA is the time elapsed between the onset of rupture and gain of proximal control.[1] As induction of general anesthesia relieves the pain, relaxes the abdominal wall musculature, and releases a sympathetic tone, resulting in cardiovascular collapse,[2,3] induction should be withheld until the incision is ready to be made. In the case of endovascular repair, femoral access and placement of a balloon occlusion catheter may be placed under local anaesthesia, prior to induction. A rapid transfusion protocol with blood products in the room, autologous blood recovery system (Cell Saver), and a body warmer should be available. In most patients, a long midline transabdominal incision from the xiphoid process just above the symphysis is made.[2,3] In selected patients, including those with ileostomy/urinary stoma or a contained type IV thoracoabdominal aneurysm, left flank incision through the 9th or 10th intercostal space may be a better option depending on the extent of the aneurysm and the patient's body habitus.

PROXIMAL CONTROL

Proximal control is best achieved at the supraceliac level in patients with extensive retroperitoneal hematoma. In patients with small to moderate size hematoma under spinal cord ischemia, blunt finger dissection at the infrarenal neck after mobilizing the ligament of Treitz is performed. Left renal vein is mobilized upwards and a vascular clamp

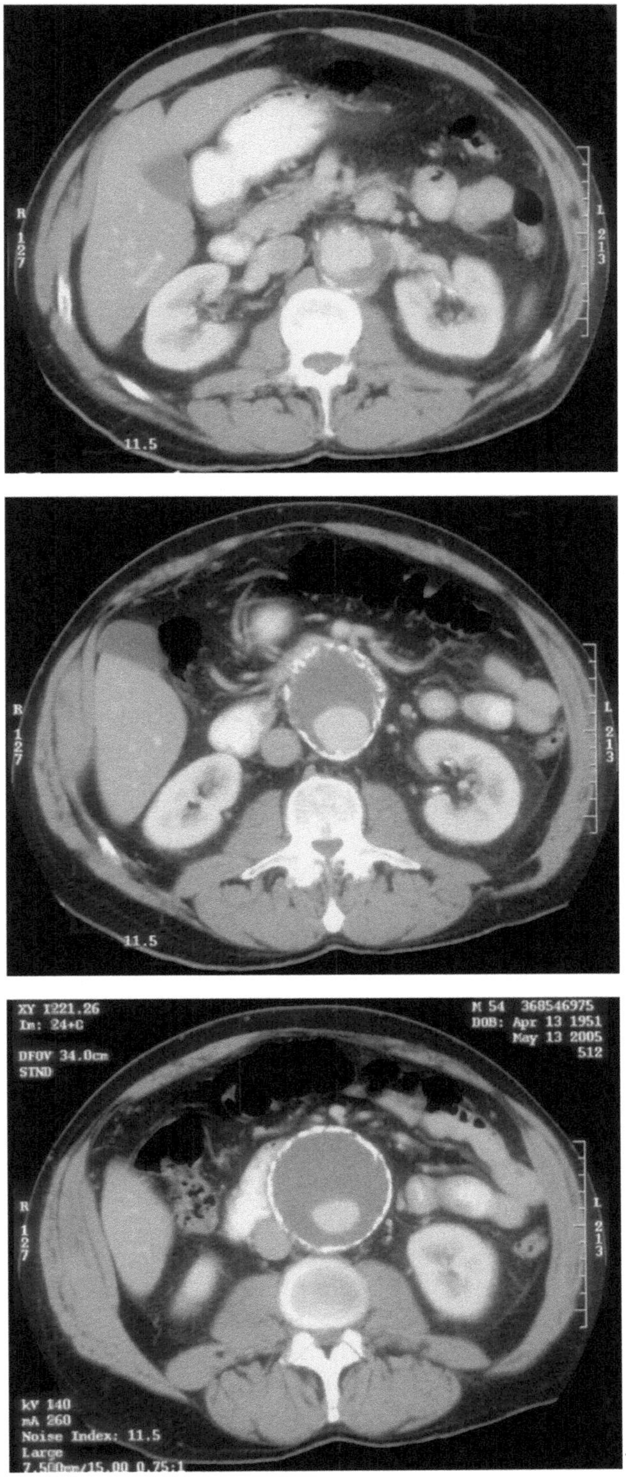

Figures 19.1–19.3 Showing juxtarenal AAA with contained rupture near the origin of the left renal artery.

is applied to aortic neck. Other methods to occlude proximal aorta including insertion of a #28 Foley catheter with 30 mL balloon. Pruitt aortic occlusion catheter on insertion of two fingers (index and middle finger) into the aortic neck are other helpful techniques to obtain proximal control.[2,5] Proactive administration of platelets and plasma in addition to packed red cells as part of the massive transfusion protocol is important during the operative reconstruction.

Exposure of the supraceliac aorta has been described in Chapter 17. After obtaining proximal control, volume status of the patient is optimized by the anesthesia team by administration of large volumes of crystalloid and blood products. If the patient has a small to moderate size hematoma with stable blood pressure, the author generally directs a smaller dose of heparin (75 international units per kilogram) to be administered by the anesthesia team with serial monitoring of ACT. In the patient with a large retroperitoneal hematoma and shock, the author generally withholds heparin administration until after proximal anastomosis is completed. After obtaining proximal control, distal control is obtained by clamping the iliac arteries; if common iliac arteries are aneurysmal, the origin of the external and hypogastric artery are clamped separately. Circumferential mobilization of the aortic neck and iliac artery is not necessary, nor is it necessary to pass a Silastic loop as this maneuver increases the chance of major venous injury. Following anterior and lateral dissection of the aortic neck and iliac arteries, a vascular clamp can be applied, following compression of the arteries between the index and middle finger. A Silastic vessel loop is placed around the inferior mesenteric artery. The anastomoses are performed as mentioned in the chapter 20 on complications of unruptured AAA.

Most complications of ruptured AAA are similar to those in the chapter 17; however, certain complications are far more common and will be described in detail.

COMPLICATIONS

ABDOMINAL COMPARTMENT SYNDROME (ACS)

ACS is a serious complication following open or endovascular repair of ruptured AAA. ACS develops as a result of increased intra-abdominal pressure secondary to massive fluid administration associated with ongoing hemorrhage and reperfusion of splanchnic bed. As a result of increased intra-abdominal pressure, there is decreased venous return due to compression of the inferior vena cava resulting in decreased cardiac output.[7] As a result of increased intra-abdominal pressure, the kidneys are compressed. With associated decrease in cardiac function, there is decrease in renal blood flow and oliguria. There is increase in airway pressure with decrease in pulmonary compliance secondary to compression of the diaphragm. ACS develops in 20% of patients following open AAA repair for ruptured aneurysm. Using intra-abdominal pressure measurements from an indwelling Foley catheter,

50% of patients develop intra-abdominal pressure greater than 20 mmHg; of those, approximately 20% develop multiple organ dysfunction or failure. Medical therapy includes neuromuscular blockage, positive PEEP, albumin, and furosemide. If left untreated, ACS results in 100% mortality secondary to multiple organ dysfunction or failure. In patients developing ACS, correction of coagulopathy is very important in the first 24 hours. Following 24 hours of repair, decompressive laparotomy should be considered in patients with stable hemoglobin and hematocrit. In certain patients with abdominal compartment syndrome, the abdomen should be kept open avoiding adhesions between the intestines and the abdominal wall. Vacuum-assisted wound closure followed by delayed primary fascial closure is often necessary.[7] Care should be taken to prevent formation of bowel fistula with proper coverage of exposed intestines.[7]

MULTISYSTEM ORGAN FAILURE

Because of the associated hypotension and ischemia reperfusion injury in patient presenting with ruptured AAA, multisystem organ failure may occur in 1–3% of patients and is associated with 50–70% mortality, significant morbidity and ICU stay.[1–3,5,6]

SPINAL CORD ISCHEMIA

The incidence of spinal cord ischemia following repair of ruptured AAA varies from 0.26–0.74%. The incidence of spinal cord ischemia following repair of thoracoabdominal aneurysm is significantly higher and is caused by imbalance of oxygen demand and oxygen delivery produced by aortic occlusion. Perfusion and oxygen delivery to the spinal cord during the period of aortic occlusion at the time of significant reduced blood flow remains the most important factor in protecting the spinal cord.

AORTIC GRAFT INFECTIONS

Aortic graft infections are often difficult to diagnose as the patient may present with nonspecific symptoms such as generalized weakness, malaise, anorexia, back pain, and unexplained weight loss. Occasionally, the patient may present with overt sepsis.[8] The laboratory and diagnostic studies are often nonspecific but may include leukocytosis with a shift to the left, elevated C-reactive protein and sedimentation rate. Blood culture may not give positive results. Common pathogens include *Staphylococcus aureus* and *Staphylococcus epidermidis*. *Staphylococcus epidermidis* infection produces biofilm and attracts foreign bodies like prosthetic graft. Biofilm contains a large number of persistent cells that protect the microorganism against neutrophil-dependent killing and complement system inactivation via deposition of C3b and immunoglobin G. Imaging studies such as CTA aid in confirming the diagnosis and help in evaluating the extent of infection.

Findings of graft infection include enhancement of perigraft tissue, stranding of soft tissues, gas bubbles, and formation of pseudoaneurysm. Nuclear scan with tagged white blood cells may also be helpful in establishing the diagnosis of graft infection.

MANAGEMENT

The patient should be started on intravenous antibiotics and physiologically optimized. Eradication of infection involves excision of the prosthetic graft and complete debridement of surrounding infected tissues. In certain situations, graft preservation has been successful with antibiotics, local wound care, and eventual soft tissue coverage with muscle flaps.[8] This approach is suitable in patients with low-grade infection without involvement of anastomosis and peripherally located infections. This treatment plan is not feasible for intra-abdominal graft infections. Options for arterial reconstruction can be broadly classified into either

a. Extra-anatomic bypass (axillobifemoral bypass graft or bilateral axillofemoral bypass graft) with aortic ligation.
b. In situ arterial reconstructions using femoral vein, spiral vein graft, cryopreserved allograft, or antibiotic impregnated prosthetic graft.

OPERATIVE PRINCIPLES

General anesthesia with hemodynamic monitoring is performed, and warming devices should be used in all patients. Either a transperitoneal midline approach or a left flank retroperitoneal approach can be used depending upon the operative plan. Transperitoneal approach is more commonly used and useful if axillofemoral graft is to be performed. Use of a left flank retroperitoneal approach avoids a hostile abdomen with satisfactory exposure of the descending thoracic and upper abdominal aorta. Disadvantages include difficult exposure of the right distal common iliac artery and the right femoral artery.[8]

After obtaining proximal and distal control of the aorta and iliac arteries at the noninfected site, individual visceral branches of the aorta may need to be controlled along with proximal control of the aorta above the diaphragm.[8] If the infection requires debridement above the visceral arteries, then the visceral cold perfusion techniques may be necessary to perfuse visceral arteries. During dissection, extreme care should be exercised to prevent injuries to the ureters, bowel, and major veins.[8] Prior to aortic crossclamping, the patient should be anticoagulated. Aggressive debridement of surrounding tissues following removal of the graft is necessary. Sonification of the graft to allow for prolonged culture times to identify slow-growing bacteria with a biofilm are often necessary. Following debridement, in situ arterial reconstruction or ligation of the aorta is performed.[8] A pedicle of greater omentum based on the left gastroepiploic artery is constructed and brought through an avascular area toward the left side of the transverse mesocolon and graft coverage is provided.

Bilateral axillofemoral graft with aortic ligation has been considered a standard therapy for aortic graft infections involving infrarenal aorta. The advantages of this approach include the ability to stage a prolonged and difficult operation in high-risk patient by performing the arterial reconstruction in one setting and the graft extirpation at the second stage. The major disadvantages of this approach include suboptimal graft patency and the potential risk of aortic stump rupture. In addition, if the aortic graft needs to be removed first in patients with bleeding secondary to aortoenteric fistula, this approach can lead to prolonged limb ischemia times. If the common femoral arteries are free of infection, distal anastomosis is performed to the common femoral artery. If there is involvement of common femoral artery, distal anastomosis is performed to superficial femoral artery or the profunda femoris artery. The reported operative mortality for this approach can be as high as 40%. There is significant risk for development of axillofemoral graft infection. The risk of aortic stump blowout can be as high as 25%.[8]

IN SITU AORTIC RECONSTRUCTION

Creation of a new aortoiliac system with the femoral vein has an important place in the arterial reconstruction in the presence of aortic graft infection. The femoral vein (greater than 6 mm in diameter) is harvested from the origin of the deep femoral vein to the popliteal vein.[8] The vein is harvested via longitudinal incision along the lateral aspect of the sartorius muscle. The sartorius muscle is retracted medially. The whole length of the femoral vein from its confluence with the deep femoral vein distally to above the knee popliteal vein with the division of the tendon of the adductor magnus muscle if necessary is performed. The branches of the superficial femoral and the popliteal artery are preserved. The valves in the femoral vein are excised by everting the vein. The vein is distended with heparinized saline. Most patients will require bifurcated reconstruction. Both femoral veins are harvested and then anastomosed to each other in a side-to-side fashion proximally to create a vein graft. The autogenous vein reconstruction may allow for a short duration of antibiotic treatment regimen. This reconstruction compares favorably with other methods of reconstruction in terms of late mortality.[8] Disadvantages include prolonged operative time, which can be reduced by use of second surgical team. The mismatch between the diameter of the aorta and the femoral vein is another disadvantage. This type of reconstruction should not be performed in unstable patients with ongoing hemorrhage or sepsis. During follow-up vein graft stenosis due to intimal hyperplasia and aneurysmal degeneration can occur. Leg swelling, deep venous thrombosis, and compartment syndrome with need for fasciotomy have been reported.

SPIRAL VEIN GRAFTS

Spiral vein grafts are reconstructed by harvesting the greater saphenous vein, splitting it longitudinally, and then suturing it over a 24-French chest tube with monofilament polypropylene suture. Prolonged operative time and degenerative changes in the vein graft are some of its disadvantages.

CRYOPRESERVED ALLOGRAFTS

As an alternative to in situ aortic graft placement, cryopreserved allograft helps in avoiding placing a prosthetic graft in the infected field. These grafts are expensive, have to be obtained from the manufacturer, and may not be available in an emergency situation. The graft is thawed before suturing in a standard fashion with lumbar arteries oriented anteriorly. There is a small risk of early perforation of the graft.

ANTIBIOTIC-TREATED GRAFT

Dacron graft pretreated with gelatin can be easily impregnated with an antibiotic, which is then soaked in rifampin in dosage of 600 mg reconstituted in 50 mL saline solution. The graft is soaked for 5–30 minutes. Excessive solution is drained off before implantation. Rifampin-treated Dacron grafts are readily available in any desired size. There is minimal risk of aortic stump disruption and a better graft patency extra-anatomic bypass graft. Limb loss is uncommon, and 5 year survival is between 40–50%. However, there is a risk of reinfection (up to 22%). Reinfection is more common with methicillin-resistant *Staphylococcus aureus*. Reinfection is reduced by radical debridement and use of an omental wrap.

SECONDARY AORTOENTERIC FISTULA

1. It is one of the most dreaded complication of AAA repair and occurs in 0.5–1.2% of all aortic reconstructions. Important consideration of the management of patient with secondary aortoenteric fistula include hemodynamic status – stable or unstable from ongoing active life-threatening hemorrhage.[8]

2. Risk to the patient from major operation, which can be technically challenging.
3. Location of the distal anastomosis (distal aorta, common iliac, external iliac, or femoral arteries).
4. Status of the aortic neck as determined by CTA of the abdomen and pelvis. To determine if there is adequate aortic neck length for a new proximal aortic anastomosis, the communication is between a previously placed aortic graft and the third or fourth portion of the duodenum. The patient usually presents 2–3 years following initial AAA repair with gastrointestinal (GI) bleeding. The GI bleeding may manifest as melena initially (herald bleed). Initial massive bleeding is uncommon. The patient may present with sepsis in up to 50% of instances. The communication between the GI tract and the prosthetic graft can involve the anastomosis (true AEF) or the graft body or the limb (prosthetic enteric erosion). In the aortoenteric fistula, the bleeding is from the aorta, while in the prosthetic enteric erosion bleeding is from the edge of the bowel wall. About 25% of patients may present with sepsis. Esophagogastric duodenoscopy with attention to the distal portions of the duodenum is necessary, though it is extremely uncommon to visualize the graft material on endoscopy. CTA image demonstrates perigraft fluid, thickening of the bowel wall with inflammation and fat stranding. Air in the periprosthetic area and pseudoaneurysm formation may also be present. In a hemodynamically stable patient after confirmation of the diagnosis or a strong suspicion of the diagnosis, surgeon may choose two different management options.
   A. Staged or bilateral axillofemoral graft followed by infected aortic graft excision.
   B. Excision of the aortic graft with inline aortic graft reconstruction with following conduits.
5. Femoral vein.
6. Cryopreserved arterial allograft.
7. Rifampin-impregnated Dacron graft. Prior to inline replacement, radical debridement of inflammatory tissue around the graft along with coverage of the proximal anastomosis, and the omental pedicle flap is necessary. In general, staged extra-anatomic grafting and graft excision is recommended in patients with multiple comorbidities.

The patient should be on broad spectrum antibiotics due to polymicrobial nature of the infection. Through a long midline incision, supraceliac exposure of the aorta is obtained (Chapter 17), and proximal control is obtained after systemic heparinization and mannitol infusion is started. Distal control is obtained at the iliac or femoral artery level. A new inline graft should be proposed before exposing the site of aortoenteric communication. If bleeding is encountered at the site of the fistula, proximal and distal clamps are immediately applied. As the infrarenal segment of the aorta is exposed, the proximal clamp is moved from supraceliac to infrarenal location to reduce visceral and renal ischemia time. Depending upon the inflammatory changes in the aorta below the renal arteries, suprarenal clamping may be more appropriate. Proximal perirenal aorta is debrided and proximal aortic anastomosis is performed. The opening in the bowel wall is isolated with saline-soaked lap sponges. Vascular clamp is moved distal to proximal anastomosis to check for hemostasis. Debridement of remaining periaortic tissue is completed. Complete excision of the infected graft is performed. Distal anastomosis is performed to the iliac arteries beyond the previously performed distal anastomosis. The duodenal defect is debrided and closed transversely by interrupted sutures in two layers. In most instances, the defect is relatively small.

If the infected graft extends distal to the femoral arteries, groin incisions are performed first with exposure of the graft and superficial deep femoral artery origins, although new tunnels in the retroperitoneum are ideal, but in practice are difficult to accomplish without risking injury to the iliac veins and the ureters. Sartorius muscle rotation flaps are created after transecting the muscle at its origin from the anterior superior iliac spine. This promotes coverage of the new groin anastomosis. Wound VAC is applied for both open groin incisions.

In high-risk patients, bilateral axillofemoral bypass followed by graft excision is safer. This approach reduces the extent of the abdominal portion of the operation and decreases ischemia-reperfusion injury associated with prolonged pelvic and lower extremity clamp time. After performance of bilateral axillobifemoral bypass graft, the patient should undergo staged excision of the graft, repair of the defect in the duodenum, and closure of the aortic stump in 0–3 days later. The aortic stump is closed in two layers with 3-0 interrupted Prolene sutures and a horizontal mattress second layer of continuous suture. In most patients, distal anastomosis of axillofemoral graft is performed to the deep femoral arteries. Incisions should be placed lateral to the sartorius and in a relatively clean area. Endovascular repair is also an option as a bridge to definitive repair in extremely high-risk patients.

In a hemodynamically unstable patient, the patient can be taken immediately from the ER to the hybrid operating room. Percutaneous access under ultrasound guidance is performed followed by placement of a large sheath in the femoral artery. A proximal aortic balloon occlusion catheter is then advanced to obtain proximal control. If endovascular repair is feasible, then this should be considered as a bridge to definitive repair. If not, a midline incision is made and proximal supraceliac control is obtained. If there is limited contamination, rifampin-soaked Dacron graft reconstruction can be performed after debridement. If the patient's condition is poor, ligation of the aorta, removal of the graft, and debridement followed by extra-anatomic grafting is more appropiate.[8]

Case Example 1

Late graft infections with aortoduodenal fistula following open repair of contained rupture of abdominal aortic aneurysm

A 54-year-old male presented to the emergency room with severe abdominal and back pain. Emergent CTA of the abdomen showed contained rupture (fat stranding) near the left renal artery posteriorly (Figures 19.1–19.3). Patients' comorbidities included hypertension, heavy nicotine use and alcohol abuse. He was known to have chronic bilateral superficial femoral artery occlusion with stable claudication. Patient was taken to the operating room emergently and was found to have a small contained hematoma in the juxta renal aspect of the aorta on the left side. Exposure for proximal control of the aorta included ligation of the left renal vein, which was performed close to the inferior vena cava. Proximal control of the aorta was obtained at the suprarenal level. Following clamping of the common iliac arteries for distal arterial control, the aneurysm sac was opened. The aneurysm sac contained a large amount of greyish brown ("muddy") thrombus from which a sample was sent for culture. An aorto-bilateral common iliac reconstruction was performed using a bifurcated (20 mm × 10 mm) knitted Dacron graft.

Despite a prolonged postoperative course, the patient eventually met criteria for discharge and was discharged on the 12th day after initial repair. Patient was seen at follow-up with diminished appetite and generalized weakness presented after 3 years with fever, chills, melena as well as acute ischemia of right lower extremity of 6 hours duration. CTA of the abdomen showed infected graft with gas bubbles around the graft and occlusion of the right limb and nonfunctioning right kidney (Figures 19.4 and 19.5). Patient was taken to the operating room in an emergent fashion. GI endoscopy was not performed as patient became hypotensive. Patient was explored through the midline transperitoneal approach. A secondary aortoenteric fistula was identified involving the aortic graft and the fourth portion of the duodenum. The infected graft was excised with ligation of the aorta. Repair of the duodenal fistula (involving the 4th portion of the duodenum) was performed primarily in two layers. Lower extremity perfusion was reestablished with an axillobifemoral graft arterial reconstruction. Cultures of the involved tissue grew both gram-positive and gram-negative microorganisms. Patient died on the fourth postoperative day from multisystem organ failure.

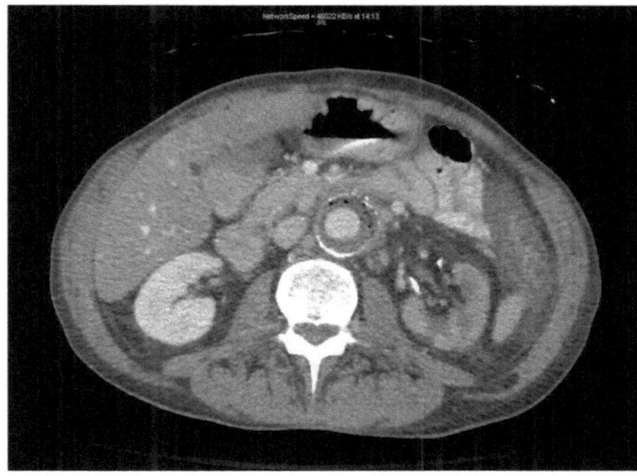

Figure 19.4 Showing gas around the aortic graft indicative of graft infection.

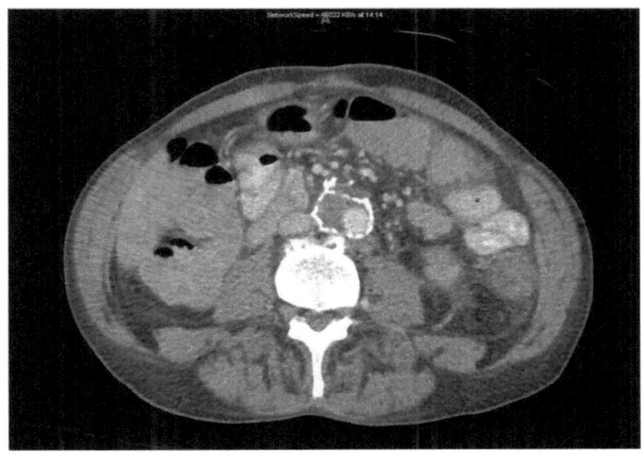

Figure 19.5 Occlusion of the right limb aorto-biiliac graft.

REFERENCES

1. Hans SS, Huang RR. Results of 101 ruptured abdominal aortic aneurysm repairs from a single surgical practice. Arch Surg. 2003;138(8): 898–901. doi:10.1001/archsurg.138.8.898
2. Hans S. Open Ruptured AAA Repair In Hans S, Shepard A, Weaver M, et al (Ed.), Endovascular and Open Vascular Reconstruction: A Practical Approach. Taylor & Francis Group, LLC: Boca Raton, FL; 2017: 205–211.
3. Noel AA, Gloviczki P, Cherry KJ Jr., et al. Ruptured abdominal aortic aneurysms: The excessive mortality rate of conventional repair. J Vasc Surg. 2001;34(1): 41–46. doi:10.1067/mva.2001.115604
4. Johansson PI, Stensballe J, Rosenberg I, Hilslov TL, Jorgensen L, Secher NH. Proactive administration of platelets and plasma for patients with a ruptured abdominal aortic aneurysm: Evaluating a change in transfusion practice. *Transfusion*. 2007;47(4): 593–598. doi:10.1111/j.1537-2995.2007.01160.x

5. Eslami MH, Messina LM. Ruptured AAA: Open surgical management. Semin Vasc Surg. 2010;23(4): 200–205. doi:10.1053/j.semvascsurg.2010.10.001
6. Cho JS, Kim JY, Rhee RY, et al. Contemporary results of open repair of ruptured abdominal aortoiliac aneurysms: Effect of surgeon volume on mortality. J Vasc Surg. 2008;48(1): 10–17; discussion 17-18. doi:10.1016/j.jvs.2008.02.067
7. Bjorck M. Management of the tense abdomen or difficult abdominal closure after operation for ruptured abdominal aortic aneurysms. Semin Vasc Surg. 2012;25(1): 35–38. doi:10.1053/j.semvascsurg.2012.03.002
8. Robinson WP, Schanzer A, Li Y, et al. Derivation and validation of a practical risk score for prediction of mortality after open repair of ruptured abdominal aortic aneurysms in a US regional cohort and comparison to existing scoring systems. J Vasc Surg. 2013;57(2): 354–361. doi:10.1016/j.jvs.2012.08.120
9. Nypaver T. Primary and Secondary Aortoenteric Fistula In Hans S, Shepard A., Weaver M., et al (Ed.), Endovascular and Open Vascular Reconstruction: A Practical Approach. Taylor & Francis Group, LLC: Boca Raton, FL; 2017: (257–262).

20

Complications of open thoracoabdominal aortic aneurysm repair

DANIEL KIM AND JAHAN MOHEBALI

Open repair of thoracoabdominal aortic aneurysms (TAAA) remains a significant undertaking for both patient and operative team, even in experienced, high-volume centers.[1–5] The extent of aneurysm and subsequent repair is categorized according to Crawford's eponymous classification and has significant implications for both intraoperative conduct and postoperative complications as described in his benchmark series.[6] Because more extensive repair (Extent II > Extent I > Extent III) results in greater intraoperative disruption of perfusion and consequent physiologic derangement, it is intuitively associated with greater adverse outcomes, specifically, paraplegia, renal failure, gut ischemia, and death. Conversely, in experienced hands, the least extensive Type IV repairs have mortality comparable with standard open abdominal aortic reconstruction.[2] As such, numerous intraoperative adjuncts and postoperative management techniques have been described to minimize the adverse physiologic effects of repair associated with more extensive aneurysms. The principles of successful repair consequently hinge upon two overarching goals:

1. Replacement of all aneurysmally degenerated aorta to prevent future rupture and need for re-intervention.
2. Mitigating the metabolic effects of decreased end-organ oxygen delivery during and after repair.

This chapter will begin with a brief description of the author's approach to the overarching conduct of the open repair of TAAA, including the role of various global perfusion strategies. Organized by affected organ system, the next section will hone in on the exact technical steps necessary to minimize adverse outcomes while also covering the various intraoperative adjuncts used to decrease the effects of ischemia in these vascular beds. The last section will review our standard postoperative management of open TAAA patients through the initial ICU period and is organized into a standard "organ systems" approach to facilitate application of this information to direct bedside care of patients.

OVERALL OPERATIVE CONDUCT

PERFUSION STRATEGY

Choosing a perfusion strategy, including no perfusion strategy in a "clamp-and-sew" repair, is a decision that must be made in the preoperative period as it has implications for the surgical and anesthetic teams as well as the overall conduct of the operation. Because open repair of TAAA by definition implies disruption of renovisceral, spinal cord, and lower extremity blood flow during a portion of reconstruction, planning must include a strategy to decrease these ischemia times. The simplest strategy is to operate expeditiously once the proximal cross clamp is applied. As noted above, Type IV TAAA lends itself quite nicely to this technique as the risk of cord ischemia is minimal and the renovisceral segment reconstruction can be incorporated into the proximal anastomosis in the form of a generous bevel that encompasses the ostia of these vessels +/− the left renal artery.[2] Because most patients can tolerate a supraceliac clamp time and period of total mesenteric ischemia that is less than 20–30 minutes, the clamp-and-sew technique is effective in experienced hands.[2] In Type IV cases requiring a more complex and lengthy reconstruction, an alternative strategy should be pursued.

More extensive open TAAA repair is accomplished by dividing the aneurysm into sections separated between vascular clamps and repairing the segments sequentially. Applying a clamp-and-sew strategy to these aneurysms means that the distal sections remain ischemic throughout the repair of the more proximal segments. Thus, expediency and simple reconstructive strategy for branches (i.e., inclusion patches and bevels), become paramount. Cases where individual bypasses, targeted endarterectomies, and compromised aortic tissue (degeneration following acute or chronic dissection; connective tissue disorder) are required do not lend themselves to this approach without a substantial increase in patient morbidity and mortality.

Not surprisingly, improved outcomes in more extensive and/or complicated repairs can be achieved by maintaining blood flow to end-organs during proximal reconstruction. Because sequential clamping only isolates one segment of the aorta at a time, perfusion to any portion of the distal circulation will supply blood to all end-organs outside the isolated segment. This concept is referred to as distal aortic perfusion (DAP) and can be either passive, in the form of a shunt, or active in the form of mechanical circulatory support. DAP provides an added crucial benefit in cases of high thoracic aortic cross-clamping: left ventricular afterload reduction. Afterload reduction helps to mitigate the acute increase in myocardial stroke work and consequent demand ischemia to the patient.

Furthermore, DAP has a two-fold mitigation effect on paraplegia risk. Cord perfusion is dependent on cerebrospinal perfusion pressure, which is the mean aortic pressure minus the cerebrospinal fluid (CSF) pressure. Because the sudden increase in left ventricular afterload increases central venous pressure, which is transmitted to CSF pressure, DAP helps to avoid these pressure spikes in the CSF. By simultaneously augmenting distal aortic pressure and keeping CSF pressure down, DAP can substantially decrease paraplegia rates (Cambria Lancaster paper, Safi paper).[7,8]

The simplest form of DAP is passive shunting, first described by Gott in 1968 using a heparin-coated polyvinyl chloride (PVC). A similar effect can be achieved by sewing a temporary, non-tunneled, 10 mm Dacron graft from the left axillary artery to the left common femoral artery. It is the author's preference to use this technique in urgent/emergent cases as it is expedient and establishes distal aortic perfusion even before entering the chest and abdomen. The technique is particularly useful when the left pleural space is particularly hostile, as can occur in re-operative settings. With this passive strategy, however, blood flow through the shunt can only be regulated by the pressure gradient across the clamped portion of the aorta. As such, DAP can only be increased by driving up the proximal aortic pressure, most often, pharmacologically.

Active shunting in the form of mechanical circulatory support can be separated into full cardiopulmonary bypass and partial bypass techniques. The most commonly used partial bypass technique for open TAAA repair is left atrial-femoral bypass (Figure 20.1). An intake/drainage cannula is placed into the left atrium either directly through a pursestring in the left atrial appendage or through the left inferior pulmonary vein. The arterial return cannula is placed in the left common femoral artery but can also be placed into an iliac artery or directly into the distal aorta/aneurysm. A simple centrifugal pump propels the blood through the circuit; because it draws oxygenated blood, no membrane oxygenator is necessary,

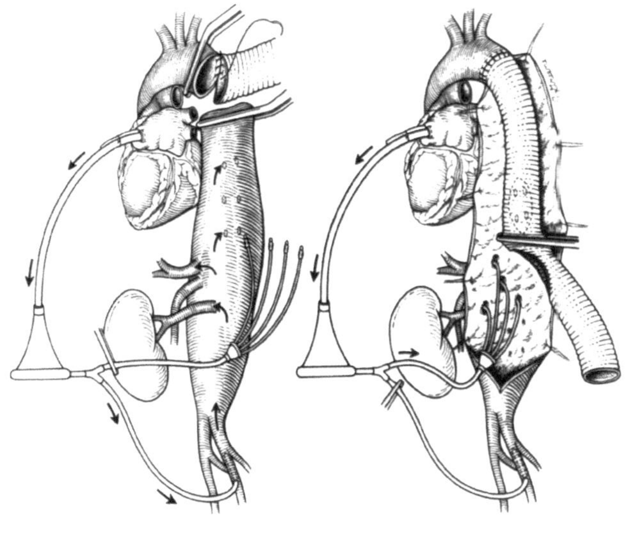

Figure 20.1 Left atrial-femoral bypass providing distal aortic perfusion during extensive open thoracoabdominal aortic aneurysm repair. (Conrad MF, Cambria RP. Contemporary management of descending thoracic and thoracoabdominal aortic aneurysms: endovascular versus open. *Circulation* 2008; 117:841–852.)

allowing for lower heparin doses than would be required with full cardiopulmonary bypass. Because left-atrial femoral bypass pulls pre-load from the left heart, it also serves to reduce left ventricular afterload.

Conversely, full cardiopulmonary bypass employs a membrane oxygenator and can therefore draw blood directly from the systemic venous circulation. This is most commonly accomplished by directing a long venous cannula through the femoral vein and up into the inferior vena cava near the atrio-caval junction. After passing through the membrane oxygenator, the blood is again returned to the distal circulation through the femoral artery.

An adjunct to full cardiopulmonary bypass is deep hypothermic circulatory arrest (DHCA). The technique allows for the complete cessation of circulation and operating in a bloodless field. Because the risks of this technique include pulmonary and cerebrovascular complications, which are not insignificant, it is the author's preference to employ DHCA only in cases where aortic tissue is compromised (acute dissection, connective tissue disorder), when the distal arch cannot be clamped, or in cases of catastrophic bleeding as described by Safi et al.[9] Conversely, because hypothermia has protective effects for ischemic tissues, some surgeons routinely employ this technique for TAAA repair.[4]

As described above, each strategy has benefits and disadvantages. While our institution has previously demonstrated that mechanical circulatory support proves beneficial in extensive aneurysm repairs, more recent and ongoing work seem to support the fact that at high-volume, experienced centers, there is a trend toward equivalence across strategies.[7,10,11] Furthermore, the causal effects of perfusion strategy alone are difficult to disentangle from the effects of the various other adjuncts (described in subsequent sections) employed in open TAAA repair.

PREOPERATIVE ADJUNCTS AND ANESTHESIA

The associated hemodynamic shifts and alterations in cardiac afterload that occur during repair make extensive planning and communication with an experienced anesthesia team absolutely crucial. As described above, this becomes even more important for extensive aneurysms or in cases where DAP will be employed. It is our practice to clearly discuss the operative plan, including the number of visceral bypasses, positions of aortic cross-clamps, anticipated end-organ/regional aortic ischemic times, perfusion strategy, as well as organ-specific adjuncts prior to the case with both the anesthesiology and surgical tech/nursing teams.

For extent I–III TAAAs, a CSF drain and radial arterial line are placed in the preoperative holding area. Placement of the arterial line into the right arm is preferred, as placement into the left arm may result in a dampened signal once the patient is positioned.

In the operating room, the patient's airway is secured with a double-lumen endotracheal tube for extent I–III aneurysms, which require extensive entry into the left hemithorax and left lung isolation to expose the proximal descending thoracic aorta. After the patient is asleep, somatosensory motor-evoked potential monitoring (SSMEVP) probes are secured, and a central line, typically in the right internal jugular vein, with pulmonary artery (Swan-Ganz) catheter is placed. The anesthesia team is reminded that any paralytics used during induction and exposure should be short-acting as to not interfere with SSMEVP once the aortic cross clamp is placed later in the case. A nasogastric tube is placed in supine position. Finally, a right femoral arterial line is placed sterilely by a member of the surgical team. This is performed with micropuncture access under ultrasound guidance followed by insertion of a 4 or 5F sheath over a 3J wire. The sheath is sutured to the skin and the prepped area is covered with a piece of Ioban to maintain sterility in the rare event when access to the right groin is required during the operation.

POSITIONING

Exposure of the thoracoabdominal aorta in its entirety requires visualization of both the supra- and infradiaphragmatic aorta. To accomplish this, the patient is positioned such that the point of maximal bed flexion, the so-called "break in the bed," lies midway between the inferior costal margin and the anterior superior iliac spine for a type IV aneurysm. As the aneurysm becomes more extensive and proximal, this "break" is moved cephalad such that it is positioned at around the 6th or 7th interspace for Type I aneurysms. The patient is turned into the right lateral decubitus position with the shoulders anywhere from 60 degrees to completely perpendicular to the bed. The left arm is supported over the right arm with an arm board (Figure 20.2). Now the bed is

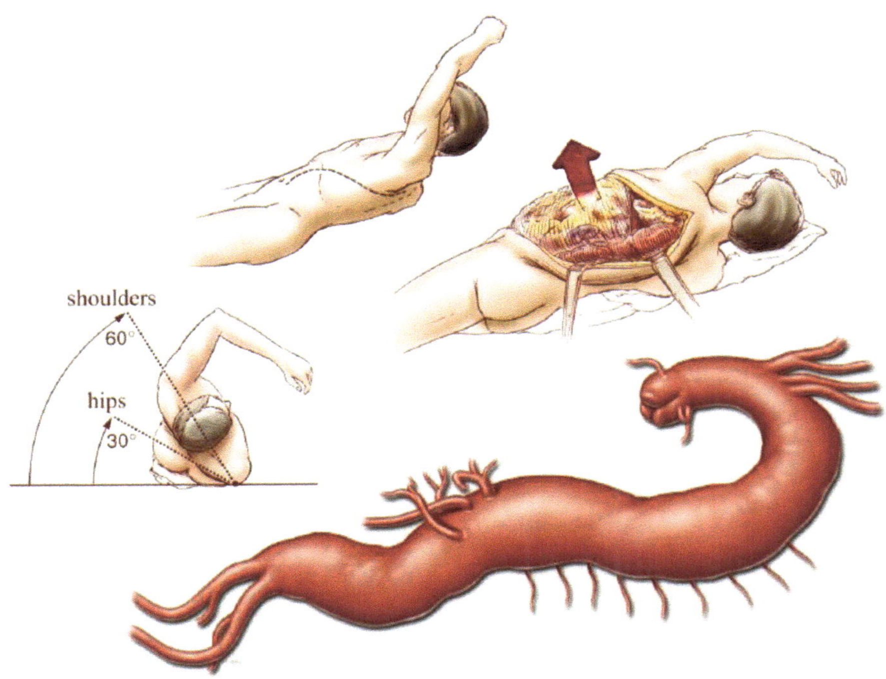

Figure 20.2 Thoracoabdominal aortic aneurysm repair with a branched graft. (de la Cruz KI, LeMaire SA, Weldon SA, Coselli JS. Thoracoabdominal aortic aneurysm repair with a branched graft. Ann Cardiothorac Surg, 2012 Sep;1(3):381–93.)

"broken" to the desired flexion/extension angle. The left hip is extended and the right is slightly flexed with pillows placed in between to avoid pressure points. Now a suction bean bag device is activated to maintain this position. Finally, the hips are allowed to fall back toward the table such that the torso spirals along its axis from the decubitus to supine position moving cephalad to caudad. This can be facilitated by abruptly pulling up on a draw sheet placed beneath the patient's hips while ensuring the shoulder stay perpendicular to the table. The maneuver allows the torso to "untwist" once the thoracoabdominal incision is made. Once appropriate padding is placed, the patient is belted into position and a final check of all monitoring lines, lower extremity pulse volume recordings, and SSMEVP is repeated to ensure that nothing became dislodged by positioning.

EXPOSURE AND SURGICAL APPROACH

Our typical approach is to alter the interspace of entry based on the extent of aneurysm (Figure 20.3) as follows: Extent I and II, top of the 6th rib (5th interspace); Extent III, top of the 8th rib (7th interspace); Extent IV, top of the 9th or 10th rib (8th or 9th interspace). The standard thoracoabdominal incision consists of a left thoracotomy that crosses the costal margin and transitions to a paramedian left laparotomy terminating just below the level of the umbilicus or more distal in the case of iliac involvement. The thoracotomy skin incision is made at roughly the same level as the interspace of entry except for type I and II aneurysms when the incision must be kept below the tip of the scapula. In these cases, an upper dermocutaneous flap is fashioned with the Bovie cautery by undermining along the superficial fascia to the scapula tip. The tip is released from the serratus anterior and bluntly yet gently separated from the rib cage with a Davidson scapula retractor. Divided edges of the serratus and latissimus (if partially transected) can be marked with long sutures for later re-approximation. Sliding a hand underneath the scapula allows for counting of the interspaces. Once the appropriate space has been confirmed, the intercostal muscles are carved off the superior portion of the rib with the cautery so as to avoid the neurovascular bundle, taking care not to violate the parietal pleura. Once the pleura is visualized, the left lung is deflated to allow safe entry into the left hemithorax sharply through the pleura to avoid inadvertent thermal injury to the lung. The thoracotomy is developed to the costal margin. On the abdominal side, the fascia is scored where the costal margin will be transected. The diaphragm is freed from the underside of the margin by passing a Kelly clamp, and the margin is sharply transected with heavy scissors.

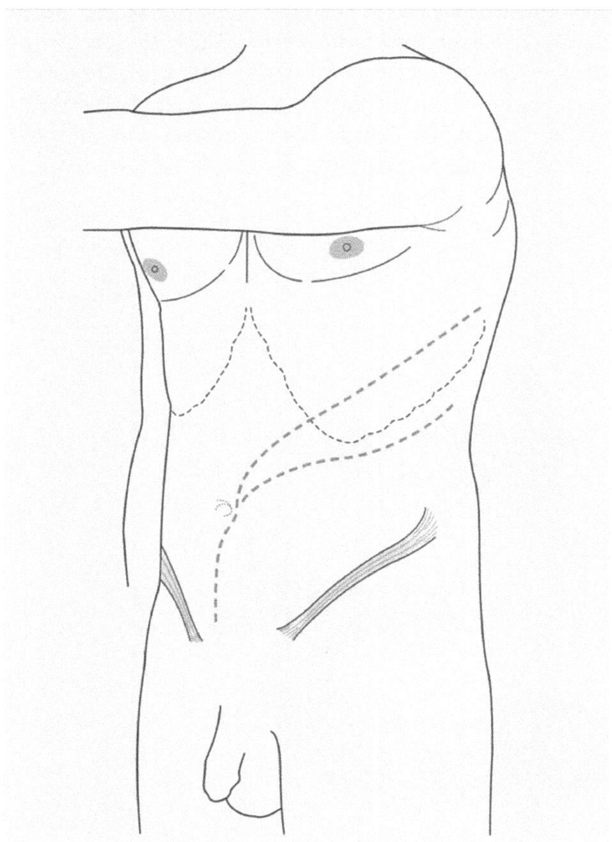

Figure 20.3 Variation in thoracotomy component of thoracoabdominal incision depending on aneurysm extent. (Modified from Hallett and Mills with permission from Elsevier. Comprhensive Vascular and Endovascular Surgery; 2004.)

The abdominal portion of the exposure can be approached from a retroperitoneal or transperitoneal approach. While the retroperitoneal approach helps to keep the viscera out of the way, thereby facilitating exposure and reducing insensible and thermal losses, it inhibits direct visualization of bowel perfusion in cases where individual visceral vessel reconstruction may be necessary. For retroperitoneal exposure, the surface of the diaphragm can be followed to the pre-peritoneal plane, which is then followed to the retroperitoneal by sweeping the peritoneal sac off the underside of the abdominal wall and the diaphragm. If the transperitoneal approach is used, the left white line of Toldt must be taken down to enter the retroperitoneal plane. Gerota's fascia is scored with the Bovie cautery deep to this, and the kidney is reflected up and out of its bed to complete the left medial visceral rotation (Mattox maneuver). In cases of a retroaortic left renal vein or when access to the more distal SMA is necessary, the kidney can be left down (modified Mattox maneuver). Once the viscera or peritoneal sac have been reflected, it is the author's preference to use a self-retaining Omni retractor system to maintain appropriate exposure. The diaphragm is then divided circumferentially along its costal insertions to avoid the central tendon and phrenic nerve, leaving enough of a cuff along the rib for later re-approximation. Marking stitches placed during division facilitate closure later.

With the left kidney mobilized anteriorly, there is frequently a renal lumbar vein that will tether the left renal vein toward the spine. The renal lumbar vein is suture ligated and serves as a marker for the approximate location of the left renal artery, which should be sharply mobilized from surrounding tissue and encircled with a vessel loop. The artery is then dissected back to its aortic origin to identify the correct plane of aortic exposure. Once the wall of the aneurysm is cleared at the left renal take-off, dissection should advance cephalad with division of the left Crus, which crosses the aorta just above the artery. This completes the division of the diaphragm previously initiated from the costal margin.

Exposing the descending thoracic aorta begins with division of the inferior pulmonary ligament, which is facilitated by putting the collapsed left lower lobe on traction using a Duval lung clamp. Single-lung ventilation is critical when descending thoracic aortic exposure is necessary. The inferior pulmonary ligament is divided to the hilum, stopping short of the left inferior pulmonary vein, which can be further exposed and isolated for left-atrial femoral bypass cannulation. Rotating the deflated left lung medially will allow for division of the mediastinal pleura to the distal aortic arch for extent I and II aneurysms. When gaining control of the aorta at this level, care should be taken to avoid injury to the recurrent laryngeal nerve, the pulmonary artery, and the esophagus. In the case of the latter, and NG tube or trans-esophageal echo probe is extremely helpful for identification. If distal arch clamping or zone 2 clamping is required, division of the ligamentum arteriosum may be necessary.

Once the proximal clamp site is circumferentially controlled, dissection of the visceral segment can be continued by sequentially identifying the celiac and SMA and controlling them with vessel loops (Figure 20.4). In most cases, right renal artery access is difficult and not necessary. Instead, the vessel can be controlled from within the aneurysm once it is opened. When DAP is planned, sequential circumferential clamp sites should be developed to facilitate retrograde perfusion of renovisceral and segmental arteries.

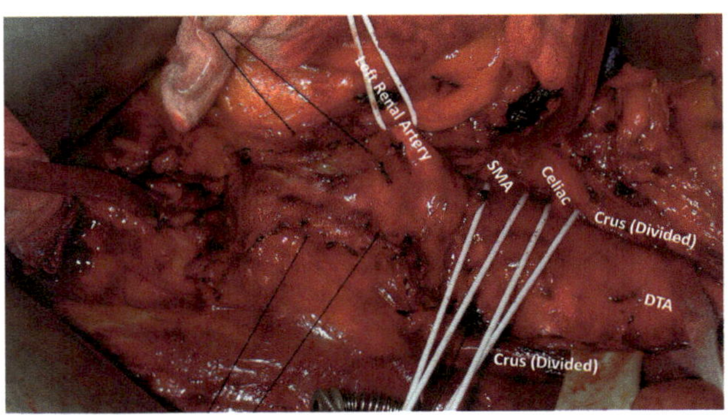

Figure 20.4 Exposure of the visceral aortic segment begins with identification and control of the left renal artery, which is reflected upward following the left medial visceral rotation. The artery is dissected back to its aortic origin, and then the peri-aortic plane is developed proximally to identify the SMA, celiac, and descending thoracic aorta (DTA).

ANASTOMOSES AND REPAIR

In fashioning our graft, we use a gelatin-impregnated, woven, Dacron graft. Our preferred technique for addressing the renovisceral segment, anatomy permitting, follows Crawford's inclusion technique, which evolved from the need for expediency during clamp-and-sew reconstruction.[11] This method attempts to incorporate the ostia of the visceral and renal arteries into the minimum amount of anastomoses. For extent II and III aneurysms, a tailored ellipse is cut into the side of the graft, and an inclusion patch of the native aorta involving the celiac, SMA, and right renal arteries is sewn from within the aneurysm (Figure 20.5A).[11] The suture line is fashioned such that the celiac and right renal arteries are at the apices of the ellipse. Topologically, the left renal artery is most commonly reconstructed by means of a separate sidearm off the graft. When substantial interostial distance would result in the incorporation of unacceptable amounts of residual native aortic tissue within the patch, or in cases where the reconstruction is being performed for connective tissue disease, individual bypasses to all renovisceral vessels are performed. If bypasses are planned, side arms are sewn to the main Dacron tube graft in a fashion tailored to the individual patient's anatomy. For extent I aneurysms, our preferred visceral segment reconstruction is a generous distal beveled anastomosis of the main aortic graft with the heel coursing around the ostium of the celiac artery and a sidearm for the left renal artery (Figure 20.5B). The mirror image of this construct is used for extent IV aneurysms, where the proximal aortic anastomosis now becomes the bevel with the heel coursing around the right renal artery ostium and the toe taken up behind the celiac (Figure 20.5C). Again, the left renal artery is reconstructed by means of a separate side-arm. Further details of individual renovisceral reconstruction are addressed in the respective complications section.

Prior to clamping, the patient is appropriately heparinized based on perfusion strategy and use of mechanical circulatory support. The spinal drain is opened and set to a pressure of 10 mmHg. For extent I–III aneurysms, the proximal anastomosis should be performed end-to-end to a completely transected aorta, avoiding a Creech technique, which risks injury to the esophagus in this location. In patients with connective tissue disorder, we reinforce all anastomoses with a felt strip. The distal anastomosis is typically sewn to the infrarenal aorta or the aortic bifurcation using a Creech technique on the backwall. If iliac aneurysms are present, a bifurcated graft to the iliac or femoral vessels may be necessary.

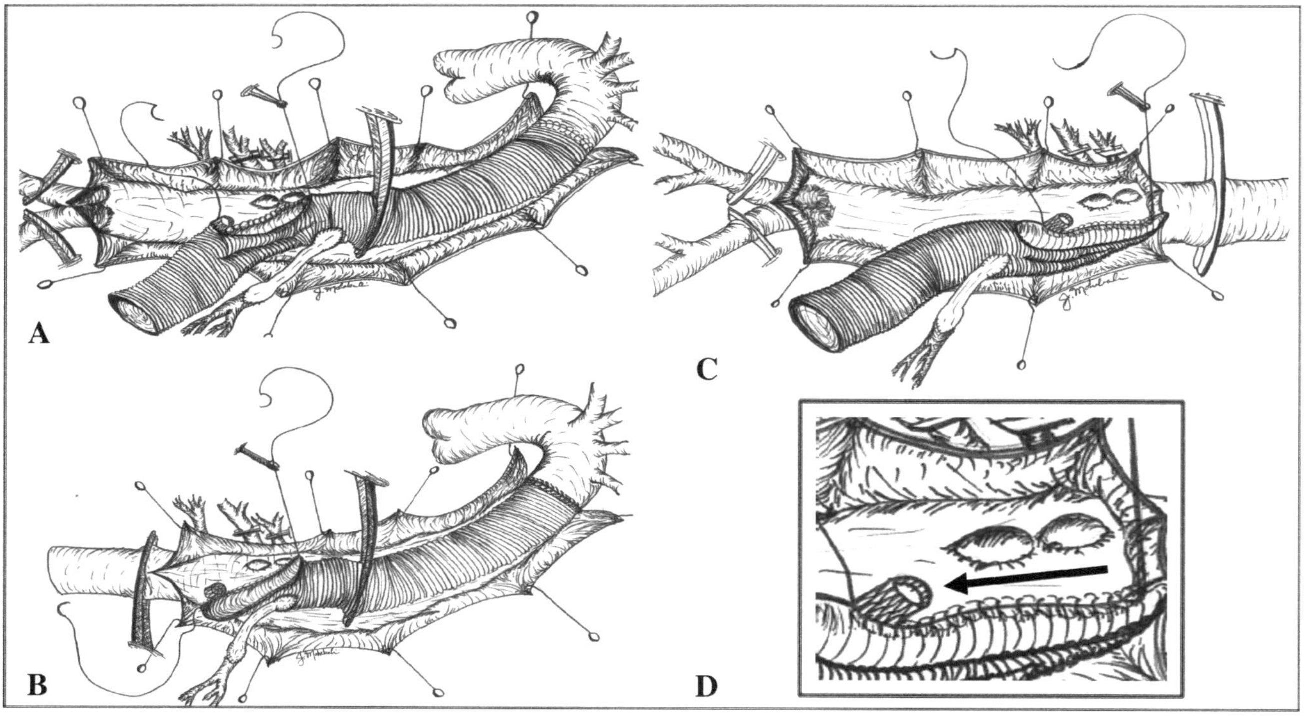

Figure 20.5 (A) Preferred method for reconstruction of the reno-visceral segment with the right renal, SMA and celiac incorporated into a single inclusion patch sewn from within the aneurysm. (B) For extent I repair, the renovisceral vessels can be incorporated into a long, beveled distal anastomosis. (C) For extent IV repair, the renovisceral vessels are incorporated into a proximal beveled anastomosis. (D) A trans-aortically deployed balloon-expandable stent into the right renal artery orifice can help prevent ostial collapse/coaptation from the suture line and also treat any disease. Note that for all panes in this figure, the left renal artery bypass is depicted completed in its final resting position whereas in reality, this bypass is completely following the major renovisceral reconstruction.

Once the proximal anastomosis and thoracic aorta have been addressed, attention is brought to the visceral segments. Again, if feasible, the celiac, SMA, and right renal arteries are fashioned into a single inclusion button. The suture line will include the edge of the vessel orifice when able. Ostial endarterectomy can be carefully performed if necessary. A balloon-expandable stent can also be deployed into the origin of the right renal artery to prevent anastomotic compromise (Figure 20.5D). If there is a large separation between the celiac and SMA, the celiac can be amputated and fashioned into a separate Carrell patch. Once the inclusion patch is sewn to the graft, the proximal clamp is moved distally to allow blood flow to the visceral vessels. A left renal artery bypass is performed typically with a 6 mm PTFE graft. If an inclusion patch is unable to be performed, or if the patient has an underlying connective tissue disorder, separate bypasses are done to the celiac and SMA in sequential fashion to limit the ischemic time.

Whenever feasible, the aortic clamp is moved down to restore blood flow to the vessels as they are reattached to the graft. After the aortic repair is complete, protamine sulfate is administered to reverse the effects of heparin. Every effort is made to have the patient euthermic. All suture lines and anastomosis are evaluated for hemostasis. The aortic aneurysm wall and peritoneum is reapproximated over the graft when possible. If this is not possible, an omental flap is fashioned for coverage. In the chest, a Goretex graft can be used to avoid direct graft to lung contact. Two chest tubes (one straight, one angled) are placed prior to closing the chest.

SPECIFIC COMPLICATIONS

Because the major complications associated with open TAAA repair (paraplegia, renal failure, mesenteric malperfusion, myocardial infarction) primarily result from intraoperative or postoperative end-organ ischemia, their respective rate of occurrence is proportional to the oxygen demands and baseline metabolic rates of the at-risk tissue as well as the degree to which blood flow is interrupted to these vascular beds. This in turn, is greatly affected by collateral blood supply. Thus, the overarching principles in decreasing these complications hinges upon augmenting perfusion and, in turn, oxygen delivery, and/or temporarily decreasing metabolic rate during repair. Oxygen delivery is guided by the following equation:

$$\begin{aligned}&\textit{Arterial Oxygen Delivery}\\&= \textit{Cardiac Output} \times \{\textit{Oxygen Bound to Hemoglobin}\\&+ \textit{Oxygen Dissolved in Blood}\}\end{aligned}$$

$$DaO_2 = HR \times SV \times \left[\left(1.39 \times Hgb \times SpO_2\right) + \left(0.003 \times PaO_2\right)\right]$$

Careful review demonstrates that the only variables which can be manipulated to augment delivery include (from left to right) heart rate, stroke volume, hemoglobin concentration, oxygen saturation, and the partial pressure of oxygen in the blood. The following sections cover organ-specific adjuncts that often work in concert with one or more of the global perfusion strategies (DAP, DHCA) discussed previously to either maximize oxygen delivery or to decrease metabolic demand for oxygen.

PARAPLEGIA

Perhaps the most devastating complication after open TAAA repair is paraplegia secondary to spinal cord ischemia. The patients most at risk for this complication are those with extensive aneurysmal disease (type I–II), presence of dissection, and acuity of presentation.[12–14,15] Historically, the spinal cord injury rate following open TAAA has been reported to be upwards of 20%.[16] As such, a variety of intraoperative and postoperative adjuncts have been developed and subsequently evolved in efforts to combat this dreaded outcome, which has also been shown to decrease long-term survival.[14] As noted above, these techniques include augmented perfusion via collateral vessels (DAP, reimplantation of segmental arteries, CSF drainage), and decreasing metabolic oxygen demand (regional epidural cooling, corporeal hypothermia associated with DHCA). However, based on the current literature, only CSF drainage has been shown to reduce spinal cord ischemia rates. Nevertheless, most experienced surgeons will employ one or more of these adjuncts routinely so, the exact causal mitigative effects of each one individually cannot be disentangled from the others. Although the data are heterogenous, the combined effects can decrease the risk of permanent paraplegia to the single digits even in extensive TAAA repair.[15,16]

The main arterial supply of the spinal cord is by three longitudinal arteries (anterior spinal artery and the two posterolateral spinal arteries). These are supplemented by arterial inflow from the subclavian artery, the thyrocervical and costocervical trunks, the segmental arteries (intercostals and lumbars), and the internal iliac arteries, all of which contribute to a collateral network of vessels that supplies the cord.[17] This collateral network concept has been described and confirmed by multiple thought leaders in the field including Wynn, Acher, Griepp, Backes, and Jacobs.[15,18,19] The concept has been further substantiated in the endovascular realm by Eagleton et al.[20] Unfortunately, unlike in endovascular repair, which primarily disrupts segmental blood flow, proximal aortic cross-clamping in open TAAA repair inherently affects multiple downstream inflow sources to the collateral network (intercostals, lumbars, internal iliacs, left subclavian in distal arch cases). As expected, a more proximal cross-clamp exacerbates this effect. Furthermore, a longer cross-clamp time was also associated with greater paralysis as described in Crawford's inceptive series (36) and confirmed by numerous subsequent authors and studies.[5–7,21,22] Intuitively then, providing additional inflow to the collateral network should mitigate this effect. Indeed, using hydrogen perfusion studies, Svensson proved that DAP in the form of left-atrial femoral bypass maintained blood flow to the cord during creation of the proximal anastomosis.[12] These results were further supported by Dr. Safi's group, who demonstrated that aortic cross-clamp time and extent I aneurysmal disease were no longer significant predictors of paraplegia when left heart bypass (LHB) or cardiopulmonary bypass (CPB) were employed.[23]

Cord perfusion is also dependent on CSF pressure, which opposes arterial inflow (cerebrospinal perfusion pressure = mean aortic pressure – cerebrospinal fluid pressure). Thus, in addition to augmenting collateral network mean arterial pressure, decreasing CSF pressure also decreases paraplegia risk. Crawford et. al performed the first randomized controlled trial of CSF drainage and concluded that there was no difference between the study patients and controls.[24] However, only 50ccs of CSF were drained, and the main criticism of that study remained that patients were not adequately drained to impact their spinal cord perfusion pressure.[24] Since then, Svensson and Coselli have both demonstrated CSF drainage to have a significant effect on the reduction of paralysis.[25,26] A recent meta-analysis demonstrated that CSF fluid drainage decreased the spinal cord ischemia rate by nearly half in their pooled analysis. The overall number needed to treat was 14, with an absolute risk reduction of 7%, which is similar to the systematic review performed by Cina et al. that showed a NNT of 11, with an absolute risk reduction of 9%.[16,27] However, this benefit did not continue to late presentations of spinal cord ischemia and may be related to reperfusion-type injury.

CSF drainage is not without its own set of complications that can be equally devastating and morbid. These include catheter fracture, postural headache, neuraxial hematoma, intracranial hemorrhage, meningitis, failed CSF drainage, and even death.[28] The overall CSF complication rate, however, has been reported at a rate of 1.5–5% at experienced centers.[3] Because of this risk-benefit ratio, we routinely employ spinal drainage for all extent I–III aneurysms, but not for type IV aneurysms, which have demonstrated paraplegia rates similar to open juxta and suprarenal repair at our institution.[2] To further minimize complications, it is the authors' preference to cancel and reschedule the operation for a later date if a traumatic tap with substantial bloody drainage occurs as the risk of neuraxial hematoma following heparinization is felt to be too high. During the procedure, constant closed loop communication with the anesthesia team to ensure ongoing free drainage of CSF, particularly following the application of the aortic cross clamp, is paramount. Postoperative care of the drain begins at the time of transfer off the operating table where meticulous care ensures that inadvertent dislodging is avoided. Additionally, any time the patient is moved or brought out of a completely flat and supine position, the drain must be clamped to avoid excessive rapid drainage and consequent intracranial hemorrhage.

Cryopreservation of cellular tissue has been employed for decades. Similarly, it has been shown that hypothermia can reduce metabolic rate and oxygen demand in nervous tissue.[15] Based on this principle, in 2000, Cambria and Davison developed a method for regional spinal cord hypothermia with epidural cooling that was successful in 97% of patients in their series, with a spinal cord ischemia rate of 7% overall (type I/II 12%, all other types, 2.3%) in the setting of a clamp-and-sew technique with selective intercostal reimplantation.[29] While we no longer employ this technique routinely, we do continue to use mild permissive corporeal hypothermia (32–34°C) during repair. Deep hypothermic circulatory arrest has been used to hypothetically decrease rates of paralysis, but this is typically only used in TAAA operations that involve the distal arch or to avoid cross clamping aorta affected by connective tissue disease.[15]

The open TAAA technique of regional cooling with a clamp-and-sew technique has largely evolved toward one with distal aortic perfusion with SSMEVP monitoring (Figure 20.6). Routine reimplantation of the intercostal arteries had previously been a strategy for neuroprotection but has been shown to increase operative times and blood loss.[26,30,31] SSMEVP evolved from the desire to have real-time data on the status of spinal cord circulation during the operation. This is based on the collateral network concept of cord circulation has previously discussed by Griepp et al.[18] Most such collaterals arise caudal to the distal aortic clamp (i.e., from the pelvic and hypogastric arteries).[19] Normal SSMEVP have a strong negative predictive value, and patients without signal loss are unlikely to emerge post-procedure with a neurologic deficit.[32] Lancaster et al. indicated that SSMEVP monitoring along with distal aortic perfusion via atrial femoral bypass (AFB) was an independent predictor of improved perioperative death and paraplegia rates as well as long-term survival in patients undergoing extent I–III TAAs.[7] AFB is begun by cannulating the left atrium through the left inferior pulmonary vein and the arterial return is typically via the left common femoral artery. Bypass is initiated with flows of

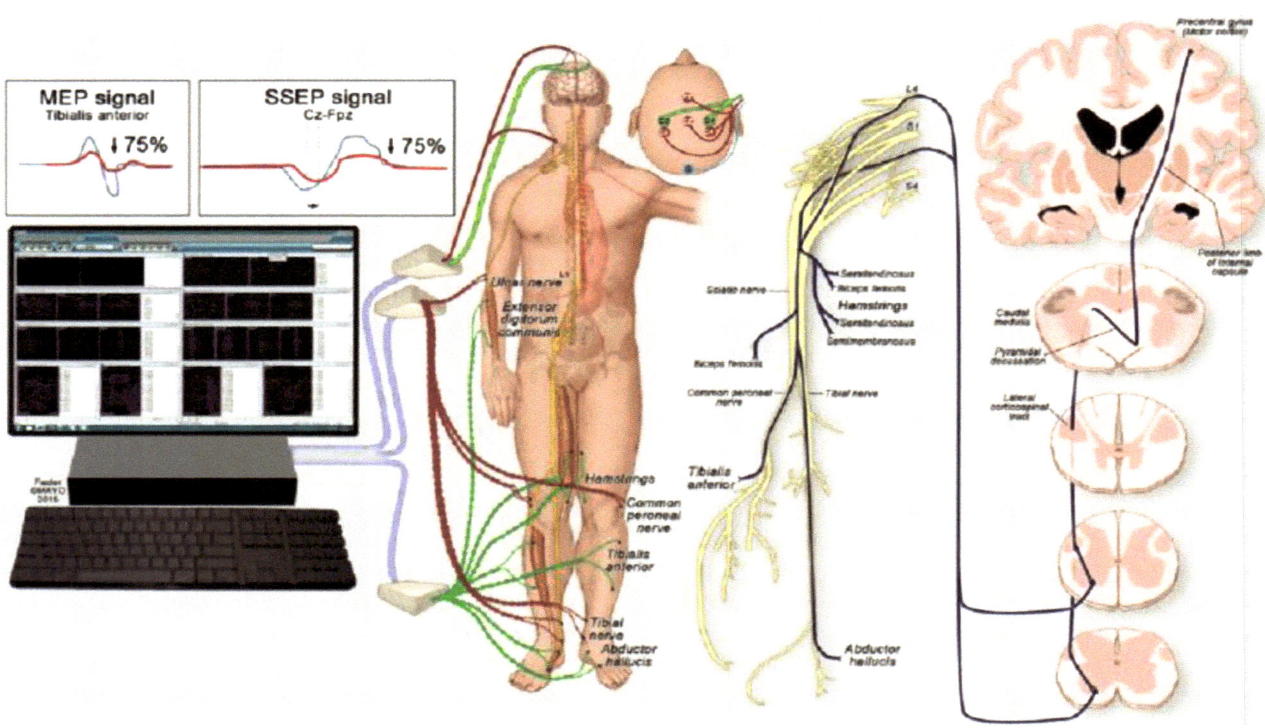

Figure 20.6 Somatosensory motor-evoked potential monitoring relies on motor stimuli sent from the motor cortex and detected in the extremities, and sensory stimuli evoked in the extremities and detected in the sensory cortex. (Banga P, de Souza LR, Oderich GS. Neuromonitoring, cerebropsinal fluid drainage, and selective use of iliofemoral conduits to minimize risk of spinal cord injury during complex endovascular aortic repair. *J Endovasc Ther*, December 2015; 23(1):139–149.)

500 mL/min and gradually increased until distal perfusion (per previously placed right femoral a-line) reaches at least 60 mmHg. SSMEVPs are monitored by a dedicated neurologist familiar with the procedure and available to troubleshoot technical issues such as patient response to anesthetic agents and electrode failure. At our institution, a sudden drop in SSMEVP amplitude (occurring within 2–10 minutes) or a sustained progressive drop (within 10–40 minutes) of > 75% from baseline is considered significant.[33] If these changes do not respond to an increase in perfusion pressure, then intercostal reconstruction via an inclusion button is performed. If the SSMEVPs are unchanged, then the intercostal arteries are oversewn.

Postoperatively, the patient is typically kept intubated (less so with type IV TAAA) and resuscitated in the surgical intensive care unit. Once the patient has achieved hemodynamic stability and euthermia, the sedation is lightened to obtain a baseline neurologic examination. This exam is particularly focused on the sensory and motor function of the lower extremities given the significant risk of paraplegia/paralysis with open TAAA repairs. The exam should elicit contraction of the hip flexors and rectus femoris muscles to raise the knee of the bed. Patients with spinal cord ischemia may still be able to move their toes if sacral sparing is present. Furthermore, symmetry in the exam should be maintained in both strength and sensation. If the patient is unable to follow commands after sedation is weaned, a stat CT head is obtained to rule out any intracranial process. The spinal drain is kept in place for 3–4 days. It is clamped during any times of patient positioning or transport. The goal of the drain is to maintain spinal cord perfusion pressures greater than 60 mmHg. This generally corresponds as a CSF pressure < 10 mmHg. Therefore, the spinal drain is kept at a pressure of 10 mmHg and allowed to drain 15–20 cc of CSF per hour. The drain can be raised or lowered from the zero/reference point (patient's right atrium) in order to control the flow from the drain. The rate of CSF drainage must be regulated, as excessive drainage has been associated with intracranial hemorrhage.[34]

In the setting of a delayed neurologic deficit, several maneuvers can be employed. Increasing the mean arterial pressure (MAP) is first-line therapy. Increases in MAP are done until symptoms resolve or the ceiling of a tolerable MAP is reached. The next step involves lowering the CSF pressure by maintaining the spinal drain to a pressure of less than 5 mmHg. If drain malfunction is suspected, reinsertion can be performed in the intensive care unit under sterile conditions.

In the setting of a blood-tinged or bloody CSF and no neurologic deficits, our protocol is to stop the drainage and correct any coagulopathy and platelet deficits. After correction of the coagulopathy, the CSF is drained to determine if the CSF has cleared. If the CSF does not clear, then the decision is made to remove the drain and replace it if necessary. If the patient develops any neurologic findings such as an altered mental status or focal deficits, then a stat CT scan is performed to exclude an intracranial hemorrhage. Patients at risk for this complication are those with pre-existing intracranial pathology, coagulopathy, or patients with an increased rate of drainage from their spinal drain. In the setting of intracranial hemorrhage, neurosurgical evacuation may be necessary.

Our institution routinely caps the spinal drain prior to removal to evaluate for any development of neurologic sequelae. Removal of the spinal drain is performed in the setting of no neurologic sequalae and, if possible, off all vasopressors. If no symptoms develop, the drain is removed. CSF leak is a rare occurrence. Initial treatment consists of conservative measures, such as bed rest, limiting the patient's head less than 30 degrees, and hydration. If there is no resolution within 24 hours, then a blood patch is performed.

Pulmonary

Pulmonary-related complications remain the most common complication after open repair of TAAAs and can be expected to be present in at least one-third of patients.[1,12,35] Patients with descending thoracic aorta and TAAA are at high risk for pulmonary complications due to their typical comorbidities (COPD, high prevalence of cardiovascular disease, smoking history, increased age).[35,36] Adding to these comorbidities is the need for single-lung ventilation as well as large thoracoabdominal incisions, which are associated with postoperative pain and the potential impact on pulmonary outcomes.

Preoperatively, the patient's overall health and nutritional status contribute to the risk of pulmonary complications. A low albumin level is associated with respiratory failure, with the morbidity increasing at an exponential rate as the albumin levels fall below 3.5 g/dL. In addition, patients with a greater than 10% weight loss over the previous 6 months are at an increased risk of pulmonary complications.[5,35,37]

During the repair, division of the diaphragm has previously been associated with a higher probability of prolonged ventilatory support. However, preservation of the diaphragm has been associated with a significant decrease in hospital stay by an average of 4 days.[38] Preservation of the diaphragm is an independent predictor of weaning from the ventilator in < 72 hours.[39] At our institution, after the costal margin is divided with a heavy Mayo scissors, the diaphragm is divided circumferentially along its costal insertions. Marking stitches are places at intervals along its division to aid in reconstruction. Division of the diaphragm in this manner avoids the phrenic nerve attachments into the diaphragmatic muscle. In extent IV TAAA repairs, minimal diaphragmatic division is necessary. If necessary, partial division of the diaphragm can be performed for improved retraction and visualization.

The left phrenic nerve arises from the cervical nerve roots of C3 to C5 and descends anteriorly between the pericardium and mediastinal pleura. It then penetrates the diaphragm on the lateral border of the heart. Injury to the phrenic nerve can cause a diaphragmatic palsy resulting in a paresis of the left hemi-diaphragm. The left vagus nerve crosses the distal arch and the recurrent laryngeal nerve will be seen coursing from it and dividing under the arch at the ligamentum arteriosum. Left vocal cord paralysis is another commonly described complication related to open TAAA repairs. In Coselli's series, the overall rate was 15.4%, but was higher (26.1%) in extent I repairs.[5] This is similar to Wong and colleagues, results of vocal cord paralysis with an overall rate of 18.3%. Understandably, the rates of left vocal cord paralysis was approximately 30% for extent I and II TAAA and almost non-existent for extent III and IV TAAA (1% and 0%, respectively).[40] Injury to the left recurrent laryngeal nerve can occur during exposure, aortic clamping, or suturing, especially when working near the left subclavian artery. Left vocal cord paralysis has a significant impact on a patient's protection of airway. This injury should be suspected in patients with a hoarse voice and can be confirmed by direct flexible laryngoscopy. Treatment can be provided by direct cord medialization or polytetrafluoroethylene injections. Collaboration with otolaryngologists and the speech pathologists will be instrumental in the treatment of this morbidity.

Every precaution is taken to avoid unnecessary trauma to the lung itself. Keeping the majority of the dissection extrathoracic also precludes the need for a double-lumen tube. Most importantly, the utmost effort should be toward avoiding intraoperative and postoperative hypoxemia. Conrad et al. demonstrated the highest odds ratio (4.0) of spinal cord ischemia as related to any pulmonary complication.[14]

Two chest tubes (apical and angled) are placed at the conclusion of the open TAAA repair. The angled chest tube should be left in place for 5–7 days or until the patient has been adequately diuresed. Gentle diuresis typically occurs on the second postoperative day when the intense inflammatory response to the operation begins to subside. We encourage early cessation of bed rest (when able) and frequent incentive spirometry use.

Tracheostomy after open TAAA occurs in 4–9% of patients. Etz and colleagues evaluated pulmonary complications of descending and TAAA repairs. Independent predictors of pulmonary complications include a preoperative BUN greater than 24 mg/dL and a ruptured aneurysm. After univariate analysis, a history of COPD, creatinine greater than 2.5 mg/dL pre- or postoperatively, and transfusions were associated with pulmonary failure.[35] Interestingly, the presence of tracheostomy did not correlate with mortality in their series. The authors state that this may be explained by placing tracheostomies early in patients with significant pulmonary comorbidities, with the intent to improve their pulmonary care and mobility. This is reflected in our practice, as an early tracheostomy will aid in a patient's pulmonary toilet and decrease their dependency on the ventilator.

Cardiovascular

Preoperative evaluation of any active cardiac disease should be done to rule out any evidence of unstable angina, recent MI (or reversible areas of myocardial ischemia), acute heart failure, symptomatic valvular heart disease, or significant arrythmias. In these cases, a multidisciplinary discussion should be performed to address these issues in the setting of the patients aortopathy. Evaluation the patient's functional capacity should be performed as part of their preoperative appointment. This is done by measuring their metabolic equivalents (MET) and can be used to estimate their activities of daily living. Functional status is a predictor of mortality in patients with aortic aneurysms and can be used to guide preoperative testing.[41] Patients with < 4 METs should have their clinical cardiac risk factors assessed, and be considered for additional cardiac testing.

From an operative standpoint, the clamp-and-sew technique, as advocated by Crawford, emphasized simplicity and expediency.[42] Since then, several adjuncts have emerged to limit the amount of ischemia to end organs during the aortic cross clamp. Atrial femoral bypass and hypothermic circulatory arrest remain two primary methods of distal aortic perfusion during cross clamping of the aorta. There are three main functions of distal aortic perfusion. The first is left ventricular offloading, which helps decrease the profound physiologic derangements associated with cross clamping. Cross clamping leads to an acute rise in left ventricular preload and afterload which subsequently results in an increase in left ventricular wall stress, and myocardial oxygen demand.[10] The second is to aid in the control of proximal hypertension. The third advantage is a reduction in organ ischemia. Crawford, in his benchmark series, demonstrated that a prolonged cross-clamp time was correlated with an early death, even after multivariate analysis.[42] Cross clamping without afterload reduction can cause an increase in central venous pressure and CSF pressure contributing to a decrease in overall spinal cord perfusion.[43,44] In addition, Mohebali et al. demonstrated a significant decrease in operative mortality, pulmonary complications, and acute renal failure when using extracorporeal bypass for distal aortic perfusion.[10] Svensson's evaluation of left atrial femoral bypass proved that blood supply was maintained when the aorta was cross clamped.[12,25] Subsequent studies have shown that left heart bypass does reduce the risk of paraplegia and paralysis.[1,45] Use of extracorporeal bypass for type III is more variable (and dependent on anatomy), and rarely needed for type IV TAAAs. The main disadvantages for distal aortic perfusion are the requirement of heparin, and the activation of the coagulation as well as inflammatory cascade.

When preparing for open TAAAs, particularly when expecting to use adjuncts for distal aortic perfusion, a femoral arterial line (preferably right-sided) is required to adjust the bypass flow rate. Left heart bypass is composed of a circuit consisting of an inflow cannula proximal to the aortic clamp, a centrifugal pump, and an outflow cannula within the distal aorta or femoral artery. The proximal inflow cannula is typically in the left atrial appendage or left pulmonary vein. As previously discussed, bypass is initiated with flows of 500 mL/min and gradually increased until distal perfusion reaches at least 60 mmHg. Distal perfusion can be adjusted per SSMEVP or urine output.

Deep hypothermic circulatory arrest with total cardiopulmonary bypass also establishes distal aortic perfusion. Some authors champion this approach to decrease the overall metabolic demands of the spinal cord, kidneys and viscera, while others have seen a high rate of pulmonary complications and no reduction in the rates of spinal cord ischemia or acute kidney injury.[9] Currently, this technique preferably in situations when proximal control is not achievable. This is typically due to the presence of rupture, aneurysm location/size, or dissection. In addition, total cardiopulmonary bypass for the treatment of TAAAs can be done in the setting of simultaneous aortic arch repair. Finally, cardiopulmonary bypass may be beneficial in the setting of connective tissue disorders, as it will allow the surgeon to avoid undo clamp injuries to the aorta.[4,46]

Gastrointestinal

Mesenteric ischemia is a dreaded complication during and after open TAAA repair with a reported 2.5% incidence and 62% mortality.[47] Mortality is substantially higher if the ischemia is not discovered and corrected intraoperatively or immediately postoperatively.[11] The exact manifestation of ischemia also varies based on the vascular distribution involved. Celiac malperfusion may vary from clinically non-significant to fulminant hepatic failure, pancreatitis, and duodenal necrosis depending on the individual patient's collateral anatomy and baseline vascular disease. SMA malperfusion most commonly manifests as bowel ischemia. As described earlier, our preferred technique for visceral reconstruction is incorporation within an inclusion patch (extent II and III), or within the distal (extent I), or proximal (extent IV) anastomoses. Additionally, we address any significant intrinsic branch vessel disease that may compromise reconstruction at the time of the operation. This may include trans-aortic orificial eversion endarterectomy and/or stenting.[11] In these cases, particular care must be taken to ensure that treatment does not result in a distal dissection within the branch vessel. Intraoperatively, a trans-peritoneal thoracoabdominal exposure provides the advantage of direct visualization and assessment of the bowel following reconstruction, though a robust Doppler signal in the celiac and SMA is also adequate. In general, revascularization of the IMA followed the same posture as abdominal aortic aneurysm repair in that adequate backbleeding typically obviates targeted revascularization. It should be noted, however, that SMA malperfusion, may consequently manifest as colonic ischemia if the IMA is not revascularized.

Postoperatively, clinical signs of mesenteric ischemia may be nonspecific and include abdominal pain, prolonged ileus, melena, hematochezia, fever, or abdominal distension. Intubation and sedation over the first 24–48 postoperative hours exacerbates that challenge of making a diagnosis based solely on exam. Furthermore, other findings such as prolonged ileus, melena, hematochezia, and fever may not manifest for days, necessitating a high index of suspicion to make the diagnosis. In many cases, a rapidly escalating vasopressor or inotrope requirement, worsening metabolic acidosis, and rising serum lactate despite adequate volume resuscitation must raise the suspicion of mesenteric ischemia both intra- and postoperatively. A normal lactate, however, does not definitively rule out ischemia.[48] Bedside mesenteric duplex can be extremely helpful if flow through the celiac and SMA can be definitively detected, however, an equivocal result secondary to poor visualization should prompt expeditious re-exploration in the immediate postoperative period if there is adequate clinical suspicion. In general, it is the authors' preference to re-explore rather than obtain axial imaging in the immediate postoperative period, as the latter approach offers no means of intervention, may delay diagnosis and/or intervention, and additionally adds to the risk of acute kidney injury because of contrast nephropathy following renal ischemia. When suspicion for ischemia arises days following a successful initial postoperative course, axial imaging becomes increasingly relevant as it also allows for some assessment of bowel involvement. Colonoscopy or flexible sigmoidoscopy during this period also can be helpful to diagnose ischemic colitis.

In addition to dilutional coagulopathy and surgical blood loss, visceral (particularly hepatic) ischemia, has been implicated in perioperative coagulopathic bleeding.[12,49] As expected, there is a higher incidence of mesenteric ischemia after performing an open TAAA with a clamp-and-sew technique without any adjuncts to limit visceral ischemia. Safi and colleagues had previously shown that visceral perfusion (provided by distal aortic perfusion) was a statistically significant predictor of decreased postoperative alkaline phosphatase, prothrombin time (PT) and partial thromboplastin time (PTT).[8] Visceral perfusion, in effect, mitigates the rise in liver ischemic-related lab values seen, particularly after open type II TAAA.[8] Previous studies have documented the coagulopathy and metabolic derangements that occur after 30 minutes of a supraceliac aortic clamp.[50,51] For the proximal beveled anastomosis previously described for type IV TAAA, if anatomically feasible, the authors clamp the aorta in an angled fashion between the celiac and SMA in such a way as to maintain antegrade flow through the celiac while simultaneously allowing the toe of a beveled proximal anastomosis to be carried up behind the celiac.

If this is not possible, the proximal anastomosis must be completed within 20–30 minutes to avoid the detrimental effects of total mesenteric ischemia. In type IV cases where the celiac and SMA require a more complex reconstruction than simple inclusion into a proximal vessel, a bifurcated Dacron graft can be sewn onto the healthy distal descending thoracic aorta with a side-biting clamp in place to maintain antegrade flow to the reno-visceral vessels and lower extremities. Next, the distal anastomoses to the celiac and SMA can be completed sequentially so as to avoid any complete mesenteric ischemia time. With these anastomoses completed, the aorta can be cross-clamped distal to the bifurcate graft, maintaining antegrade perfusion to the celiac and SMA and effectively downstaging the operation to a juxtarenal reconstruction.

For more extensive aneurysms (I–III, V) distal aortic perfusion or in-line mesenteric shunting is necessary to avoid prolonged visceral ischemia. Passive perfusion via a temporary axillary-femoral bypass or active mechanical perfusion in the form of cardiopulmonary or left atrial-femoral bypass provide visceral perfusion via antegrade flow during sequential aortic clamping, or via antegrade flow from side-arm perfusion catheters. Deep hypothermic circulatory arrest mitigates the effects of visceral ischemia. While complete circulatory arrest without cerebral perfusion is poorly tolerated for periods longer than 30 minutes, corporeal arrest following completion of the proximal anastomosis (restoration of flow to the arch vessels) can be tolerated for up to 1.5 hours without significant clinical effect.

Passive in-line mesenteric shunting provides another visceral ischemia-mitigating adjunct in extensive aneurysm resection when distal aortic perfusion is not available or feasible (clamp-and-sew technique). This technique was first described in animal experiments by Cohen and colleagues.[52] At our institution, in-line mesenteric perfusion was previously described by Cambria et al.[53] A 10 mm Dacron side-arm graft is attached to the main aortic prosthesis distal to the planned proximal thoracic anastomosis and a 12-18F single stage venous cannula is attached to this with an intercept connector and sterile Zip Ties (Figure 20.7). Once the proximal aortic anastomosis is completed, the graft is clamped distal to the sidearm and the venous cannula is placed into the SMA or celiac ostium, immediately initiating passive shunting into the mesentery. Adequate perfusion through the shunt can be confirmed with Doppler and also by assessing backbleeding from the non-shunted visceral vessel. In addition, a reduction in systemic arterial pressure or an increase in end-tidal CO_2 is typically observed after initiation of in-line mesenteric perfusion.[53] The inclusion button can then be completed around the actively shunting catheter, which is removed before tying down the final suture and restoring mesenteric flow via the aortic graft. This technique reduces total visceral ischemia time to that necessary to complete the proximal aortic anastomosis. If individual bypasses are planned, then a bifurcated graft

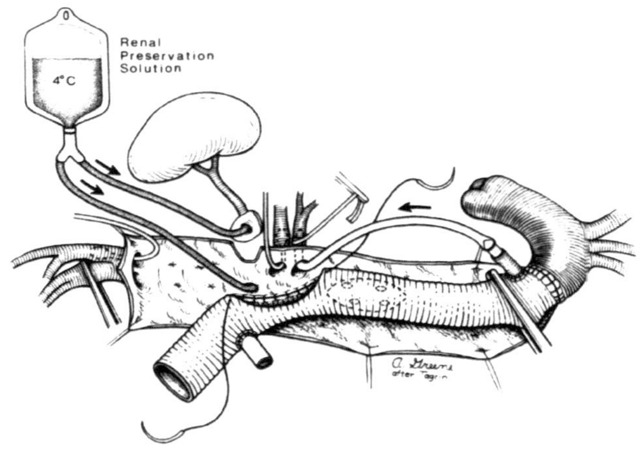

Figure 20.7 In-line mesenteric shunting during more extensive repair can be provided by a pre-sewn sidearm to the main aortic graft which is attached to a cannula inserted directly into the celiac or SMA ostium following completion of the proximal anastomosis. Direct trans-ostial administration of hypothermic renal preservation fluid is also depicted. (Conrad MF, Cambria RP. Contemporary management of descending thoracic and thoracoabdominal aortic aneurysms: endovascular versus open. *Circulation* 2008; 117:841-852.)

is employed in place of a single sidearm with the shunt attached to one of the limbs. Following completion of the proximal aortic anastomosis, shunting is again initiated through one of the limbs and the other limb is anastomosed to the non-shunted vessel. Once this anastomosis is complete, antegrade visceral perfusion is established through the graft and the shunt is removed to allow for completion of the remaining visceral anastomosis. In cases where backbleeding is poor, suggesting inadequate collateral flow, the second anastomosis can be completed around the shunt, which is again removed prior to tying down the final suture.

Late nonischemic GI complications associated with open TAAA repair arise primarily from graft-enteric fistulas and are associated with substantial morbidity and mortality.[54,55] Fortunately, with proper technique, the vast majority are preventable. Proximally, the thoracic aorta is intimately associated with the esophagus. This relationship becomes even more pronounced in the setting of aneurysmal degeneration, and the risk of fistula formation is further compounded by the lack of an esophageal serosal layer. As such, it is our practice to ensure proper intraoperative identification of the esophagus with either a nasogastric tube or transesophageal echo probe. As opposed to other anastomoses where a Creech technique may be employed, the thoracic aorta is always circumferentially transected and cleared of surrounding tissue to avoid inadvertent incorporation of the esophagus in the suture line. In addition, we routinely place either an NGT or a transesophageal probe to help us locate the esophagus during our thoracic dissection. When feasible, the aneurysm sac can be closed over the aorta; however, tremendous care should be taken to ensure that suture bites are well away from the esophagus itself. Similarly, in the abdomen, care should be taken to avoid inadvertent incorporation of the duodenum into an inclusion button or distal aortic anastomosis employing Creech technique. This is particularly important when the exposure is entirely extraperitoneal as the duodenum may not be clearly visualized in these situations and care should be taken to sweep the peritoneal sac off the back of the aorta prior to suturing. Aneurysmal aortic wall and retroperitoneal fat should be closed over the graft reconstruction when anatomically possible. In patients where there is insufficient tissue for coverage, we are very pro-active in fashioning a pedicled omental flap for coverage. The authors' standard approach is to mobilize the omentum off the transverse colon and stomach, taking care to preserve the gastro-epiploic arcade along the greater curvature of the stomach through the entire width of the flap. The left gastro-epiploic artery serves as the pedicle, and the entire flap can be tunneled through the back of the lesser sac, lateral to the tail of the pancreas and splenic hilum, which allows it to lay nicely in the retroperitoneum over the graft. Depending on the amount of omentum harvested, the flap can provide thoracic graft coverage as well, though care should be taken to avoid an excessively tight diaphragmatic crus and aortic hiatus reconstruction so as to avoid ischemia and congestion to the thoracic portion of the flap.

Renal

Acute renal failure contributes substantially to the morbidity and mortality after open TAAA repair.[56] Progression to dialysis-dependent renal failure has been reported in 1.5–10.7% of patients after an elective repair, with mortality approaching 25–40% for these patients.[57] Open TAAA reconstruction applies considerable physiologic stress to the kidneys in several ways, though the most salient driver of postoperative renal dysfunction is ischemia time.[58] Even during periods of presumably adequate perfusion, hypotension, either intra- or postoperative, as well as existing renal artery stenosis, blood product transfusion, and thromboembolic events may contribute to impaired renal function. Fortunately, even though acute kidney injury is common after supra-renal aortic clamping, most patients eventually regain function in the longer term postoperatively.[57]

Similar to the effects of regional epidural cooling historically performed for spinal cord protection, cooling the renal parenchyma reduces the rate of oxygen consumption and metabolic demands of the kidney. Koksoy et al. described a significantly lower incidence of renal morbidity in patients given renal cold solutions during their open TAAA, even showing superior results when compared with normothermic blood perfusion.[59] Wynn and Acher also showed substantial benefit with a 4° renal perfusion solution to induce profound renal hypothermia and demonstrated that extent of aneurysm was no longer a predictor of postoperative renal failure, even when employing a simple clamp-and-sew method in these patients.[57] Our renal cold solution involves a mixture of 4°C lactated Ringer's solution with mannitol (25 g/L) and methylprednisolone (1 g/L) directly into the renal arteries using a 12F single-stage venous cannula (Figure 20.7). An initial 300 cc bolus is given and can be followed with a continuous infusion via Pruitt perfusion catheter for more extensive and prolonged reconstructions.

Our preferred reconstruction technique for the renovisceral segment has been described in the previous sections. Notably, when sewing the inclusion button for extent II and III repair or the proximal bevel of an extent IV reconstruction, we temporarily "stent" the right renal ostium open by allowing the 12F renal cold cannula to remain in place as the suture line courses around. In 2005, we described trans-aortic stenting of the right renal artery with a Palmaz Blue™ 6 mm stent deployed directly into the right renal artery ostium in cases of pre-existing disease or when there was compromise/collapse of the orifice secondary to encroachment of the suture line (Figure 20.8).[60,61] The author has slightly modified this technique to utilize a 6 × 22 iCAST covered stent, which is deployed into the artery and then incorporated into the suture line of the main aortic graft. This modification has a theoretical benefit of addressing any aneurysmal degeneration at the renal ostium and should facilitate branch-fenestrated endografting that may be necessary in the long term if the visceral segment patch degenerates. In situations of unfavorable topology when incorporating the right renal artery would result in an unacceptable amount of residual aortic tissue, the vessel can be reconstructed via a separate inclusion button or bypass. Its posterolateral position, however, makes sidearm reconstruction particularly challenging. Previously, to address this, we employed a GORE® hybrid vascular graft with the expanded PTFE end sewn into the main aortic graft following deployment of the self-expanding stent into the vessel.[61] As these grafts have been discontinued, we now construct our own hybrid graft utilizing a GORE® Viabahn and ePTFE graft. The ePTFE graft is punctured several centimeters away from one end with a starter needle and wire. The wire is advanced into the renal artery. The GORE® Viabahn is advanced over the wire and is positioned with one half within the renal artery and one half within the ePTFE graft to bridge the gap and is then fully deployed. The Viabahn is sutured to the renal artery ostium with 6-0 prolene in four quadrants to secure it. The puncture site in the ePTFE is primary closed, and the free end of the graft is then pulled to length and sewn into the main aortic graft.

The left renal artery is almost always reconstructed via a separate bypass because of standard ostial topology (Figure 20.5). The authors' preference is to utilize a ringed ePTFE graft (8 mm whenever possible, 6 mm for smaller vessels). The pitfall of this bypass is the potential for

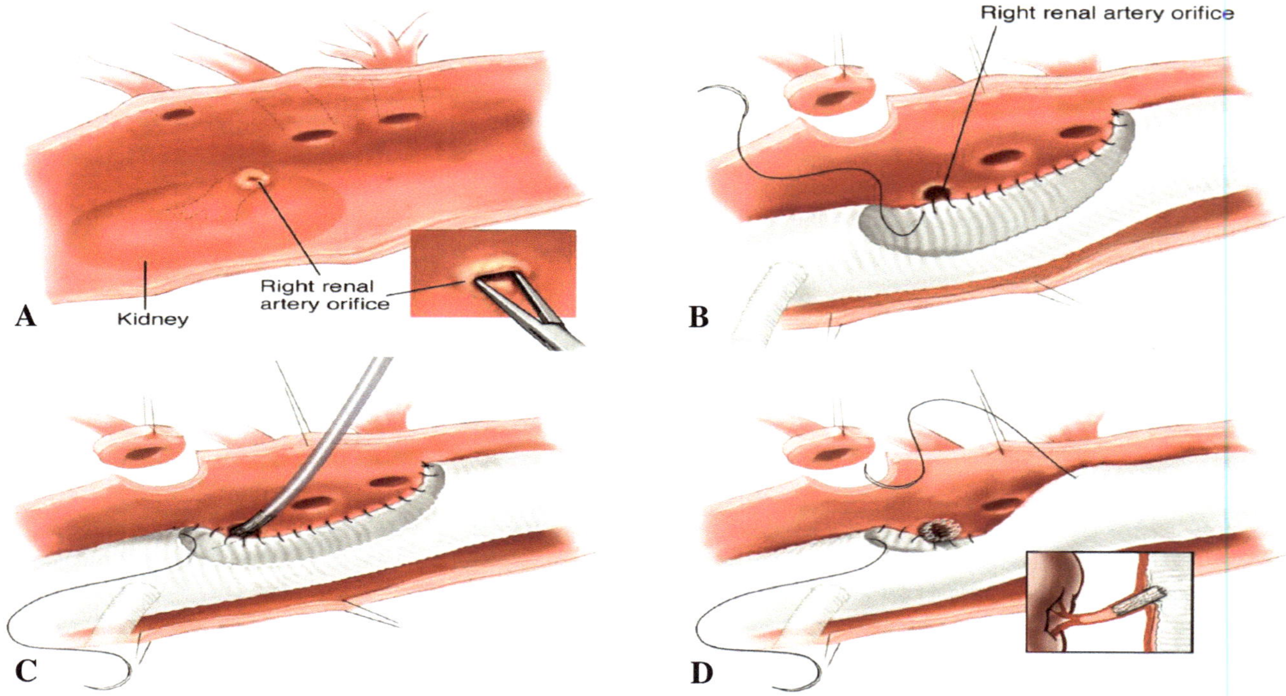

Figure 20.8 Steps in transaortic stenting of the right renal artery during en-bloc reconstruction of the renovisceral segment. (Patel R, Conrad MF, Paruchuri V, Kwolek CJ, Cambria RP. Balloon expandable stents facilitate right renal artery reconstruction during complex open aortic aneurysm repair. *J Vasc Surg* 2010;51(2):310-315.)

kinking of the graft when the kidney rests in its anatomical position. To circumvent this, the bypass graft is fashioned in either an extremely short or long length. Overall 5-year patency of the renal arteries were 96–97% regardless of the reconstructive technique used.[11] However, success also depends on employing adjunctive orificial endarterectomy and/or stenting to address intrinsic disease (reported between 15% and 45% in patients undergoing open TAAA repair) at the time of reconstruction.[11,62]

Assessment of urine output begins immediately following reconstruction. There is often a delay in urine production following large renal cold boluses as the kidney must rewarm before gaining function. Additionally, intraoperative compression of ureters by retractors may contribute to oligoanuria. Postoperatively, urine output is strictly monitored and helps guide resuscitative efforts. We aim for a urine output of at least 0.5–1 cc/kg/hr. If the patient is completely anuric (despite adequate resuscitation as measured by markers of perfusion) by the time of ICU arrival, there should be suspicion for renal artery reconstruction compromise or failure. An immediate bedside renal artery duplex confirming flow through the reconstruction or even pulsatile flow at the renal hilum alone can be reassuring. In equivocal cases, it is the author's preference to take an aggressive posture toward expedited evaluation and possible salvage with immediate angiography. In many cases, a kink or flow-limiting dissection beyond the distal anastomosis can be salvaged endovascularly. Open re-exploration is reserved for angiographically confirmed reconstruction failure that cannot be salvaged by endovascular means. If open revision is necessary, additional renal cold perfusate should be administered.

Hematologic

Patients undergoing open repairs of TAAA are prone to bleeding diathesis due to a number of factors. Large blood losses, insensible losses, massive transfusions resulting in dilutional coagulopathy as a result of inadequate factor/platelet transfusion and citrate toxicity, hypothermia, extracorporeal circulation, impaired liver synthetic function as a result of hepatic ischemia, acidemia, and systemic heparinization all contribute to this coagulopathy. A proactive approach to address anemia and thrombocytopenia during the case may lead to improved outcomes rather than reacting to laboratory values drawn during the case. It is our preference to resuscitate in a one-to-one-to-one manner (one unit packed cells, one six pack platelets, one unit fresh frozen (FF)) as described in the trauma literature, particularly in cases of substantial blood turnover. Again, active and ongoing discussion with the anesthesia team throughout the operation is imperative as the surgeon can report not only blood loss, but the quality of clot formation in the operative field when gaining hemostasis toward the end of the operation.

Patient body temperature must be considered throughout the operation. While mild permissive hypothermia is beneficial, care should be taken to avoid a run-away state where rewarming becomes incredibly challenging. This is particularly important during clamp-and-sew or passive shunting cases where the warmer from a mechanical circulatory support circuit is not available. In these cases, warmed blood transfusion with a Belmont device is very useful. An underbody Bair hugger in addition to raising the operative theater's room temperature can also help with a patient's hypothermia, though the Bair hugger must be turned off prior to cross clamping in order to avoid thermal burns if no distal perfusion is maintained. Finally, an eye toward appropriate calcium repletion is crucial as the citrate in stored blood will bind and reduce serum calcium levels, which are necessary for appropriate clotting factor function.

Postoperative bleeding may result in a return to the operating room, which is associated with additional morbidity and mortality.[63] First-line treatment in the ICU should be to achieve normothermia. We routinely initiate a fresh frozen plasma drip at 50 cc/hr for the first 12–24 hours postoperatively to assist with coagulopathy, particularly when there has been liver ischemia intraoperatively. Strict blood pressure control should be enforced to balance the risk of suture line bleeding with the risk of spinal cord and other end-organ ischemia which may contribute to ongoing acidemia and coagulopathy. The typical blood pressure goal is a MAP between 80–90 mmHg. A lower blood pressure goal can be tolerated in patients with evidence of bleeding or patients with connective tissue disorders, though our preference is a posture toward early and aggressive re-exploration for bleeding as prolonged postoperative hypotension may substantially increase the risk of spinal cord injury. In many cases, occult splenic injury resulting from the left medial visceral rotation is the culprit and necessitates rapid splenectomy. Cryoprecipitate consists of von Willebrand factor, factor VIII, factor XIII and fibrinogen.

From a coagulopathy standpoint, thrombelastography (TEG) is a useful adjunct to help guide resuscitative efforts. TEG is a rapid point-of-care test that measures the entire coagulation cascade. TEG can also be adjusted for temperature and can reveal the effect of hypothermia on a patient's coagulopathy. Overall, TEG has been shown to help guide management of coagulopathic bleeding and reduce the need for transfusions in the setting of TAAA,[64] but is not readily available at all institutions. It may also help guide an earlier return to surgical re-exploration if no identifiable coagulopathy is present in the setting of postoperative bleeding.

Infectious disease

The incidence of prosthetic aortic graft infections has been reported as 0.6–6%, with an associated mortality of 20–24%.[62,65–67] Most cases of open aortic graft infections occur within the initial postoperative period. The bulk of aortic graft infections are caused by gram-positive bacteria.[68] The primary effort of combating graft infections during open TAAA begins with sterile technique and perioperative antibiotics. Antibiotics are administered within one hour of skin incision. Meticulous attention is paid at the time of closure. Furthermore, close attention to postoperative wound care is conducted, particularly at the posterior aspect of the thoracoabdominal incision. This portion of the wound is typically covered to avoid constant abrasion from the patient's body against the bed. As noted in the GI section above, a late complication of open TAAA repair is enteric-graft fistulae, which often present with GI bleeding and/or symptoms of graft infection. A full discussion of the medical and surgical management techniques of these complex and highly morbid challenging conditions is beyond the scope of this chapter; however, ensuring inadvertent esophageal and small bowel injury during the operation, as well as appropriate soft tissue coverage of implanted grafts as described earlier, is of paramount importance.

REFERENCES

1. Patel VI, Lancaster RT, Conrad MF, Cambria RP. Open surgical repair of thoracoabdominal aneurysms - the Massachusetts General Hospital experience. Ann Cardiothorac Surg. 2012;1(3): 5.
2. Patel VI, Ergul E, Conrad MF, et al. Continued favorable results with open surgical repair of type IV thoracoabdominal aortic aneurysms. J Vasc Surg. 2011;53(6): 1492–1498. doi:10.1016/j.jvs.2011.01.070
3. Estrera AL, Sandhu HK, Charlton-Ouw KM, et al. A Quarter Century of Organ Protection in Open Thoracoabdominal Repair: Ann Surg. 2015;262(4): 660–668. doi:10.1097/SLA.0000000000001432
4. Kouchoukos NT, Kulik A, Castner CF. Outcomes after thoracoabdominal aortic aneurysm repair using hypothermic circulatory arrest. J Thorac Cardiovasc Surg. 2013;145(3): S139–S141. doi:10.1016/j.jtcvs.2012.11.077
5. Coselli JS, LeMaire SA, Preventza O, et al. Outcomes of 3309 thoracoabdominal aortic aneurysm repairs. J Thorac Cardiovasc Surg. 2016;151(5): 1323–1338. doi:10.1016/j.jtcvs.2015.12.050
6. Crawford ES. Thoraco-abdominal and abdominal aortic aneurysms involving renal, superior mesenteric, celiac arteries. Ann Surg. 1974;179(5): 763–772. doi:10.1097/00000658-197405000-00032
7. Lancaster RT, Conrad MF, Patel VI, Cambria MR, Ergul EA, Cambria RP. Further experience with distal aortic perfusion and motor-evoked potential monitoring in the management of extent I-III thoracoabdominal aortic anuerysms. J Vasc Surg. 2013;58(2): 283–290. doi:10.1016/j.jvs.2013.01.042

8. Safi HJ, Miller III CC, Yawn DH, et al. Impact of distal aortic and visceral perfusion on liver function during thoracoabdominal and descending thoracic aortic repair. J Vasc Surg. 1998;27(1): 145–153. doi:10.1016/S0741-5214(98)70301-5
9. Safi HJ, Miller III CC, Subramaniam MH, et al. Thoracic and thoracoabdominal aortic aneurysm repair using cardiopulmonary bypass, profound hypothermia, and circulatory arrest via left side of the chest incision. J Vasc Surg. 1998;28(4): 591–598. doi:10.1016/S0741-5214(98)70081-3
10. Mohebali J, Carvalho S, Lancaster RT, et al. Use of extracorporeal bypass is associated with improved outcomes in open thoracic and thoracoabdominal aortic aneurysm repair. J Vasc Surg. 2018;68(4): 941–947. doi:10.1016/j.jvs.2017.12.072
11. Mohebali J, Latz C, Cambria R, et al. The Long-term Fate of Renal and Visceral Vessel Reconstruction After Open Thoracoabdominal Aortic Aneurysm Repair. *Present Soc Vasc Surg Annu Meet June 2019 Prelim Accept Publ* J Vasc Surg. 2019.
12. Svensson LG, Crawford ES, Hess KR, Coselli JS, Safi HJ. Experience with 1509 patients undergoing thoracoabdominal aortic operations. J Vasc Surg. 1993;17(2): 357–368; discussion 368–370.
13. LeMaire SA, Miller CC, Conklin LD, Schmittling ZC, Coselli JS. Estimating group mortality and paraplegia rates after thoracoabdominal aortic aneurysm repair. Ann Thorac Surg. 2003;75(2): 508–513. doi:10.1016/s0003-4975(02)04347-3
14. Conrad MF, Crawford RS, Davison JK, Cambria RP. Thoracoabdominal Aneurysm Repair: A 20-Year Perspective. Ann Thorac Surg. 2007;83(2): S856–S861. doi:10.1016/j.athoracsur.2006.10.096
15. Wynn MM, Acher CW. A Modern Theory of Spinal Cord Ischemia/Injury in Thoracoabdominal Aortic Surgery and Its Implications for Prevention of Paralysis. J Cardiothorac Vasc Anesth. 2014;28(4): 1088–1099. doi:10.1053/j.jvca.2013.12.015
16. Khan NR, Smalley Z, Nesvick CL, Lee SL, Michael LM. The use of lumbar drains in preventing spinal cord injury following thoracoabdominal aortic aneurysm repair: An updated systematic review and meta-analysis. J Neurosurg Spine. 2016;25(3): 383–393. doi:10.3171/2016.1.SP INE151199
17. Melissano G, Bertoglio L, Rinaldi E, Leopardi M, Chiesa R. An anatomical review of spinal cord blood supply. J Cardiovasc Surg (Torino). 2015;56(5): 699–706.
18. Griepp RB, Griepp EB. Spinal cord perfusion and protection during descending thoracic and thoracoabdominal aortic surgery: The collateral network concept. Ann Thorac Surg. 2007;83(2): S865–869; discussion S890-892. doi:10.1016/j.athoracsur.2006.10.092
19. Backes WH, Nijenhuis RJ, Mess WH, Wilmink FA, Schurink GWH, Jacobs MJ. Magnetic resonance angiography of collateral blood supply to spinal cord in thoracic and thoracoabdominal aortic aneurysm patients. J Vasc Surg. 2008;48(2): 261–271. doi:10.1016/j.jvs.2008.03.015
20. Eagleton MJ, Shah S, Petkosevek D, Mastracci TM, Greenberg RK. Hypogastric and subclavian artery patency affects onset and recovery of spinal cord ischemia associated with aortic endografting. J Vasc Surg. 2014;59(1): 89–94. doi:10.1016/j.jvs.2013.07.007
21. Conrad MF, Ergul EA, Patel VI, et al. Evolution of operative strategies in open thoracoabdominal aneurysm repair. J Vasc Surg. 2011;53(5): 1195–1201.e1. doi:10.1016/j.jvs.2010.11.055
22. Safi HJ, Bartoli S, Hess KR, et al. Neurologic deficit in patients at high risk with thoracoabdominal aortic aneurysms: the role of cerebral spinal fluid drainage and distal aortic perfusion. J Vasc Surg. 1994;20(3): 434–444; discussion 442–443. doi:10.1016/0741-5214(94)90143-0
23. Safi HJ, Miller CC, Huynh TTT, et al. Distal aortic perfusion and cerebrospinal fluid drainage for thoracoabdominal and descending thoracic aortic repair: 10 years of organ protection. Ann Surg. 2003;238(3):372–380; discussion 380–381. doi:10.1097/01.sla.0000086664.90571.7a
24. Crawford S, Svensson G, Hess KR, et al. A prospective randomized study of cerebrospinal fluid drainage to prevent paraplegia after high-risk surgery on the thoracoabdominal aorta. 13(1):11.
25. Svensson LG, Hess KR, D'Agostino RS, et al. Reduction of neurologic injury after high-risk thoracoabdominal aortic operation. Ann Thorac Surg. 1998;66(1): 132–138. doi:10.1016/s0003-4975(98)00359-2
26. Coselli JS, LeMaire SA, Köksoy C, Schmittling ZC, Curling PE. Cerebrospinal fluid drainage reduces paraplegia after thoracoabdominal aortic aneurysm repair: Results of a randomized clinical trial. J Vasc Surg. 2002;35(4): 631–639. doi:10.1067/mva.2002.122024
27. Cinà CS, Abouzahr L, Arena GO, Laganà A, Devereaux PJ, Farrokhyar F. Cerebrospinal fluid drainage to prevent paraplegia during thoracic and thoracoabdominal aortic aneurysm surgery: A systematic review and meta-analysis. J Vasc Surg. 2004;40(1): 36–44. doi:10.1016/j.jvs.2004.03.017
28. Youngblood SC, Tolpin DA, LeMaire SA, Coselli JS, Lee V-V, Cooper JR. Complications of cerebrospinal fluid drainage after thoracic aortic surgery: A review of 504 patients over 5 years. J Thorac Cardiovasc Surg. 2013;146(1): 166–171. doi:10.1016/j.jtcvs.2013.01.041

29. Cambria RP, Davison JK, Carter C, et al. Epidural cooling for spinal cord protection during thoracoabdominal aneurysm repair: A 5-year experience. J Vasc Surg. 2000;31(6): 1093–1102. doi:10.1067/mva.2000.106492
30. Acher CW, Wynn MM, Mell MW, Tefera G, Hoch JR. A quantitative assessment of the impact of intercostal artery reimplantation on paralysis risk in thoracoabdominal aortic aneurysm repair. Ann Surg. 2008;248(4): 529–540. doi:10.1097/SLA.0b013e318187a792
31. Safi HJ, Miller CC, Carr C, Iliopoulos DC, Dorsay DA, Baldwin JC. Importance of intercostal artery reattachment during thoracoabdominal aortic aneurysm repair. J Vasc Surg. 1998;27(1): 58–66; discussion 66-68. doi:10.1016/s0741-5214(98)70292-7
32. Keyhani K, Miller CC, Estrera AL, Wegryn T, Sheinbaum R, Safi HJ. Analysis of motor and somatosensory evoked potentials during thoracic and thoracoabdominal aortic aneurysm repair. J Vasc Surg. 2009;49(1): 36–41. doi:10.1016/j.jvs.2008.08.005
33. Simon M, Borges L, Hart E, Grottkau BE, Peck M, Conrad MF. Intraoperative neurophysiologic monitoring and mapping of the spinal cord. In: Intraoperative Neurophysiology: A Comprehensive Guide to Monitoring and Mapping. Demos Medical; 2010: 177–266.
34. Estrera AL, Sheinbaum R, Miller CC, et al. Cerebrospinal Fluid Drainage During Thoracic Aortic Repair: Safety and Current Management. Ann Thorac Surg. 2009;88(1): 9–15. doi:10.1016/j.athoracsur.2009.03.039
35. Etz CD, Di Luozzo G, Bello R, et al. Pulmonary Complications After Descending Thoracic and Thoracoabdominal Aortic Aneurysm Repair: Predictors, Prevention, and Treatment. Ann Thorac Surg. 2007;83(2): S870–S876. doi:10.1016/j.athoracsur.2006.10.099
36. Smetana GW, Lawrence VA, Cornell JE, American College of Physicians. Preoperative pulmonary risk stratification for noncardiothoracic surgery: Systematic review for the American College of Physicians. Ann Intern Med. 2006;144(8): 581–595. doi:10.7326/0003-4819-144-8-200604180-00009
37. Cartin-Ceba R, Sprung J, Gajic O, Warner DO. The Aging Respiratory System: Anesthetic Strategies to Minimize Perioperative Pulmonary Complications. In: Silverstein JH, Rooke GA, Reves JG, McLeskey CH, eds. Geriatric Anesthesiology. Springer New York; 2008: 149–164. doi:10.1007/978-0-387-72527-7_11
38. Huynh TTT, Miller CC, Estrera AL, Sheinbaum R, Allen SJ, Safi HJ. Determinants of hospital length of stay after thoracoabdominal aortic aneurysm repair. J Vasc Surg. 2002;35(4): 648–653. doi:10.1067/mva.2002.121566
39. Engle J, Safi HJ, Miller CC, et al. The impact of diaphragm management on prolonged ventilator support after thoracoabdominal aortic repair. J Vasc Surg. 1999;29(1): 150–156. doi:10.1016/s0741-5214(99)70356-3
40. Wong DR, Parenti JL, Green SY, et al. Open repair of thoracoabdominal aortic aneurysm in the modern surgical era: Contemporary outcomes in 509 patients. J Am Coll Surg. 2011;212(4): 569–579; discussion 579-581. doi:10.1016/j.jamcollsurg.2010.12.041
41. Endicott KM, Emerson D, Amdur R, Macsata R. Functional status as a predictor of outcomes in open and endovascular abdominal aortic aneurysm repair. J Vasc Surg. 2017;65(1): 40–45. doi:10.1016/j.jvs.2016.05.079
42. Crawford ES, Crawford JL, Safi HJ, et al. Thoracoabdominal aortic aneurysms: Preoperative and intraoperative factors determining immediate and long-term results of operations in 605 patients. J Vasc Surg. 1986;3(3): 389–404. doi:10.1067/mva.1986.avs0030389
43. Kahn RA, Stone ME, Moskowitz DM. Anesthetic consideration for descending thoracic aortic aneurysm repair. Semin Cardiothorac Vasc Anesth. 2007;11(3): 205–223. doi:10.1177/1089253207306098
44. Schepens M, Dossche K, Morshuis W, et al. Introduction of adjuncts and their influence on changing results in 402 consecutive thoracoabdominal aortic aneurysm repairs. Eur J Cardio-Thorac Surg. 2004;25(5): 701–707. doi:10.1016/j.ejcts.2004.01.033
45. Coselli JS, LeMaire SA. Left heart bypass reduces paraplegia rates after thoracoabdominal aortic aneurysm repair. Ann Thorac Surg. 1999;67(6): 1931–1934. doi:10.1016/S0003-4975(99)00390-2
46. Kulik A, Castner CF, Kouchoukos NT. Outcomes after thoracoabdominal aortic aneurysm repair with hypothermic circulatory arrest. J Thorac Cardiovasc Surg. 2011;141(4): 953–960. doi:10.1016/j.jtcvs.2010.06.010
47. Achouh PE, Madsen K, Miller CC, et al. Gastrointestinal complications after descending thoracic and thoracoabdominal aortic repairs: A 14-year experience. J Vasc Surg. 2006;44(3): 442–446. doi:10.1016/j.jvs.2006.05.018
48. Abboud B, Daher R, Boujaoude J. Acute mesenteric ischemia after cardio-pulmonary bypass surgery. World J Gastroenterol. 2008;14(35): 5361. doi:10.3748/wjg.14.5361
49. Cohen JR, Angus L, Asher A, Chang JB, Wise L. Disseminated intravascular coagulation as a result of supraceliac clamping: Implications for thoracoabdominal aneurysm repair. Ann Vasc Surg. 1987;1(5): 552–557. doi:10.1016/S0890-5096(06)61439-8

50. Gertler JP, Cambria RP, Brewster DC, et al. Coagulation changes during thoracoabdominal aneurysm repair. J Vasc Surg. 1996;24(6): 936–943; discussion 943–945. doi:10.1016/s0741-5214(96)70039-3
51. Illig KA, Green RM, Ouriel K, et al. Primary fibrinolysis during supraceliac aortic clamping. J Vasc Surg. 1997;25(2): 244–251; discussion 252–254. doi:10.1016/s0741-5214(97)70346-x
52. Cohen JR, Schroder W, Leal J, Wise L. Mesenteric shunting during thoracoabdominal aortic clamping to prevent disseminated intravascular coagulation in dogs. Ann Vasc Surg. 1988;2(3): 261–267. doi:10.1016/S0890-5096(07)60012-0
53. Cambria RP, Davison JK, Giglia JS, Gertler JP. Mesenteric shunting decreases visceral ischemia during thoracoabdominal aneurysm repair. J Vasc Surg. 1998;27(4): 745–749. doi:10.1016/S0741-5214(98)70242-3
54. Schoell T, Manceau G, Chiche L, et al. Surgery for secondary aorto-enteric fistula or erosion (SAEFE) complicating aortic graft replacement: a retrospective analysis of 32 patients with particular focus on digestive management. World J Surg. 2015;39(1): 283–291. doi:10.1007/s00268-014-2750-5
55. Baril DT, Carroccio A, Ellozy SH, et al. Evolving strategies for the treatment of aortoenteric fistulas. J Vasc Surg. 2006;44(2): 250–257. doi:10.1016/j.jvs.2006.04.031
56. Patel VI, Lancaster RT, Ergul E, et al. Postoperative renal dysfunction independently predicts late mortality in patients undergoing aortic reconstruction. J Vasc Surg. 2015;62(6): 1405–1412. doi:10.1016/j.jvs.2015.07.084
57. Wynn MM, Acher C, Marks E, Engelbert T, Acher CW. Postoperative renal failure in thoracoabdominal aortic aneurysm repair with simple cross-clamp technique and 4°C renal perfusion. J Vasc Surg. 2015;61(3): 611–622. doi:10.1016/j.jvs.2014.10.040
58. Kudo FA, Nishibe T, Miyazaki K, et al. Postoperative renal function after elective abdominal aortic aneurysm repair requiring suprarenal aortic cross-clamping. Surg Today. 2004;34(12): 1010–1013. doi:10.1007/s00595-004-2871-9
59. Köksoy C, LeMaire SA, Curling PE, et al. Renal perfusion during thoracoabdominal aortic operations: cold crystalloid is superior to normothermic blood. Ann Thorac Surg. 2002;73(3): 730–738. doi:10.1016/s0003-4975(01)03575-5
60. Patel R, Conrad MF, Paruchuri V, Kwolek CJ, Cambria RP. Balloon expandable stents facilitate right renal artery reconstruction during complex open aortic aneurysm repair. J Vasc Surg. 2010;51(2): 310–315. doi:10.1016/j.jvs.2009.04.079
61. Setacci F, Pecoraro F, Chaykovska L, et al. The Gore Hybrid Vascular Graft in renovisceral debranching for complex aortic aneurysm repair. J Vasc Surg. 2016;64(1): 33–38. doi:10.1016/j.jvs.2015.12.059
62. Clouse WD, Marone LK, Davison JK, et al. Late aortic and graft-related events after thoracoabdominal aneurysm repair. J Vasc Surg. 2003;37(2): 254–261. doi:10.1067/mva.2003.62
63. Cinà CS, Clase CM. Coagulation disorders and blood product use in patients undergoing thoracoabdominal aortic aneurysm repair. Transfus Med Rev. 2005;19(2): 143–154. doi:10.1016/j.tmrv.2004.11.003
64. Rahe-Meyer N, Solomon C, Winterhalter M, et al. Thromboelastometry-guided administration of fibrinogen concentrate for the treatment of excessive intraoperative bleeding in thoracoabdominal aortic aneurysm surgery. J Thorac Cardiovasc Surg. 2009;138(3): 694–702. doi:10.1016/j.jtcvs.2008.11.065
65. O'Connor S, Andrew P, Batt M, Becquemin JP. A systematic review and meta-analysis of treatments for aortic graft infection. J Vasc Surg. 2006;44(1): 38–45. doi:10.1016/j.jvs.2006.02.053
66. Kieffer E, Sabatier J, Plissonnier D, Knosalla C. Prosthetic graft infection after descending thoracic/thoracoabdominal aortic aneurysmectomy: management with in situ arterial allografts. J Vasc Surg. 2001;33(4): 671–678. doi:10.1067/mva.2001.112314
67. Vogel TR, Symons R, Flum DR. The incidence and factors associated with graft infection after aortic aneurysm repair. J Vasc Surg. 2008;47(2): 264–269. doi:10.1016/j.jvs.2007.10.030
68. Hodgkiss-Harlow KD, Bandyk DF. Antibiotic Therapy of Aortic Graft Infection: Treatment and Prevention Recommendations. Semin Vasc Surg. 2011;24(4): 191–198. doi:10.1053/j.semvascsurg.2011.10.013

21

Complications of open repair of juxtarenal aortic aneurysm

MARK F. CONRAD

Abdominal aortic aneurysms (AAA) develop through a complex process involving a combination of genetic and environmental factors. Approximately 80% are degenerative, 15–20% are secondary to chronic dissection and the remaining have other etiologies such as infection or aortitis. The classification of abdominal aortic aneurysms is based upon their proximity to the renal arteries and the location of the clamp site required for repair. A true juxtarenal abdominal aortic aneurysm (JAAA) begins at or above the lowest renal artery and can extend up to the level of the superior mesenteric artery (SMA), but the aortic diameter is normal at the level of the celiac artery. Open repair of a JAAA will require clamping above at least one renal artery with resultant ischemia to one or both kidneys during creation of the proximal anastomosis. JAAA make up approximately 15% of all AAA.[1] A type IV thoracoabdominal aneurysm (TAAA) is more extensive with an upper limit at the crus of the diaphragm. Repair of these aneurysms requires a supraceliac clamp and graft reconstruction itself extends to the celiac axis. This chapter will focus on the open repair of JAAA.

The critical concern with JAA is rupture, which has traditionally been associated with a high mortality. A recent review of the Medicare population showed that the annual rupture rate in 2008 was half that of 1995 and the operative mortality decreased from 44% to 36%.[2] The strongest predictor of rupture is aneurysm size. Natural history studies have shown that the risk of rupture is negligible in JAAA less than 5 cm, equivalent to the risks associated with open surgery in the 5–6 cm range, and, increases substantially when the diameter exceeds 6 cm and/or the rate of interval growth is ≥10 mm per year. These findings are true in men, but women have been shown to have a four-fold increase in the risk of rupture at a given size compared to men.[3] These observations have led to the acceptance of 6.0 cm for men and 5.5 cm for women as a generally appropriate size threshold for recommendation of surgical intervention for JAAA and symptomatic aneurysms should be repaired emergently regardless of size.[4] Other risk factors for rupture include increasing patient age, female gender, pain (including atypical pain), a history of chronic obstructive pulmonary disease (COPD), symptoms attributable to the aneurysm, and dissection developing within a degenerative aneurysm.

PREOPERATIVE PLANNING

MEDICAL EVALUATION

The 5-year survival after open JAAA repair is 70% even at centers of excellence with low perioperative mortality.[5] Patient selection for open repair of JAAA is predicated upon weighing the likelihood of aneurysm rupture against the risk of surgery as conferred by the patient's medical history and active comorbidities. An accurate assessment of associated comorbid conditions is mandatory to guide appropriate decision making with respect to recommending open surgical repair. Patients with active cardiac disease, capacity-limiting COPD, and renal failure are at highest risk for postoperative complications and death after open JAAA repair, and long-term mortality in this cohort of patients is driven by cardiovascular and pulmonary disease regardless of the method of repair. The patient's functional capacity should be determined, and SVS guidelines recommend that anyone who is not capable of moderate activity (MET < 4) should undergo noninvasive stress testing with dipyridamole thallium scanning or the equivalent thereof to assess perioperative myocardial ischemic potential.[6] In addition, all patients should have a 12-lead ECG within 30 days of surgery, and patients with a history of symptoms suggestive of heart failure should have an assessment of left ventricular function. Because smoking is a major driver of aneurysm growth, it is common for patients to have pulmonary issues; it is estimated that 7–13% of patients with a treatable JAAA will have COPD.[4,5] Indeed, the severity of the COPD and ability to optimize pulmonary functional capacity prior to surgery predicts perioperative outcomes.[6] Therefore, when significant impairments of pulmonary reserve are expected, the patient should undergo preoperative pulmonary function studies and consult with a pulmonologist for optimization of medical therapy. Patients with preoperative renal insufficiency do poorly after open JAAA repair. Recent studies have shown that if the eGFR is < 30 mL/min or the patient is on dialysis, the 30-day mortality is over 10% and 2-year survival is only 33%.[7] This significantly changes the risk–benefit ratio of open repair and is an important factor to consider in patient selection. For patients with mild disease, strategies such as preoperative hydration and holding ACE inhibitors and angiotensin receptor antagonists on the day of surgery have been shown to reduce hypotension during the procedure that could promote acute kidney injury during the postoperative period.[8] Finally, advanced age is an important component only in as much as it is accompanied by overall fragility and impaired functional status, which have both been shown to predict mortality. However, functional age is more important than stated age and we have successfully treated patients in their late 90's with open JAAA repair.

IMAGING

Associated vascular diseases and comorbid conditions are commonplace in patients presenting for treatment of JAAA. Synchronous aneurysms typically involving the descending thoracic aorta have been observed in 10–30% of patients being evaluated for JAAA and are more common in women.[9,10] Therefore all patients should undergo baseline cross-sectional imaging of the chest, abdominal, and pelvic aorta at the time of initial diagnosis. In contemporary practice, a dynamic, fine-cut, contrast-enhanced CT scan with or without helical reconstruction is the preferred imaging modality and provides (1) accurate assessment of aneurysm size and extent, (2) a baseline study to which future images may be compared, and (3) Important anatomic information such as the anatomy and topography of the visceral segment, relationship of the left renal vein to the aorta (anterior or posterior), the presence of thrombus and atherosclerosis, and appropriate areas for clamping. Other abnormalities such as the horseshoe or pelvic kidney, duplicated or left-sided IVC and inflammatory aneurysms can also be identified with CTA (Figure 21.1).

Accurate assessment of the size of JAAA is contingent upon measurement in the appropriate perpendicular plane. Three-dimensional reconstruction of the abdominal and visceral aorta with determination of the centerline of flow ensures that any cross-sectional measurement will be perpendicular to the aortic axis. The quality of current CT scanners with three-dimensional reconstruction is exceptional; in our practice, this has become the image modality of choice for the evaluation and treatment of JAAA.

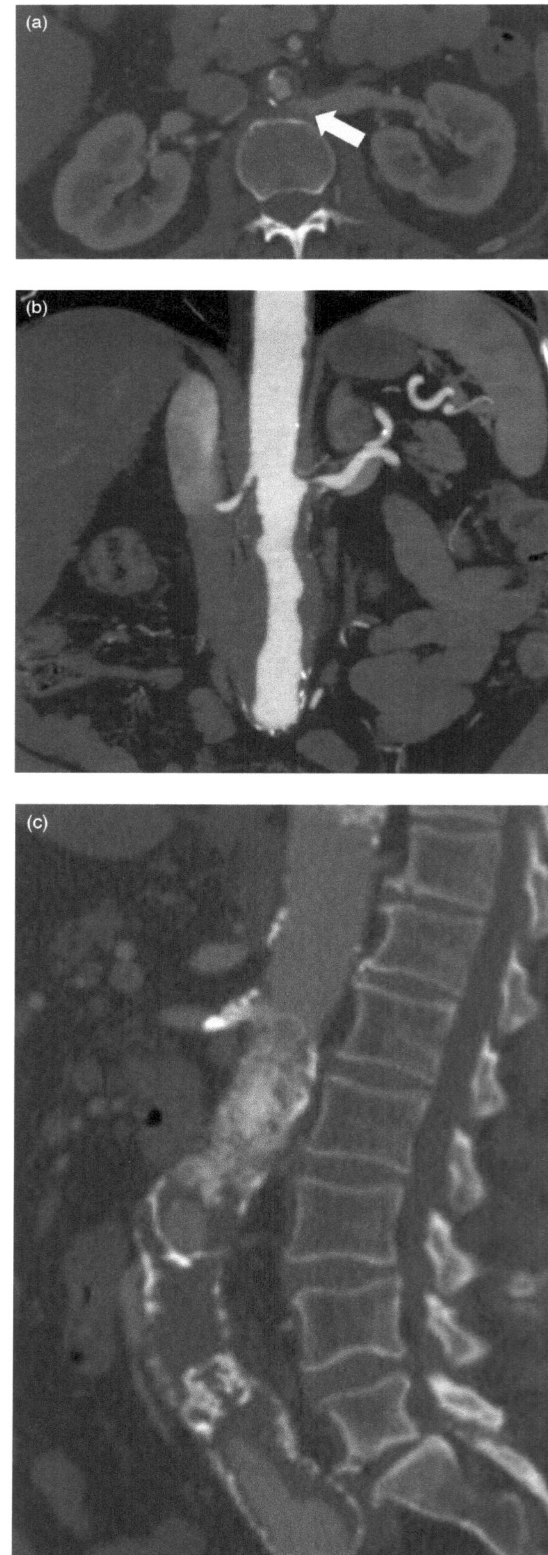

Figure 21.1 (a) CTA showing retroaortic renal vein (arrow). (b) Three dimensional reconstruction of renal arteries with thrombus extending to the level of the renal arteries. (c) CT reconstruction showing highly calcified visceral segment that would lead to clamping above the celiac artery.

SURGERY

OPERATIVE APPROACH

All open aortic surgery should be performed under general anesthesia. It is preferable for the anesthesia team to evaluate the patient prior to the day of surgery, so that appropriate time for developing an anesthetic plan, lines, and other means of hemodynamic monitoring is allowed. The use of an epidural for pain control in the postoperative period is useful. In addition, arrangements should be made for autotransfusion given the unavoidable amount of intraoperative blood loss.

The juxtarenal aorta can be approached from a trans-peritoneal or retroperitoneal incision (Figure 21.2). The benefits of the trans-peritoneal approach include easy access to iliac artery aneurysms, a universal familiarity among surgeons, and shorter times to achieving proximal control of the aorta. However, it is less ideal for patients who have had previous abdominal surgery, have a horseshoe kidney or known inflammatory aneurysm. In addition, the presence of the upper abdominal organs can limit access to the superior visceral segment of the aorta. A left retroperitoneal incision provides easy access to even the supra-celiac aorta and is preferred for patients who are obese, have had prior surgery, or require a high clamp site. However, access to the right renal and common iliac arteries can be challenging with this approach, and these patients are better approached from the front. A recent comparison of the two approaches to open AAA repair in the National Surgical Quality Improvement Program (NSQIP) found no difference in 30-day outcomes on multivariable analysis.[11]

TRANS-PERITONEAL APPROACH

The patient is positioned supine on a standard operating room table with both arms extended. The area from the nipple line to mid thighs should be included in the prep

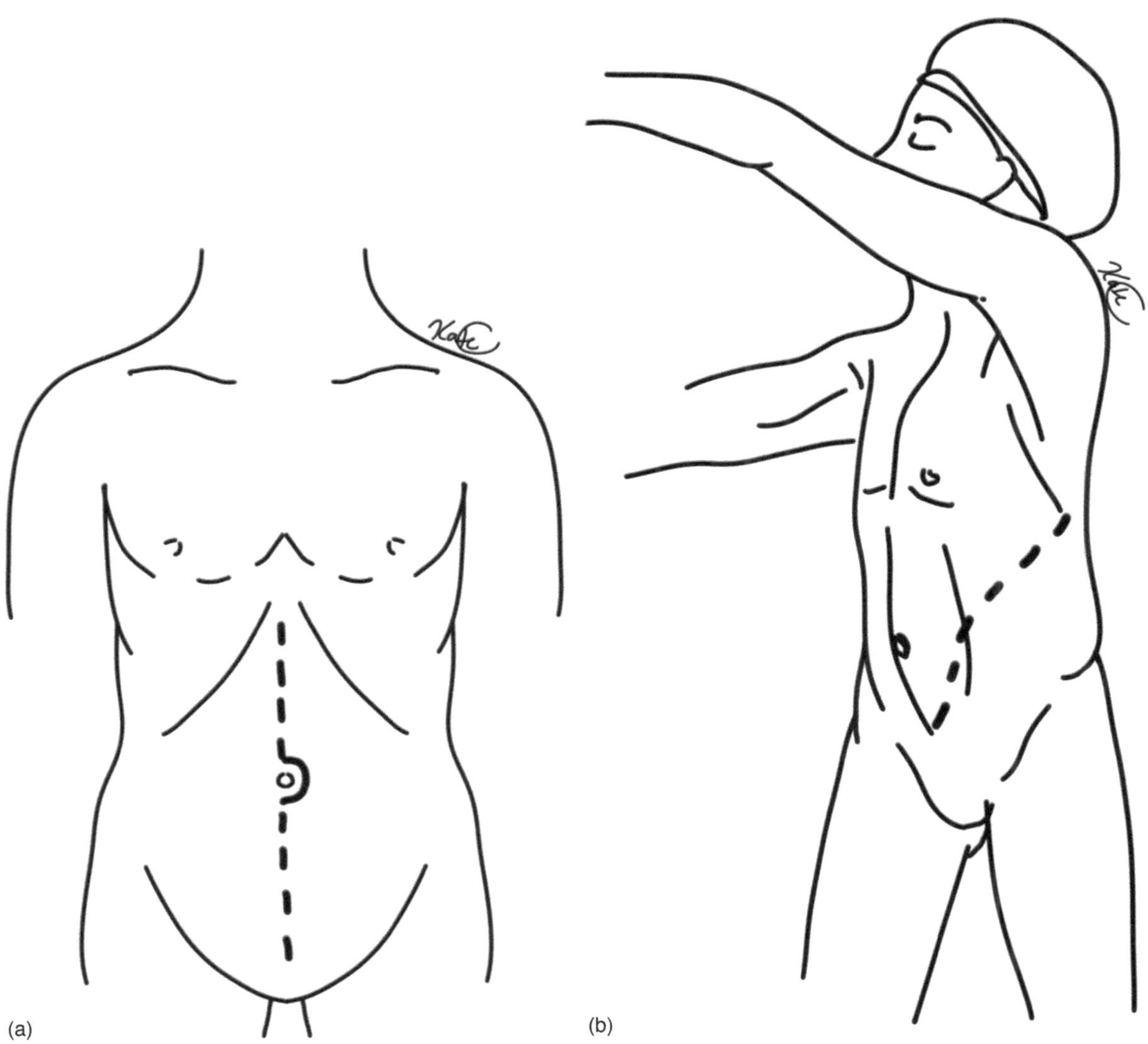

Figure 21.2 (a) Incision for transperitoneal approach to the aorta. (b) Incision for retroperitoneal approach to the aorta.

field, to allow exposure for a high incision, as well as the groins should access to the femoral vessels be needed. The hair is clipped and a towel is placed over the perineum. Any previous incisions within the prep field are marked. A Steri drape or Ioban is used to secure the drapes in position. Once in position, check PVRs and/or distal pulses for reference after the repair is complete.

A generous midline incision from the xiphoid to the pubis is made and dissected until the peritoneal cavity is entered. It may be necessary to extend the incision cephalad lateral alongside the xiphoid if higher exposure is needed or in emergent situations such as a rupture where immediate supraceliac control is needed. A self-retaining retractor system should then be positioned. We prefer the Omni retractor as the open configuration of the system does not limit the width of exposure. The greater omentum and transverse colon are brought cephalad and packed away in a moistened towel or lap pad on top of the patient's chest. The small bowel should be retracted to the right and packed within a separate moistened towel. The small bowel is gently placed behind a self-retaining retractor, taking care not to compromise the SMA. This exposes the ligament of Treitz, which can be divided along the jejunum to the level of the aorta. Reposition the retractor to allow as much small bowel to be out of the field as possible, and take down the ligament of Treitz with electrocautery, taking care not to injure the bowel. The inferior mesenteric vein is identified and ligated during this dissection. This allows access to the infrarenal aorta, where the overlying retroperitoneal tissue can be dissected free. Depending on how much aorta is needed for an adequate cuff of the proximal anastomosis, an anterior renal vein may need to be mobilized cephalad, with ligation of the gonadal and/or adrenal vein for better exposure.

The supraceliac aorta can be exposed from the transperitoneal approach. The left lobe of the liver is retracted laterally by taking down the triangular ligament. Next, the gastrohepatic ligament is divided and the gastroesophageal junction is exposed. This can be accomplished expeditiously by palpating for the nasogastric tube and applying caudal traction. Division of the gastrohepatic ligament must be done with the thought that a replaced left hepatic artery may be coursing beneath this structure. The esophagus can be retracted to the patient's left, and this maneuver will expose the aorta. An aortic compressor can be used in extreme circumstances; however dissection of the aorta circumferentially and surrounding the aorta with a shoestring if the patient's condition allows is preferable. This exposure, while useful when urgent supraceliac control is needed, will not allow access to the visceral segment of the aorta. In order to gain this exposure, a right or left medial visceral rotation should be incorporated into the dissection. The use of a right medial visceral rotation will allow access to the right renal artery, as well as placing the SMA on 90 degree tension and is useful for clearing a clamp site in those patients with a juxtarenal aneurysm who have very little room between

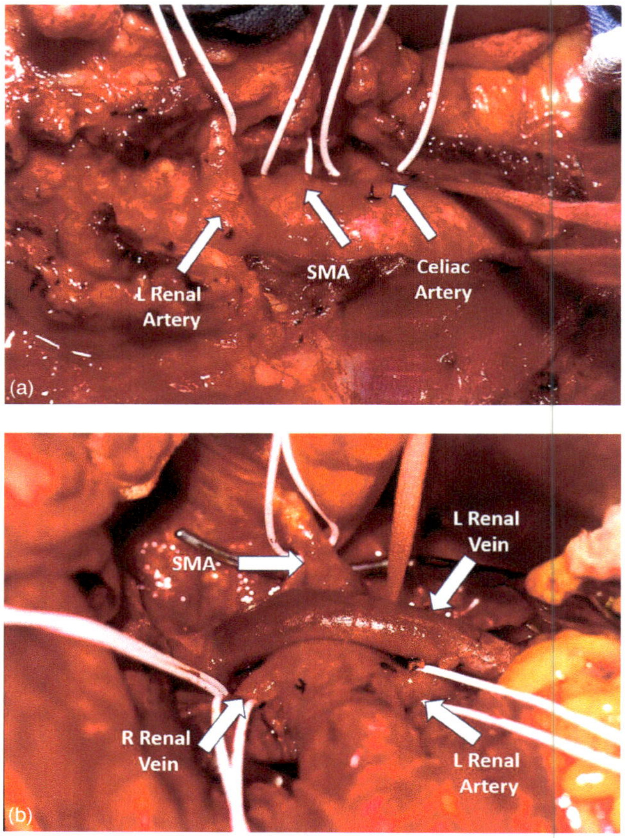

Figure 21.3 (a) Retroperitoneal exposure of the aorta. The left kidney is up, and the left renal artery is visible. The origin of the SMA and celiac arteries are easily exposed here by dividing the crus of the diaphragm. (b) Anterior exposure of the aorta. The left renal vein is mobilized and the SMA is exposed just superior to the left renal vein.

the renals and SMA. The use of a left medial visceral rotation also allows for exposure to the entire visceral segment of the aorta, as well as the left renal artery. Care in this approach must be made to avoid injury to the spleen and tail of the pancreas (Figure 21.3).

RETROPERITONEAL APPROACH

The patient is positioned in the lateral position with the left side up at an approximately 60 degree angle. Extend the right arm on an arm board, being sure to leave room for an Omni or other self-retaining retractor post. The upper, left arm should be placed on another arm board and padded to prevent neural injury. The bed should be flexed at the patient's flank to open up the area between the ribs and the anterior superior iliac spine. Position the legs so that the lower leg is straight and the upper leg is bent. Use two pillows as padding between legs. A bean bag can be inflated to keep the patient in place, and use thick cloth tape over the hip to secure the patient on his/her side. Ideally the patient should be placed on a bean bag, however blanket rolls can be used anteriorly and posteriorly to further secure the patient. Be sure to allow access to prep from the spine posteriorly to the umbilicus anteriorly, and from the nipple line to the groins. All bony prominences and pressure points should be well padded to avoid injury. Use clippers to remove hair within the prep area. Prep from the axilla and nipple line to the upper thigh. Mark all previous incisions and use a Steri drape or Ioban over the entire prepped area to secure the drapes. Once in position, check (pulse volume recordings) PVRs and/or distal pulses.

If the clamp position is at the SMA or just above the celiac trunk, a 9th (over the 10th rib) interspace retroperitoneal incision will provide adequate exposure. Carry the incision from the posterior axillary line to the anterior border of the rectus. Divide the transversalis fascia and enter the retroperitoneal space down to but not violating Gerota's fascia. It is possible to stay entirely within a retroperitoneal plane; however, if the peritoneum is violated, the abdominal contents can be packed away with retractors or the peritoneum can be repaired with a running 3-0 running chromic suture. The aorta may be approached via an anterorenal (colloquially referred to as "leaving the kidney down") or retrorenal plane ("taking the kidney up"). Generally, the aorta is approached via a retrorenal approach unless there is a renal vein running posterior to the aorta. As the retroperitoneal dissection continues, the left ureter should be identified and swept toward the midline and placed behind a retractor to avoid injury during dissection of the aorta. The renal artery is identified and dissected back to its origin to identify the aorta.

The renal artery should be cephalad to the vein, and once this is identified it can be used as a landmark and dissected back to the aorta. The renal lumbar vein should be identified and ligated to avoid injury and excessive bleeding. Once the origin of the renal artery is identified, a right angle can be placed along the surface of the aorta and the overlying retroperitoneal tissue divided with electrocautery. It is imperative here to get on the aorta and stay on the aorta to avoid excessive bleeding from the retroperitoneal tissue. The aorta is exposed to the bifurcation and can be dissected circumferentially here if a clamp site is planned, however, the left iliac vein can course posterior to the bifurcation and should be avoided. It is often easier to expose an area of the left common iliac artery for clamping and control the right common iliac artery with an occlusion balloon from within. It is unwise to gain circumferential control of the iliacs in this situation as the iliac veins are often adherent to the posterior aspect of the artery and are easily injured, leading to rapid exsanguinating blood loss. Identify and isolate the IMA with a vessel loop. Pay particular attention to identifying and not injuring the ureters, which will eventually cross anterior to the iliac vessels. If necessary and if the incision is placed along a higher rib space, the dissection can be carried caudal to expose the entire visceral segment (Figure 21.3).

ANEURYSM REPAIR

A proximal clamp site should be chosen based upon axial imaging that allows adequate room for aneurysm repair while minimizing ischemia to the visceral segment of the aorta. A review of the National Surgical Quality Improvement Program (NSQIP) database showed that the mortality and incidence of postoperative renal dysfunction was significantly higher with supraceliac clamping when compared to supra-renal clamp placement.[12] Once the clamp is placed, the aorta is opened and bleeding lumbar arteries are ligated. With the aorta open, the proximal extent of the aneurysm can be identified as a ring of normal tissue at the top of the aneurysm. The traditional teaching has been to remove all aneurysmal tissue to prevent anastomotic degeneration over time. However, in cases where the aneurysm ends at the level of the renal arteries, a plication technique has been advocated.

Removal of all aneurysm tissue in a JAAA repair requires a beveled anastomosis with bypass to the left renal artery. The aortic prosthesis is prepared by attaching a 6 mm polytetrafluoroethylene (PTFE) side-arm graft that will serve as the conduit for left renal artery reconstruction. For most aneurysms, a Dacron graft is the preferred conduit because it handles well and is easy to suture. However, a PTFE conduit can be used to repair mycotic aneurysms because of its decreased susceptibility to infection. At this point, the surgeon begins the clamping sequence in close cooperation with the anesthesiologist. The left renal artery is ligated and transected. The renal cold solution (approximately 300 cc of a mixture of normal saline with 19 g mannitol and 500 mg of methylprednisolone per liter at 4°C) is then injected into the artery using a soft catheter, and the continuous renal cold drip is started. The suture line of the beveled graft is begun at the level of the right renal artery and the back wall is completed first. It is important to take full-thickness bites of the aorta here to avoid bleeding when the clamp is removed. As the posterior aspect of this suture line continues around the inferior border of the right renal artery, we exchange the 6F perfusion catheter for a 12F perfusion catheter to temporarily stent the origin of the right renal artery. The catheter is gently agitated up and down as the suture line moves around the renal artery orifice to ensure that it is not compromised by generous suture bites as they pass outside of the aorta. Recently, we have used a 6 × 15 or 6 × 18 balloon-expandable stent to ensure that the suture line does not compromise right renal artery flow. The stent is placed under direct vision after the proximal suture line is beyond the orifice of the artery. Just prior to completing the suture line, a single flush of the proximal aortic cross-clamp is performed in order to ensure that no clot or debris has built up above the clamp. Reconstruction of the left renal artery is now accomplished with a separate side-arm graft of 6 mm PTFE. This provides a direct deliberate anastomosis in end-to-end fashion while allowing flexibility to deal with

(a) (b)

Figure 21.4 (a) Plicated aneurysm cuff technique, in which the aneurysm cuff is plicated on itself and cuff is sewn to the graft up to the level of the renal arteries. (b) Beveled anastomosis with left renal artery bypass technique, in which a beveled anastomosis incorporating the right renal artery origin is used with subsequent left real artery bypass.

the spectrum of occlusive lesions, multiple renal arteries, and other wrinkles that may be encountered. It is important to orient this side-arm graft so that it will not kink when the left renal artery is returned to its anatomic position. Some surgeons advocate the use of a single inclusion button that contains the renal arteries and the visceral vessels. This often requires the inclusion of too great an area of the native, aneurysmal aorta, unless the aneurysm is small in the visceral artery segment. A single, pristine left renal artery and orifice may be directly reimplanted and the clamp is then advanced to a position inferior to the origin of the left renal artery graft prior to completing the distal aortic anastomosis (Figure 21.4).

The plication technique does not involve a bypass to the left renal artery. After clamping, the aneurysm is opened and lumbar arteries are ligated as in the previous description. The proximal aneurysm is tied off, leaving a small cuff of aneurysm to sew to. The anastomosis is created in an endoaneurysmal or Creech fashion where the suture passes through the aortic wall twice so that the aneurysmal wall folds on itself, thus creating a native tissue pledget ring. This can be accomplished with interrupted or continuous sutures as necessary (Figure 21.4). In a recent comparison of both anastomotic techniques, there was no difference in mortality or anastomotic aneurysmal degeneration at 5 years.[13]

We make every effort to perform tube type of reconstructions to the aortic bifurcation unless there is gross aneurysmal disease of the proximal common iliac arteries. After reestablishment of flow to the lower extremities and verification of adequate lower extremity perfusion by intraoperative pulse volume recordings, Doppler signals in the left renal, celiac, and superior mesenteric vessels are checked in addition to palpation of the superior mesenteric artery pulse in the root of the mesentery. Careful inspection of the inferior aspect of the aneurysm sac is necessary to detect backbleeding lumbar vessels, which can be a source of significant postoperative hemorrhage.

The redundant aneurysm sac is then sutured securely over the aortic graft. The left kidney is returned to its anatomic position and perinephric fat suffices to provide adequate coverage of the aortic graft in the region of the visceral aortic segment. Prior to closure, renal artery reconstructions are interrogated one final time.

PROCEDURE-RELATED COMPLICATIONS

MORTALITY

The operative mortality after open JAAA is similar to infra-renal repair at high-volume centers. A review of our experience showed that the 30-day mortality was 2.5%.[14] This is in line with two meta-analyses of the literature that reported a mortality in the range of 2.0–4.0%.[1,15] The main predictors of poor outcomes in the perioperative setting include steroid use and baseline renal insufficiency, but several series have shown no predictors in multivariate models.[1,14,16] Long-term survival after JAAA repair has not been well described but in our experience, it is similar to patients who undergo infra-renal AAA repair. In our most recent series of 200 patients, the 5-year actuarial survival was 74% with age, elevated creatinine and steroid use serving as negative predictors.[14]

RENAL FAILURE

The most common complication after open JAAA repair is development of postoperative renal dysfunction secondary to acute tubular necrosis. Indeed, up to 65% of patients will experience some degree of renal decline after open JAAA repair, but, thankfully, most of these are transient and mild.[17] In a review of 1,256 patients undergoing open JAAA repair, Jongkind et al. reported an 18% incidence of perioperative renal insufficiency and 3.3% rate of new-onset dialysis.[1] While in our own series, the rate of early dialysis was 2%, with one patient recovering renal function prior to discharge.[14] For most patients, the development of postoperative renal dysfunction is related to a combination of factors including the duration of warm renal ischemia (> 30 minutes), baseline renal function, intraoperative hypotension, and age.

The significant effect that chronic renal insufficiency has on longevity and quality of life cannot be overemphasized. Whereas, it is well recognized that dialysis dependent renal failure is a predictor of mortality, chronic renal insufficiency with a decreasing GFR < 60 mL/minute is also associated with an increased risk of death from any cause.[18] In the complex aortic literature, the relationship between baseline creatinine and postoperative complications is well documented, and a series from the Mayo Clinic showed that a Cr > 1.5 was predictive of postoperative mortality, myocardial infarction, and need for dialysis after open JAAA repair.[16] To wit, the association between preoperative renal dysfunction and postoperative complications should weigh heavily on the decision of whether a patient is a good candidate for open JAAA repair.

Outcomes of JAAA repair are closely correlated with postoperative renal complications; accordingly, operative adjuncts intended to protect the kidneys are often employed. Pre-clamp infusion of mannitol, furosemide, dopamine, or fenoldopam have been used with variable success. Mannitol is thought to be a free radical scavenger and is usually given in a dose of 1 g/kg 15 minutes prior to placing the supra-renal cross clamp. Furosemide is a diuretic that is thought to protect the kidney by reducing renal tubular oxygen demand. Both of these agents are used regularly without level one evidence of benefit. Fenoldopam is a selective dopamine receptor agonist that causes dilation of renal arterial beds, and several studies have shown that, when given in a dose of 0.1 mg/kg/min, it can help preserve overall renal function during aortic cross clamping. Finally, preservation of kidney function through the infusion of a renal cold solution has been supported by a firm literature base. Our approach involves direct installation of renal preservation fluid (lactated Ringer's solution with 25 g mannitol/L and 1 g/L methyl prednisolone at 4°C) into the renal ostium during ischemia. If the left renal artery is transected prior to placing the proximal aortic clamp, 250 mL of the renal cold solution is instilled into the artery followed by a continuous drip through a 6Fr perfusion balloon-tipped catheter. Once the aorta is opened, renal cold is infused in the right renal artery through the ostium, which should be coursing down and away from the surgeon. Experience has shown that such an infusion will result in a rapid decline of renal parenchymal temperature to 15°C after the bolus infusion. During the continuous infusion, renal core temperatures remain in the 25°C range and can be monitored by direct temperature probes in the renal cortex.

RESPIRATORY FAILURE

Both smoking and the presence of COPD are associated with an increased risk of developing aneurysmal degeneration of the aorta. So, it is no surprise that respiratory complications including prolonged intubation, reintubation, and pneumonia can occur with an incidence as high as 20% after JAAA repair.[11] Several studies have shown that the presence of COPD does not necessarily increase the perioperative morbidity after open JAAA repair, but failure to optimize COPD patients will.[19,20] A large series of JAAA from the Mayo Clinic reported a 16% rate of pulmonary complications and cited patient age, and factors associated with renal and visceral ischemic time as major predictors.[16] Interestingly, COPD was not a predictor of postoperative respiratory failure despite being present in 35% of the surgical cohort. Medical interventions that can decrease the risk of postoperative pulmonary complications include smoking cessation at least 2 weeks prior to surgery and the administration of bronchodilators in patients with a history of symptomatic COPD or abnormal pulmonary function tests.[23]

The best operative approach to reduce pulmonary complications remains a topic of debate. Several early studies showed that the retroperitoneal approach led to a reduction of pulmonary complications,[21,22] but a recent NSQIP review found the opposite result.[11] In our experience, the retroperitoneal approach leads to fewer respiratory complications, and, in our most recent series of JAAA repair, the combined pneumonia and reintubation rate was less than 10%.[14] Indeed, in patients with patients with marginal respiratory reserve, we favor the retroperitoneal over the transperitoneal approach.

BLEEDING

Open repair of JAAA can be a big undertaking and there are several steps of the operation that have the potential to produce rapid, exsanguinating hemorrhage if not executed with deliberate precision. The first potentially dangerous maneuver is clearing the retroperitoneal tissue off of the aorta. When coming from the retroperitoneal approach, you must first find the left renal artery and use this as a landmark. If the kidney is up, the renal lumbar vein will be just caudal to the artery and should be identified and ligated. Inadvertent transection of this vein can lead to massive bleeding as the distal end retracts towards the spine. If this vein (or any other) is injured, it is important not to begin grabbing with your forceps as this will often make the injury larger. The key is to dissect the vein free, identify the tear or transected end and then control the bleeding. The next move with the potential to create audible bleeding is obtaining proximal control of the aorta. It is important to stay on the aorta when dissecting circumferentially; if it does not go easily, do not force things. There is a risk of injury to lumbar arteries and veins in the area as well as the inferior vena cava, which can be adherent to the aorta. Both of these injuries are difficult to control and need to be dissected free of surrounding tissue prior to repair to avoid making things worse. Finally, there is a risk of injury to the common iliac veins if one attempts to gain circumferential distal control. Indeed, many surgeons just dissect out the anterior portion of the iliacs in order to avoid injuring an adherent iliac vein. If an injury occurs, do not make it worse by grabbing the area! Control the bleeding with digital pressure, dissect the vessel completely, and then repair it primarily. If the bleeding is too brisk, consider clamping and transecting the iliac artery to expose the vein. Ultimately, the best way to avoid this complication is with careful and deliberate dissection.

Upon completion of an open JAAA repair, the patient can be at increased risk for continued bleeding. It is important to look for bleeding lumbar arteries after the distal clamps are removed as repressurization can make previously hemostatic vessels bleed. Also, the aneurysm sac edge should be inspected as this can be a source of postoperative hemorrhage. It is also important to inspect the anastomoses very well as minor bleeding can become major if the blood pressure spikes postoperatively. The final place to inspect is the spleen. Seemingly minor capsular tears can lead to splenic blowout and hemorrhage in the postoperative period, and we have a low threshold for splenectomy in these cases.

COLON ISCHEMIA

A rare but devastating complication after open JAAA repair is the development of bowel ischemia. This has been reported to occur in around 0.5% of patients after elective repair and is more common after rupture. Despite its rare occurrence, the development of colon ischemia has a mortality > 50% in most studies, such that early identification is essential.[14,16] Patients will present with hypotension, acidosis, and a lactate that does not correct with resuscitation, and an early, bloody bowel movement is an ominous sign but only occurs about one third of the time. The best way to prevent this complication is by assessment of IMA backbleeding prior to ligation. If the IMA is large or has no bleeding when transected (signifying a disruption in collateral flow), then it should be re-implanted prior to the end of the case. If ischemia is suspected, the patient should be evaluated with a flexible sigmoidoscope, preferably in the ICU. If full-thickness ischemia is identified, the patient needs to return to the operating room for re-exploration, resection and diversion with a colostomy to prevent soilage of the graft. All patients with ischemic colitis should be placed on broad-spectrum antibiotics, and less severe cases can be treated with antibiotics alone.

ANEURYSM DEGENERATION

Unlike FEVAR, open JAAA repair has a very low late graft-related complication rate, but patients should undergo surveillance at least every 5 years.[24,25] In our most recent experience, 30% of patients were found to have additional noncongruent aneurysms on long-term surveillance. Half of these were in the descending thoracic aorta and ultimately required either TEVAR or open repair.[14] There is also a risk of developing aneurysmal degeneration of the proximal or distal anastomosis. This has been reported to occur in 1–6% of patients depending on the length of follow-up.[23] Such aneurysmal degeneration is often treated with endovascular techniques because re-operative aortic surgery can be a highly challenging and morbid undertaking.

REFERENCES

1. Jongkind V, Yeung KK, Akkersdijk GJ, Heidsieck D, Reitsma JB, Tangelder GJ, Wisselink W. Juxtarenal aortic aneurysm repair. J Vasc Surg. 52(3):760–7.
2. Schermerhorn ML, Bensley RP, Giles KA, Hurks R, O'Malley AJ, Cotterill P, Chaikof E, Landon BE. Changes in abdominal aortic aneurysm rupture and short term mortality 1995–2008. Ann Surg. 2012;256(4): 651–658.
3. The UK Small Aneurysm Trial Participants. Long-term outcomes of immediate repair compared with surveillance of small abdominal aortic aneruysms. N Engl J Med. 2002; 346: 1445–52.
4. Brown PM, Zelt DT, Sobolev B. The risk of rupture in untreated aneurysms: The impact of size, gender and expansion rate. J Vasc Surg. 2003;37: 280–4.
5. Conrad MF, Crawford RS, Pedraza JD, Brewster DC, LaMuraglia GM, Corey M, Abbara S, Cambria RP. Long-term durability of open abdominal aortic aneurysm repair. J Vasc Surg. 2007;46(4): 669–75.
6. Chaikof EL, Dalman RL, Eskandari MK, Jackson MB, Lee WA, Mansour MA, Mastracci TM, Mell M, Murad MH, Nguyen LL, Oderich GS, Patel MS, Schermerhorn ML, Starnes MW. The society for vascular surgery practice guidelines on the cure of patients with an abdominal aortic aneurysm. J Vas Surg. 2018;67(1): 1–77.

7. Yuo TH, Sidaoui J, Marone LK, Avgerinos ED, Makaroun MS, Chaer RA. Limited survival in dialysis patients undergoing intact abdominal aortic aneurysm repair. J Vasc Surg. 2014;60: 908–13.
8. Bertrand M, Godet G, Meersschaert K, Brun L, Salcedo E, Coriat P. Should the angiotensin II antagonists be discontinued before surgery? Anesth Analg. 2001;92: 26–30.
9. Wallinder J, Georgiou A, Wanhainen A, Bjorck M. Prevalence of Synchronous and Metachronous Aneurysms in Women with Abdominal Aortic Aneurysm. Eur J Vasc Endovasc Surg. 2018;56(3): 435–440.
10. Chaer RA, Vasoncelos R, Marone LK, Al-Koury G, Rhee RY, Cho JS, Makaroun MS. Synchronous and Metachronous Thoracic Aneurysms in Patients with Abdominal Aortic Aneurysms. J Vasc Surg. 2012;56(5): 1261–5.
11. Buck DB, Ultee KJH, Zettervall SL, Soden PA, Darling J, Wyers M, van Herwaarden JA, Schermerhorn ML. Transperitoneal Versus Retroperitoneal Approach for Open Abdominal Aortic Aneurysm Repair in the Targeted Vascular National Surgical Quality Improvement Program. J Vasc Surg. 2016;64: 585–91.
12. Varkevisser RRB, de Guerre LEMV, Swerdlow NJ, Dansey K, Latz CA, Liang P, Li C, Verhagen HJM, Schermerhorn ML. The Impact of Proximal Clamp Location on Peri-Operative Outcomes Following Open Surgical Repair of Juxtarenal Abdominal Aortic Aneurysms. Eur J Vasc Endovasc Surg. 2020;59: 411–418.
13. Wang, LJ, Tsougranis GH, Tanious A, Chang DC, Clouse WD, Eagleton MJ, Conrad MF. The removal of all proximal aneurysmal aortic tissue does not affect anastomotic degeneration after open juxtarenal aortic aneurysm repair. J vasc Surg. 2020;71: 390–9.
14. Tsai S, Conrad MF, Patel VI, Kwolek CJ, LaMuraglia GM, Brewster DC, Cambria RP. Durability of Open Repair of Juxtarenal Abdominal Aortic Aneurysms. J Vasc Surg. 2012;56: 2–7.
15. Tallarita T, Sobreira ML, Oderich GS. Results of Open Pararenal Abdominal Aortic Aneurysm Repair: Tabular Review of the Literature. Ann Vasc Surg. 2011;24: 143–149.
16. West CA, Noel AA, Bower TC, Cherry KJ, Gloviczki P, Sullivan TM, Kalra M, Hoskin TL, Harrington JR. Factors Affecting Outcomes of Open Surgical Repair of Pararenal Aortic Aneurysms: A 10-Year Experience. J Vasc Surg. 2006;43: 921–8.
17. Saratzis A, joshi S, Benson RA, Bosanquet D, Dattani N, Batchelder A, Fisher O, Ioannidou E, Brown MJ, Imray CH. Acute Kidney Injury in Aortic Intervention: Findings from the Midlands Aortic Renal Injury Cohort Study. Eur J Vasc Endovasc Surg. 2020;59: 899–909.
18. Go AS, Chertow GM, Fan D, McCulloch CE, Hsu CY. Chronic kidney disease and the risks of death, cardiovascular events, and hospitalization. The New England journal of medicine. 2004;351(13): 1296–305.
19. Axelrod DA, Henke PK, Wakefield TW, Stanley JC, Jacobs LA, Graham LM, Greenfield LJ, Upchurch GR. Impact of Chronic Obstructive Pulmonary Disease on Elective and Emergency Abdominal Aortic Aneurysm Repair. J Vasc Surg. 2001;33(1): 72–76.
20. Upchurch GR, Proctor MC, Henke PK, Zajkowski P, Riles EM, Ascher MS, Eagleton MJ, Stanley JC. Predictors of Severe Morbidity and Death after Elective Abdominal Aortic Aneurysmectomy in Patients with Chronic Obstructive Pulmonary Disease. J Vasc Surg. 2003;37(3): 594–599.
21. Leather RP, Shah DM, Kaufman JL, Fitzgerald KM, Chang BB, Feusted PJ. Comparative analysis of retroperitoneal and transperitoneal aortic replacement for aneurysm. Surg Gynecol Obstet. 1989;168: 387–93.
22. Peck JJ, McReynolds DG, Baker DH, Eastman AB. Extraperitoneal approach for aortoiliac reconstruction of the abdominal aorta. Am J Surg. 1986;151: 620–3.
23. Chaikof EL, Brewster DC, Dalman RL, Makaroun MS, Illig KA, Sicard GA, Timaran CH, Upchurch GR, Veith FJ. The Care of Patients with an Abdominal Aortic Aneurysm: The Society for Vascular Surgery Practice Guidelines. J Vasc Surg. 2009;50(8s): 1s–49s.
24. Kalman PG, Rappaport DC, Merchant N, Clarke K, Johnston KW. The value of late computed tomographic scanning in identification of vascular abnormalities after abdominal aortic aneurysm repair. J Vasc Surg. 1999;29(3): 442–50.
25. Mantoni M, Neergaard K, Christoffersen JK, Lambine TL, Baekgaard N. Long-term computed tomography follow-up after open surgical repair of abdominal aortic aneurysms. Acta Radiol. 2006;47(6): 549–53.

SUGGESTED READINGS

Chaikof EL, Brewster DC, Dalman RL, Makaroun MS, Illig KA, Sicard GA, Timaran CH, Upchurch GR, Veith FJ. The Care of Patients with an Abdominal Aortic Aneurysm: The Society for Vascular Surgery Practice Guidelines. J Vasc Surg 2009; 50(8s): 1s-49s.

Tsai S, Conrad MF, Patel VI, Kwolek CJ, LaMuraglia GM, Brewster DC, Cambria RP. Durability of Open Repair of Juxtarenal Abdominal Aortic Aneurysms. J Vasc Surg 2012; 56: 2–7.

Buck DB, Ultee KJH, Zettervall SL, Soden PA, Darling J, Wyers M, van Herwaarden JA, Schermerhorn ML. Transperitoneal Versus Retroperitoneal Approach for Open Abdominal Aortic Aneurysm Repair in the Targeted Vascular National Surgical Quality Improvement Program. J Vasc Surg 2016; 64: 585–91.

22

Complications of open repair of splanchnic aneurysms

BJOERN D. SUCKOW AND DAVID H. STONE

Splanchnic artery aneurysms, while somewhat uncommon, are identified in contemporary practice with increased frequency in light of widely utilized advanced imaging techniques. Accordingly, these lesions, both true and false aneurysms alike, once diagnosed will often require definitive surgical management. The widespread adoption and evolution of catheter-based techniques and therapies have significantly impacted the therapeutic management of visceral aneurysms. Nevertheless, there are instances when an open surgical approach remains both prudent and the treatment of choice. Accordingly, specific complications and morbidities remain associated with an open surgical repair paradigm and should be considered when choosing treatment.

All considered, aneurysms of the celiac artery and its respective branches constitute more than 80% of visceral segment aneurysms, though more infrequent splanchnic lesions will be considered herein as well.

SPLENIC ARTERY ANEURYSMS

PRESENTATION

Splenic artery aneurysms are the most common of the splanchnic aneurysms and account for roughly 60% of such lesions encountered in practice.[1,2] It has been speculated by autopsy studies that the incidence of splenic aneurysms may be as high as 10% among older patient cohorts.[3] It has been repeatedly determined that splenic aneurysms are more prevalent among women, with a 4:1 prevalence ratio compared to men.[4,5] Often noted to be of saccular morphology in the mid or distal segments of the splenic artery (Figure 22.1), it is typically recommended that aneurysms greater than 2 cm be considered for treatment as well as when diagnosed in pregnant women or female patients of child-bearing age who wish to become pregnant.[5]

In general, there are four underlying conditions that may predispose patients to developing splenic artery aneurysms. (1) Medial fibrodysplasia and its ensuing impact on the media's smooth muscle cells can lead to aneurysm formation in the splenic artery. While more common as an underlying etiology for renal artery-induced hypertension, medial fibrodysplasia can directly impact the integrity of the splenic arterial wall. (2) Modulations in reproductive hormones during gestation can lead to presumptive altered-flow dynamics in the splenic artery and predispose toward aneurysm formation. (3) Portal hypertension and/or splenomegaly may predispose to splenic aneurysm formation among patients with cirrhosis who may experience increased splenic flow and elevated estrogen levels. (4) Localized arteritis, which may ensue in the setting of pancreatitis or polyarteritis nodosa among others, may predispose to splenic aneurysmal degeneration.

Splenic artery aneurysms are usually asymptomatic. Symptoms, when present, often include vague epigastric pain, left upper quadrant pain, or back pain. Hemodynamic demise or frank shock may occur in the setting of free rupture. At times, initial bleeding from a ruptured splenic aneurysm may be contained in the lesser sac leading to transiently stable hemodynamics. Alternatively, the patient may become subsequently unstable when free rupture consequently transpires via extravasation of blood from the lesser sac via the foramen of Winslow or the pars flacida of the gastrohepatic omentum.[6]

Given the observed role in reproductive hormone physiology and splenic artery aneurysms, their presence during pregnancy warrants particular attention. There is an increased risk of rupture during pregnancy, which carries a significant associated morbidity and mortality for both the mother and fetus. Accordingly, when diagnosed during pregnancy, splenic aneurysms will require therapeutic attention depending on when during the gestational period the diagnosis is established.[6]

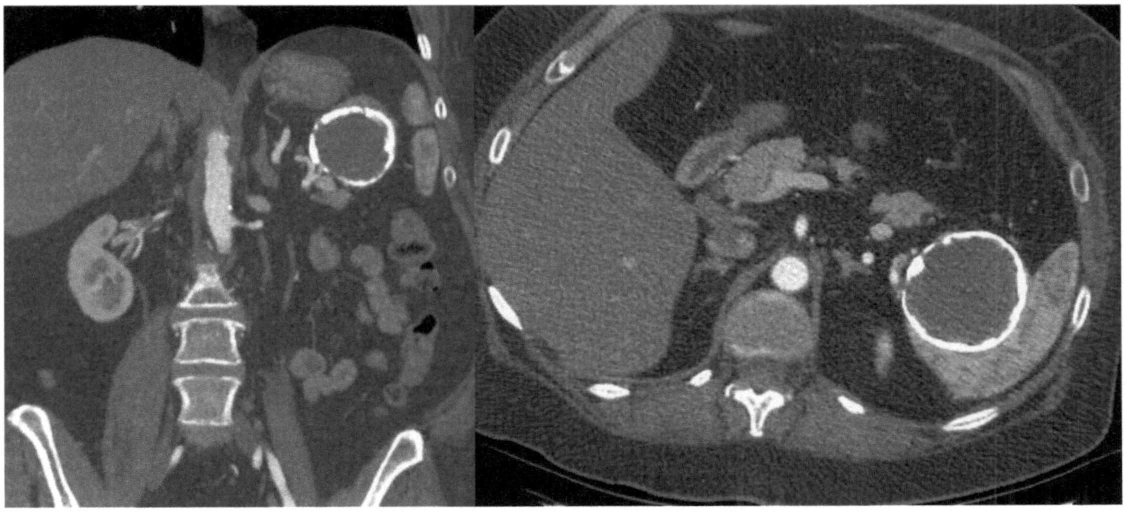

Figure 22.1 Splenic artery aneurysm.

OPERATIVE MANAGEMENT

The advent and evolution of endovascular therapies has largely supplanted an "open first" approach in managing splenic artery aneurysms. These will often include either a coil/embolization strategy, using a cyanoacrylate glue or some type of coil packing. A stent graft approach can be utilized as well, though at times can be limited in utility due to splenic artery tortuosity.[7] However, open repair remains a viable approach in the definitive treatment of splenic aneurysms, in both elective and ruptured settings and when a cathether-based approach is not feasable. Open treatment may involve exclusion of the aneurysm with proximal and distal ligation, or ligation with interval reconstruction. Splenectomy is reserved with or without distal pancreatectomy for more distal and hilar lesions which preclude ligation or reconstruction. Exposure is usually accomplished by mobilizing the splenocolic ligament and splenic flexure away from the abdominal wall.

Results of an open surgical approach remain good with high survival and relatively low complication rates. Marrone et al. documented 1- and 5 year survival to be 100% and 92%, respectively.[8] A large meta-analysis documented the outcomes of a large group of splenic aneurysms repaired via an open approach, documenting fewer long-term complications and reinterventions as compared to a catheter-based paradigm.[9] Alternatively, the same review demonstrated endovascular repair to be the more cost-effective option with better quality-adjusted life years from the patient perspective.[10] Complications from an open surgical approach can include overwhelming post-splenectomy infection, and thus it is important for surgeons to consider vaccination when a splenectomy occurs as part of the treatment approach. Thankfully, this remains a rare event. In addition, post-splenectomy left upper quadrant abscess formation is a possible, though rare, clinically observed complication. An open technique can additionally lead to pancreatitis as a sequelae if pancreatic manipulation or distal pancreatectomy is necessary during the operation. This can often lead to subsequent pseudocyst formation, which may require additional endoscopic or surgical management.[11,12] Potential splenic infarction may occur if the aneurysm is ligated proximally and distally, though this remains unusual as the short gastric vessels will more commonly provide adequate collateral flow to justify a splenic preservation operative approach.

HEPATIC ARTERY ANEURYSMS

PRESENTATION

Hepatic artery aneurysms are the second most common splanchnic aneurysm and constitute roughly 13–20% of visceral artery aneurysms.[13,14] The overwhelming majority (80%) of hepatic artery aneurysms are anatomically situated in an extrahepatic location (Figure 22.2), with the remainder situated in the extrahepatic space or within the liver parenchyma itself. Nearly two-thirds of hepatic aneurysms form in the common hepatic artery, one-quarter in the right hepatic artery, and approximately 5% in the left.[15,16] The anatomic relationship of the aneurysm in regard to the gastroduodenal artery will carry associated technical implications when considering operative intervention. Unlike splenic artery aneurysms, there is no known association with pregnancy. However, other underlying conditions such as arteritis, arterial dysplasia, or trauma may play a role in aneurysm formation. The majority of these lesions are detected incidentally on imaging performed for alternative indications. Most hepatic

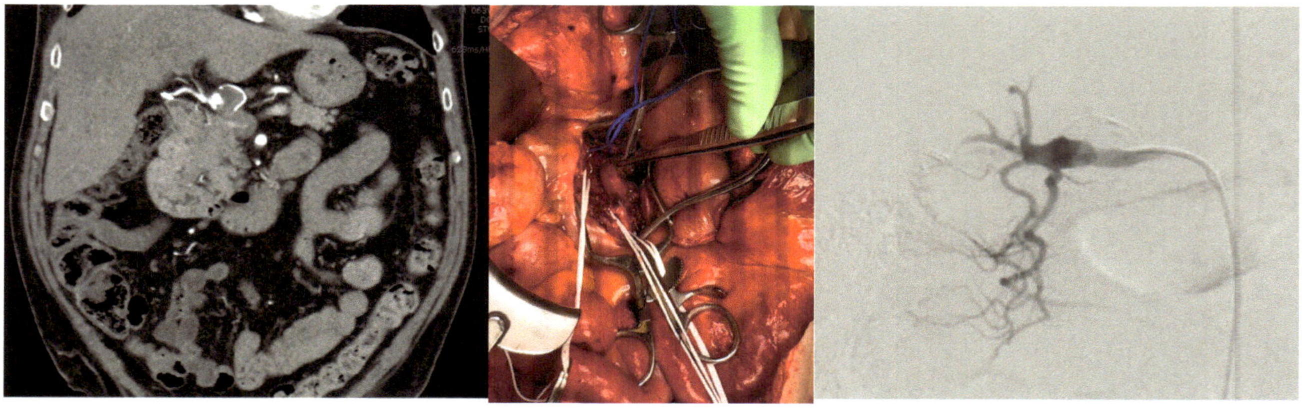

Figure 22.2 Hepatic artery aneurysm.

artery aneurysms remain asymptomatic, though it is felt that rupture may approach 25% in larger lesions.[17] In this setting, hepatic aneurysms greater than 2 cm, pseudoaneurysms, or symptomatic aneurysms should be repaired. When symptomatic, abdominal discomfort, and back pain may ensue. In rarer instances, hemobilia, jaundice, and/or GI bleeding may occur.[13,18]

OPERATIVE MANAGEMENT

Like splenic aneurysms, catheter-based therapeutic approaches have become utilized where appropriate and when anatomically feasible. Often, however, open surgical approaches are frequently employed for the treatment of these lesions and carry with them certain potential complications and/or morbidities. Exposure can usually be accomplished comfortably via a generous right subcostal or bilateral subcostal incision versus an upper midline approach. Often, if the aneurysm is proximal to the gastroduodenal artery (GDA), the aneurysm can be ligated, with collateral flow precluding the need for in-line reconstruction. If the aneurysm extends into the proper hepatic artery, reconstruction will often be required with careful attention to avoiding branch ligation, which can potentially lead to hepatic necrosis if somewhat distal. Additional complications to consider associated with open hepatic aneurysm repair include gall-bladder necrosis. Specifically, if the right hepatic artery is ligated, cholecystectomy should be considered given the potential for this complication.[19] Additionally, consideration should be given to the potential pitfalls of hepatic artery ligation in patients with baseline liver dysfunction or cirrhosis who may not be able to compensate via portal flow.[20] Furthermore, there is obvious appeal for a catheter-based approach for treating intraparenchymal lesions; however, hepatic resection is possible, though it will be associated with all of the associated inherent pitfalls of hepatectomy and should be carefully considered weighing a patient's comorbidity profile and physiologic fitness for resection.[21]

CELIAC ARTERY ANEURYSMS

PRESENTATION

Celiac artery aneurysms are rare, comprising less than 4% of splanchnic artery aneurysms, and are most commonly detected concomitantly with other splanchnic or aortic aneurysms (40% of the time).[2,13,22] Historically, celiac artery aneurysms were primarily caused by a presumptive infectious etiology (syphilis); in the contemporary era, they are most often caused by medial degeneration and/or atherosclerosis.[23] There appears to be no association between pregnancy and celiac artery aneurysms. However, a significant percentage of aneurysms are noted to develop in the setting of post-stenotic dilation from median arcuate ligament compression. Therefore, a modest number of celiac artery aneurysms may be encountered in younger patients.[24] The majority of celiac artery aneurysms are diagnosed incidentally on imaging. Rupture rates are reported between 10–20% with an associated mortality risk of 50%.[23,25] Unfortunately, aneurysm size, morphology, calcification, and etiology are not associated with rupture risk (likely a phenomenon of low incidence), and therefore traditional consensus criteria recommended treatment of all diagnosed celiac artery aneurysms unless prohibited by patient comorbidities.[25,26] Several modern series, however, report no rupture among patients with celiac artery aneurysms measuring less than 2.5 cm diameter.[13,26] In our practice, we have reserved treatment for celiac artery aneurysms which measure greater than 2.5 cm, and, have not encountered any ruptured celiac artery aneurysms less than that size.

OPERATIVE MANAGEMENT

Open surgical treatment remains a durable and viable approach to celiac artery aneurysm repair. Endovascular techniques usually include embolization and/or exclusion of the celiac artery because the short length of the celiac trunk limits complete stent graft exclusion of most aneurysms. Successful endovascular repairs therefore rely on adequate collateral blood supply to the viscera, specifically the liver. Open repair can similarly comprise simple ligation of the celiac trunk if sufficient collateral blood flow exists. Ligation without arterial reconstruction has been reported in roughly 30% of cases, but it should be avoided in patients with liver disease as well as in those with limited collateral networks to the stomach (prior splenectomy).[1,23] Other surgical options include ligation or aneurysmectomy with surgical bypass (aortoceliac or hepatorenal), or aneurysmorrhaphy in cases of small saccular lesions. Direct exposure of the celiac trunk is performed via upper midline laparotomy or bilateral subcostal incisions. The gastrohepatic ligament is divided, followed by division of the median arcuate ligament and right crus of the diaphragm. A retroperitoneal left thoracoabdominal incision may be preferable in cases of a hostile abdomen and allow for better aortic and peri-aortic exposure, however, it limits more distal access to the hepatic artery.

Complications from open repair of a celiac artery aneurysm include esophageal injury during dissection of the crura, which can be mitigated by placement of a nasogastric tube. If no arterial reconstruction is performed, there remains a risk of hepatic ischemia, while gastric ischemia is rare unless in situations of poor collateral blood supply. Arterial reconstruction is traditionally performed with an antegrade aortoceliac bypass of prosthetic conduit. Patency rates are poorly described given the low frequency of celiac aneurysms. However, primary patency of antegrade aortoceliac bypass for occlusive disease ranges from 82% at 3 years to 70% at 5 years and can be inferred to be similar or potentially superior in patients without associated atherosclerotic disease.[27,28] Dissection of the distal celiac trunk, especially into the proximal splenic or hepatic vessels, may result in pancreatitis postoperatively. Left hepatic lobe damage can incur from retractor placement and we recommend mobilization of the left lobe by dividing the triangular and coronary ligaments. Routine abdominal operative complications of postoperative ileus, myocardial infarction in elderly patients, and bleeding from dissection or anastomoses should be considered as well.

SUPERIOR MESENTERIC ARTERY ANEURYSMS

PRESENTATION

Aneurysms of the superior mesenteric artery (SMA) account for 6% of splanchnic artery aneurysms and are more common among males.[13] They usually occur in the proximal 5 cm of the SMA, although more distal aneurysms have been described (Figure 22.3). Unlike other splanchnic artery aneurysms, the etiology for SMA aneurysms remains predominantly mycotic (60%). *Staphylococcus* and *Streptococcus* species are most common and usually result from intravenous drug use or bacterial endocarditis. SMA aneurysms are frequently symptomatic, unlike other splanchnic artery aneurysms. Their associated symptoms are likely due to their frequent underlying infectious etiology and their consequential impact on intestinal perfusion, potentially leading to bowel ischemia. Due to the higher resistance bed of the small bowel compared to other splanchnic vessels, SMA aneurysms more frequently present with thrombosis and acute ischemia (Figure 22.4). Other etiologies for SMA aneurysms include medial degeneration, connective tissue disease, polyarteritis nodosa, and pancreatitis. Patient symptoms with SMA aneurysms commonly include abdominal pain, weight loss, post-prandial pain, fevers, nausea, and vomiting.[1,29–31] Rupture rates for SMA aneurysms range from 38–50% and are associated with a mortality of up to 90% due to bleeding and bowel ischemia.[29] Repair is indicated in symptomatic, mycotic, or SMA aneurysms measuring over 2.5 cm.[13,29]

OPERATIVE MANAGEMENT

Endovascular treatment options for SMA aneurysms have been described and usually involve a combination of stent graft exclusion with or without coil or glue embolization of side-branches to prevent endoleak.[32] However, due to the frequent mycotic etiology of SMA aneurysms,

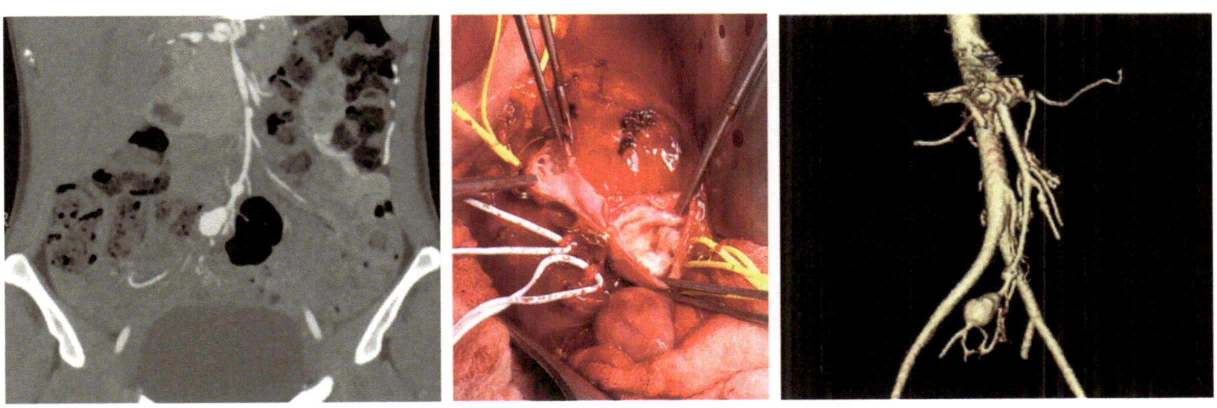

Figure 22.3 Superior mesenteric artery (SMA) aneurysm.

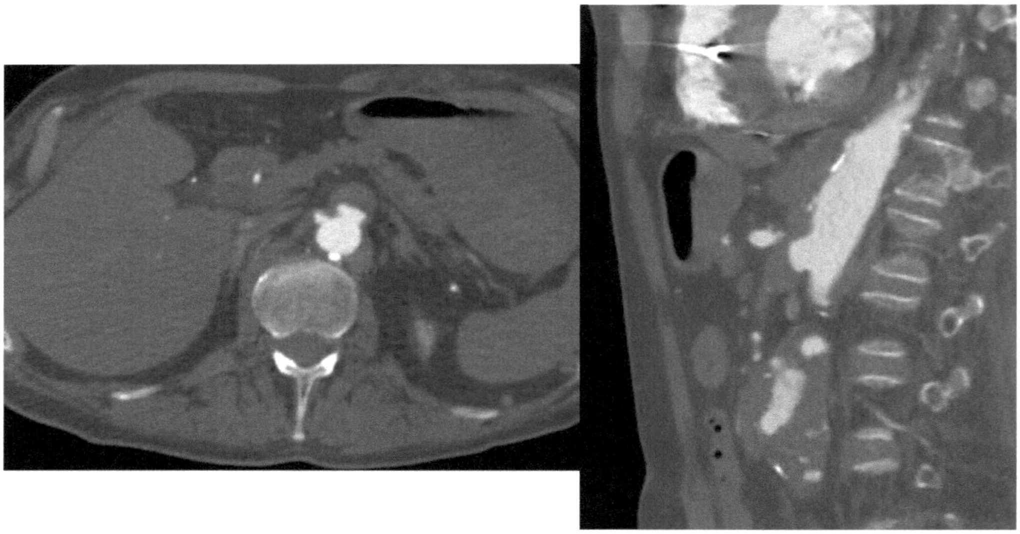

Figure 22.4 Thrombosed SMA aneurysm.

stent grafting is often discouraged in those cases given the potential for chronic infection of the implanted prothesis. Further, significant ischemia of portions of the intestine may arise from SMA branch occlusion to obtain exclusion of the aneurysm. Open surgical treatment usually consists of aneurysmectomy with arterial reconstruction or aneurysmorrhaphy. Unlike other splanchnic artery aneurysms, ligation of SMA aneurysms is rarely a viable option given their frequent proximal location and resultant potential for bowel ischemia. Branch SMA aneurysms, though rare, may be suitable for ligation and require adjunctive partial small bowel resection. Most SMA aneurysms are repaired via midline laparotomy and direct anterior exposure within the small bowel mesentery with dissection down to its root and involved branches for vascular control. A retroperitoneal lateral approach may be suitable for exposure if the SMA aneurysm is located proximally and a bypass from the aorta to the proximal SMA is required for arterial reconstruction. Aneuresmectomy with interposition graft placement is commonly used for proximal main SMA vessel aneurysms. More distal SMA aneurysms that involve multiple side-branches may be better suited to aneurysmorrhapy with plication and/or patch angioplasty to preserve blood flow to the small bowel branches, especially important branches such as the middle colic artery.

Complications of open SMA aneurysm repair relate to the location of the aneurysm along the SMA axis and the extent of repair required. Bowel ischemia and need for bowel resection is related to incident presentation (occlusion or mycosis) and the ability to preserve or re-establish bowel perfusion. Given the high likelihood of a mycotic etiology and/or bowel ischemia requiring resection, we advocate against the use of prosthetic bypass/interposition graft or prosthetic patch if aneurysmorrhaphy is performed. If the underlying etiology is from intravenous drug abuse or bacterial endocarditis, recurrent SMA aneurysms may develop unless the underlying condition is addressed. Patients with vasculitis may also present with multifocal SMA aneurysms (Figure 22.4) or may develop metachronous de novo aneurysms at a later time. Therefore, surveillance imaging of these patients is warranted.[29,31,33] More routine surgical complications such as postoperative ileus, adhesion-related bowel obstruction, bowel stricture from ischemia, pancreatitis from dissection around the proximal SMA, and myocardial infarction also apply and should be considered during the postoperative period following open SMA aneurysm repair.

REFERENCES

1. Shanley CJ, Shah NL, Messina LM. Uncommon splanchnic artery aneurysms: pancreaticoduodenal, gastroduodenal, superior mesenteric, inferior mesenteric, and colic. Ann Vasc Surg. 1996;10(5): 506–15.
2. Shanley CJ, Shah NL, Messina LM. Common splanchnic artery aneurysms: splenic, hepatic, and celiac. Ann Vasc Surg. 1996;10(3): 315–22.
3. Bedford PD, Lodge B. Aneurysm of the splenic artery. Gut. 1960;1: 312–20.
4. Messina LM, Shanley CJ. Visceral artery aneurysms. Surg Clin North Am. 1997;77(2): 425–42.
5. Dave SP, Reis ED, Hossain A, Taub PJ, Kerstein MD, Hollier LH. Splenic artery aneurysm in the 1990s. Ann Vasc Surg. 2000;14(3): 223–9.
6. Stanley JC, Veith F, Wakefield TW. Current Therapy in Vascular and Endovascular Surgery, Fifth Edition. Elsevier Saunders; 2014.
7. Lakin RO, Bena JF, Sarac TP, Shah S, Krajewski LP, Srivastava SD, et al. The contemporary management of splenic artery aneurysms. J Vasc Surg. 2011;53(4): 958–64; discussion 65.

8. Marone EM, Mascia D, Kahlberg A, Brioschi C, Tshomba Y, Chiesa R. Is open repair still the gold standard in visceral artery aneurysm management? Ann Vasc Surg. 2011;25(7): 936–46.
9. Hogendoorn W, Lavida A, Hunink MG, Moll FL, Geroulakos G, Muhs BE, et al. Open repair, endovascular repair, and conservative management of true splenic artery aneurysms. J Vasc Surg. 2014;60(6): 1667–76 e1.
10. Hogendoorn W, Lavida A, Hunink MG, Moll FL, Geroulakos G, Muhs BE, et al. Cost-effectiveness of endovascular repair, open repair, and conservative management of splenic artery aneurysms. J Vasc Surg. 2015;61(6): 1432–40.
11. Cadili A, de Gara C. Complications of splenectomy. Am J Med. 2008;121(5): 371–5.
12. Weledji EP. Benefits and risks of splenectomy. Int J Surg. 2014;12(2): 113–9.
13. Corey MR, Ergul EA, Cambria RP, English SJ, Patel VI, Lancaster RT, et al. The natural history of splanchnic artery aneurysms and outcomes after operative intervention. J Vasc Surg. 2016;63(4): 949–57.
14. Arneson MA, Smith RS. Ruptured hepatic artery aneurysm: case report and review of literature. Ann Vasc Surg. 2005;19(4):540–5.
15. Abbas MA, Fowl RJ, Stone WM, Panneton JM, Oldenburg WA, Bower TC, et al. Hepatic artery aneurysm: factors that predict complications. J Vasc Surg. 2003;38(1): 41–5.
16. Luebke T, Heckenkamp J, Gawenda M, Beckurts KT, Lackner K, Brunkwall J. Combined endovascular-open surgical procedure in a great hepatic artery aneurysm. Ann Vasc Surg. 2007;21(6): 807–12.
17. Busuttil RW, Brin BJ. The diagnosis and management of visceral artery aneurysms. Surgery. 1980;88(5): 619–24.
18. Pasha SF, Gloviczki P, Stanson AW, Kamath PS. Splanchnic artery aneurysms. Mayo Clin Proc. 2007;82(4): 472–9.
19. Iseki J, Tada Y, Wada T, Nobori M. Hepatic artery aneurysm. Report of a case and review of the literature. Gastroenterol Jpn. 1983;18(2): 84–92.
20. Madding GF, Kennedy PA. Hepatic artery ligation. Surg Clin North Am. 1972;52(3): 719–28.
21. Salcuni PF, Spaggiari L, Tecchio T, Benincasa A, Azzarone M. Hepatic artery aneurysm: an ever present danger. J Cardiovasc Surg (Torino). 1995;36(6): 595–9.
22. Hossain A, Reis ED, Dave SP, Kerstein MD, Hollier LH. Visceral artery aneurysms: experience in a tertiary-care center. Am Surg. 2001;67(5): 432–7.
23. Graham LM, Stanley JC, Whitehouse WM, Jr., Zelenock GB, Wakefield TW, Cronenwett JL, et al. Celiac artery aneurysms: historic (1745-1949) versus contemporary (1950-1984) differences in etiology and clinical importance. J Vasc Surg. 1985;2(5):757–64.
24. Jimenez JC, Rafidi F, Morris L. True celiac artery aneurysm secondary to median arcuate ligament syndrome. Vasc Endovascular Surg. 2011;45(3): 288–9.
25. Stanley JC, Wakefield TW, Graham LM, Whitehouse WM Jr, Zelenock GB, Lindenauer SM. Clinical importance and management of splanchnic artery aneurysms. J Vasc Surg. 1986;3(5): 836–40.
26. Stone WM, Abbas MA, Gloviczki P, Fowl RJ, Cherry KJ. Celiac arterial aneurysms: a critical reappraisal of a rare entity. Arch Surg. 2002;137(6): 670–4.
27. Jimenez JG, Huber TS, Ozaki CK, Flynn TC, Berceli SA, Lee WA, et al. Durability of antegrade synthetic aortomesenteric bypass for chronic mesenteric ischemia. J Vasc Surg. 2002;35(6): 1078–84.
28. Scali ST, Ayo D, Giles KA, Gray S, Kubilis P, Back M, et al. Outcomes of antegrade and retrograde open mesenteric bypass for acute mesenteric ischemia. J Vasc Surg. 2019;69(1): 129–40.
29. Stone WM, Abbas M, Cherry KJ, Fowl RJ, Gloviczki P. Superior mesenteric artery aneurysms: is presence an indication for intervention? J Vasc Surg. 2002;36(2): 234–7; discussion 7.
30. Lorelli DR, Cambria RA, Seabrook GR, Towne JB. Diagnosis and management of aneurysms involving the superior mesenteric artery and its branches–a report of four cases. Vasc Endovascular Surg. 2003;37(1): 59–66.
31. Kordzadeh A, Watson J, Panayiotopolous YP. Mycotic aneurysm of the superior and inferior mesenteric artery. J Vasc Surg. 2016;63(6): 1638–46.
32. Tulsyan N, Kashyap VS, Greenberg RK, Sarac TP, Clair DG, Pierce G, et al. The endovascular management of visceral artery aneurysms and pseudoaneurysms. J Vasc Surg. 2007;45(2): 276–83; discussion 83.
33. Zilun L, Henghui Y, Yang Z, Mian W, Guangqi C, Shenming W. The Management of Superior Mesenteric Artery Aneurysm: Experience with 16 Cases in a Single Center. Ann Vasc Surg. 2017;42: 120–7.

SUGGESTED READINGS

Corey MR, Ergul EA, Cambria RP, English SJ, Patel VI, Lancaster RT, et al. The natural history of splanchnic artery aneurysms and outcomes after operative intervention. J Vasc Surg. 2016;63(4):949-57.

Hogendoorn W, Lavida A, Hunink MG, Moll FL, Geroulakos G, Muhs BE, et al. Open repair, endovascular repair, and conservative management of true splenic artery aneurysms. J Vasc Surg. 2014;60(6):1667-76.e1.

23

Complications of open repair of renal artery aneurysms

CHLOÉ A. POWELL AND DAWN COLEMAN

Renal artery aneurysms are rare with an incidence of about 0.1% in the general population. When discovered during autopsy, studies reveal an incidence of 0.01–0.09%, whereas in angiographic and computed tomography studies, the incidence varies from 0.3% to 2.5%.[1] The demographics of those who develop renal artery aneurysms include persons in the sixth decade of life with a female predominance.[1] Renal artery aneurysms are also associated with fibromuscular dysplasia due to the multiple stenotic and post-stenotic dilated lesions along the renal artery.[2] In the rare case, Ehlers-Danlos syndrome type IV, which affects type III collagen, can be contributory due to the increased fragility of the artery.[3]

CLASSIFICATION

Renal artery aneurysms are classified by their morphology and location, which can determine the treatment approach. Roughly 90% of true aneurysms are extraparenchymal with the majority being saccular in nature, which occur at artery bifurcations.[1,4,5] About 75% of saccular renal artery aneurysms occur at first-or second-order bifurcations. Renal artery aneurysms may also be fusiform and are usually the result of post-stenotic dilation in the setting of athersclerotic disease.[5,6] Intralobar aneurysms are often associated with congenital and connective tissue diseases.[5]

CLINICAL PRESENTATION/ MANIFESTATION

Most renal artery aneurysms are asymptomatic and typically found incidentally on imaging for unrelated conditions.[4] Of those that develop symptoms, hypertension is the most common.[7] The relationship between renal artery aneurysms and hypertension is ill-defined; however, there are many hypotheses. Hypertension may be the result of renin-mediated vasoconstriction in the setting of renal artery stenosis, which can cause post-stenotic fusiform aneurysms. Other mechanisms for hypertension include distal thrombus embolization or propagation and the resultant artery occlusion leading to segmental parenchymal ischemia, compression of adjacent renal artery branch leading to renin-mediated hypertension, or flow turbulence altering hemodynamics. Other symptoms include flank pain and hematuria. The most dreaded manifestation of renal artery aneurysm is rupture resulting in life-threatening hemorrhage. These patients typically present with acute flank or abdominal pain and hypotension.[5,8] The associated mortality in renal artery aneurysm rupture is about 10%. Among survivors of aneurysm rupture, 90% have a loss of the kidney. The mortality of aneurysm rupture is significantly greater in the pregnant population where it is associated with a 50% maternal mortality and 75% fetal mortality.

DIAGNOSTIC WORKUP

RAAs are mostly discovered incidentally when imaging is acquired for an unrelated reason. The primary modality for diagnosis of renal artery aneurysms is computed tomography angiography (CTA). The advantages of CTA is that it is noninvasive and fast.[8] Though CTA is widely used, digital subtraction angiography remains the gold standard; digital subtraction angiography remains the gold standard, although is is associated with complication risks that include access-site bleeding as an example. Other imaging modalities can supplant catheter based arteriography. Other imaging options include magnetic resonance angiography and duplex ultrasonography.[1,5]

SURGICAL MANAGEMENT

Historic indications for intervention included aneurysm size > 2 cm, women of childbearing age or those who are currently pregnant, medically refractory hypertension, symptoms including pain and hematuria, and rupture. The size threshold for repair remains controversial, however, with some advocating elective repair at larger sizes (i.e., > 3 cm) in light of the benign natural history of slow to null growth.[53]

Open surgery offers low morbidity and mortality, and long-term patency. The approach taken is dependent on the aneurysm location, size, and morphology. Solitary saccular aneurysms can be resected with either primary closure if the aneurysm neck is small or with patch angioplasty using autologous or prosthetic material. Fusiform aneurysms or large segmental aneurysms can be treated by aneurysmectomy with bypass. Aortorenal bypass is the most common; however, if the aorta is heavily calcified, one may need to consider more indirect bypass options including iliorenal, hepatorenal, or spleno-renal bypass.[4,5,9] Complex distal or intrarenal aneurysms that involve multiple arterial segments require exposure of the renal hilum and warm ischemia time can be prolonged. In these circumstances, extracorporeal reconstruction allows for the necessary exposure and the kidney can be maintained with cold perfusion. After ex vivo surgery, the kidney can either be autotransplanted in its original location or into the iliac fossa. Total nephrectomy, which was once the standard of care, especially for complex distal branch aneurysms, is most often performed in the setting of renal artery aneurysm rupture where the patient is hemodynamically unstable and the warm ischemia time is prolonged.[8]

COMPLICATIONS

TECHNICAL

Graft choice

Conduit choice is important when planning open operative management of renal artery aneurysms. The options are autologous conduit, which includes saphenous vein or hypogastric artery, or synthetic conduit.[10] Saphenous vein is the most commonly used bypass conduit at about 75%; however, it risks aneurysmal dilation over time, so hypogastric artery is often favored for children and young adults in an effort to avoid late degeneration.[10] Synthetic conduit may include Dacron or polytetrafluorethylene (PTFE) when distal renal targets are appropriately sized (> 4 mm).[11] Autogenous tissue is often favored due to its resistance to infection, ease of handling for branched renal artery aneurysm repair, and long term durability.[12] Earlier review of complications from saphenous bypass grafts for renal artery reconstruction demonstrated 0–1% required revision.[13,14] Traditionally, saphenous vein grafts were thought to have superior primary patency rates in comparison to PTFE; however, patency rates may be comparable. English et al. demonstrated a 4-year patency rate of 96% with saphenous vein.[10] Pfieffer et al. similarly reported a patency rate of 95% with an average follow-up of 99 months, whereas a large analysis by Paty et al. showed a primary graft patency of 92% at 108 months with PTFE.[15,16]

Early Graft Failure

When either acute thrombosis or stenosis occurs, it requires urgent intervention to avoid renal compromise. Acute occlusion of the bypass graft in the perioperative period is usually the result of technical failure resulting from dissection flaps, graft kinking/twisting, or anastomotic constrictions. An end-to-end anastomosis with a generous spatulation of the graft and artery can lessen the risk for stricture.[13] Revascularization for stenosis, alternatively, may intel placement of an interposition graft or a vein patch angioplasty across the constricted area. Alternatively, the surgeon may opt to repair the area of stenosis via endovascular techniques, particularly if re-operation would pose a significant risk given the patient's comorbidities. Transluminal angioplasty with or without stenting has been shown to resolve anastomotic stenosis.[17,18]

Thrombosis of a renal artery bypass graft may be secondary to kinking of the graft; if vein conduit is used, the presence of valves in the region of the anastomosis may lead to stagnation of blood flow and thrombus formation. In this setting, re-operation with graft thrombectomy, repair of any technical defects, and/or a redo bypass may be warranted.[19] Though re-operation to address acute occlusion is ideal, it can be fraught with significant morbidity. There have been cases where non-surgical alternatives have been employed to address acute graft failure from thrombosis. Options for revascularization include direct thrombolysis or percutaneous thrombectomy. Thrombolysis, though likely to restore patency, has many disadvantages.[19] The duration of lytic therapy can be lengthy, taking several hours to days; if perfusion to the kidney is compromised for that duration, the kidney might be rendered non-functional. In patients who have recently undergone major abdominal surgery, thrombolysis also poses a high bleeding risk, thus its use in the perioperative setting is limited.[19] Percutaneous thrombectomy is advantageous because it can retrieve fresh thrombus readily without enduring the bleeding risk and it does not necessarily preclude re-operation if it proves to be unsuccessful.[19] In the event of failed revascularization, nephrectomy may be inevitable.[9,20]

LATE COMPLICATIONS

Graft dilation and aneurysm formation

Over time saphenous vein graft may demonstrate dilation, which has been reported to occur in 20–40% of vein grafts used in aortorenal bypasses; however, progression to a true aneurysm is less common.[21,22] Aneurysmal degeneration in vein grafts has been reported in 5–6% of cases followed with arteriography.[21,22] The mechanism for dilation remains unclear. Travis et al. hypothesized that the dilation may be due to the low-resistance, high-velocity flow that occurs with aortorenal bypasses, similar to that which leads to dilation of vein in arteriovenous fistula maturation for hemodialysis.[12] In some cases the aneurysmal change is poststenotic.[13] Dilation also occurs in arterial conduit, but it is less common.[23] Complications of aneurysmal change include distal embolization of thrombotic debris resulting in renal infarction and rupture. Aneurysmal rupture would most certainly be catastrophic; however, there have only been two case reports in the literature of late rupture of an aortorenal vein graft.[12,24] Lavigne et al. presented a case of a 42-year-old woman who had undergone a saphenous vein aortorenal bypass graft at the age of 23 who was found to have a 6 cm aneurysm of the graft. Rupture of the graft led to emergent exploration and ultimately nephrectomy due to hemodynamic instability.[24] The other case report by Travis et al. is of a 75-year-old woman who had undergone a saphenous vein aortorenal bypass graft 22 years prior and subsequently developed a 6 cm aneurysm. Intraopertively, the aneurysm ruptured. She underwent resection of the aneurysm with placement of a PTFE bypass graft.[12]

Management of aneurysmal vein graft is typically via open surgical technique. Plication of the aneurysmal graft has been performed as a means to limit further dilation.[13] Alternatively, the aneurysmal portion may be excised and replaced with synthetic graft.[25] In the advent of endovascular approaches for the management of aneurysm formation of native renal artery, there are cases where these techniques have also been applied to aneurysmal aortorenal vein bypass graft. Novotny et al. reported the case of a 77-year-old man who had undergone bilateral venous aortorenal bypass grafts 30 years previously and developed a stenosis of the proximal anastomosis and 4.2 cm aneurysm of the left renal bypass graft. A self-expandable stent graft was placed in the aneurysm, which also dilated the stenosis. At 3 months, CT angiography confirmed stent patency and complete thrombosis of the aneurysm sac.[26] In another case report, a 31-year-old woman with Takayasu arteritis underwent an aortorenal saphenous vein bypass graft 5 years previous. She developed a 1.5 cm aneurysm of the vein graft, which was addressed with embolization. 12 month follow-up with CTA demonstrated no recurrence of the aneurysm.[27]

Pseudoaneurysms are also rare complications of renovascular reconstruction.[28] Unlike true aneurysms, which involve dilation of all three layers of the vessel wall, pseudoaneurysms result from injury to at least one of the layers of the arterial wall forming a hematoma that then becomes encapsulated from the reactive fibrosis that occurs in the surrounding connective tissue.[29] Pseudoaneurysms are usually secondary to vessel injury, faulty suture line, or infection.[30] In the setting of renovascular reconstruction, pseudoaneurysms occur at the site of the anastomosis. They may be asymptomatic and found on surveillance imaging or symptomatic presenting with hypertension, hematuria, worsening renal function, or, depending on the site of the reconstruction, flank pain or abdominal pain.[30] The indications for repair include a symptomatic pseudoaneurysm, size > 2.5 cm, showing significant growth, or one caused by infection.[30] Options for repair include open surgery or endovascular repair. Endovascular repair with coils, stents, or thrombotic agents are alternatives.[30] There is always risk, regardless of operative technique, of possible loss of the kidney.

Prosthetic graft infection and enteric fistualization

One of the primary concerns with the use of synthetic conduit for renal artery reconstruction is graft infection. In general, vascular graft infection is rare with an incidence of 1–5%, though the sequelae can be devastating.[31] The leading cause of graft infections is contamination at the time of the index procedure.[32] The second most common cause is spread from a contiguous site.[31] Other etiologies include contamination from bacteremia (rare) or enteric erosion where aortoenteric fistula may lead to graft infection or vice versa.[31,32]

Aortoenteric fistula following abdominal aortic repair is a rare complication with an incidence of 0.36 to 1.6%, but is a well-documented phenomenon.[33,34] Enteric fistualization following renal artery bypass with synthetic graft is less common.[1] Similarly when left untreated, it is nearly fatal. Of the various bypass options for renal artery revascularization, enteric fistulization is reported primarily in patients who have undergone aortorenal bypass.[35–39] Gastrointestinal bleeding is the most common presenting symptoms with over 50% of patients experiencing a herald bleed. Other symptoms include abdominal pain, back pain, general malaise, retroperitoneal abscess, shock, sepsis, septic embolization, or graft occlusion.[40,41] Management involves resuscitation and hemodynamic support where appropriate, broad spectrum antibiotic therapy to include coverage of enteric flora, and surgical repair. The mainstay of treatment is excision of the graft and resection of the affected portion of the intestine.[40] Open repair is associated with significant operative mortality ranging from 40% to 50%; within the last two decades endovascular techniques have been employed as a means to bridge unstable patients. In the long term, endovascular repair has been associated with higher rates of recurrent infection and bleeding.[41–43] Additionally, the use of endovascular techniques for aortoenteric fistulas have been in patients who had undergone primary repair of abdominal aorta or thoracic aorta pathology and not necessarily renal artery reconstructions.

PERIPROCEDURAL COMPLICATIONS

Intraprocedural rupture and hemorrhage

Renal artery aneurysm rupture intraoperatively is potentially life threatening. If the bleeding can be controlled in a short period of time and the relevant anatomical exposures for renal artery reconstruction can be made, it may be reasonable to continue with kidney salvage. However, if the patient is hemodynamically unstable, or if the warm ischemia time would result in kidney failure, nephrectomy is the operation of choice.[44]

In general, management of intraoperative hemorrhage is a concerted effort between the surgical and anesthesia teams. The primary tenet of early hemorrhage control is rapid control of the source of bleeding. In the case of rupture, the approach detailed above may allow for hemorrhage control; however, during major open intra-abdominal surgery, there are numerous potential sources of bleeding from injury to other arterial or venous structures, the anastomosis of the reconstructed vessels, adjacent organs, or generalized microvascular bleeding. Bleeding from vessels requires obtaining proximal and distal control followed by either restoration of flow via a conduit or, intentional ligation of the offending vessel. Topical hemostatic agents that are collagen- or fibrin-based derivatives may be efficacious in anastomotic bleeding or more generalized microvascular bleeding.[45]

It is prudent in the midst of addressing hemorrhage that the lethal triad of coagulopathy, hypothermia (temperature < 34°C), and acidosis (pH < 7.2) be avoided as it carries a significant risk of mortality.[46] Resuscitation for hemorrhage should be guided by the magnitude and rate of blood loss, evidence of organ ischemia, and intravascular volume status rather than an absolute transfusion threshold. Initial resuscitation may be with crystalloid; however, blood products should be given. For massive hemorrhage, a packed red blood cells to platelets to fresh frozen plasma ratio should be 1:1:1 as it reduces mortality (ie: massive transfusion protocol).[47,48] Additionally, resuscitative efforts can be tailored toward the degree of coagulopathy that is present. Viscoelastic methods such as thromboelastography (TEG) and rotational elastometry (ROTEM) can be useful point of care diagnostic tools to reduce the number of transfusions.[49]

Renal perfusion

Prolonged warm ischemia time, greater than 30–40 minutes, can result in poor renal function and the development of acute tubular necrosis and acute kidney injury, which may lead to temporary or permanent dialysis. When prolonged warm ischemia is anticipated, adjuncts to decrease the metabolic rate of the kidney and preserve function should be considered. Two common techniques for renal artery perfusion include ex vivo and in situ cold renal perfusion. For the ex vivo technique, the kidney is completely mobilized from Gerota's fascia and freed from the surrounding structures. The ureter is left intact and mobilized to the level of the pelvic brim and the periureteral collaterals are controlled with elastic loops. Once mobilization is complete and before the renal artery and vein are ligated, the patient is systemically heparinized. The renal vein is divided at its juncture with the vena cava. The kidney is placed in a plastic sling, immersed in ice slush and the kidney is flushed with commercially available perfusate that has been chilled to 4C. In the in situ technique, the renal vein is left intact and a venotomy is made before cold perfusion of the kidney. Similar to the ex vivo technique, surface hypothermia is maintained by immersing the kidney in ice. Regardless of technique, the kidney should be flushed until it appears asanguineous and the venous effluent is clear. The remainder of the hilar dissection is performed and before the final division of the renal artery branches is performed, the kidney is once again perfused with perfusate.[10,50] Most perfusates use cold crystalloid, either lactated Ringer's or 0.9% normal saline. They may also use various additives including mannitol, prostacyclin E, methylprednisolone, or heparin.[1,51] There is no intrinsic benefit of ex vivo compared to in situ cold renal perfusion with respect to preservation of renal function.[15] Instead, the decision should be dictated by the exposure that most easily facilitates repair.

Complex renal artery aneurysms involving multiple branches may not be conducive to in vivo revascularization because of suboptimal exposure, which increases the risk for prolonged renal ischemic time. In those circumstances, ex vivo reconstruction is advantageous. A nephrectomy is performed, after which the kidney is perfused with renal preservation solution. Following reconstruction, the kidney may be autotransplanted to the iliac fossa or to its original site.[51,52]

Surveillance postprocedure

Patients who have had renal artery aneurysm repairs should be monitored closely. Yearly renal artery duplex ultrasounds are used to monitor the patency of the reconstruction and detect any technical problems that necessitate early corrective intervention, whether open or endovascular. Abnormal findings on duplex ultrasound are confirmed with CT, magnetic resonance angiography, or diagnostic angiography.[9] Majority of patients (58%–75%) who undergo repair of renal artery aneurysm repair are either cured or experience significant improvement in their blood pressure.[15,53]

Persistent or recurrent hypertension may be the result of renal parenchymal disease or failures of the primary reconstruction. The imaging techniques described above can help identify the latter, which might require open surgical or endovascular intervention.[13,54]

REFERENCES

1. Coleman DM, Stanley JC. Renal artery aneurysms. J Vasc Surg. 2015 Sep;62(3): 779–85.
2. Poutasse EF. Renal artery aneurysms. J Urol. 1975 Apr;113(4): 443–9.
3. Mattar SG, Kumar AG, Lumsden AB. Vascular complications in Ehlers-Danlos syndrome. Am Surg. 1994 Nov;60(11):827–31.
4. StanleyJC, Rhodes EL, Gewertz BL, Chang CY, Walter JF, Fry WJ. Renal artery aneurysms. Significance of macroaneurysms exclusive of dissections and fibrodysplastic mural dilations. Arch Surg Chic Ill 1960. 1975 Nov;110(11): 1327–33.
5. González J, Esteban M, Andrés G, Linares E, Martínez-Salamanca JI. Renal Artery Aneurysms. Curr Urol Rep. 2014 Jan;15(1): 376.
6. Poutasse EF. Renal artery aneurysms: their natural history and surgery. J Urol. 1966 Mar;95(3): 297–306.
7. Dzsinich C, Gloviczki P, McKusick MA, Pairolero PC, Bower TC, Hallett JW, et al. Surgical management of renal artery aneurysm. Cardiovasc Surg Lond Engl. 1993 Jun;1(3):243–7.
8. Calligaro KD, Dougherty MJ. Renal artery aneurysms and arteriovenous fistulae. In: Sidawy AN, Perler BA, editors. Rutherford's Vascular Surgery and Endovascular Therapy. 9th ed. Philadelphia: WB Saunders; 2019. p. 1696–703.
9. Henke PK, Cardneau JD, Welling TH, Upchurch GR, Wakefield TW, Jacobs LA, et al. Renal artery aneurysms: a 35-year clinical experience with 252 aneurysms in 168 patients. Ann Surg. 2001 Oct; 234(4): 454–62; discussion 462–463.
10. English WP, Pearce JD, Craven TE, Wilson DB, Edwards MS, Ayerdi J, et al. Surgical management of renal artery aneurysms. J Vasc Surg. 2004 Jul;40(1): 53–60.
11. Steuer J, Bergqvist D, Björck M. Surgical Renovascular Reconstruction for Renal Artery Stenosis and Aneurysm: Long-Term Durability and Survival. Eur J Vasc Endovasc Surg Off J Eur Soc Vasc Surg. 2019 Apr;57(4): 562–8.
12. Travis JA, Hansen KJ, Miller PR, Dean RH, Geary RL. Aneurysmal degeneration and late rupture of an aortorenal vein graft: case report, review of the literature, and implications for conduit selection. J Vasc Surg. 2000 Sep;32(3): 612–5.
13. Stanley JC, Whitehouse WM, Zelenock GB, Graham LM, Cronenwett JL, Lindenauer SM. Reoperation for complications of renal artery reconstructive surgery undertaken for treatment of renovascular hypertension. J Vasc Surg. 1985 Jan;2(1): 133–44.
14. Hansen KJ, Deitch JS, Oskin TC, Ligush J, Craven TE, Dean RH. Renal artery repair: consequence of operative failures. Ann Surg. 1998 May;227(5): 678–89; discussion 689–690.
15. Pfeiffer T, Reiher L, Grabitz K, Grünhage B, Häfele S, Voiculescu A, et al. Reconstruction for renal artery aneurysm: operative techniques and long-term results. J Vasc Surg. 2003 Feb;37(2): 293–300.
16. Paty PS, Darling RC, Lee D, Chang BB, Roddy SP, Kreienberg PB, et al. Is prosthetic renal artery reconstruction a durable procedure? An analysis of 489 bypass grafts. J Vasc Surg. 2001 Jul; 34(1): 127–32.
17. Garfinkel HB, Rohr RE, Rottenberg RW. Angioplasty of a stenotic aorto-renal artery saphenous vein bypass graft to a single kidney. Am J Kidney Dis Off J Natl Kidney Found. 1984 Sep;4(2): 171–4.
18. Kusakabe M, Sasaki H, Sato J, Akahane M, Miyata T, Ohtomo K. Percutaneous transluminal renal angioplasty with stenting for stenotic venous bypass grafts: report of two cases. SpringerPlus. 2013;2: 456.
19. Rivitz SM, Kaufman JA, Cambria RP, Geller SC. Percutaneous aspiration thrombectomy of an acutely occluded aortorenal bypass graft. AJR Am J Roentgenol. 1995 Feb;164(2): 455–8.
20. Robinson WP, Bafford R, Belkin M, Menard MT. Favorable outcomes with in situ techniques for surgical repair of complex renal artery aneurysms. J Vasc Surg. 2011 Mar;53(3): 684–91.
21. Dean RH, Wilson JP, Burko H, Foster JH. Saphenous vein aortorenal bypass grafts: Serial arteriographic study. Ann Surg. 1974 Oct;180(4): 469–78.
22. Stanley JC, Ernst CB, Fry WJ. Fate of 100 aortorenal vein grafts: characteristics of late graft expansion, aneurysmal dilatation, and stenosis. Surgery. 1973 Dec;74(6): 931–44.
23. Lye CR, String ST, Wylie EJ, Stoney RJ. Proceedings: Aortorenal arterial autografts: late observations. J Cardiovasc Surg (Torino). 1976 Feb;17(1): 84–5.
24. Lavigne J, Keppenne V, Limet R. Late rupture of a saphenous vein aortorenal graft. J Vasc Surg. 1999 Apr;29(4): 722–3.
25. Bath J, Cho J-S. Aneurysm of a 32-year-old aortorenal saphenous vein bypass graft. Ann Vasc Surg. 2012 Nov;26(8): 1128.e7–1128.e10.

26. Novotný J, Peregrin JH, Stríbrná J, Janousek R. Treatment of venous aortorenal bypass graft aneurysm using a stent-graft. Cardiovasc Intervent Radiol. 2010 Feb;33(1): 177–81.
27. Hu H, Chen X, Wu Z, Zhao J, Huang B, Ma Y, et al. Aneurysmal Degeneration of an Aortorenal Bypass for Takayasu Renal Artery Stenosis: A Novel Endovascular Intervention. Ann Vasc Surg. 2018 May;49: 316.e1–316.e4.
28. Dimitroulis D, Bokos J, Zavos G, Nikiteas N, Karidis NP, Katsaronis P, et al. Vascular complications in renal transplantation: a single-center experience in 1367 renal transplantations and review of the literature. Transplant Proc. 2009 Jun;41(5): 1609–14.
29. Ngo TC, Lee JJ, Gonzalgo ML. Renal pseudoaneurysm: an overview. Nat Rev Urol. 2010 Nov; 7(11): 619–25.
30. Che H, Men C, Yang M, Zhang J, Chen P, Yong J. Endovascular repair of a transplant renal artery anastomotic pseudoaneurysm using the snorkel technique. J Vasc Surg. 2014 Oct;60(4): 1052–5.
31. Wilson WR, Bower TC, Creager MA, Amin-Hanjani S, O'Gara PT, Lockhart PB, et al. Vascular Graft Infections, Mycotic Aneurysms, and Endovascular Infections: A Scientific Statement From the American Heart Association. Circulation. 2016 15;134(20): e412–60.
32. Swain TW, Calligaro KD, Dougherty MD. Management of infected aortic prosthetic grafts. Vasc Endovascular Surg. 2004 Feb;38(1): 75–82.
33. Champion MC, Sullivan SN, Coles JC, Goldbach M, Watson WC. Aortoenteric fistula. Incidence, presentation recognition, and management. Ann Surg. 1982 Mar;195(3): 314–7.
34. Hallett JW, Marshall DM, Petterson TM, Gray DT, Bower TC, Cherry KJ, et al. Graft-related complications after abdominal aortic aneurysm repair: Reassurance from a 36-year population-based experience. J Vasc Surg. 1997 Feb;25(2): 277–84; discussion 285–286.
35. Shaigany A, Gillespie L, Mock JP, Vassarhelyi L, Danovitch SH. Aortoenteric fistula. A complication of renal artery bypass graft. Arch Intern Med. 1976 Aug;136(8): 930–2.
36. Howard RJ, Leonard JJ, Howard BD. Renal artery-cholecystoduodenal fistula. A late complication of dacron patch angioplasty for renal artery stenosis. Arch Surg Chic Ill 1960. 1978 Jul; 113(7): 888–90.
37. Keeffe EB, Krippaehne WW, Rösch J, Melnyk CS. Aortoduodenal fistula: complication of renal artery bypass graft. Gastroenterology. 1974 Dec;67(6): 1240–4.
38. Hobson JD. Endoscopic diagnosis of a bleeding fistula between a grafted renal artery and the duodenum. Gastrointest Endosc. 1976 Nov;23(2): 86–7.
39. Campbell HC, Ernst CB. Aortoenteric fistula following renal revascularization. Am Surg. 1978 Mar;44(3): 155–8.
40. Armstrong PA, Back MR, Wilson JS, Shames ML, Johnson BL, Bandyk DF. Improved outcomes in the recent management of secondary aortoenteric fistula. J Vasc Surg. 2005 Oct;42(4): 660–6.
41. Bergqvist D, Björck M. Secondary arterioenteric fistulation–a systematic literature analysis. Eur J Vasc Endovasc Surg Off J Eur Soc Vasc Surg. 2009 Jan;37(1): 31–42.
42. Kakkos SK, Papadoulas S, Tsolakis IA. Endovascular management of arterioenteric fistulas: A systemic review and meta-analysis of the literature. J Endovasc Ther Off J Int Soc Endovasc Spec. 2011 Feb;18(1): 66–77.
43. Antoniou GA, Koutsias S, Antoniou SA, Georgiakakis A, Lazarides MK, Giannoukas AD. Outcome after endovascular stent graft repair of aortoenteric fistula: A systematic review. J Vasc Surg. 2009 Mar;49(3): 782–9.
44. Orion KC, Abularrage CJ. Renal artery aneurysms: movement toward endovascular repair. Semin Vasc Surg. 2013 Dec;26(4): 226–32.
45. Chee YE, Liu SE, Irwin MG. Management of bleeding in vascular surgery. Br J Anaesth. 2016 Sep;117 Suppl 2: ii85–94.
46. Cosgriff N, Moore EE, Sauaia A, Kenny-Moynihan M, Burch JM, Galloway B. Predicting life-threatening coagulopathy in the massively transfused trauma patient: hypothermia and acidoses revisited. J Trauma. 1997 May;42(5): 857–61; discussion 861–862.
47. Zink KA, Sambasivan CN, Holcomb JB, Chisholm G, Schreiber MA. A high ratio of plasma and platelets to packed red blood cells in the first 6 hours of massive transfusion improves outcomes in a large multicenter study. Am J Surg. 2009 May;197(5): 565–70; discussion 570.
48. Duchesne JC, Hunt JP, Wahl G, Marr AB, Wang Y-Z, Weintraub SE, et al. Review of current blood transfusions strategies in a mature level I trauma center: were we wrong for the last 60 years? J Trauma. 2008 Aug;65(2): 272–6; discussion 276–278.
49. Inaba K, Rizoli S, Veigas PV, Callum J, Davenport R, Hess J, et al. 2014 Consensus conference on viscoelastic test-based transfusion guidelines for early trauma resuscitation: Report of the panel. J Trauma Acute Care Surg. 2015 Jun;78(6): 1220–9.

50. Bhamidipati CM, Coselli JS, LeMaire SA. Perfusion techniques for renal protection during thoracoabdominal aortic surgery. J Extra Corpor Technol. 2012 Mar;44(1): P31–37.
51. Crutchley TA, Pearce JD, Craven TE, Edwards MS, Dean RH, Hansen KJ. Branch renal artery repair with cold perfusion protection. J Vasc Surg. 2007 Sep;46(3): 405–12; discussion 412.
52. Dean RH, Meacham PW, Weaver FA. Ex vivo renal artery reconstructions: indications and techniques. J Vasc Surg. 1986 Dec;4(6): 546–52.
53. Klausner JQ, Lawrence PF, Harlander-Locke MP, Coleman DM, Stanley JC, Fujimura N, et al. The contemporary management of renal artery aneurysms. J Vasc Surg. 2015 Apr;61(4): 978–84.
54. Ekeström S, Liljeqvist L, Nordhus O, Tidgren B. Persisting hypertension after renal artery reconstruction. A follow-up study. Scand J Urol Nephrol. 1979;13(1): 83–8.

24

Complications of open repair of femoral and popliteal aneurysms

FARAH MOHAMMAD AND MITCHELL WEAVER

DIAGNOSIS PREVENTION AND MANAGEMENT

Degenerative aneurysms of the femoral-popliteal arterial segments are encountered much less frequently by the vascular surgeon than aneurysms involving the aorta and iliac arterial segments, and the same goes for their repair and complications of those repairs. While open repair of aneurysms involving the femoral and popliteal arteries is generally straight forward and associated with very acceptable results when performed in an elective setting, these operations, like all vascular surgical operations, may be accompanied by complications which usually fall into the categories of loss of graft patency/limb ischemia, wound complications/infection, and in late follow-up progression of disease. In order to prevent complications and provide the best outcome for the patient when they do occur, there are several steps that can be taken: ensuring the initial operation is performed for an appropriate indication, the patient is medically optimized for the operation, the conduct of the operation is performed in the appropriate manner, and when complications do occur they are promptly recognized and treated.

INDICATIONS FOR INITIAL REPAIR

The natural history and true incidence of aneurysm in the femoral-popliteal arterial segments is not as well defined as for aortic aneurysms. Degenerative popliteal artery aneurysms (Figure 24.1) are the most common type of true peripheral aneurysm, with degenerative femoral aneurysms being significantly less prevalent, most often limited to the common femoral artery or involving the proximal origins of the superficial or deep femoral artery. Isolated superficial femoral or deep femoral artery aneurysms are less common. It is recommended that all patients fit for surgery who have a symptomatic femoral or popliteal aneurysm undergo repair. Symptoms may be acute limb-threatening ischemia from arterial thrombosis, thromboembolism or, very rarely rupture, or chronic symptoms of ischemia manifested as claudication or tissue loss, which may have an insidious onset due to chronic silent embolization. Aneurysms may also present with symptoms from local compression of the nerve or vein causing pain, paresthesia, or limb swelling.[1–3]

Asymptomatic aneurysms found incidentally on an imaging study or as a pulsatile mass on physical exam may also present for evaluation. Ideal management of these aneurysms is less clear. Multiple reports find that up to 35% of patients with popliteal artery aneurysms will develop ischemic complications in follow-up, and those presenting with symptoms may require an amputation up to 25% of the time, which as lead to a traditional size criteria of ≥ 2.0 cm to consider elective repair popliteal artery repair.[1–3] The size criteria for femoral artery aneurysms (Figure 24.2) has traditionally been ≥ 2.5 cm, however a recent study suggested that the size for elective femoral aneurysm repair should be increased to ≥ to 3.5 cm.[4] Additional factors that are considered when contemplating aneurysms repair should include the presence of thrombus, as significant thrombus in a low-risk patient may justify repair at a smaller diameter, as lack of thrombus in a high-risk patient may justify watchful waiting in a larger aneurysm. Distal arterial runoff should also be considered as distal arterial occlusions may be evidence of chronic embolization in an otherwise asymptomatic patient. Ambulatory/functional status as well as overall health status and comorbidities should also weigh in the

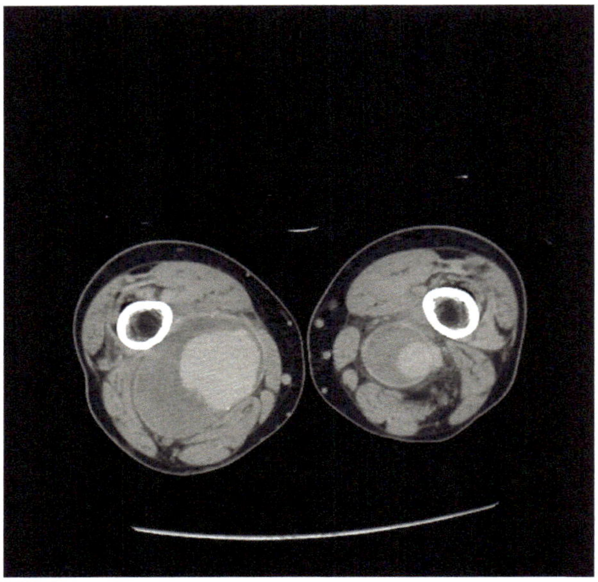

Figure 24.1 Computed tomography angiogram demonstrating bilateral large popliteal artery aneurysms.

decision as a nonambulatory high-risk patient's risk benefit ratio of undergoing elective and preventive procedure needs to be thoroughly considered.

For popliteal artery aneurysms specifically, a greater degree of distortion or angulation of the artery may increase risk of thrombosis and should be considered when deciding to intervene. One additional scenario to specifically mention is the completely thrombosed popliteal artery aneurysm in an asymptomatic patient or even one with claudication. These patients do not automatically require surgical intervention, with indications for invasive intervention being the same as claudication from atherosclerotic peripheral vascular occlusive disease.

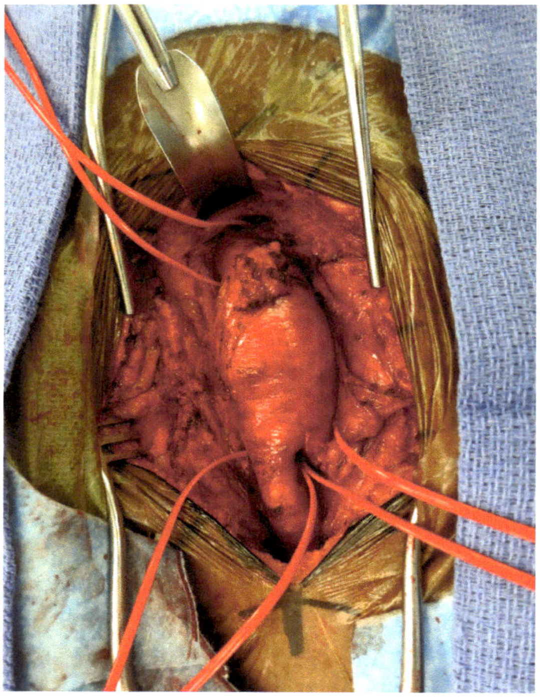

Figure 24.2 Intra-operative photograph of common femoral artery aneurysm.

FEMORAL ANEURYSM REPAIR AND COMPLICATIONS

Initial repair of common femoral artery aneurysms is generally straightforward and performed through a longitudinal incision overlying the artery. Generally adequate proximal exposure can be obtained with retraction of the inguinal ligament and exposure of the distal external iliac artery. In rare occasions where more proximal exposure is required, an oblique supra inguinal incision can be made with dissection carried down to develop the retroperitoneal space exposing the external iliac artery. If the aneurysm is isolated to the common femoral artery endpoint, a sewing ring may be obtained distally at the common femoral artery bifurcation. If the proximal portions of either or both the superficial or deep femoral arteries are involved, a reconstruction with a direct bypass to one with reimplantation or short jump graft to the other artery, if both are patent. Patients are systemically heparinized prior to arterial clamping. Using a technique similar to abdominal aortic aneurysm repair where the back wall is not resected may theoretically decrease injury to surrounding structures if suitable to do so. Reconstructions are usually performed with a prosthetic graft of either polytetrafluoroethylene (PTFE) (Goretex) or polyethylene terephthalate (Dacron), which allow for good size match and have been shown to have excellent patency; however, an adequate size vein graft may also be used. Isolated aneurysms of either the superficial femoral or deep femoral artery also may be repaired with resection or ligation of the artery and interval bypass.

Operative outcomes have generally been quite favorable with low morbidity and mortality. A recent review by Lawrence et al. of 182 patients with 236 degenerative femoral aneurysms undergoing 177 open repairs and 3 endovascular repairs (isolated superficial femoral aneurysms) reported very low early mortality of 2 patients (one myocardial infarction and one multi-organ failure). Complications reported were infection (6%), bleeding (2%), and seroma (3%). No early or late limb loss was reported.[4] The short length and likely satisfactory inflow and outflow arteries likely explain the excellent patency and limb preservation of these bypass. Thus, if such bypass was complicated by early graft thrombosis, one's first concern would be to ensure no technical error in the anastomosis or failure to arterial disease in the inflow or out flow artery. Management of wound complications is further discussed in Chapter 26, "Complications of Axillofemoral, Femoral-Femoral and Ilio-Femoral Grafts: Diagnosis, Prevention, and Management."

POPLITEAL ANEURYSM REPAIR AND COMPLICATIONS

Considerations for open repair of popliteal aneurysms include approaches that may be medial or posterior and conduit that may be vein or a prosthetic graft. The medial approach (Figure 24.3) is the most common approach reported, with advantages including its familiarity to most surgeons, and the versatility it allows for proximal and distal exposure. This is important in cases where the aneurysm extends proximally with involvement of the superficial femoral artery, or in cases in which there is a more distal/tibial artery target as the outflow vessel. The medial approach also allows for ready access to the great saphenous vein. With the medial approach, the artery is ligated proximal and distal to the aneurysm with interval bypass. An attempt to ligate all side branches of the aneurysm should be made to prevent continued pressurization and growth of the aneurysm sac. This may also, in larger aneurysms, require opening of the aneurysm sac with ligation of branches internally to depressurize the sac. The medial approach typically requires longer bypass lengths and, especially if there is any compromise to the runoff (Figure 24.4), greater saphenous vein conduits are preferred.

The posterior approach (Figure 24.5) is performed through an S or step incision over the popliteal artery aneurysm, taking care to avoid a perpendicular incision across the knee crease. This dissection stays medial to the major nerves and veins in approaching the artery. This approach is ideal for very localized popliteal artery aneurysms, especially in cases of nerve or vein compression, as this approach allows for complete excision of the aneurysm and decompression of the space. However, proximal and distal exposure is severely limited. Proximal extent of exposure is to the adductor canal, and the distal extent of exposure by this approach is usually to about the anterior tibial artery. With this exposure, there is usually lack of ready access to an appropriately sized vein, which is the author preferred conduit; however, this approach also allows for typically very short bypasses for which the use of prosthetic grafts in this position for this indication have been reported to have satisfactory results. A recent meta-analysis by Phair et al. including 7 studies with 1427 patients (338 posterior and 1089 medial approaches) suggests superiority of posterior approach over medial approach for patency, aneurysm exclusion, and need for re-operation; the authors however acknowledge that high level comparative data were not present as the studies were observational and not randomized.[5]

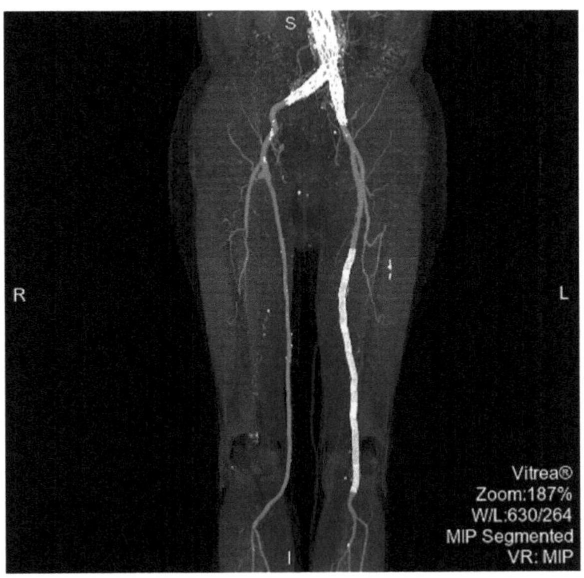

Figure 24.3 Computed tomography angiogram in patient with history of bilateral popliteal artery aneurysms. The right lower extremity demonstrates a bypass from the common femoral artery to the below-knee popliteal artery with in situ greater saphenous vein for repair of right popliteal artery aneurysm. The left lower extremity demonstrates an endovascular repair of the left popliteal artery aneurysm. Note the aorta bi-iliac endograft which was placed for repair of an aortic aneurysm.

Overall, there are very acceptable results for the elective repair of popliteal artery aneurysms, with outcomes significantly better than when repaired under emergent conditions. Overall, long-term patency appears to be better with vein grafts than with prosthetic grafts as a series by Huang et al. examined the patency of 336 grafts after popliteal artery aneurysm repair with 242 vein graft and 94 prosthetic grafts. This series demonstrated significantly better primary and secondary patency at 5 years for vein grafts (94% and 85%) versus prosthetic graft, (63% and 50%).[6] Dawson et al. in a review of the literature found 2,445 PPA in 1673 reporting patency at 5 years of 77% to 100% for vein grafts vs 29% to 74% for prosthetic grafts and with this concluded that the type of conduit, the presence of symptoms, and the quality of the runoff correlated with operative results.[1] Other series however find more favorable results for prosthetic grafts, including Pulli et al. reporting a series of 152 repairs, 118 PTFE grafts (71.5%) and 34 vein grafts (79.9%) in which no difference in patency was found at 60 months[7] and Beseth et al. reviewed a series of 30 repairs via posterior approach 25 PTFE and 5 Dacron grafts in patients with popliteal artery aneurysm, median follow-up of 21.5 months. Twenty-five patients had two- or three-vessel runoff. The 2-year primary and secondary patency were 92.2% and 95.8%, respectively, with limb salvage of 100%.[8] These patients had good runoff and presumably very short bypasses.

Morbidity and mortality for popliteal aneurysms is generally reported to be quite low. As with all vascular reconstruction complications, they typically fall into systemic complications, wound/infectious complications, and graft failure/limb ischemia complications. Systemic complications can best be avoided by proper patient selection, ensuring that cardiopulmonary status is optimized,

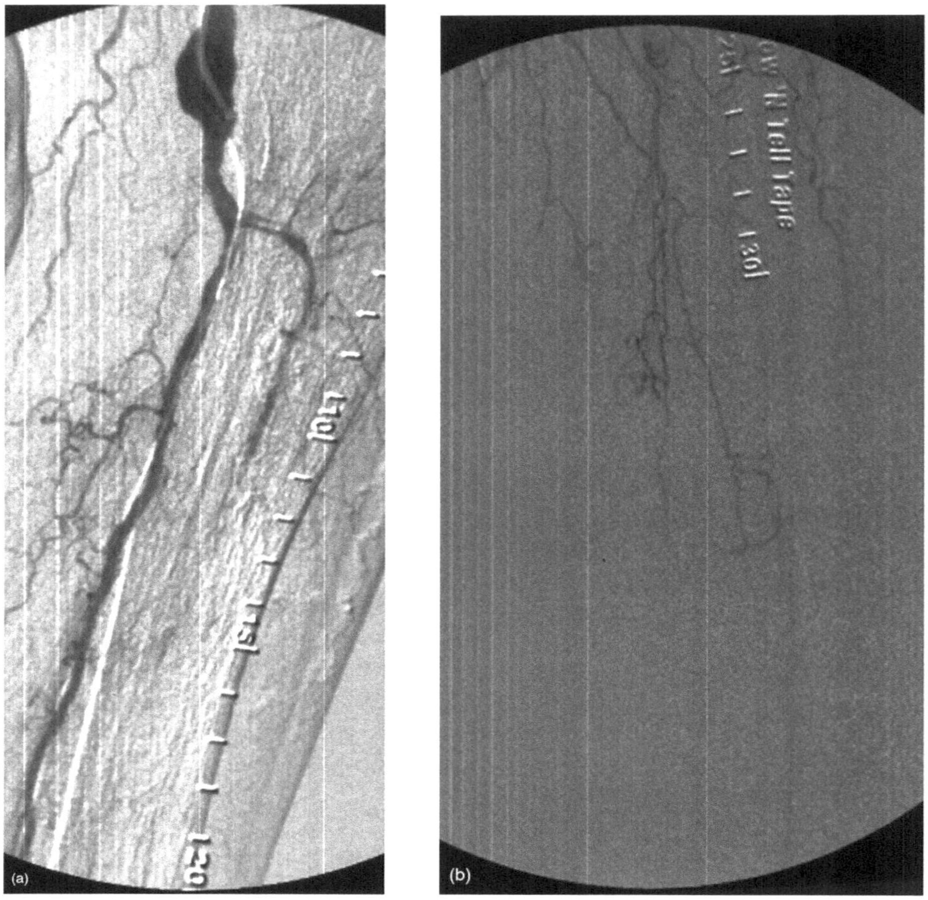

Figure 24.4 Digital subtraction angiograms in patient presenting with left lower extremity ischemia and thrombosed popliteal artery aneurysm (a) Following catheter-directed thrombolysis, a single vessel tibial artery (peroneal artery) is recovered, but still with severely compromised tibial vessel runoff. (b) Prior to catheter-directed thrombolysis, no tibial are vessels visualized.

cessation of smoking by smokers, and optimization of comorbidities such as hypertension, dyslipidemia, chronic obstructive pulmonary disease, and anemia. Wound complications are best avoided with proper tissue handling and meticulous wound closure. Strategies aimed at reducing wound infections include ensuring appropriate perioperative antibiotic administration, appropriate skin prep, maintaining a normothermic patient, and avoiding blood loss. Prosthetic graft infection typically requires graft excision and re-do bypass via an uninfected field. For further discussion of management of wound and infection see Chapter 26, "Complications of Axillofemoral, Femoral-Femoral and Iliofemoral Grafts: Diagnosis, Prevention, and Management."

In cases of early graft failure, the bypass should be inspected for technical error, which could include a proximal or distal anastomotic complication, or a twisting or kinking of the graft. The inflow artery should be evaluated for adequate flow and to ensure that there are no proximal hemodynamically significant lesions that would be affecting it, along with assessment of the outflow artery, as low flow and poor runoff may be etiologies of early graft thrombosis. The anastomoses should be examined for technical defects. The bypass conduit should also be examined for twist, kinks, or sites of possible compression thoughout its course. In the case of vein conduit, the vein should be examined for any abnormal segment or retained valves. The patient should also be anticoagulated, and a hypercoagulable state or thrombogenic conduit should be considered. Thrombectomy may be performed by gently passing a balloon catheter, and possibly also locally instilling a thrombolytic such as tissue plasminogen activating factor. Once flow is restored in the graft, the graft, as well as the arteries proximal and distal to it, may be further interrogated with digital subtraction angiography (using multiple projections if no obvious defect is found) or duplex ultrasound. If the conduit is believed to be the factor leading to failure, if the original graft was prosthetic, and there is satisfactory quality vein, consider redoing the bypass with vein. If original bypass was with vein which is now felt to be of poor quality, consider redoing bypass with better quality vein if available or with a prosthetic conduit.

In cases of late graft failure, treatment depends on degree of symptoms. Late graft failure may present as

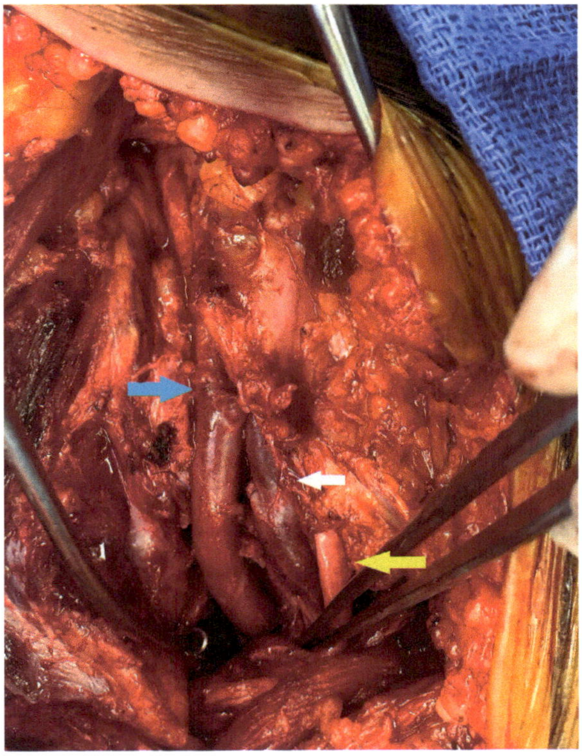

Figure 24.5 Intraoperative photograph of posterior approach to popliteal artery aneurysms. Red arrow is pointing to anastomosis between native artery and vein graft which is medial. The blue arrow is directed at the popliteal vein, and the yellow arrow is directed at the nerve.

insidiously as a decrease in ankle brachial indices on routine follow-up and/or a return to preoperative ischemic symptoms, to profound acute limb ischemia. Patients presenting with acute limb ischemia are evaluated using Rutherford criteria[9] for acute limb ischemia, which involves evaluation of sensory function, motor function, and presence or absence of pedal Doppler signals. Those patients with neurologic deficit require more urgent intervention for hope of achieving limb salvage. On the other hand, a patient with no symptoms or minimal symptoms of claudication may only require observation.

The diagnosis of graft occlusion can be typically made on physical exam by loss of graft as well as distal pulses, and can be confirmed with duplex ultrasound. Both CT angiography as well as catheter-based angiography can confirm graft occlusion as well as add additional assessment of inflow and outflow arteries. In appropriate candidates, catheter-directed thrombolysis may be initiated at the time of catheter-directed angiography if the graft thrombosis is believed to be relatively acute. This allows for possible salvage of the graft and possible exposure of an underlying lesion that led to the graft, which can then be treated in order to prevent recurrent thrombosis. Additional treatment options would include an attempt at surgical graft thrombectomy, and after assessing for an underlying culprit lesion that can be treated, or performing a redo bypass after identifying appropriate inflow and outflow arteries as well as adequate conduit.

An additional late complication of popliteal artery aneurysm repair performed by ligation and interval bypass can be continued growth of the aneurysm. This is caused by continued arterial pressurization of the aneurysm sac via genicular branches of the popliteal artery that were not ligated at the time of surgery. Continued aneurysm growth may lead to neuropathic symptoms like nerve compression, swelling from venous compression, and pain. Treatment involves either excision of the aneurysm or exploration of the aneurysm with evacuation of its contents and over-sewing any bleeding branches from within the aneurysm sac.

REFERENCES

1. Dawson I, Sie RB, van Bockel JH. Atherosclerotic popliteal aneurysm. British journal of surgery. 1997;84(3): 293–9.
2. Szilagyi DE, Schwartz RL, Reddy DJ. Popliteal arterial aneurysms. Their natural history and management. Archives of surgery (Chicago, Ill: 1960). 1981;116(5): 724–8.
3. Vermilion BD, Kimmins SA, Pace WG, Evans WE. A review of one hundred forty-seven popliteal aneurysms with long-term follow-up. Surgery. 1981;90(6): 1009–14.
4. Lawrence PF, Harlander-Locke MP, Oderich GS, Humphries MD, Landry GJ, Ballard JL, et al. The current management of isolated degenerative femoral artery aneurysms is too aggressive for their natural history. Journal of vascular surgery. 2014;59(2): 343–9.
5. Phair A, Hajibandeh S, Hajibandeh S, Kelleher D, Ibrahim R, Antoniou GA. Meta-analysis of posterior versus medial approach for popliteal artery aneurysm repair. Journal of vascular surgery. 2016;64(4): 1141–50.e1.
6. Huang Y, Gloviczki P, Noel AA, Sullivan TM, Kalra M, Gullerud RE, et al. Early complications and long-term outcome after open surgical treatment of popliteal artery aneurysms: is exclusion with saphenous vein bypass still the gold standard? Journal of vascular surgery. 2007;45(4): 706–13; discussion 13–5.
7. Pulli R, Dorigo W, Troisi N, Innocenti AA, Pratesi G, Azas L, et al. Surgical management of popliteal artery aneurysms: Which factors affect outcomes? Journal of vascular surgery. 2006;43(3): 481–7.
8. Beseth BD, Moore WS. The posterior approach for repair of popliteal artery aneurysms. Journal of vascular surgery. 2006;43(5): 940–4; discussion 4–5.
9. Rutherford RB. Clinical staging of acute limb ischemia as the basis for choice of revascularization method: when and how to intervene. Seminars in vascular surgery. 2009;22(1): 5–9.

25

Complications of open aortofemoral bypass

ELIZABETH A. BLAZICK

While not as common as infrainguinal occlusive disease, atherosclerotic occlusive aortoiliac disease remains a common cause of lower extremity ischemic symptoms in middle age and elderly patients. Though aortoiliac occlusive disease alone is rarely the cause of critical limb ischemia due to sufficient collateral circulation, it can result in disabling claudication involving the hips, buttocks, thighs, and calves. Critical limb ischemia may develop when this disease pattern develops in conjunction with infrainguinal disease. In males, this can also lead to impotence as a result of internal pudendal artery hypoperfusion. The triad of Leriche's syndrome is described as impotence, thigh and buttock claudication, and decreased femoral pulses, and should warrant a search for aortoililac occlusive disease. Aortoililac plaque can also be the cause of the microembolization of atherosclerotic debris to the terminal vessels in the feet, causing "blue toe syndrome" and leading to significant pain and potentially tissue loss despite adequate resting perfusion pressures and sometimes intact distal pulses.

Typically, patients with aortoiliac occlusive disease alone who present with claudication are younger than those patients presenting with infrainguinal disease, though they carry many of the same risk factors including tobacco use, diabetes, hypercholesterolemia, and hypertension. Open aortoililac revascularization can be considered in patients with severe, lifestyle-limiting claudication who have been medically optimized in terms of their other comorbidities. Revascularization should also be pursued for any patient with critical limb ischemia or any evidence of atheroembolic event.

Preoperative workup traditionally included formal diagnostic angiogram, however that has largely been replaced by noninvasive axial imaging, including CTA or MRA to delineate the extent of the disease. The Trans-Atlantic Intersociety Consensus (TASC II) document has helped dictate first-line therapy depending on extent of disease. Percutaneous balloon therapy is often sought as first-line therapy in patients with TASC A or B lesions (focal, short segment lesions 3–10 cm, unilateral or bilateral). Open revascularization is generally reserved for those with long segment occlusions or diffuse disease.[1] With the advancement of endovascular techniques and equipment, aortobifemoral bypass (ABF), which had long been considered the gold standard for aortoiliac occlusive disease, is increasingly now reserved for more complex patients. This impact has been two-fold in consideration of perioperative complications: surgeons are performing a lower volume of open surgery, and those surgeries are reserved for patients with more demanding anatomy, often in the setting of previous percutaneous failure. This trend in the management of aortoiliac occlusive disease makes awareness of the complications of ABF of the utmost importance for any surgeon performing this procedure, to both mitigate the risk and appropriately identify and manage any complication that may occur.

BRIEF TECHNICAL SUMMARY

Preoperative planning is critical for the performance of an expedient and successful operation. Attention should be paid to the proximal extent of the disease, both to identify an appropriate clamp zone as well as identify suitable aorta to serve as the proximal anastomosis. The location of the left renal vein should be noted as anterior or posterior to the aorta to avoid inadvertent injury during dissection or clamping. The proximal anastomosis can be performed in an end-to-end or end-to-side fashion. Most surgeons favor the end-to-end anastomosis and reserve end-to-side only for those individuals who lose perfusion of an important branch, such as a hypogastric or inferior mesenteric artery (IMA), that is perfused only by in-line flow from the aorta and cannot be perfused by retrograde flow from the femoral anastomosis, as in the case of

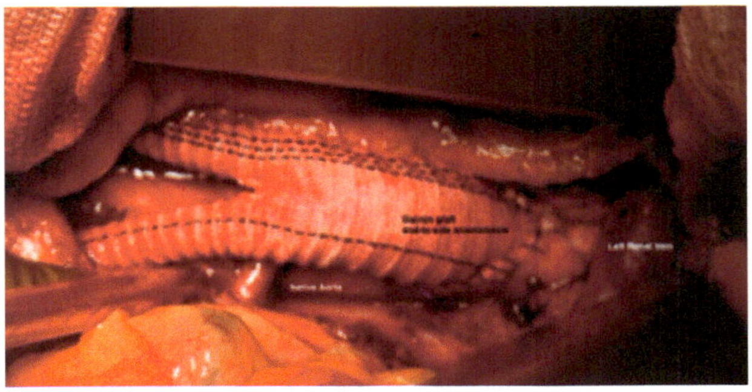

Figure 25.1 End-to-side aortic anastomosis at the level of the renal vessels. Note the graft is trimmed to ensure a short main body.

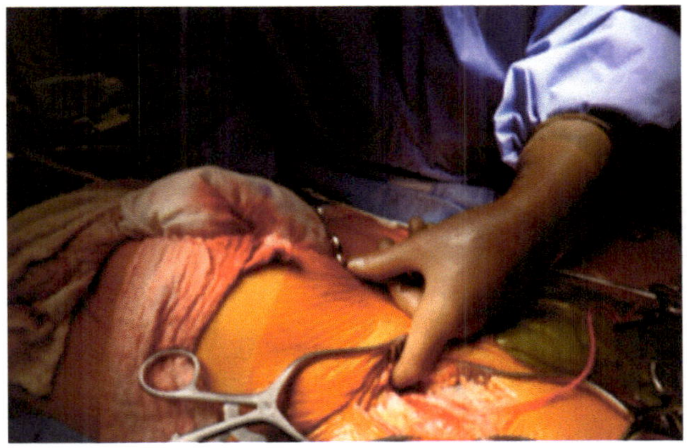

Figure 25.2 Creation of the tunnel using blunt dissection with fingers.

external iliac artery occlusion (Figure 25.1). The femoral vessels should be carefully studied on imaging to determine if further reconstruction, including endarterectomy or profundoplasty, will be required at the time of surgery. Generally, the size of the graft should be based on the size of the femoral arteries to avoid significant size mismatch at these anastomoses.

The patient is positioned supine and prepped from nipples to knees bilaterally. Traditionally, both groins are dissected first to avoid insensate heat loss from the open abdominal incision; however, our experience has suggested that length of surgery correlates with higher infection risk in exposed infrainguinal incisions, therefore our practice is to begin with a midline incision to expose the aorta. In patients with multiple abdominal operations, a retroperitoneal approach may be utilized. The transverse colon is reflected superiorly and wrapped in a moist towel. The ligament of Treitz is taken down with electrocautery, and the inferior mesenteric vein is typically ligated. The small bowel is reflected to the patient's right and contained within a moist towel and using the fence or similar large, broad retractor for the Omni or Bookwalter. The renal vein (if anterior) is identified and carefully dissected out, and encircled with a silastic vessel loop. The renal arteries are then dissected out and encircled with vessel loops. The IMA is ligated. At this point, we will dissect out the femoral vessels, taking care to ligate the bridging vein over the external iliac to prevent injury during tunneling. Making sure to avoid the ureters, the tunnel is carried out using blunt dissection with the operator's fingers directly on top of the iliac vessels to ensure the tunnel is posterior to the ureter (Figure 25.2). Once the tunnel is made, a Penrose drain is passed through to mark the course of the tunnels, and the patient is heparinized.

When doing an end-to-end anastomosis, if the cross clamp can be applied below the renal vessels, there is no need for interruption of renal flow. However, if the proximal extent of disease is at the level of the renal vessels, a clamp zone, even temporarily, must be cleared suprarenally. The renal vessels are occluded using circumferential loops or bulldog clamps to prevent embolization, and then the aortic cross clamp is applied. The aorta is transected taking care to ensure enough space to move the aortic clamp infrarenally and still leave enough of a cuff to sew the anastomosis. A segment of the infrarenal aorta is excised distally to ensure the graft can be positioned in a straight, anatomic position. Using a Penfield or similar device, the aortic stump can be circumferentially endarterectomized if needed. At this time, the renal arteries should be flushed; the aorta can be reclamped below the renal vessels and then the suprarenal clamp is removed to minimize renal ischemia time. If the proximal anastomosis is to be end-to-side, the aortotomy is usually made at or just distal to the level of the renal vessels using an aortic punch. The bifurcated Dacron graft is then trimmed to ensure a short main body, and the anastomosis is completed with 3-0 Prolene (Figure 25.1).

Once the proximal anastomosis is completed and hemostatic, the tunneling clamp is the passed under the Penrose drains, and each limb of the graft is grasped and carried through the tunnels, again taking care not to injure the ureter or any bridging veins. The limbs are pulled with enough tension to avoid kinking or redundancy, and the end-to-side anastomosis is carried out, along with femoral endarterectomy and patching if needed. Closure is standard multilayer for the abdomen and groins.[2–6]

MORTALITY AND COMPLICATIONS

Overall, the mortality rate of elective ABF has been quoted from 1–3.6%,[7–9] though complication rates can run as high as 20%. Furthermore, mortality increases with concomitant complication, with mortality as low at 0.5% with no complications, 10% with one major complication, and up to 36% with three or more major complications. Complication and mortality were significantly higher in patients with increasing age, presence of tissue loss, baseline renal insufficiency (threefold-risk of death), and coronary heart disease (two-fold risk of death). There was no statistically significant difference in complications in patients with hypertension, tobacco abuse, surgical approach (midline vs retroperitoneal), diabetes or BMI. Medical complications (cardiac, pulmonary, etc.) are far more common (15%) than surgical complications (8.2%).[7] Prevention and treatment of medical complications are largely mitigated with appropriate patient selection preoperatively and meticulous anesthetic and perioperative management, thus the remainder of this chapter will focus on surgical complications.[10–13]

COMPLICATIONS

1. Thrombosis/graft failure
2. Graft infection
3. Hemorrhage
4. Nonvascular laparotomy complications (ventral hernia, bowel obstruction)
5. Intestinal ischemia
6. Groin complications (lymphocele, hematoma, local wound infection/dehiscence)
7. Aortoenteric fistula/erosion
8. Ureteral injury/obstruction
9. Sexual dysfunction
10. Chylous ascites
11. Anastomotic pseudoaneurysm

THROMBOSIS/GRAFT FAILURE

Description and incidence

The aortobifemoral bypass has excellent early and late patency. Several studies have shown 85–92% patency at 5 years and 70–75% at 10 years.[9,14–16] Nevertheless, graft thrombosis is the most commonly encountered late complication of this operation. Early graft thrombosis is more likely to be the result of embolism, technical error such as kinking, external compression of the graft, anastomotic narrowing, or inadequate distal runoff. Late thrombosis is likely related to progression of atherosclerotic disease.

Prevention/avoidance

There is no difference in long-term patency between end-to-end vs end-to-side proximal anastomosis. In fact, the graft-femoral anastomosis is the key technical component of the operation to help prevent graft thrombosis and is the most important determinant of late graft patency. It is crucial that there be unimpeded flow into the profunda femoris, and this must be confirmed at the time of surgery (Figure 25.3). If there is stenotic disease of the profunda, a concomitant profundoplasty should be performed, or the graft-femoral anastomosis should be carried down onto the profunda past the orifical disease. Some authors

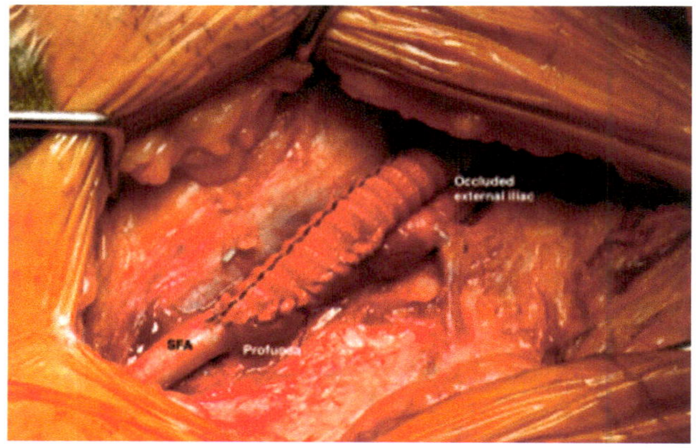

Figure 25.3 Femoral anastomosis, ensuring adequate outflow down the profunda.

suggest that all graft-femoral anastomosis should be performed in this fashion to prevent against future progression of atherosclerotic disease or "functional" profunda obstruction from the anastomosis.[6,17]

Bilateral limb thrombosis or complete graft occlusion is much rarer than single-limb thrombosis, and is generally due to an inflow problem. This can be avoided by placing the proximal anastomosis in close proximity to the renal vessels, which will avoid progressive atherosclerotic lesions in the native aorta above the anastomosis compromising inflow.

Treatment

Early graft thrombosis often requires operative intervention for thrombectomy and repair of the underlying technical issue, or infrainguinal intervention to improve outflow. A late unilateral limb thrombosis can be treated percutaneously with catheter-directed thrombolysis or via open thrombectomy. Often even with successful thrombolysis, an outflow stenosis is uncovered as the cause of the thrombosis, necessitating open revision.[18] Open approach with thrombectomy may be preferable, as a stenosis at the distal anastomosis can be revised at the time of thrombectomy, therefore relegating the patient to a single operation instead of multiple procedures. While initial thrombectomy can be accomplished with a standard Fogarty embolectomy catheter, use of a specialized corkscrew adherent clot or graft thrombectomy catheter is useful for removal of fibrinous, more adherent clot material than an elastomeric balloon alone may not clear. This should be done under fluoroscopic guidance and with a low threshold for balloon occlusion of the contralateral limb to prevent embolic debris inadvertently flushing down the other limb. If thrombectomy is unsuccessful, a femoral-femoral bypass may be needed as a "bail out" to revascularize the affected leg, and the patient should be widely prepped accordingly whenever a unilateral thrombectomy is being performed.

Often unilateral limb thrombosis clinically presents as claudication due to aforementioned collateral flow to the leg, but up to a quarter of patients will present with acute critical limb ischemia. In this case, concomitant infrapopliteal disease is often present, and should be interrogated preoperatively. In this subset of patients, additional infrainguinal bypass may necessary at the time of thrombectomy.

Bilateral or complete graft occlusion as previously stated is often due to an inflow problem, and therefore consideration should be taken for in situ graft replacement or axillobifemoral bypass rather than bilateral thrombectomies via the groin.

Long-term implications/outcomes

Long-term patency after revision has been quoted at 68% with an 85% limb salvage rate in patient who present with critical limb ischemia.[18]

GRAFT INFECTION

Description and incidence

Aortic graft infection is a rare (0.2–5%)[19] but devastating complication. Infection is generally attributed to be a result of inoculation of bacteria from elsewhere in the patient at the time of surgery. This is most often from the skin, and can also be seeded in the postoperative periods as a result of skin breakdown.[7,20] Even more rare, contact between the graft and the gastrointestinal tract can result in infection; this is discussed further in the section on aortoenteric fistula. Graft infection is notoriously difficult to diagnose, though if missed and allowed to propagate can lead to systemic sepsis, and when involving either the femoral or aortic anastomosis can cause breakdown, pseudoaneurysm, or hemorrhage. Though it can occur at any time in the postoperative period, the average time from original surgery to symptomatic infection ranges from 41 to 62 months. There is a high rate of mortality (40%), limb loss (11%), and reinfection (18%) if not treated adequately.[21]

Prevention and avoidance

Concomitant or nosocomial infection, particularly blood stream septicemia, urinary tract infection, and development of wound infection are strong predictors of later graft infection. In addition, advanced age has been identified as an independent factor associated with graft infection.[20,21] For this reason, preoperative workup should pay particular attention to any source of infection, and if the patient's clinical condition allows, surgery should be delayed until the infection can be adequately treated. Postoperatively, meticulous incisional care to avoid wound breakdown is imperative.

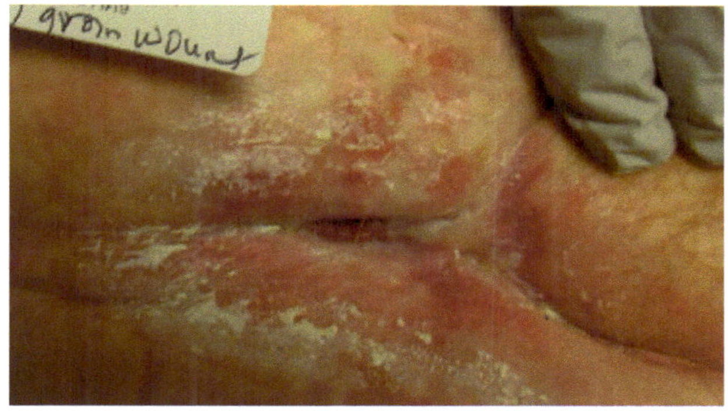

Figure 25.4 Groin incision demonstrating mild erythema and a chronically draining sinus tract in a patient with an underlying *Staphylococcal* graft infection.

Treatment

Patients with a graft infection can present with fulminant sepsis; many more indolent infections can be difficult to diagnose. Patients may exhibit abdominal or back pain or tenderness. The incisions, particularly the groin where the graft is closer to the skin, may demonstrate erythema or a draining sinus tract (Figure 25.4). Laboratory values may demonstrate a leukocytosis or elevated inflammatory markers. Imaging usually demonstrates fluid or gas around the graft (Figure 25.5 and Figure 25.6).

In addition to antibiotics, the mainstay of treatment of the infected aortic graft is complete graft excision and debridement of local infected tissue. Once completed, there are several reconstructive options: extra-anatomic bypass and several methods of inline bypass with cryopreserved (cadaveric) allograft, bovine pericardium, rifampin-bonded prosthetic, and autogenous vein via the neo-aortoiliac system (NAIS procedure). There are advantages and disadvantages to all methods, and there is no single "best approach" for an infected aortic graft. Rather, the treatment should be based on the virulence of the infection, urgency of the operation (i.e., ruptured infected pseudoaneurysm versus indolent infection), and the overall fitness and comorbidities of the patient.

Extraanatomic bypass has long been regarded as the gold standard for reconstruction after excision of infected aortoiliac grafts. The oft-cited benefit of this technique is that this allows the new graft material to be tunneled distant to the infected site, theoretically decreasing risk of reinfection. Disadvantages of this technique include the need to oversew and leave a pressurized aortic stump at what was the proximal anastomosis of the former ABF. In order to do this, the native aortic tissue must be debrided to healthy tissue, and is often oversewn multiple times with Prolene suture. Some authors advocate reinforcing the suture line with a strip of felt pledget if the aortic wall is attenuated, though this requires the risk of leaving a foreign body behind in an infected field. An omental flap should be left in place to bolster and exclude the stump from the bowel. Distal reconstruction can be performed

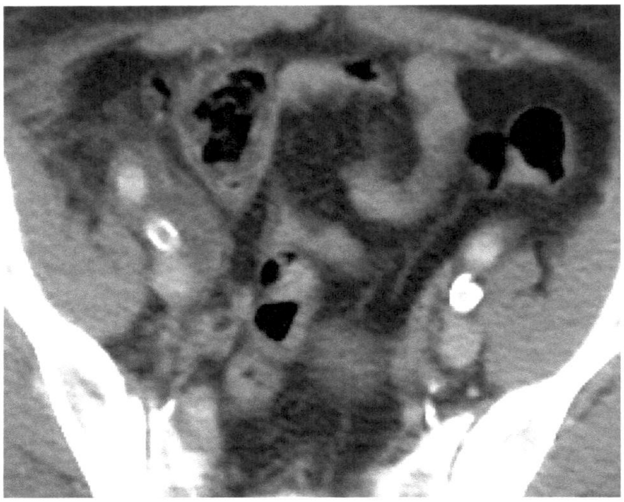

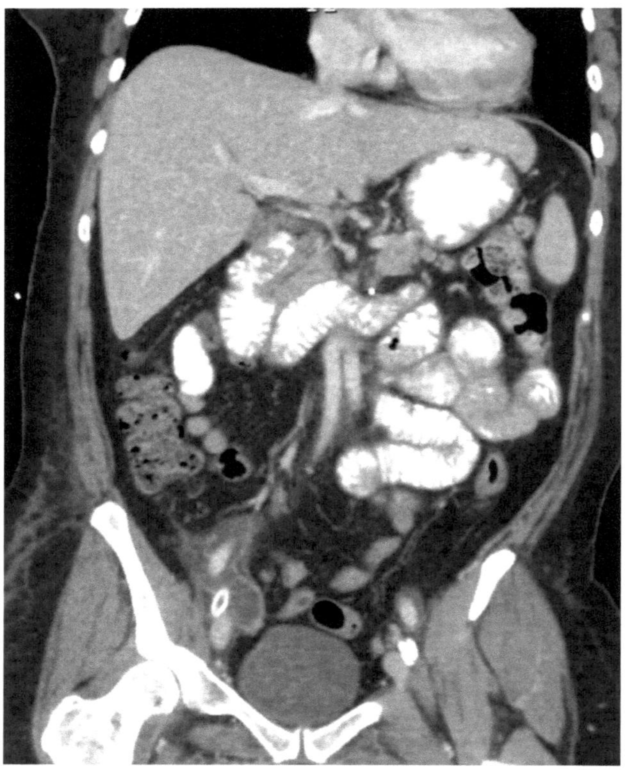

Figure 25.5 and 25.6 CT scan demonstrating a rim-enhancing fluid collection around the right limb of an infected aortobifemoral bypass 1 month after placement.

to the profunda artery or even the popliteal to avoid reconstruction in the contaminated groin. A muscle flap should be used for coverage of the anastomosis.

Cryopreserved allograft reconstruction is one of the quickest ways of reconstruction and, of the methods mentioned, has one of the lowest rates of reinfection, only slightly worse than autogenous vein. Its use is often limited by availability and limited sizes or lengths of cadaveric grafts, particularly in an urgent or emergent situation, as most facilities do not have these immediately available and must pre-order an appropriate graft. Fashioning a graft out of bovine pericardium may be a better option when cryopreserved allograft is not immediately available and has shown similarly low reinfection rates.[22] Antibiotic-impregnated Dacron graft, usually prepared intraoperatively by soaking the graft in a solution 1200 mg of rifampin diluted in 20 mL normal saline is another option, particularly in patients with infection from a low virulence bacteria.

Use of autogenous vein in the NAIS procedure, usually by harvesting the bilateral femoral veins, which are then spliced together proximally in order to create a bifurcated venous graft, is the most resistant to reinfection (< 2%) but is by far the most invasive and laborious reconstruction, which may preclude this from being an ideal option in frail or unstable patients. This generally is performed by two surgical teams, one performing the "clean" venous harvest and subsequent graft construction, while the other team performs the graft excision and debridement either concomitantly or sequentially. Once the lower extremity harvest incisions are closed, the neoaortoiliac venous graft is implanted in situ. NAIS has a high long-term patency rate ranging from 75–91% at 5 years.[23,24]

Graft preservation may be a consideration for a limited subset of circumstances. Patients who present with focal infection, such as limited to one groin or limb, low virulence bacteria, and no signs of systemic sepsis, have been treated successfully without total graft excision. On the other end of the spectrum, frail patients or those with a hostile abdomen who would have a prohibitively high risk of mortality with complete graft excision may also be considered for graft-preservation therapy. Management still generally involves serial surgical debridement of the infected site, segmental vascular reconstruction ideally with venous conduit, consideration of use of antibiotic impregnated beads, and long-term parenteral antibiotics use. Intraoperative culture data are paramount, and more virulent organisms such as *Pseudomonas* should be considered for the standard complete graft excision.[23,25]

Long-term implications/outcomes

Prognosis is largely dependent on the site and extent of graft involvement, the urgency of the re-operation to control the sepsis, and the underlying condition of the patient.[26] Antibiotic use should be guided by intraoperative cultures and should be continued for at least 6 weeks postoperatively but may be needed long-term or even lifelong in certain situations.

Reinfection can occur in up to 25% of these patients, and long-term surveillance is mandatory.[27] While it was initially felt that extraanatomic bypass would have a low risk of reinfection given its distant location from the infected field, this has not necessarily borne out in the literature with reinfection rates as high as 27%.[28] Thrombosis of the revascularization can be seen more commonly when done for graft infection and can lead to limb loss in up to a third of patients.[29]

One of the greatest risks of long-term morbidity and mortality is blowout of the aortic stump in those patients who undergo extraanatomic bypass, which can be seen in up to 23% of patients. For many surgeons, this has made in situ reconstruction via any of the described methods a more attractive option, and studies suggest a lower mortality rate in patients who underwent inline reconstruction with antibiotic-soaked graft than in those who underwent extraanatomic bypass.[30]

Up to 22% of patients who were operated on for aortoenteric fistula were found to have graft infections with Staphylococcal species or underlying biofilm, suggesting a role that untreated indolent infection may have played a role in development of the fistula. The bacterial speciation suggests more of a causative role rather than an effect of GI colonization.[31]

HEMORRHAGE

Description and incidence

Early postoperative hemorrhage is a relatively rare complication, with an incidence of 1–2%.[2,4] Longitudinal studies have shown that intraoperative blood loss with ABF has increased, likely due to increased operative complexity and decreased surgeon experience with open revascularization as endovascular treatment of aortoiliac disease has increased in prevalence, thus reserving open surgery for the more complex cases or prior revascularization failure.[20] Last, postoperative hemorrhage (> 28 days) is usually a result of aggressive graft infection, resulting in anastomotic breakdown.

Prevention and avoidance

Intraoperative hemorrhage is best avoided by familiarity of the anatomy, and in particular assessment of venous structures both on preoperative imaging and knowledge of at-risk venous structures. Most patients undergo a preoperative CT scan, and knowledge of anomalous retroaortic renal vein or anomalous IVC (left-sided or duplicate) is imperative to avoid injury during dissection or clamping. Other areas where venous structures are at risk of injury during dissection include the inferior mesenteric, adrenal, gonadal, lumbar, and iliac veins.

Preoperative medication for patients on antiplatelet or anticoagulation should be managed on a case by case basis. Aspirin has been shown to decrease postoperative mortality and is generally continued through surgery, though it is associated with a slightly higher risk of hemorrhagic complications. Data from cardiac surgery literature have shown a significant increase in hemorrhagic complications in patients on clopidogrel, and unless absolutely contraindicated, it is recommended this drug be stopped at least 7 days preoperatively. Patients who are fully anticoagulated for mechanical valves, atrial fibrillation, pulmonary embolism, or deep venous thrombosis on warfarin or a novel anticoagulant should have this stopped preoperatively; however, those with a mechanical valve or high CHA2D2-VASC score should be considered for heparin bridging.[32]

Awareness of bleeding diathesis preoperatively and appropriate dosing of anticoagulation intraoperatively are imperative. If an extensive aortic endarterectomy is required and the wall of the aortic cuff appears attenuated, preemptive placement of a felt pledget ring may be helpful. Alternatively, a cuff of graft 1–2 cm in width may be reserved after trimming the main body and slid over the suture line after completion to act as a circumferential bolster; however, this can only be slid into place before re-pressurizing the graft. Upon completion of the aortic anastomosis, clamping one limb of the graft and instilling heparinized saline via an asepto syringe to check for bleeding points on the proximal anastomosis can allow for repair without blood loss. Repair sutures should not be placed under pressure and therefore done with the aortic clamp in place. Meticulous repair of the anastomosis should be sought, as multiple episodes of clamping and reclamping can lead to hemodynamic lability and predispose to other complications, such as cardiac dysfunction.

Treatment

Aggressive postoperative management in the ICU or similarly high level of care is needed to identify hemodynamic changes early that are suggestive of hemorrhagic decompensation. Coagulopathy should be assessed for by monitoring PTT, PT, INR, platelet count and fibrinogen levels, rather than hematocrit, which may not be an acute indicator of bleeding. There is often a dilutional coagulopathy seen in these patients, and coagulopathic correction should be dictated based on these results. Ideally, coagulopathy, hypothermia, and acidosis should be corrected prior to return to the operating room if patient stability allows.

Long-term implications/outcomes

There are little data available on long-term outcomes after re-exploration for bleeding after aortoiliac reconstruction.

NONVASCULAR LAPAROTOMY COMPLICATIONS

Description and incidence

Complications related to the laparotomy incision and intra-abdominal dissection include incisional wall hernia and late small bowel obstruction. Incisional wall hernia, where intrabdominal contents protrude through a fascial defect associated with the incision (Figure 25.7), occurs in up to 10% of all patients undergoing abdominal surgery.

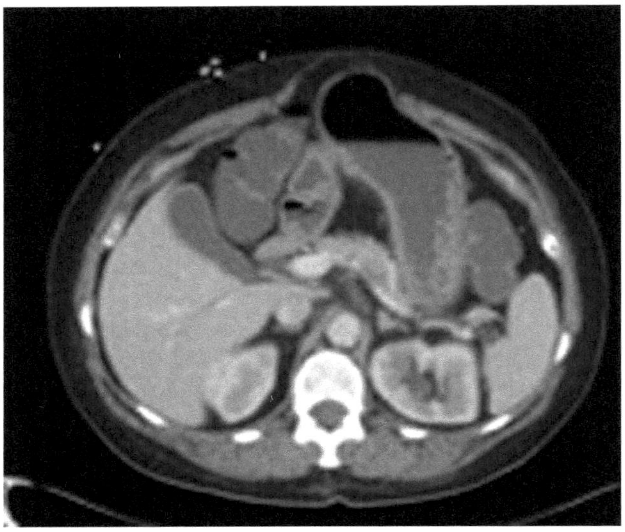

Figure 25.7 Ventral hernia containing part of the stomach in a patient who previously underwent aortobifemoral bypass.

Incidence is higher in patients undergoing vascular surgery and is well described in patients after open aneurysm repair, occurring in more than 30% of that population, but this occurs with lower frequency (3–20%) in patients treated for aortoiliac occlusive disease.[33,34] It has been postulated that collagen defects associated with aneurysmal disease predisposed this subset of patients to a higher rate of incisional hernia.

Small bowel obstruction (SBO) can be seen at any time after open intraabdominal surgery, usually as result of adhesive disease or more uncommonly related to an internal hernia. SBO is seen in 7.5% of patients after ABF, with 4.6% of patients requiring operative intervention for the obstruction.

Prevention and avoidance

There are extensive data in the general surgery literature on the avoidance and prevention of hernia. A recent meta-analysis specific to patients undergoing aortic surgery showed decreased hernia formation in those patients who were closed with a suture:wound length ratio of more than 4:1 and in those who underwent closure with mesh. There was no difference between midline and retroperitoneal incision.[35] In high-risk patients, particularly those who have previously undergone abdominal wall repair, pre-emptive involvement with a general surgeon skilled in complex repair of abdominal wall defects may be helpful.

Treatment

Primary indications for hernia repair generally include size, pain, or incarceration of bowel or omentum. There any many options for surgical repair, including primary repair, component separation, and use of mesh or other prosthetics in either an open or laparoscopic approach. Often a combination of component separation and mesh are used for optimal results.

Long-term implications/outcomes

Outcomes and recurrence for ventral hernia depends on the size of hernia and the type of repair. Recurrence after component separation or mesh repair is approximately 20%, with slightly lower rates using a laparoscopic approach or a combination of mesh and component separation.[36]

While subset analysis for patients undergoing aortoiliac surgery is lacking, large population studies of patients who develop SBO after abdominal surgery showed those who underwent operative intervention of SBO had a lower risk of recurrence (13%) versus those who were managed medically (21%).[37]

INTESTINAL ISCHEMIA

Description and incidence

Patients with extensive aortoiliac disease are predisposed to atherosclerotic disease in other vascular beds, including the mesenteric vessels. Interruption of vital collaterals during surgery can predispose patients to mesenteric ischemia. Risk factors for patients with mesenteric ischemia include advanced age, underlying cardiac disease including arrhythmias, low cardiac output, valvular disease, and intra-abdominal malignancy.[38,39c] Intestinal ischemia occurs in 2–3% of aortic reconstructive cases,[40] and the most common distribution is the rectosigmoid colon.

Prevention and avoidance

Due to the high rate of intestinal ischemia in patients with underlying cardiac disease, a meticulous preoperative workup and optimization of cardiac pathology should be sought before consideration of ABF surgery. Additionally, in patients with a high burden of mesenteric atherosclerotic disease, a staged approach may be appropriate. This author has had success in staging mesenteric revascularization several weeks to months before ABF in patients with symptoms of chronic mesenteric ischemia and lower extremity claudication in an effort to mitigate this risk as well as allow the patient to improve nutritional status before undertaking aortoililac revascularization.[41]

Intraoperatively, any attempt to preserve flow to a patent hypogastric artery should be done, as in patients with occlusive disease the blood supply of the colon is dependent on collaterals from the SMA and hypogastric vessels. If the IMA is patent, a proximal end-to-side anastomosis may be considered, or after completion of an end-to-end anastomosis IMA reimplantation should be performed. Intraoperative hypotension should be avoided.

Treatment

Diagnosis requires a high index of suspicion as initial signs and symptoms can be vague and nonspecific. In the case of embolic disease, the onset can be significant and acute, whereas occlusive disease from underlying atherosclerotic burden can be more insidious. Clinically, the patient may exhibit abdominal tenderness and distention, and the most common sign is diarrhea. Lab values, including leukocytosis, elevated lactate, or metabolic acidosis are nonspecific and, when due to intestinal ischemia, can be a late finding. Duplex sonography is sensitive (> 92%),[42] however technically this can be of limited value depending on the skill of the operator and the presence of intraabdominal gas and bandages. Whereas catheter angiography has long been considered the gold standard of diagnosis, CTA has begun to supplant traditional angiography as the test of choice due to the noninvasive nature and ease of obtaining this test while still providing a specificity of 94% and sensitivity of 96%.[43] In patients with suspected colonic ischemia, there should be a low threshold for sigmoidoscopy.

Ischemia involving only the mucosa can often be managed nonoperatively with bowel rest in patients who are stable, with reassuring and improving clinical exam and labs. This generally results in mucosal sloughing, which improves in days. Unstable patients, those with worsening acidosis, physical exam, or those who show erosive or gangrenous changes on sigmoidoscopy should promptly return to the operating room for exploration and anticipated bowel resection.

Long-term implications/outcomes

Transmural colonic ischemia has a high mortality rate, as high as 80–100% if not property treated, thus stressing the need for a high index of suspicion and expedited management if the concern for bowel ischemia exists.

GROIN COMPLICATIONS (LYMPHOCELE, HEMATOMA, LOCAL WOUND INFECTION/DEHISCENCE)

Description and incidence

Groin complications are seen in a fifth of patients, and will require an operative intervention in 6.8% of the cohort in a recent report. Most of these will occur within the first 3 months. Several patient factors have been implicated in predisposing to a groin complication, such as increased BMI, diabetes, and the presence of a previously operated groin.[44,45]

The most common complication is a seroma/lymphocele, which are terms often used interchangeably in both definition and treatment paradigm, though there is a slight difference. A seroma occurs when there is dead space and/or a reaction to a foreign body, such as the graft. The inflammatory response within the surrounding tissues leads to a transudate of serous fluid, which has a straw-colored appearance and consistency to similar pleural or peritoneal fluid. A lymphocele occurs specifically when lymphatic channels are not appropriately ligated or cauterized during dissection of the groin, resulting in a nonepithelialized collection of lymph. Clinically they can appear the same—a soft, ballotable bulge in the groin, usually without overlying skin changes. This can easily be distinguished from a hematoma as the hematoma appears more heterogeneous and dense on imaging, whereas a lymphocele or seroma appears cystic. A lymphatic fistula can develop if the lymphocele develops a cutaneous communication, manifesting as the drainage of crystal clear fluid from a small sinus, usually in the incision. The amount of fluid can be voluminous or only a few drops expressed with movement or manipulation depending on the size of the draining lymphatic channels.

Hematoma, well described elsewhere, is the collection of blood and is generally a result of inadequate hemostasis at the time of surgery (Figures 25.8 and 25.9).

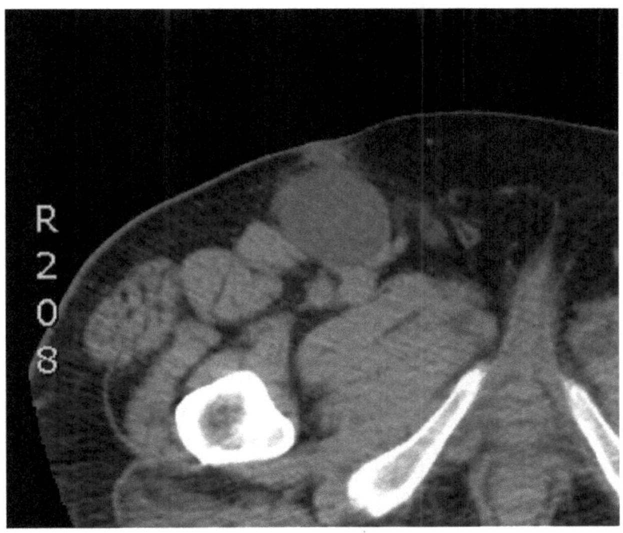

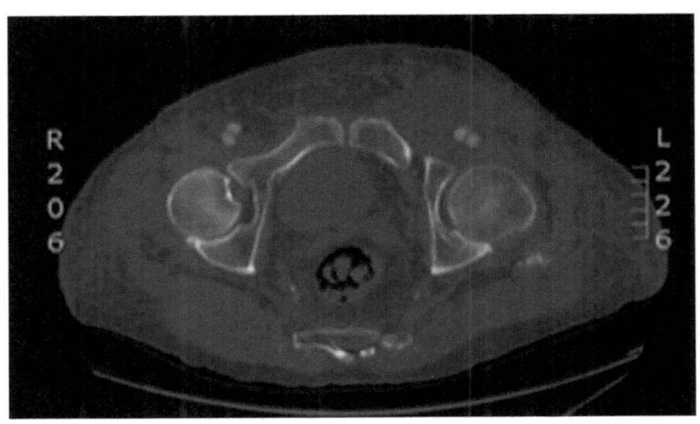

Figures 25.8 and 25.9 Figure 25.8 shows a groin lymphocele, which is well circumscribed and homogenous. A hematoma, in Figure 25.9, is more heterogeneous in appearance and has significant stranding in the surrounding tissues.

Surgical wound dehiscence can be superficial or deep, and management is often dictated by the presence of concomitant infection and depth of involvement, particularly in regards to the underlying graft and vessels. The Szilagi classification is often used, with type I limited to skin necrosis, superficial wound dehiscence, and/or local infection. Type II includes deep wound dehiscence and fat necrosis, whereas Type III involves the underlying graft.

Prevention and avoidance

Previous authors have postulated that a transverse groin incision is protective for complications rather than a longitudinal incision.[46] However, this may be a technical challenge for those patients who require extensive femoral endarterectomy, and more recent data show no difference in lymphocele formation, and limited evidence that transverse incisions are protective against infection.[47] Still, it may be somewhat protective in those patients with appropriate habitus who based on preoperative imaging, will need no or limited endarterectomy.

Meticulous dissection, including using a combination of electrocautery and suture ligation for any visible vessels or lymph channels, is mandatory. It has been postulated that use of the harmonic scalpel may provide superior lymphatic seal during groin dissection, and while data in the vascular literature is limited, this has not been consistently borne out in the oncology literature when groin dissection is done specifically for lymphadenectomy.[48,49] Any obvious pooling of clear lymphatic fluid during operation should be suture ligated. Groin closure should be in multiple layers.

Groin complications are noted to be more common in infrainguinal reconstructions than in aortofemoral reconstructions. Early limb movement, infection, and reoperation have been noted to be a risk factor in groin complications, particularly seroma or lymphocele. Placing patients on limited activity restrictions should be considered, particularly for those with prior groin exposures.[50]

Many types of dressing, including gauze, silver-impregnated, and cyanoacrylate glue, have been used, however no one has consistently been proven to be superior. Much attention has been paid to the use of a topical negative-pressure wound therapy system placed at the time of surgery in an effort to decrease wound complications. A self-contained dressing consisting of a sponge and occlusive dressing is placed over a closed incision and connected to a portable vacuum device that maintains a subatmospheric pressure, which is thought to help decrease fluid within the underlying wound bed, maintain apposition of skin edges and, and allow minimal external contamination. These are applied at the time of skin closure and maintained in place until postoperative day 5–7. These types of dressing have been shown to drop the rate of incision dehiscence and surgical site infection from previously published rates as high as 20% to 5–11%. There was no difference in the rate of other groin incision complications, however most trials did not specifically attempt to measure this variable.[51–54]

Treatment

Small seromas or those which are asymptomatic can be safely observed and may resolve spontaneously. Larger seromas, especially those in conjunction with skin breakdown, should have a lower threshold for operative intervention. The previous incision is generally reopened and the fluid collection drained. Interrogation for a source of lymphatic drainage should be done carefully and ligated if found. Injection of isosulfan or methylene blue in the foot preoperatively may help identify lymphatic channels. The wound is copiously irrigated, and some advocate the use of betadine to incite an inflammatory response and act as a sclerosant. The tissue edges are oversewn using monofilament absorbable suture, and the reapproximated carefully, minimizing dead space. If there is a large defect or infection is suspected, closure with a muscle flap may be necessary. Lymphoceles that develop remote from the initial operation must raise the concern for underlying graft infection and should be worked up as such, including intraoperative culture of the fluid.

Treatment of a wound dehiscence depends on the depth and amount if tissue involved. Superficial dehiscence can be managed with local wound care on an outpatient basis. Antibiotics are often not needed unless there is cellulitis, purulence, or other signs of local infection. Deeper dehiscence into the fat layer but without exposed graft should be debrided in the operating room, both for patient comfort and to determine the extent of graft involvement. Negative-pressure wound vac therapy is helpful in patients with Szilagi Type II wounds, though caution with these systems must be undertaken if there is potentially exposed graft or vessel.

Long-term implications/outcomes

Sixty percent of these complications are diagnosed after initial hospital discharge, and they are the most common reason for hospital readmission and a significant source of financial burden on the healthcare system. Wound complications lengthens the overall recovery from weeks to months, and puts patient at risk for graft infection and thromboses.[50]

AORTOENTERIC FISTULA/EROSION

Description and incidence

In patients with previous aortic surgery, fistulization, or erosion can develop between the graft and the gastrointestinal tract in 0.36–1.6% of patients with an average onset of 2 to 6 years after surgery.[28,55,56] Classically, the most common site for fistulization to develop is between the proximal suture line and distal duodenum, however graft enteric erosion can occur at any point, usually due to pressure necrosis of the bowel segment from the pulsating, high-pressure graft. The primary difference between the two conditions is that massive hemorrhage can occur with fistulization, whereas erosion may have a more insidious onset, similar to graft infection as bacteria can translocate from the gastrointestinal lumen to the graft material.[57]

Aortoenteric fistula (AEF) often presents with a "herald bleed" that may be self-limiting due to vasospasm and thrombus formation, but if untreated it will progress to massive GI exsanguination, which can happen hours to months later. Still, GI bleeding has only been noted in 73% of patients. Other presentations include sepsis, back or abdominal pain, thrombosis, or peritonitis.[56]

Prevention and avoidance

It has been postulated that an end-to-side anastomosis predisposes for an aortoenteric fistula; however, this has not been shown to be a clinically significant predictor.[58] Ensuring that closure of the retroperitoneum fully covers the graft, including the proximal anastomosis, is imperative. In thin patients or those who do not have sufficient retroperitoneum to sufficiently exclude the graft from the bowel, a pre-emptive omental flap placement may be necessary.

Treatment

A high index of suspicion for AEF must be present in any patient with a history of aortic surgery presenting with gastrointestinal hemorrhage, even in a stable patient where bleeding may clinically have stopped. Workup is predicated on the stability of the patient at the time of presentation, and goals of treatment include control of bleeding, excision of infected graft and tissue, management of bowel sepsis, and revascularization.

Massive hemorrhage mandates activation of a massive transfusion protocol and urgent surgical exploration as well as the administration of broad-spectrum antibiotics for presumed GI violation. The patient should be widely prepped, including the chest and legs in case extra-anatomic bypass or lower extremity venous harvest is needed. If possible, proximal control with balloon occlusion should be obtained. Once proximal and distal aortic control is obtained, the bowel should be dissected off the aorta. A small bowel defect can be repaired primarily, otherwise segmental resection is required. This should be completed after the vascular repair is complete and inline flow restored. Vascular repair will depend on the amount of contamination; if this is minimal, an in situ repair with femoral vein, cadaveric aorta, or rifampin-soaked graft can be safely performed. In the case of local sepsis, the graft should be excised, the aortic stump oversewn, and extra-anatomic bypass performed. An omental flap should be constructed to lay between the bowel and aortic repair or stump.

A stable patient allows for further diagnostics which can aid in treatment planning. CTA has become the preferred initial test, as this can show concerning findings such as air around the graft, loss of soft tissue planes between the bowel and aorta, and perigraft fluid collections, and it has the highest detection rate of AEF of all available modalities. This also helps more definitively show the extent and anatomy of the fistula. Contrast extravasation is not typically seen, and should not be considered an exclusion of the diagnosis of AEF. An EGD is also a necessary test, predominantly to evaluate for other sources of GI bleeding, as the direct visualization of graft material is not seen in the majority of cases. For a diagnostic study, the fourth portion of the duodenum must be visualized and should be performed by an experienced endoscopist who is instructed about the concern of underlying AEF, as EGD risks manually disrupting an overlying clot providing tamponade and resulting in exsanguination.

Endovascular repair has been attempted, particularly in sick patients who were felt to be poor operative candidates, however this is associated with high rates of recurrent infection and bleeding and is generally advocated as a tool to bridge unstable patients to definitive surgical excision.[57]

Long-term implications/outcomes

Left untreated, AEF is universally fatal, and even with expeditious management the average fatality rate is 30–40%, with some studies as high as 86%. Though long-term implications and considerations such as recurrent infection and aortic stump blowout are similar to those with graft infection, patients with AEF have a worse outcome than those with graft infection alone, with a 50% mortality rate at 3 years.[58]

URETERAL INJURY/OBSTRUCTION

Description and incidence

Ureteral injury occurs < 1% of the time, and is generally associated with three technical facets of the operation: dissection near the iliac vessels, creation of the tunnel, and closure of the retroperitoneum. Injuries typically involve the distal ureter.

Graft limbs that are inadvertently placed superficial to the ureter during the tunneling process may lead to ureteral compression, or in rare cases a ureteroarterial fistula, an extremely rare complication limited to case reports in the literature. A secondary form of ureteral obstruction may develop even with properly placed graft limbs, likely related to postoperative inflammatory response.

Prevention and avoidance

Adherence to meticulous surgical technique is imperative for avoidance of this injury. Dissection should be minimized near the iliac bifurcation where the ureters frequently cross the vessels. Identification of the ureters and frequent visualization during operative maneuvers in the pelvis are key. Preoperative placement of ureteral stents has not been shown to be protective against ureteral injury in other high-risk, nonvascular pelvic surgery, though this has not been specifically studied in vascular patients.[60]

Tunneling of the graft limb from the abdominal incision to the femoral incision must be done with as much direct vision as possible, ideally using blunt dissection with the surgeon's fingers to ensure the tunnel is directly overlying the iliac artery to ensure the graft will lie deep to the ureter.

Treatment

If a ureteral injury is identified intraoperatively, prompt involvement of a urologist is needed. Contusions without obvious violation of the lumen may be treated with ureteral stent only. Distal ureteral injuries can be dealt with by direct reimplantation of the ureter into the bladder or with a psoas hitch procedure. Small (< 3 cm) defects may allow a uretero-ureterostomy. Ureteral stenting to protect ureteral repair is often mandated, though patient positioning for aortobifemoral bypass does not usually allow for intraoperative cystoscopy, and this may need to be performed at the conclusion of the case prior to awakening from anesthesia.[61]

Most (50–70%) ureteral injuries are not identified at the time of surgery. Patients who develop flank pain, peritonitis, or other nonspecific signs of infection early in the postoperative course such as fever or leukocytosis should be suspected of having a ureteral injury. CT scan may demonstrate a retroperitoneal fluid collection suggestive of a urinoma, and if there is a high index of suspicion, CT can be protocolized to be performed with delayed scans to provide a CT-intravenous pyelogram, which, if positive, will demonstrate enhancement of the fluid collection suggestive of contrast leak from the injury. These patients may require long-term ureteral stenting and nephrostomy tube placement in addition to urologic surgical repair.[62]

Incidentally discovered asymptomatic postoperative hydroureter/hydronephrosis can often be managed conservatively, and spontaneous resolution is often seen (Figures 25.10 and 25.11). In patients who develop symptoms, such as pain, persistent infection, or deterioration in renal function, surgical management can include balloon dilation, ureterolysis, or ureter transection and re-anastomosis in a position superficial to the graft. In the rare instance when spontaneous massive hematuria is seen and a uretero-graft fistula is suspected, concomitant placement of a ureteral stent and graft endoprosthesis has been successfully described.[63]

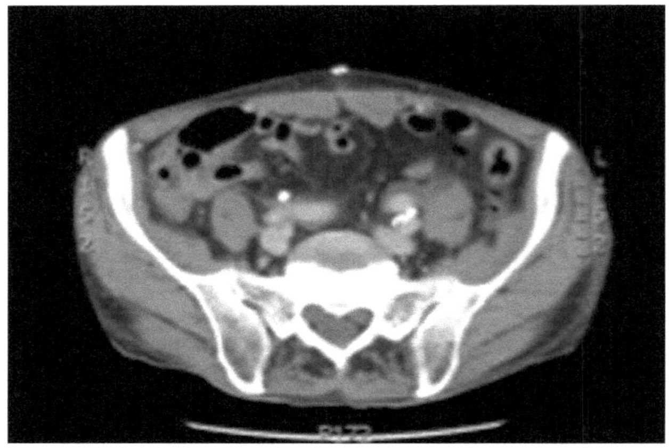

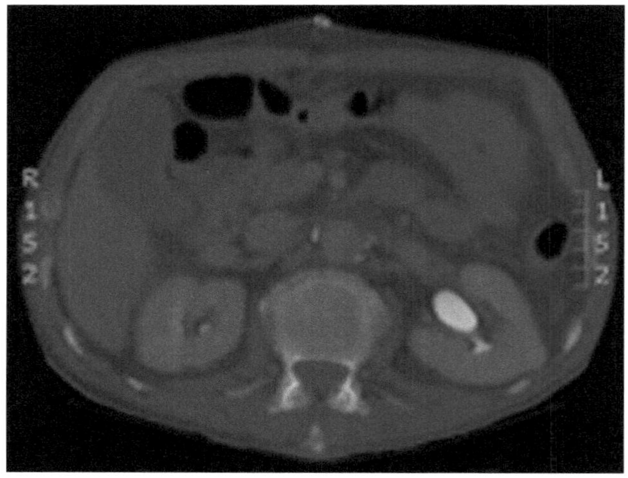

Figures 25.10 and 25.11 CT with delayed images to show the urologic structures demonstrates the left ureter deep to the ABF limb. It is in the correct position superficial to the graft on the right. Hydronephrosis resulting from this is seen in Figure 25.11. Repeat imaging 1 month later showed resolution of the hydronephrosis.

Long-term implications/outcomes

Ureteral obstruction in the absence of documented injury may develop in < 5% of patients.[64] Long-term outcomes in patients with ureteral injuries are excellent if the injury is identified and repaired at the time of injury. Ten percent of patients who require a ureteroureterostomy will develop a stricture. In patients who require a ureteral implantation, reflux may occur, but this typically does not lead to issues with infection or renal function deterioration in adults, unlike in the pediatric population. In those patients with urologic complications significant enough to warrant later surgical intervention, 55% went on to develop a graft complication (thrombosis, infection, fistula), so heightened surveillance for such issues should be undertaken by the vascular surgeon.[65]

SEXUAL DYSFUNCTION

Description and incidence

Erectile dysfunction (ED) has been reported in up to 80% of patients with occlusive aortoiliac disease; however, there are many nonvascular causes in this patient population for ED including age, hormonal, neuropathic, diabetes, medication, urologic, or alcohol/hepatic causes. Five to fifteen percent of patients with ED are primarily from inadequate pelvic perfusion.[10,13] While up to 60% of patients report some deterioration of penile function (including those who reported some decreased function preoperative), 25–37% of patients develop new erectile dysfunction after ABF, which is thought to be iatrogenic.[32,66,67]

Retrograde or "dry" ejaculation has been reported to occur in 3–9% of patients undergoing aortoiliac surgery in contemporary studies. For antegrade ejaculation to occur, the bladder neck must close, and this is reliant upon the T11 to L3 sympathetic nerve fibers, which anatomically are located along the aortic bifurcation and within the tissues to the left of the distal aorta and left common iliac aorta.

Prevention and avoidance

Due to the myriad causes, it is imperative for the surgeon to assess patency of hypogastric patency as well as document an accurate history of erectile function preoperatively, both to ascertain if penile function is present and thus can be preserved or if pelvic vasculature can be altered to maintain this. It is also worthwhile to determine the importance of penile function and plans for potential further childbearing to the patient. Consideration for a formal urologic evaluation of impotence can be undertaken in select patients to better determine if ED is vasculogenic or the result of another etiology. This consultation is important for proper education and to set patient expectations about the risk of aortic surgery on erectile function and the potential for retrograde ejaculation.

Intraoperatively, preservation of at least one preoperatively patent hypogastric artery is important in maintaining erectile function. In patients with occluded external iliac vessels and patent hypogastric artery, an end-to-side anastomosis should be performed or a patent hypogastric artery should be reimplanted. Minimal dissection in the area of the aortic bifurcation and left common iliac artery should be done to minimize risk of retrograde ejaculation.

Treatment

While vasculogenic impotence may be iatrogenic, impotence is generally not responsive to oral phosphodiesterase inhibitors. Intracavernosal injection with a combination of vasoactive material (alprostadil, papaverine, and phentolamine) has shown efficacy of up to 89% in patients who are nonresponders to oral therapy and after other pelvic surgeries. Surgical implantation of a penile prosthesis also has a high success rate in patients with ED.[68]

Retrograde ejaculation is generally not surgically correctable and, if further childbearing is required, will necessitate the assistance of a urologist with expertise in infertility.

Long term implications/outcomes

Ninety-two percent of patients were not counselled about sexual dysfunction preoperatively, and 26% stated they would have refused the procedure if they had known this was a direct risk of surgery.[66]

CHYLOUS ASCITES

Description and incidence

A very rare complication of open aortic surgery, chylous ascites results from injury to the cysterna chyli during dissection of the proximal aorta causing intraperitoneal lymph leak. This is generally more common with open aortic aneurysm repair, as this generally is associated with more proximal aortic dissection but has also been seen with ABF. Chylous ascites does not usually manifest until days to weeks after surgery and presents as painless abdominal swelling or large-volume ascites on imaging (Figures 25.12 and 25.13). It is suggested by a low serum albumin, though definite diagnosis can be made by sampling the ascitic fluid, which will appear milky.

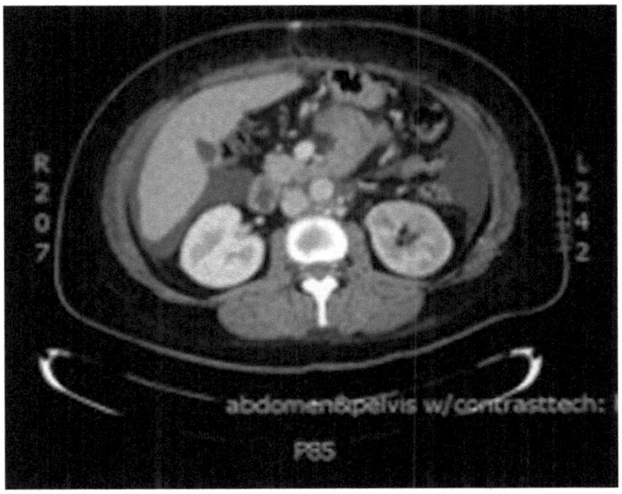

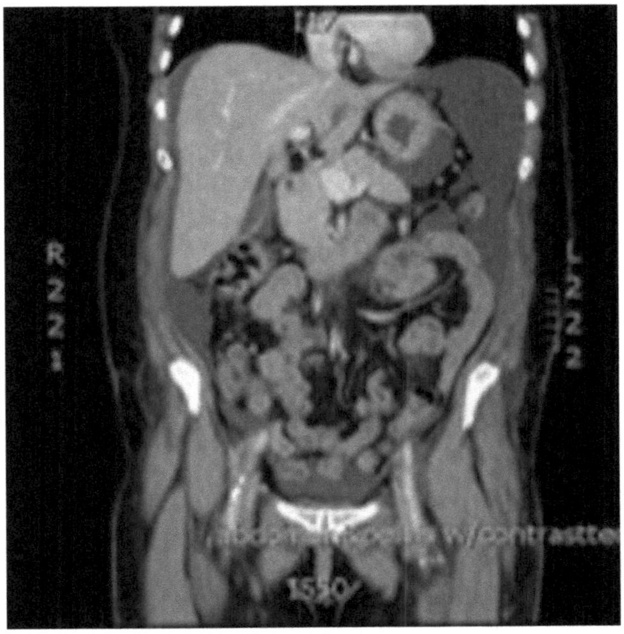

Figures 25.12 and 25.13 Chylous ascites on CT.

Microscopic analysis of the fluid reveals high triglyceride levels, low cholesterol and glucose levels, and a serum/chylous albumin gradient < 1.1.[69,70] Incidence is extremely low; however, it has been postulated that true incidence is underreported.

Prevention and avoidance

The cysterna chyli is the terminus of the thoracic duct in the abdomen, which also receives the lymph from the intestinal and lumbar lymphatic trunks. It is located in the retroperitoneal space, and most commonly in the left latero-aortic space around the level of the first two lumbar vertebrae. Extensive dissection in this area should be avoided, as it can cause disruption of these lymphatics and lead to a chyle leak.

Treatment

Published data are largely relegated to case reports, which note treatment can range from conservative management,[71–73] peritoneal-venous shunting, or open or laparoscopic ligation of lymphatic fistula, which has shown to be the most definitive.[75] Efforts on conservative treatment, sometimes for as long at 8 weeks, should be exhausted before resorting to more invasive treatments. Simple paracentesis alone is generally not successful, however when done in conjunction with diet alteration, including total parental nutrition (TPN), reduction of fat intake, or ingestion of medium-chain triglycerides for up to 3 months, is generally recommended but small reviews have not suggested that this affected outcomes.[72]

Long-term implications/outcomes

Chylous ascites from aortic surgery carries a better prognosis than when it develops after other intrabdominal surgeries. Three reported deaths in the literature were from sepsis, pulmonary embolism, and malnutrition.[74] There was no reported recurrence after open surgical ligation.[75]

ANASTOMOTIC PSEUDOANEURYSM

Description and incidence

Pseudoaneurysms (PSA) occur as a late complication, and are far more common in the femoral anastomosis (6–8.7%) than in the aortic anastomosis (2.9%). Femoral pseudoaneurysms occur bilaterally in 3% of patients.[32] They are generally a result of structural fatigue and degeneration of the fabric or tissue composing the anastomosis, while the perianastomotic fibrotic tissue prevents immediate hemorrhage and expands over time, containing the PSA. Over time, the fibrous tissue may rupture or the overlying skin integrity may degrade, leading to hemorrhage. While less common, the concern for indolent infection must always be considered (Figure 25.14).

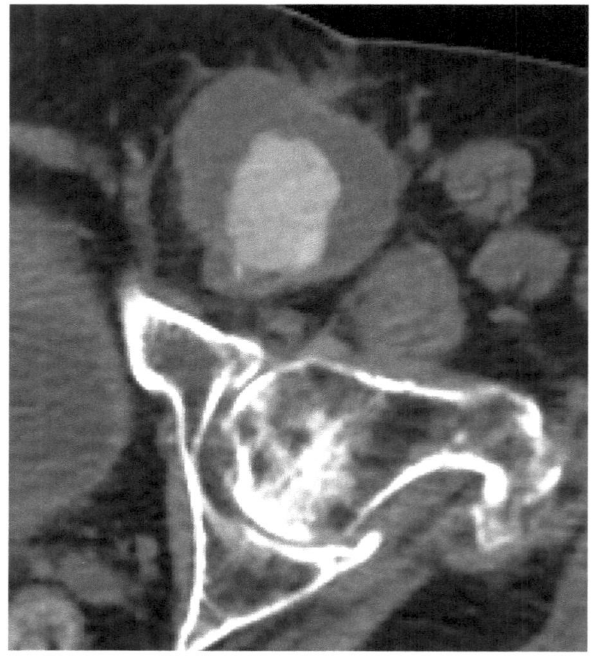

Figure 25.14 Large femoral anastomotic pseudoaneurysm which developed 2 years after aortobifemoral bypass. Repair was by interposition graft from the old graft to the profunda.

Prevention and avoidance

Avoiding undue tension when transecting the graft for the femoral anastomosis and using meticulous suturing technique is paramount. The graft must be cut to length to avoid redundancy, but not so short as to be overly taut. While the operator sews the anastomosis, the assistant should place distal traction on the graft limb so the anastomosis is not sewn under tension.

Treatment

Due to the concern of bowel involvement, aortic PSA always mandates surgical repair. If sufficient space between the renal vessels exists, endograft may be sufficient. If the anatomy precludes endovascular intervention, open surgery is required. If there is no concern for infection, the suture line may be primarily reinforced if the aortic tissue is healthy or an interposition graft can be performed to replace the original anastomosis.

Small (< 2.5 cm), asymptomatic femoral PSA, particularly in high-risk patients can be observed with frequent surveillance, however repair is indicated for those increasing in size or if they become symptomatic. Scar tissue can make dissection difficult, and proximal and distal control is usually gained as distant from the PSA as possible to avoid uncontrolled rupture. Access via the arm and use of a balloon for occlusion during dissection can be helpful, though this necessitates dissection in a heparinized field. Repair is best performed using an interposition graft with an end-to-end anastomosis to the common femoral, profunda, or SFA with profundal reimplantation depending on the integrity of the native arterial vessel. Alternatively, endovascular and hybrid techniques utilize a covered stent graft from the graft limb into the profunda in patients with an occluded SFA, or into the SFA with open reimplantation of the profundal have been described, which avoids the re-operative groin dissection.[76,77]

Because of the risk of infection, the artery and surrounding tissue should be cultured at the time of surgery.

Long-term implications/outcomes

Endovascular repair of aortic PSA has shown long-term success rates from 81–91%.[78] Repair of femoral PSA show a long-term success rate in 80–95%. Emergent repair of femoral PSA has a much higher mortality rate than elective repair (46.6% vs 0%).[28]

REFERENCES

1. Norgren L, Hiatt WR, Dormandy MR, et al. Intersociety Consensus for the Management of Peripheral Arterial Disease (TASC II). J Vasc Surg 2007; S5A.
2. Brewster DC. Aortofemoral bypass. In: Fischer JF, Bland KI, eds, Mastery of Surgery, 5th ed. Philadelphia: Wolters Kluwer/Lippincott Williams & Wilkins; 2007: 2063–2074.
3. Brewster DC. Clinical and anatomic considerations for surgery in aortoiliac disease and results of surgical treatment. Circulation 1991 Feb; 83(2 Suppl): 42–52.
4. Brewster DC. Current controversies in the management of aortoiliac occlusive disease. J Vasc Surg 1997 Feb; 25(2): 365–79.
5. Menard MT, Shah S, Belkin M. Aortoiliac Disease: Direct Reconstruction. In: Sidawy AN, Perler BA, eds, Rutherfords's Vascular Surgery and Endovascular Therapy, 9th ed. Philadelphia: Elsevier Saunders; 2019: 1397–1415.
6. Brewster DC. Aortofemoral Bypass for Atherosclerotic Aortoililac Occlusive Disease. In: Stanley JC, Veith F, Wakefield T, eds, Current Therapy in Vascular and Endovascular Surgery, 5th ed. Philadelphia: Elsevier Saunders; 2014: 418–422.
7. Bredhal K, Panduro Jensen L, Schroeder TV, et al. Mortality and complications after aortic bifurcated bypass procedures for chronic aortoiliac occlusive disease. J Vasc Surg. 2015 Jul; (62(1): 75–82.
8. Van der Akker PJ, van Schilfgaarde R, Brand R, et al. Long term results of prosthetic and non-prosthetic reconstruction for obstructive aorto-iliac disease. Eur J Vasc Surg. 1992 Jan; 6(1): 53–61.
9. DeCarlo, et al. Laparotomy- and groin-associated complications are common after aortofemoral bypass and contribute to reintervention. J Vasc Surg. 2020 Apr 10; S0741-5214(20): 30322.
10. Brewster DC. Complications of aortic and lower extremity procedures. In: Strandness DE, van Breda A, eds, Vascular Disease: Surgical and Interventional Therapy. New York: Churchill Livingstone; 1994: 1151.
11. de Vries SO, Hunink MG. Results of aortic bifurcation grafts for aortoiliac occlusive disease: a meta-analysis. J Vasc Surg. 1997;26(4): 558–69.
12. Szilagyi DE, Elliott JP Jr, Smith RF, et al. A 30-year survey of the reconstructive surgical treatment of aortoiliac occlusive disease. J Vasc Surg. 1986;3(3): 421–36.
13. Crawford ES, Bomberger RA, Glaeser DH, Saleh SA, Russell WL. Aortoiliac occlusive disease: factors influencing survival and function following reconstructive operation over a 25-year period. Surgery. 1981;90(6): 1055–67.
14. Nevelsteen A, Suy R. Graft occlusion following aortofemoral Dacron bypass. Ann Vasc Surg. 1991 Jan; 5(1): 3207.
15. Johnson WC, LoGerfo FW, Vollman RW, et al. Is axillo-bilateral femoral graft an effective substitute for aortic-bilateral iliac/femoral graft? An analysis of ten years experience. Ann Surg. 1977 Aug; 186(2): 123–9.
16. Friedman SG, Lazzaro RS, Spier LN, et al. A prospective randomized comparison of dacron and polytetrafluoroethylene aortic bifurcated grafts. Surgery. 1995 Jan; 117(1): 7–10.
17. Burguer R, Higgins RF, Cotton LT. Geometry, blood flow, and reconstruction of the deep femoral artery. Am J Surg. 1975 Jul; 130(1): 68–73.
18. Erdoes LS, Bernhard VM, Berman SS. Aortofemortal graft occlusion: strategy and timing of reoperation. Cardiovasc Surg. 1995 June; 3(3): 277–83.
19. Blom AS, Dougherty MJ, Calligaro KD., In-situ treatment of aortic graft infection with prosthetic grafts and allografts. In: Stanley JC, Veith F, Wakefield T, eds, Current Therapy in Vascular and Endovascular Surgery, 5th ed. Philadelphia: Elsevier Saunders; 2014: 418–422.

20. Herscu G, Wilson SE. Prosthetic infection: Lessons from treatment of the infected vascular graft. Surg Clin North Am. 2009 Apr; 89(2): 391–401.
21. Vogel TR, Symons R, Flum DR. The incidence and factors associated with graft infection after aortic aneurysm repair. J Vasc Surg. 2008 Feb; 47(2): 264–9.
22. Almasi-Sperling V, Heger D, Meyer A, et al. Treatment of aortic and peripheral prosthetic graft infection with bovine pericardium. J Vasc Surg. 2020 Feb; 71(2): 592–598.
23. Back, MR. Graft Infection. In: Sidawy AN, Perler BA, eds, Rutherfords's Vascular Surgery and Endovascular Therapy, 9th ed. Philadelphia: Elsevier Saunders; 2019: 588–602.
24. Chung J, Clagett GP. Neoaortoiliac System (NAIS) procedure for the treatment of the infected aortic graft. Semin Vasc Surg. 2011 Dec; 25(4): 220–6.
25. Calligaro KD, Veith FJ, Yuan JG, et al. Intra-abdominal aortic graft infection: Complete or partial graft preservation in patients at very high risk. J Vasc Surg. 2003 Dec;38(6):1199–1204.
26. Swain TW, Calligaro KD, Dougherty MD. Management of infected aortic graft. Vasc Endovascular Surg. Jan-Feb 2004; 38(1): 75–82.
27. Charlton-Ouw KM, Sandhu HK, Huang G, et al. Reinfection after resection and revascularization of infected infrarenal abdominal aortic grafts. J Vasc Surg. 2014 Mar; 59(3): 684–92.
28. O'Hara PJ, Hertzer NR, Beven EG, et al. Surgical management of infected abdominal aortic grafts: Review of a 25-year experience. J Vasc Surg. 1986 May; 3(5): 725–31.
29. Quinones-Baldrich WJ, Hernandez JJ, Moore WS. Long-term results following surgical management of aortic graft infection. Arch Surg. 1991 Apr; 126(4): 507–11.
30. O'Connor s, Andrew P, Batt M, et al. A systematic review and meta-analysis of treatment for aortic graft infections. J Vasc Surg. 2006 Jul; 44(1): 38–45.
31. Armstrong PA, Back MR, Wilson JS, et al. Improved outcomes in the recent management of secondary aortoenteric fistula. J Vasc Surg. 2005 Oct; 42(4): 660–6.
32. Hunter GC, Westerband A. Noninfectious complications in vascular surgery. In: Moore WS, ed, Vascular and Endovascular Surgery A Comprehensive Review, 8th ed. Philadelphia: Elsevier Saunders; 2013: 919–956.
33. Takagi H., Sugimoto M, Kato T, et al. Postoperative incision hernia in patients with abdominal aortic aneurysm and aortoiliac occlusive disease: a systematic review. Eur J Vasc Endovasc Surg. 2007 Feb; 33(2): 177–181.
34. Altieri MS, Yang J, Jones T, et al. Incidence of ventral hernia repair after open abdominal aortic aneurysm and open aortofemoral or aortoiliac bypass surgery: An analysis of 17,594 patients in the state of New York. Am Surg. 2018 Aug 1; 84(8): 1388–1393.
35. Nicolajsen CW, Eldrep N. Abdominal closure and the risk of incisional hernia in aneurysm surgery: A systematic review and meta-analysis. Eur J Vasc Endovasc Surg. 2020; 59(2): 227–236.
36. Liang MK, Holihan JL, Itani K, et al: Ventral Hernia Management: Expert consensus guided by systematic review. Ann Surg. 2017; 265(1): 80–89.
37. Behman R, Nathens AB, Mason S, et al. Association of Surgical Intervention for Adhesive Small-Bowel Obstruction with Risk of Recurrence. JAMA Surg. 2019; 154(5): 413.
38. McKinsey JF, Gewertz BL. Acute mesenteric ischemia. Surg Clin North Am. 1997; 77(2): 307–18.
39. Wadman M, Syk I, Elmstahl S. Survival after operation for ischemic bowel disease. Eur J Surg. 2000;166(11): 872–7.
40. Steele SR: Ischemic colitis complicating major vascular surgery. Surg Clin North Am. 2007;87(5): 1099–114.
41. Makhija N, Singh R, Kiran U, et al. Mesenteric ischaemia occurring as a late complication after-aorto-femoral bypass. Indian J Anaesth. 2011;55(1): 57–60.
42. Brandt LJ, Boley SJ. AGA technical review on intestinal ischemia. Gastroenterology. 2000;118(5): 954–68.
43. Kirkpatrick ID, Kroeker MA, Greenberg HM. Biphasic CT with mesenteric CT angiography in the evaluation of acute mesenteric ischemia: Initial experience. Radiology. 2003;229(1):91–8.
44. Giles KA, Hamdan AD, Pomposelli RB, et al. Body Mass Index: Surgical Site Infections and Mortality after Lower Extremity Bypass from the National Surgical Quality Improvement Program 2005-2007. Ann Vasc Surg. 2010;24(1): 48–56.
45. Inui T, Bandyk DF. Vascular surgical site infection: Risk factors and preventive measures. Semin Vasc Surg. 2015;28(3-4): 201–7.
46. Swinnen J, Chao A, Tiwari A, et al. Vertical or transverse incisions for access to the femoral artery: a randomized control study. Ann Vasc Surg. 2010;24(3): 336–41.
47. Canteras M, Baptista-Silva JC, do Carmo Novaes F, Cacione DG. Transverse versus vertical groin incision for femoral artery approach. Cochrane Database Syst Rev. 2020 Apr 22;4: CD013153.
48. Matthey-Gié ML, Gié O, Deretti S, et al. Prospective Randomized Study to Compare Lymphocele and Lymphorrhea Control Following Inguinal and Axillary Therapeutic Lymph Node

Dissection With or Without the Use of an Ultrasonic Scalpel. Ann Surg Oncol. 2016;23(5): 1716–20.
49. Gié O, Matthey-Gié ML, Marques-Vidal PM, et al. Impact of the Ultrasonic scalpel on the amount of drained lymph after axillary or inguinal lymphadenectomy. BMC Surg. 2017;17(1): 27.
50. Kalman PG, Walker PM, Johnston KW. Consequences of groin lymphatic fistulae after vascular reconstruction. Vascular Surgery. 1991;25(3): 210–213.
51. Hasselmann J, Bjork J, Svensson-Bjork R, et al. Inguinal Vascular Surgical Wound Protection by Incisional Negative Pressure Wound Therapy: A Randomized Controlled Trial-INVIPS Trial. Ann Surg. 2020;271(1): 48–53.
52. Matatov T, Reddy KN, Doucet LD, et al. Experience with a new negative pressure incision management system in prevention of groin wound infection in vascular surgery patients. J Vasc Surg. 2013;57(3): 791–5.
53. Lee K, Murphy PB, Ingves MV, et al. Randomized clinical trial of negative pressure wound therapy for high-risk groin wounds in lower extremity revascularization. J Vasc Surg. 2017;66(6): 1814–1819.
54. Kwon J, Staley C, McCullough M, Goss S, et al. A randomized clinical trial evaluating negative pressure therapy to decrease vascular groin incision complications. J Vasc Surg 2018;68(6): 1744–1752.
55. Milner R, Minc S. Local complications: Aortoenteric Fistula. In: Sidawy AN, Perler BA, eds, Rutherfords's Vascular Surgery and Endovascular Therapy, 9th ed. Philadelphia: Elsevier Saunders; 2019: 615–623.
56. Batt M, Jean-Baptiste E, O'Connor S, et al. Early and late results of contemporary management of 37 secondary aortoenteric fistulae. Eur J Vasc Endovasc Surg. 2011;41(6): 748–57.
57. Antoniou GA, Koutsias S, Antoniou SA, et al. Outcome after endovascular stent graft repair of aortoenteric fistula: A systematic review. J Vasc Surg. 2009;49(3): 782–9.
58. Melliere D, Labastie J, Becquemin JP, et al. Proximal anastomosis in aortobifemoral bypass: end-to-end or end-to-side? J Cardiovasc Surg (Torino). 1990;31(1): 77–80.
59. McCann RL, Schwartz LB, Georgiade GS. Management of abdominal aortic complications. Ann Surg. 1993;217(6): 729–34.
60. Chou M, Wang C, Lien R. Prophylactic ureteral catheterization in gynecologic surgery: A 12-year randomized trial in a community hospital. Int Urogynecol 2009;20(6): 689–93.
61. Schapira HE, Li R, Gribetz M, et al. Ureteral injuries during vascular surgery. J Urol 1981; 125(3): 293–297.
62. Gayer G, Zissen R, Apter S, et al. Urinomas caused by ureteral injuries: CT appearance. Abdom Imaging. 2002;27(1): 88–92.
63. Borges LL, Torricelli FC, Ebaid GX, et al. Urological complications following aortoiliac graft: Case report and review of the literature. Sao Paulo Med J. 2010;128(3): 174–6.
64. Santucci RA, Doumanian LR. Upper urinary tract obstruction and trauma. In: Wein AJ, Kavoussi, Novick AC, et al, eds. Campbell-Walsh Urology, 10th ed. Philadelphia: Elsevier; 2007: p.1169.
65. Wright DJ, Ernst CB, Evans JR, Smith RF, Reddy DJ, Shepard AD, Elliot JP. Ureteral complications and aortoiliac reconstruction. J Vasc Surg. 1990;11(1): 29–35.
66. Braz AC, Castro-Ferreira R, Gonçalves Dias P, et al. Quality of life and aortobifemoral bypass: The importance of hypogastric arteries. Rev Port Cir Cardiotorac Vasc. 2016;23(3-4): 145–151.
67. Karkos CD, Wood A, Bruce IA, et al. Erectile dysfunction after open versus angioplasty aortoiliac procedures: A questionnaire survey. Vasc Endovascular Surg. 2004;38(2): 157–65.
68. Coombs PG, Heck M, Guhring P et al. A review of outcomes of an intracavernosal injection therapy programme. BJU Int. 2012;110(11): 1787–91.
69. Cárdenas A, Chopra S. Chylous ascites. Am J Gastroenterol. 2002;97(8): 1896–1900.
70. Talluri SK, Nuthakki H, Tadakamalla A, et al. Chylous ascites. North Am J Med Sci. 2011;3(9): 438–40.
71. Kara H. Chylous Ascites Developing after Open Thoracoabdominal Aortic Aneurysm Repair in a Patient with Marfan Syndrome. Braz J Cardiovasc Surg. 2019 Sep 3. [Epub ahead of print]
72. Williams RA, Vetto J, Quiñones-Baldrich W, et al. Chylous ascites following abdominal aortic surgery. Ann Vasc Surg. 1991;5(3): 247–52.
73. Galanopoulos G, Konstantopoulos T, Theodorou S, et al. Chylous Ascites Following Open Abdominal Aortic Aneurysm Repair: An Unusual Complication. Methodist Debakey Cardiovasc J. 2016;12(2): 119–121.
74. Duncan AA. Local complications: Lymphatic. In: Sidawy AN, Perler BA, eds, Rutherfords's Vascular Surgery and Endovascular Therapy, 9th ed. Philadelphia: Elsevier Saunders; 2019: 644–652.
75. Barakat HM, Shahin Y, McCollum P. Chylous ascites complicating elective abdominal aortic aneurysm repair: Case report and review of treatment options. Vasc Endovascular Surg. 2012;46(8): 682–5.
76. Derom A, Nout E. Treatment of femoral pseudoaneurysm with endograft in high risk patients. Eur J Vasc Endovasc Surg. 2005;30(6): 644–7.

77. Naddaf A, Hasanadka R, Hood D, et al. Repair of an anastomotic pseudoaneurysm with a novel hybrid technique. Ann Vasc Surg. 2020 Feb; 63: 439–442.
78. Lagana D, Carrafiello G, Mangini M, et al: Endovascular treatment of anastomotic pseudoaneurysms after aortoiliac surgical reconstruction. Cardiovasc Intervent Radiol. 2007:30: 1185–1191.

SUGGESTED READING

Menard MT, Shah S, Belkin M. Aortoiliac Disease: Direct Reconstruction. In: Sidawy AN, Perler BA, eds, Rutherfords's Vascular Surgery and Endovascular Therapy, 9th. Philadelphia: Elsevier Saunders; 2019: 1397–1415.

26

Complications of axillofemoral, femoral-femoral, and iliac-femoral grafts

Diagnosis, Prevention, and Management

FARAH MOHAMMAD AND MITCHELL WEAVER

In the current era of vascular surgery, endovascular therapies have become the primary treatment modality for aortoiliac arterial occlusive disease. In situations where endovascular interventions are unable to be successfully executed, aortobifemoral bypass graft with its favorable hemodynamic profile and durability is typically the treatment of choice. This leaves axillofemoral, femoral-femoral, and iliacfemoral grafting as lower tier option, for arterial reconstruction given their more invasive nature than endovascular techniques and poorer durability than aorta bifemoral bypass. These arterial reconstructions still have a role in situations in which endovascular techniques are not successful or applicable or for physiological or anatomical reasons, such as the patient medically unfit to undergo aorta bifemoral bypass or a hostile abdomen. Complications encountered with these operations generally fall into the categories of loss of graft patency/limb ischemia, wound complications/infection, and in late follow-up progression of disease. In order to prevent complications and provide the best outcome for the patient when they do occur, there are several steps that can be taken which include: ensuring the initial operation is performed for an appropriate indication, the patient is optimized for the operation, the conduct of the operation is performed in the appropriate manner, and, when complications do occur, they are promptly recognized and treated.

AXILLOFEMORAL GRAFT

Blaisdell and Hall performed the first axillofemoral bypass graft in 1963 for occlusive disease in patients considered to be high-risk surgical candidates.[1]

This operation is based on the ability of the axillary artery to supply adequate blood to the ipsilateral upper extremity and the ipsi- or bilateral lower extremities. This operation can be performed either alone or in a combination with femoral-femoral bypass. This alternate approach to aortoiliac reconstruction is usually reserved for frail patients with bilateral iliac artery occlusive disease, aortic graft sepsis, or hostile abdomen due to multiple prior abdominal operations, abdominal stomas, or radiation therapy.

OUTCOME AND COMPLICATIONS

The operative risk for axillofemoral bypass is lower than aorta bifemoral bypass as it avoids the physiologic stress of abdominal exploration and cross clamping of the aorta. Outcomes are dependent on the indication for the procedure, with significantly poorer results in the infection and emergent group.[2]

WOUND COMPLICATIONS

Mishall et al. report a 15% risk of wound complications.[3] Relatively common complications reported include infection, seroma, hematoma, and lymphocele formation. Wound complications are unfavorable prognostic factors for graft infection.

GRAFT INFECTION

Mutiple prior surgeries, especially redo exposures, are at higher risk for bacterial colonization thus increase the risk of graft infection.[4] The risk of graft infection has been reported to be up to 15%.[5] Graft infection has been more often observed when axillofemoral bypasses were performed for critical limb ischemia.[6] Bandyk et al. reported 10% re-infection risk after in situ prosthetic graft replacement for infected vascular grafts within the 26 month follow-up.[7]

GRAFT THROMBOSIS/PATENCY

Axillofemoral bypass's limited patency is the reason it remains an alternate approach to revascularization. 5 year patency has been reported from 35–80%.[8] Factors predicting decreased patency include operative indication of arterial occlusive disease, graft material (Dacron vs PTFE) and degree of infra-inguinal arterial occlusive disease. Initial reports of using Dacron non-supported grafts showed higher rates of thrombosis due to compression. However, multiple studies comparing Dacron to externally supported PTFE graft have not shown any significant difference.[9] Superficial femoral artery disease has been described in reports to be a predictor of worse outcomes.[3]

LIMB ISCHEMIA

Upper extremity ischemia is fortunately a rare complication. Mawatri et al. describe a risk of 2.5% of their 25% of grafts that occluded.[10] Kempczinski and Penn have also described arterial steal syndrome.[11] Rashleigh-Belcher et al. describe three cases of axillary artery thrombosis. They believe the likely cause was sharp angulation or pulling down of the artery from graft tension.[12] The residual stump of the proximal anastomosis of a non-functioning axillary femoral bypass graft may also be the source of arterial emboli to the distal ipsilateral upper extremity (Figure 26.1a, 26.1b, 26.1c); if this occurs, in addition to performing a thrombo-embolectomy of the upper extremity, the axillary anastomosis should be taken down and patch angioplasty of the artery performed to prevent further events.

ANASTOMOTIC DISRUPTION AND PSEUDOANEURYSMS

There are multiple case reports in the literature describing anastomotic disruption. If it occurs early in the postoperative period, its likely due to technical error. Late disruptions are highly concerning for infection. Failure to leave some redundancy on the graft can cause excessive tension, which can lead to disruption even after a minor trauma. There are various maneuvers described to prevent this complication. One is construction of the proximal anastomosis to the first portion of the axillary artery (medial to the pectoralis minor muscle), which undergoes less movement with movement of the arm. The graft is also tunneled

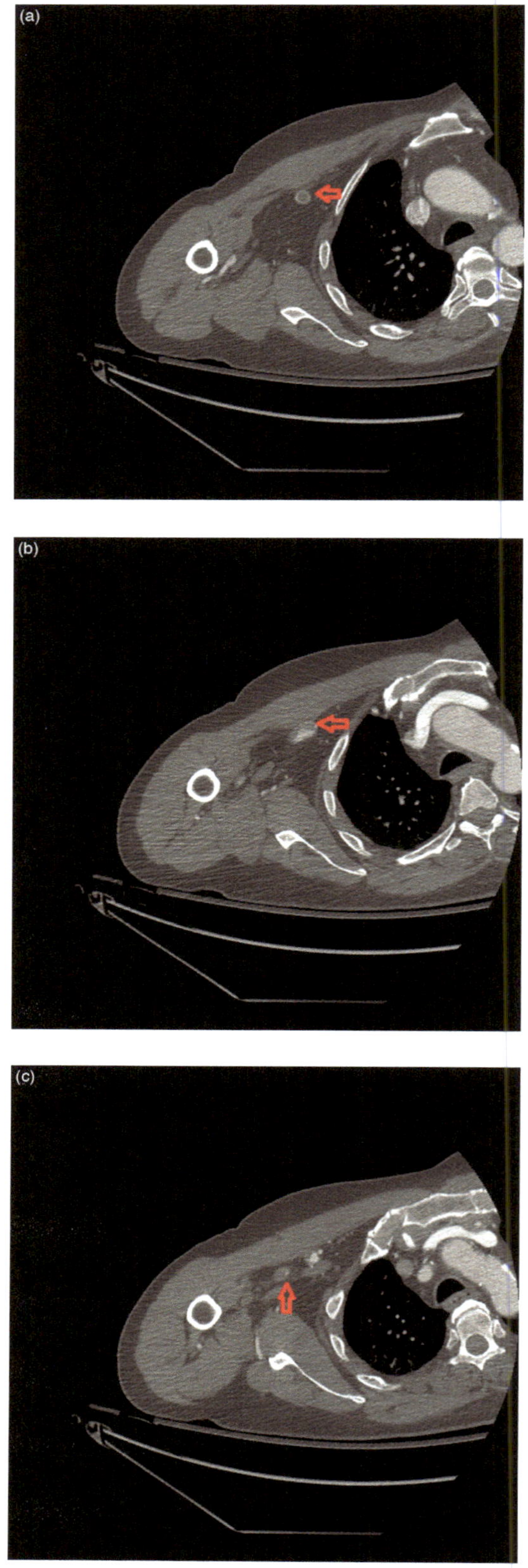

Figure 26.1 Computed tomography angiogram demonstrating: (a) (arrow) thrombosed axillofemoral bypass graft, (b) (arrow) thrombus extending from proximal anastomosis of axillofemoral bypass graft, (c) (arrow) thromboembolic occlusion of axillary artery distal to anastomosis.

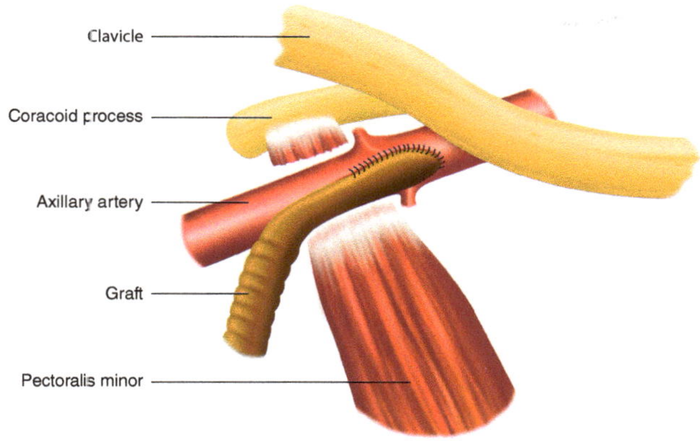

Figure 26.2 Illustration demonstrating preferred construction the proximal anastomosis of axillofemoral bypass utilizing the first portion of the axillary artery (medial to the pectoralis minor muscle). The graft is also tunneled behind the pectoralis minor muscle or, as in the illustration, muscle is divided along the artery before gently curving caudally.

behind the pectoralis minor muscle and along the artery before gently curving caudally (Figure 26.2). The anastomosis is also performed with the arm abducted to avoid tension. There is always concern for underlying infection versus technical cause if the presentation is in the subacute period though there are reports of sterile late disruption from material break down leading to pseudoaneurysms.[13]

Proximal anastomotic disruption of axillofemoral artery may be associated with forceful movements of the ipsilateral upper extremity such as arm abduction or shoulder elevation. Symptoms and signs include pain, swelling, and pulsatile mass. Confirmatory imaging, if necessary, includes duplex ultrasound and CT angiography. Surgical repair usually includes the need for supraclavicular exposure of the subclavian artery for proximal control. Endovascular techniques with balloon occlusion is another technique to consider for proximal control. The artery is then repaired with either patch angioplasty or short interposition graft. This can be followed by placement of an interposition graft between the artery and the previous graft, taking care to ensure a lack of tension on the graft.

TUNNELING AND DISSECTION INJURY

Tunneling and dissection injury specific to axillofemoral bypass include injury to the axillary artery, axillary vein and brachial plexus, as well as inadvertent entry into the peritoneal or pleural cavity during tunneling.[11] Such injuries are best avoided with careful tunneling. Entering the peritoneal cavity and creating a bowel injury can lead to catastrophic sepsis requiring resection of involved graft, repair/resection of involved bowel, and arterial reconstruction through clean uninfected planes if possible.

FEMORAL-FEMORAL BYPASS GRAFT

Vetto described the first comprehensive series of patients undergoing prosthetic femoral-femoral bypass in 1962. Femoral-femoral bypass is a good option for patients who are considered high risk for major revascularization with unilateral iliac arterial occlusive disease. The contralateral patent donor iliac system can be used for the origin of the bypass graft. It has also been described for patients undergoing aorto uni-iliac endograft placement necessitating contralateral revascularization. It is generally performed with prosthetic grafts, however autogenous may be used in cases where there is concern for infection. It is an operation of lesser magnitude than aorta bifemoral bypass and even though it is defined as technically simple by most surgeons, there are some unique technical challenges.

MORTALITY

Operative mortality should be less than 5% considering this procedure is meant to be less hemodynamically challenging versus aorta bifemoral bypass grafting. In another report, however, the mortality has been reported to be up to 10%, with even higher numbers in emergent cases.[14] This is reflective of the critically ill patient population.

GRAFT THROMBOSIS

In some studies the patency rate is reported to be up to 70% at 5 years depending on the indication for the operation.[15] Patients with critical limb ischemia do poorly compared to claudicants. Pursell et al. reports primary patency for patients with critical ischemia as 88%, 82% and 74% at 1, 3, and 5 years respectively. Respective figures for those who presented with claudication were 93, 92 and 90%.[16] Nguyen et al. reported primary patency rates of 83.7%, 73.7% and 69.8% at 1, 2, and 3 years respectively, for PTFE bypasses, and 100% for all time points for venous grafts, respectively.[17] Primary-assisted and secondary patency rates were not significantly different between the two groups.

Causes of failure may be technical or progression of disease. If there is any concern for inflow disease on the donor side, it should be addressed prior. Donor iliac angioplasty and stenting has been described as a safe option. Although there are studies that discuss the importance of minimally diseased SFA but there is sufficient data that supports the adequacy of outflow with a patent profound femoris artery.[18,19]

TUNNELING INJURY

Van Nieuwenhuizen et al. reported a case of small bowel injury due to tunneling of a femoro-femoral crossover bypass.[20] Visceral injury (e.g., bowel or bladder) while making the tunnel retro-fascial can be extremely devastating, sometimes leading to a delay in diagnosis and resultant sepsis. Similarly, Hinchliffe et al. reviewed visceral organ damage following femoro-femoral bypass.[21] At our institution we prefer finger dissection to create the tunnel to avoid this complication. Risk is higher in patients with hernia, previous pelvic surgeries, and radiation. Another technical aspect of tunneling that can lead to failure and should be avoided is kinking of the graft at the site of the anastomosis to the femoral arteries bilaterally. This can be best avoided by keeping the tunnel uniform over a larger radius arc.

INFECTION AND WOUND COMPLICATIONS

Infection may present as non-healing sinus wounds, fluid collections, exposed grafts, and anastomotic aneurysms. Pursell, in his review of 144 femoral-femoral bypasses, reports a 6% graft infection rate.[16]

ILIO-FEMORAL BYPASS

Ilio-femoral bypass is another option for high-risk patients with symptomatic unilateral iliac disease. It avoids bilateral groin exposures involved in femoral-femoral bypass grafting. Tunneling is usually straightforward; however, if proximal anastomosis is near common iliac artery bifurcation or involves the common iliac artery, care should be taken to avoid injury to the ureter as it crosses over the iliac artery, and any graft coming off of the common iliac artery should be tunneled underneath the ureter, to prevent compression of the ureter leading to hydronephrosis.

GRAFT THROMBOSIS

5 year patency can be up to 93%.[14,22] In a review by Defraigne, the primary and secondary patency rates were 94% and 100%, respectively at 1 year, and 76.7% and 95%, respectively, at 5 years.[23]

COMPLICATION SPECIFIC MANAGEMENT CONSIDERATIONS

Perigraft seroma

All prosthetic grafts can be susceptible to perigraft seromas, which are sterile fluid collections around the graft with a pseudocapsule (Figure 26.3). The exact etiology and best management of seromas are not clearly defined. Often these fluid collections will resolve with time. Aspiration may be performed to rule out infection, however the fluid will likely reoccur and aspiration itself may lead to infection of the fluid. For symptomatic patients, washout, excision of pseudo-capsule, and replacement with new graft, possibly of different material (i.e., replace Goretex with Dacron), may be a solution.

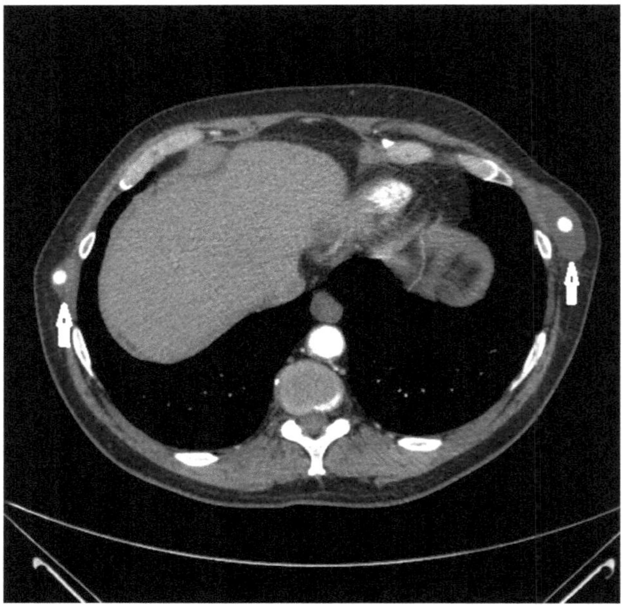

Figure 26.3 Computed tomography angiogram demonstrating fluid collections (arrows) surrouncing axillofemoral bypass grafts consistent with peri-graft seroma.

GRAFT THROMBOSIS/FAILURE

Graft thrombosis/failure both in the immediate postop period as well long term remains a significant challenge for the vascular surgeon. The underlying causes of graft failure are multifactorial. These include patient specific factors such as demographics, comorbidities, hypercoagulable states, quality of inflow and outflow vessels, as well as quality of conduit. Technical factors/errors involving the operation may lead to graft failure. Long-term progression of disease also contributes to graft failure.

Prevention of early graft failure involves preoperative assessment, including that the inflow artery is free of any upstream hemodynamically significant arterial occlusive disease and, if there is such disease present, that it is treated concomitantly. Likewise, ensure that the outflow is satisfactory. This involves in cases of "inflow operations" such as those discussed in this chapter determining whether a common femoral or profundus femoral artery endarterectomy is required in addition to the bypass. Intra-operatively, following restoration of blood flow, the distal limb should be inspected for signs of adequate perfusion, distal pulse palpated, and as well as the distal arteries insonated for the presence of Doppler signals. Further evaluation can be performed with duplex ultrasound or digital subtraction angiography.

Early graft failure typically mandates return to the operating room. Typically balloon catheter thrombectomy is first performed. Then the anastomoses should be inspected for technical error, with any findings corrected. Re-evaluation of inflow and out flow vessels adequacy should be access, and if found inadequate should be addressed. The quality of conduit material should be assessed. The graft should be evaluated for any twists or chinks. Angiography through the graft after thrombectomy may help to uncover technical defects. The patient should be anticoagulated, and hypercoagulable states should be considered.

In cases of late graft failure, treatment depends on degree of symptoms. Late graft failure may present as insidiously as a decrease in ankle brachial indices on routine follow-up and/or a return to preoperative ischemic symptoms, to profound acute limb ischemia. Patients presenting with acute limb ischemia are evaluated using Rutherford criteria[24] for acute limb ischemia, which involves evaluation of sensory function, motor function, and presence or absence of pedal Doppler signals. Those patients with neurologic deficit require more urgent intervention for hope of achieving limb salvage. On the other hand, a patient with no symptoms or minimal symptoms of claudication may only require observation.

The diagnosis of graft occlusion is typically evident on physical exam by loss of graft pulse, as well as in the case of these inflow bypasses, a femoral pulse. Graft occlusion may be confirmed using imaging studies such as duplex ultrasound, CT angiography and catheter-based angiography. Duplex ultrasound has the advantage of being noninvasive but may not be able to fully evaluate inflow and outflow vessels for operative planning. CT angiography is usually readily available and allows for imaging of not only the graft but also inflow and out flow vessels. Down sides to CT angiography include the use of radiation and IV contrast. Conventional angiography may also be useful, as at the same time in appropriate candidates catheter-directed thrombolysis may be initiated if the graft thrombosis is believed to be relatively acute and the graft is configured in such a way that allows it to be crossed with an infusion catheter. Catheter-directed thrombolysis allows for possible salvage of the graft and possible exposure of an underlying lesion that led to graft thrombosis, which can then be treated in order to prevent recurrent thrombosis (i.e., common/deep femoral artery occlusive disease requiring endarterectomy). Other treatment options include an attempt at surgical graft thrombectomy and then assessing for an underlying culprit lesion that can be treated.

Additional considerations include performing a new arterial reconstruction. Despite the fact that the patient has undergone an open extra anatomic bypass previously in the case of femoral-femoral bypass or axillary femoral bypass, the patient should be reassessed to see if they are now a candidate for either endovascular/hybrid operation with stenting of their iliac arteries, or perhaps an aorta bifemoral bypass, which may offer improved durability to the patient (Figure 26.4).

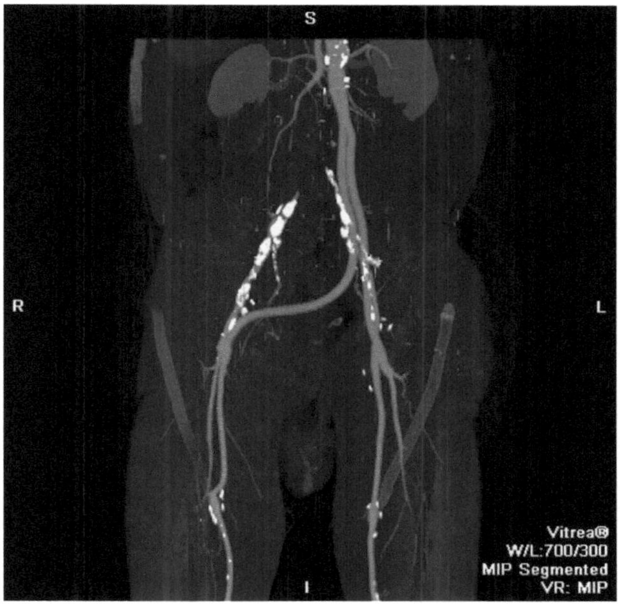

Figure 26.4 Reformatted computed tomography angiogram demonstrating re-do aorta bifemoral bypass following failed bilateral axillofemoral bypasses.

FEMORAL ANASTOMOTIC PSEUDOANEURYSM

Femoral anastomotic aneurysms (Figure 26.5) may present as an asymptomatic pulsatile mass in the groin, with symptoms such as ischemia from thrombosis, as a source of distal thrombo-embolization, as venous insufficiency,

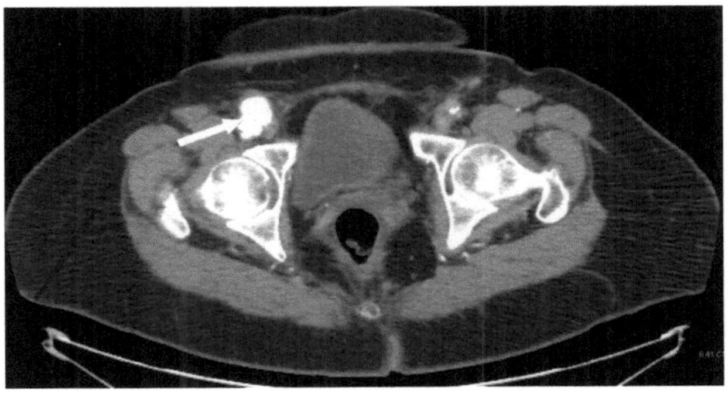

Figure 26.5 Computed tomography angiogram demonstrating: femoral anastomotic pseudoaneurysm (arrow).

DVT or femoral neuropraxia from local compression. The mere presence of a pseudoaneurysm itself may be a sign of graft infection. While all symptomatic aneurysms have an indication for repair, repair of asymptomatic aneurysm is considered once they reach a size of ≥ 2.0–2.5 cm in diameter and/or contain a significant amount of mural thrombus. Complications are uncommon in femoral anastomotic aneurysms less than 2 cm; however, larger aneurysms are associated with local complications and limb ischemia.[25,26]

Computed tomographic angiography (CTA) of abdomen, pelvis, and lower extremities is the preferred imaging modality, however other imaging modalities such as MRA, duplex ultrasound, and catheter digital subtraction angiography may also be useful. Complete imaging of all other arterial-graft anastomotic sites to rule out synchronous aneurysms should be performed. The finding of peri-anastomotic fluid and/or lack of graft incorporation noted on imaging studies should raise concern for a possible infectious process. Assessment of limb perfusion should be performed by measuring Doppler-derived ankle-brachial indices (ABIs) of both lower extremities.

The re-do nature of these operations can make them very difficult. Sharp scalpel (#15 blade) dissection is often the best method when dense scar tissue is encountered. Care should be taken not to "exarterectomize" the arterial wall. This occurs when a plane is created between the adventitia and media. Often this dissection plane appears as an easier natural dissection plane, however it will result in a residual arterial wall too weak to hold sutures. Exposure in a densely scarred operative field is frequently aided by initial identification and dissection of the proximal superficial femoral artery, which is usually associated with relatively less scar. Once this vessel has been identified, dissection can proceed more proximally.

The complicated re-do nature of these procedures, which also usually require more extensive exposure, are at increased risk for lymphatic complications.[27] Great care should be taken to ligate any structures which appear to contain lymphatic channels. Division of overlying tissues with the cautery alone is to be avoid. Attempt at control of the inflow and outflow vessels should be made before entering the aneurysm. Proximal exposure of the graft outside the groin incision should be considered for proximal control of inflow with large aneurysms. Due to the dense scar tissue often encountered with anastomotic femoral aneurysms, complete vascular control before entering the aneurysm is not always possible and in such cases balloon occlusion catheters may be useful (Figure 26.6).

Interposition of a new prosthetic graft between old graft and host artery is the most reliable repair in most cases. The aneurysm is excised and the inflow and outflow vessels are debrided back to normal arterial wall. Anastomotic sutures should be placed in normal healthy artery with good bites, creating a tension-free anastomosis.

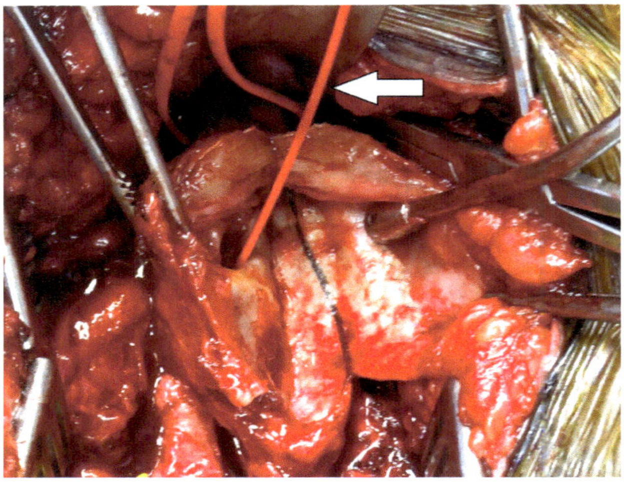

Figure 26.6 Intraoperative photograph demonstrating use of balloon catheter (arrow) for arterial control in hostile groin dissection.

Outcomes for repair of femoral anastomotic aneurysms are favorable with reported with mortality < 5% in the elective setting; however, there is significantly higher morbidity and mortality associated with emergent repairs. Recurrent femoral anastomotic aneurysms are reported in 6–19% of treated patients.[26–29]

GRAFT INFECTION

Prosthetic graft infections pose a significant morbidity and mortality risk for the patients. Patient may present with overt signs of infection such as fever or with erythema, swelling, induration, and drainage overlying the graft or surgical incisions (Figure 26.7). Supportive laboratory tests, while nonspecific, include leukocytosis with or without a left-shifted differential count and elevated inflammatory markers, such as erythrocyte

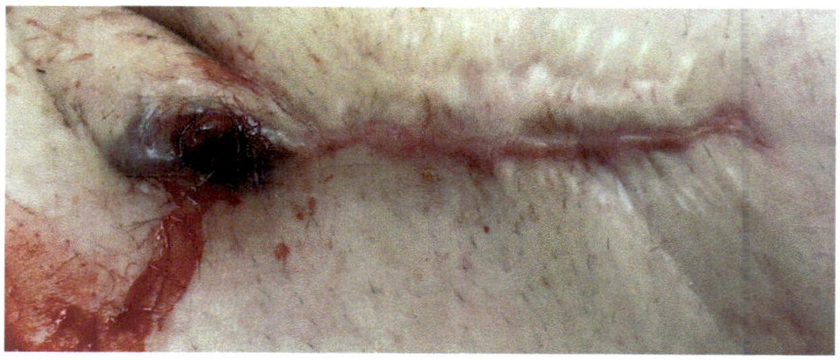

Figure 26.7 Photograph of surgical incision in groin of patient presenting with graft infection.

sedimentation rate and C-reactive protein. Blood cultures should be obtained, however they often do not yield positive results even with obvious infection. However, effort should be made to identify the offending organism. Common pathogens include *Staphylococcus aureus* and *S. epidermidis*, the latter with a penchant for foreign bodies given its biofilm-producing property.[30]

Computed tomography angiogram (CTA), which can help to confirm the diagnosis, evaluate the extent of the infection, and direct operative planning for definitive treatment. Findings consistent with graft infection include perigraft enhancement, adjacent soft tissue stranding, pockets of gas, pseudoaneurysm formation, and even frank anastomotic rupture. If the diagnosis of graft remains uncertain, a short-term follow-up CTA or a tagged white blood cell scan may further clarify the presence of infection (Figure 26.8a,b,c).

Principles include prevention or control of hemorrhage, control of infection with removal of all infected graft and debridement of all non-viable tissue as well as use of appropriate antibiotics, and insuring adequate perfusion to the extremity if possible. This may include bypassing around the infection through noninfected tissue planes, or bypassing through the same field with an autogenous conduit or cryopreserved allografts with possible muscle flap coverage. In certain situations with very virulent infections or higher risk patients, arterial ligation without arterial reconstruction may be in the patients' best interest even if it leads to limb loss, as recurrent infection and graft rupture may lead to fatal hemorrhage.

In a select group of early, low-virulent graft infections, an attempt to salvage an infected graft may be reasonable. When this strategy is selected there should be no sign of systemic infection, and the anastomosis should not be exposed. Local wound care with vacuum-assisted wound closure therapy and antibiotics has been successfully used.[31] Negative pressure wound therapy helps with creating a moist environment but at the same time suctions excessive fluid. It accelerates granulation and approximation of wounds.[32,33] Acosta et al., in his meta-analysis, reports a graft salvage rate of 83–100%.[34] Mayer, in his review of 44 patients with Szilagy grade III infections, reports a graft/native artery salvage rate of 84% with negative-pressure therapy.[35]

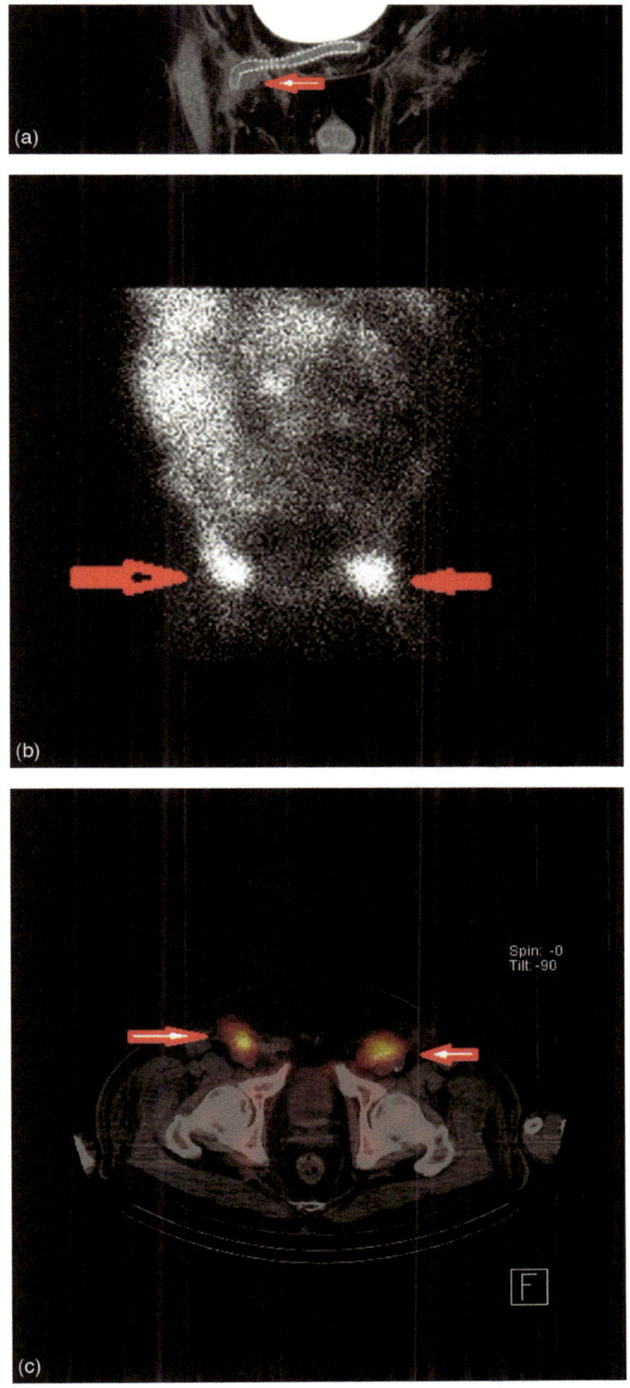

Figure 26.8 (a) Computed tomography angiogram (CTA) demonstrating fluid collection around femoral-femoral bypass graft with concern for infection. (b) Leukocyte scan demonstrating accumulation of radiolabeled leukocytes in bilateral inguinal regions(arrows). (c) Fusion imaging of the CTA and leukocyte scan demonstrating radiolabeled leukocytes around the graft.

LYMPHOCUTANEOUS FISTULAS

Lymphocutaneous fistulas following arterial reconstructions involving the femoral artery may potentially lead to much more serious complications, namely wound infection and subsequently graft infection. The underlying cause of the lymph drainage is presumably injury to lymphatics during groin dissection. No standard definition exists to describe the magnitude of the lymph fistula, nor is there a standard treatment algorithm. Suggested strategies for initial management include bed rest, antibiotics, and local wound care.[20,27,36] As an adjuvant to local wound care, the addition of negative-pressure wound therapy has been advocated. For significant lymph leaks, especially in the presence of a prosthetic graft, our practice has been early re-operation with ligation of culprit lymphatics. The addition of vascularized muscle flap coverage has also been successfully used in the treatment of lymphocutaneous fistulas.[36]

REFERENCES

1. Blaisdell FW, Hall AD. Axillary-Femoral Artery Bypass for Lower Extremity Ischemia. Surgery. 1963;54: 563–8.
2. Dickas D, Verrel F, Kalff J, Koscielny A. Axillobifemoral Bypasses: Reappraisal of an Extra-Anatomic Bypass by Analysis of Results and Prognostic Factors. World journal of surgery. 2018;42(1): 283–94.
3. Mishall PL, Matakas JD, English K, Allyn K, Algava D, Howe RA, et al. Axillobifemoral bypass: A brief surgical and historical review. Einstein J Biol Med. 2016;31(1-2): 6–10.
4. Turtiainen J, Hakala T. Surgical wound infections after peripheral vascular surgery. Scand J Surg. 2014;103(4): 226–31.
5. Passman MA, Taylor LM, Moneta GL, Edwards JM, Yeager RA, McConnell DB, et al. Comparison of axillofemoral and aortofemoral bypass for aortoiliac occlusive disease. J Vasc Surg. 1996;23(2): 263–9; discussion 9–71.
6. Ott E, Bange FC, Sohr D, Teebken O, Mattner F. Risk factors associated with surgical site infections following vascular surgery at a German university hospital. Epidemiol Infect. 2013;141(6): 1207–13.
7. Bandyk DF, Esses GE. Prosthetic graft infection. Surg Clin North Am. 1994;74(3): 571–90.
8. Martin D, Katz SG. Axillofemoral bypass for aortoiliac occlusive disease. Am J Surg. 2000;180(2): 100–3.
9. Kenney DA, Sauvage LR, Wood SJ, Berger K, Davis CC, Smith JC, et al. Comparison of noncrimped, externally supported (EXS) and crimped, nonsupported Dacron prostheses for axillofemoral and above-knee femoropopliteal bypass. Surgery. 1982;92(6): 931–46.
10. Mawatari K, Muto Y, Funahashi S, Ikeda T, Komori K, Sugimachi K. The potential risk for upper extremity thromboembolism in patients with occluded axillofemoral bypass grafts: Two case reports. Vasc Surg. 2001;35(1): 67–71.
11. Kempczinski R, Penn I. Upper extremity complications of axillofemoral grafts. Am J Surg. 1978;136(2): 209–11.
12. Rashleigh-Belcher HJ, Newcombe JF. Axillary artery thrombosis: A complication of axillofemoral bypass grafts. Surgery. 1987;101(3): 373–5.
13. Piazza D, Ameli FM, von Schroeder HP, Lossing A. Nonanastomotic pseudoaneurysm of expanded polytetrafluoroethylene axillofemoral bypass graft. J Vasc Surg. 1993;17(4): 777–9.
14. Perler BA, Burdick JF, Williams GM. Femoro-femoral or ilio-femoral bypass for unilateral inflow reconstruction? Am J Surg. 1991;161(4): 426–30.
15. Park KM, Park YJ, Kim YW, Hyun D, Park KB, Do YS, et al. Long Term Outcomes of Femorofemoral Crossover Bypass Grafts. Vasc Specialist Int. 2017;33(2): 55–8.
16. Pursell R, Sideso E, Magee TR, Galland RB. Critical appraisal of femorofemoral crossover grafts. Br J Surg. 2005;92(5): 565–9.
17. Nguyen KP, Moneta G, Landry G. Venous Conduits Have Superior Patency Compared with Prosthetic Grafts for Femorofemoral Bypass. Ann Vasc Surg. 2018;52: 126–37.
18. Todd GJ, Voorhees AB, Nowygrod R, Reemtsma K. Femorofemoral bypass for unilateral iliac artery occlusion in the presence of bilateral superficial femoral artery occlusions. J Cardiovasc Surg (Torino). 1985; 26(1): 12–4.
19. Schneider JR, Besso SR, Walsh DB, Zwolak RM, Cronenwett JL. Femorofemoral versus aortobifemoral bypass: Outcome and hemodynamic results. J Vasc Surg. 1994;19(1): 43–55; 7.
20. Van den Brande P, von Kemp K, Aerden D, Debing E, Vanhulle A, Staelens I, et al. Treatment of lymphocutaneous fistulas after vascular procedures of the lower limb: Accurate wound reclosure and 3 weeks of consistent and continuing drainage. Ann Vasc Surg. 2012;26(6): 833–8.
21. Hinchliffe RJ, Alric P, Wenham PW, Hopkinson BR. Durability of femorofemoral bypass grafting after aortouniiliac endovascular aneurysm repair. J Vasc Surg. 2003;38(3): 498–503.
22. Carsten CG, 3rd, Kalbaugh CA, Langan EM 3rd, Cass AL, Cull DL, Snyder BA, et al. Contemporary outcomes of iliofemoral bypass grafting for unilateral aortoiliac occlusive disease: A 10-year experience. Am J Surg. 2008;74(6): 555–9; discussion 9-60.
23. Defraigne JO, Vazquez C, Limet R. Crossover iliofemoral bypass grafting for treatment of unilateral iliac atherosclerotic disease. J Vasc Surg. 1999;30(4): 693–700.
24. Rutherford RB. Clinical staging of acute limb ischemia as the basis for choice of revascularization method: When and how to intervene. Seminars in vascular surgery. 2009;22(1): 5–9.
25. Ylonen K, Biancari F, Leo E, Rainio P, Salmela E, Lahtinen J, et al. Predictors of development of anastomotic femoral pseudoaneurysms after

aortobifemoral reconstruction for abdominal aortic aneurysm. American journal of surgery. 2004;187(1): 83–7.
26. Skourtis G, Bountouris I, Papacharalambous G, Mahera E, Besias N, Antoniou I, et al. Anastomotic pseudoaneurysms: Our experience with 49 cases. Annals of vascular surgery. 2006;20(5): 582–9.
27. Tyndall SH, Shepard AD, Wilczewski JM, Reddy DJ, Elliott JP, Jr., Ernst CB. Groin lymphatic complications after arterial reconstruction. Journal of vascular surgery. 1994;19(5): 858–63; discussion 63–4.
28. Markovic DM, Davidovic LB, Kostic DM, Maksimovic ZL, Kuzmanovic IB, Koncar IB, et al. False anastomotic aneurysms. Vascular. 2007;15(3): 141–8.
29. Ernst CB, Elliott JP, Jr., Ryan CJ, Abu-Hamad G, Tilley BC, Murphy RK, et al. Recurrent femoral anastomotic aneurysms. A 30-year experience. Annals of surgery. 1988;208(4): 401–9.
30. Lawrence PF. Conservative treatment of aortic graft infection. Seminars in vascular surgery. 2011;24(4): 199–204.
31. Berger P, de Bie D, Moll FL, de Borst GJ. Negative pressure wound therapy on exposed prosthetic vascular grafts in the groin. Journal of vascular surgery. 2012;56(3): 714–20.
32. Monsen C, Acosta S, Mani K, Wann-Hansson C. A randomised study of NPWT closure versus alginate dressings in peri-vascular groin infections: Quality of life, pain and cost. Journal of wound care. 2015;24(6): 252, 4–6, 8-0.
33. Zannis J, Angobaldo J, Marks M, DeFranzo A, David L, Molnar J, et al. Comparison of fasciotomy wound closures using traditional dressing changes and the vacuum-assisted closure device. Annals of plastic surgery. 2009;62(4):407–9.
34. Acosta S, Bjorck M, Wanhainen A. Negative-pressure wound therapy for prevention and treatment of surgical-site infections after vascular surgery. British journal of surgery. 2017;104(2):e75–e84.
35. Mayer D, Hasse B, Koelliker J, Enzler M, Veith FJ, Rancic Z, et al. Long-term results of vascular graft and artery preserving treatment with negative pressure wound therapy in Szilagyi grade III infections justify a paradigm shift. Annals of surgery. 2011;254(5):754–59; discussion 60.
36. Twine CP, Lane IF, Williams IM. Management of lymphatic fistulas after arterial reconstruction in the groin. Annals of vascular surgery. 2013;27(8):1207–15.

27

Complications of femoropopliteal and infrapopliteal arterial bypass

FRANK M. DAVIS AND PETER K. HENKE

It is estimated that 8 to 12 million Americans are affected by peripheral arterial disease (PAD) and the prevalence will continue to rise.[1] Infrainguinal bypass remains one of the most common open vascular operations to treat patients with PAD. In the current era, endovascular interventions are increasingly successful as stand-alone procedures. However, a significant number of patients require open bypass for lower extremity occlusive disease due to atherosclerotic burden or failure of endovascular therapy. Following open vascular reconstruction, postoperative morbidity and mortality continue to be an area of active improvement with complications occurring in up to 20% of procedures. Understanding the etiology and clinical manifestations of complications following open lower extremity revascularization is crucial for achieving the best and most durable results for PAD patients. Herein, this chapter focuses on infrainguinal bypass with brief discussion of the preoperative and operative approach to lower extremity vascular disease as well as a detailed review of perioperative morbidities with specific attention to the diagnosis and management of these complications.

INDICATIONS

Two primary indications for infrainguinal bypass remain critical limb ischemia (CLI) and claudication. For patients with CLI, defined as rest pain, tissue loss, or ankle pressure lower than 40 mmHg, only 5% will achieve limb survival at 1 year without revascularization.[2] For patients with claudication, the natural history is progressive decline in ambulatory distance before the onset of pain. Despite intensive medical management, 20–30% will develop increased disability.[3] Interventions for claudication are done to improve function in the setting of significant ongoing disability.

PREOPERATIVE ASSESSMENT AND IMAGING

Infrainguinal bypass requires a careful assessment of the extent of arterial disease as well as a detailed anatomic characterization of the inflow and outflow arteries. Generally, arteriography is the "gold standard" for most patients with CLI. However, advances in computed tomographic angiography (CTA) have led to an increasing number of patients undergoing CTAs, especially those with absent femoral pulses. Unfortunately, in the periphery, the small caliber of the infrainguinal artery and the presence of calcification in multiple vessels limit the applicability of CTA, especially in CLI patients. Preoperative imaging should identify major anatomic lesions, the inflow site, and the potential outflow vessel. In nearly all patients in whom infrainguinal bypass is indicated, suitable target arteries can be identified if diagnostic angiography is properly performed. Occasionally, duplex ultrasonography can identify suitability of the pedal targets on the foot.

The common femoral artery (CFA) is typically the inflow vessel of choice, although more distal locations such as superficial femoral, profunda, or popliteal artery may be used with equivalent patencies. Intraoperatively, if there is uncertainty about the suitability of inflow site, direct arterial pressures can be compared to a radial arterial pressure. A resting pressure gradient of > 10 mmHg is significant and a more proximal location for the site of bypass inflow should be considered. In addition, consideration of CFA endarterectomy is prudent. Regarding distal outflow target, the general principle with infrainguinal reconstruction is the distal target vessel should bypass all significant atherosclerotic disease to the most proximal limb artery that has at least one runoff artery to the foot. Thereby, the below-knee popliteal artery is the most commonly used target. Improper distal target selection can decrease long-term graft patency. Although most claudicants require only femoropopliteal bypass, a high proportion of CLI patients require tibial or pedal bypasses. Arteries distal to the outflow target should be free of hemodynamically significant disease.

Autogenous conduits provide the best patency for infrainguinal arterial reconstruction.[4] The preferred autogenous conduit is the great saphenous vein (GSV). Reversed and in situ configurations of the GSV are equally effective; however, some proponents of in situ GSV bypass suggest it provides better size matching.[5] For optimal patency, the vein should be at least 3 mm in diameter, although compressible veins between 2–3 mm in diameter can be used. Studies have shown that 5-year patency of appropriately chosen GSV conduit for above-knee bypass is > 70%,[4] while the 3-year patency for below-knee bypasses with GSV is 50–70%.[6] For patients who do not have suitable vein, a prosthetic conduit can be used. In comparison to reversed GSV grafts, PTFE have the same patency for above-knee popliteal bypasses during the first 2–3 years; however, thereafter vein grafts have superior long-term patency.[7,8] Prosthetic bypass to the below-knee popliteal artery has uniformly poor patency (54% 3-year patency of PTFE vs 61% 3-year patency for GSV).[9] Randomized trials have shown that the addition of vein cuffs significantly improves the patency of prosthetic grafts for infrageniculate bypasses (52% patency at 2 years for PTFE with vein cuff vs 29% for PTFE without cuff), with addition of warfarin.[10]

OPERATIVE TECHNIQUE

The common femoral artery is most frequently used as the inflow vessel for infrainguinal bypasses. A vertical incision is made directly over the medial third between the pubic tubercle and the anterior superior iliac spine. Adequate time should be spent ligating and cauterizing all lymphatics to reduce the risk of a lymphocele. Upon entering the femoral sheath, the common femoral artery is dissected proximally to the inguinal ligament. Distally, the common femoral artery divides into the superficial and the deep femoral artery. The lateral femoral circumflex vein crosses anterior to the deep femoral artery at the level of bifurcation. Following identification of all vessels, Silastic vessel loops are placed around each vessel to establish vessel control.

For the distal target, the above-knee popliteal artery is approached through a medial incision with the leg externally rotated and knee flexed 30°. In contrast, exposure of the infrageniculate popliteal artery is achieved through a medial incision 1–2 cm posterior to the medial edge of the tibia with the leg externally rotated and knee flexed 30°. If a distal tibial target is chosen based on the preoperative imaging, an extension of the below-knee popliteal is employed as a 10 cm incision is created 2 cm posterior to the medial edge of the tibia will allow access to the proximal anterior and posterior tibial artery. Lastly, for the peroneal artery, a vertical incision is made 2 cm behind the posterior border of the tibia in the middle third of the calf. The peroneal vessels are located deep to the posterior tibial artery on the anterior surface of the flexor hallucis longus. Once adequate exposure is obtained, the distal target is analyzed for a healthy segment with palpation, and vessel loops are placed proximally and distally.

Following exposure of the proximal and distal targets, the conduit tunnel is created. The tunneling device is passed from the femoral incision to the popliteal fossa either above or below the knee behind the sartorius muscle. The chosen conduit is marked for orientation to prevent twists, and then attached to the tunneler and pulled into position with proper positioning of the conduit checked. The proximal anastomosis is performed first in an end-to-side fashion. Regarding the distal anastomosis, care should be taken to identify a site of distal arteriotomy that is free of excessive calcification. The orientation of the graft is checked and the bulldog clamp is released to ensure pulsatile bleeding. An end-to-side anastomosis is created between the conduit and distal target using similar technique to the proximal anastomosis. Following completion of the proximal and distal anastomoses, intraoperatively a duplex Doppler provides qualitative assessment of infrainguinal bypasses by analyzing changes in velocity or spectral broadening to detect conduit defects. If there are concerns, a completion angiogram is performed using contrast injection into the hood of the proximal anastomosis.

COMPLICATIONS

The major postoperative morbidities of infrainguinal bypass include both systemic and local complications. The PREVENT III trial, with 1404 infrainguinal grafts in patients with CLI, reported perioperative systemic complications of major morbidity (17.6%), myocardial infarction (4.7%), pneumonia (1.6%), stroke (1.4%), and mortality (2.7%). A detailed review of the evaluation and management of systemic complications following vascular reconstruction has been discussed in previous chapters. In this section we will provide a review of local and graft-related complications following lower extremity revascularization including their diagnosis and management.

BLEEDING

Meticulous hemostasis during the dissection is mandatory. Investigations have demonstrated that following lower extremity open revascularization, postoperative hematoma occurs at a rate of 6.0%, but a minority require reoperation for bleeding.[11] Areas of importance for prevention of postoperative bleeding during the surgical procedure include harvesting the venous conduit and ensuring that all side branches are adequately ligated. Hemostatic clips should not be used on the venous conduit side, as they may become dislodged during tunneling. If focal bleeding is noted in the vein graft tunnel, this can be repaired by direct cut down onto the area of concern. For focal bleeding from the anastomosis, this usually requires placement of a single repair suture, but using double-pledgeted sutures are recommended for friable vessels. However, if severe bleeding is noted from the anastomosis, this may results from improper technique, failure to include all layers of the arterial wall, poor vessel integrity, or excessive tension. For this situation, the anastomosis may need to be redone to achieve hemostasis.

WOUND COMPLICATIONS

Surgical site infection and graft infection

Surgical site infection (SSI) is a common postoperative complication of lower extremity bypasses with studies demonstrating a combined rate of superficial and deep SSI occurring in approximately 11% of patients.[12] For superficial SSI, the site or sites of graft implantation should be carefully examined for any signs of inflammation. If present, the patient should receive oral antibiotics tailored toward common skin microbiota, and consideration should be given for opening and packing the involved area of the wound to heal by secondary intention. Deep SSI and graft infections occur after 0.9%–3.5% of operation, and are influenced by implant site, indication for intervention, underlying disease, and an array of patient-related risk factors. In contrast to superficial SSI developing within the perioperative period, lower extremity bypass graft infections can develop months to years after the initial operation. Virtually any microorganism can infect vascular prosthesis; however, *S. aureus* is the most prevalent pathogen and accounts for one-fourth to one half of all infections. In recent years, infections with *S. epidermidis* or gram-negative bacteria have increased in frequency. Infection with gram-negative bacteria such as *E. coli* and *Pseudomonas, Klebsiella, Enterobacter, Serratia*, and *Proteus* species can be particularly virulent. The incidence of anastomotic dehiscence and arterial rupture is high because of the ability of the organisms to produce destructive endotoxins (e.g., elastase and alkaline protease) that compromise the structural integrity of the vessel wall.

If concern exists for a deep SSI and/or graft infection, surgical incisions should be carefully inspected for erythema and draining sinuses. An elevated WBC count with a left-shifted differential count and increased erythrocyte sedimentation rate are common but nonspecific findings. Positive blood cultures are uncommon (< 5%), but when present, indicate advanced graft infection or virulent organisms. Vascular imaging is essential for the diagnosis and treatment of graft infection. Anatomic signs of graft infection, such as perigraft abscess or anastomotic aneurysm, can be accurately identified (with > 90% sensitivity) through a combination of ultrasonography, CT, magnetic resonance imaging, or arteriography. Diagnostic criteria consistent with infection include loss of normal tissue planes, collection of perigraft fluid or gas, false aneurysm, or adjacent infection of adjacent bony structures. Functional radionuclide imaging ($_{111}$In-labeled leukocytes or $_{99m}$Tc-hexametazime-labeled leukocytes) can confirm the presence of a clinically suspected graft infection when anatomic signs of perigraft infection are equivocal.

The goals of managing vascular graft infections involve initial and long-term eradication of the local and systemic septic process and maintenance of normal arterial perfusion to the involved limb tissues. Selection criteria for specific treatment modalities are based primarily on the clinical findings, extent of graft involvement, and microbiology. Important adjuncts to attain wound sterilization, especially when graft preservation is under consideration, include the use of multiple staged debridements/"washout" operative procedures to minimize residual bacterial counts, aggressive excision of involved arterial wall and perigraft tissues to healthy tissue planes, intraoperative mechanical and passive wound irrigation with cytotoxic agents, soft tissue coverage of arterial repairs with well vascularized muscle or fasciocutaneous flaps, negative-pressure wound therapy, and prolonged culture-specific antibiotics.[13–15]

Several general treatment tenets are imperative. Infection involving prosthetic biomaterials frequently requires partial or complete graft removal to eradicate the local septic process. Attempts at preservation of prosthetic grafts are appropriate only in limited circumstances. However, graft preservation is possible for most arterial infections involving autologous tissue reconstruction (vein bypass or patch). The exception is invasive infections (i.e., those producing local or systemic sepsis) caused by *Pseudomonas* species or other potentially virulent gram-negative bacteria (e.g., *Klebsiella* species, *Proteus* species, *E. coli*). MRSA is also a particularly virulent organism, associated with anastomotic dehiscence. Autologous graft excision with ex situ revascularization is recommended in this scenario.

Acceptable management for infected lower extremity bypass grafts can range from ligation and excision alone, to ligation with selective revascularization, to routine revascularization. The operation should begin with exploration of the proximal anastomosis of the involved limb, most commonly the common femoral artery. Following exposure of the bypass graft, optimal proximal vascular control should be obtained due to the friable nature of the infected arterial tissue. If purulent or an infected seroma is encountered during exposure, this should be sent for gram stain and culture in order to tailor antibiotic management in the postoperative period. Once vascular control is obtained, intraoperative test clamping of the bypass and interrogation of the extremity by Doppler can assist in assessing whether ligation will be tolerated. Persistence of a pulsatile pedal arterial signal and ankle pressure greater than 40 mm Hg with bypass occlusion may allow initial graft excision and consideration of delayed revascularization after eradication of local infection. If it is deemed that the patient can tolerate ligation, then extensive debridement of the involved tissue including skin, subcutaneous, muscle, graft, and adjacent vein is warranted in order to prevent recurrence. Following removal of the infected graft, closure of the arteriotomy can occur with the assistance of a venous patch angioplasty or cryopreserved vascular implants.

However, when limb viability cannot be ensured and arterial reconstruction is deemed necessary, it must be initiated immediately because there is a relatively short tolerance for profound ischemia. For revascularization secondary to infected lower extremity graft, important considerations include reestablishing a proximal inflow source, identifying a distal outflow target, and appropriate conduit selection. Following removal of an infected bypass graft and its proximal anastomosis, a new proximal inflow source is exposed, ideally through a clean operative field.

Selection of the proximal inflow source can include the profunda femoris artery, which may serve as a useful alternative inflow source. The mid-profunda femoris artery or distal profunda femoris artery is typically exposed by a longitudinal incision on the upper thigh, lateral to the sartorius muscle (Figure 27.1). The soft tissue is dissected until the sartorius muscle can be retracted medially. The superficial femoral artery is visualized and retracted medially as well. Dissection is carried out between the adductor magnus and the vastus medialis to expose the profunda femoris artery. Division of the lateral femoral circumflex vein overlying the profunda femoris artery may be necessary to provide adequate exposure. Additionally, the superficial femoral artery may be used as an alternate inflow source, provided it is free of proximal obstructive disease. If a vertical incision has been made in the groin, this can be extended distally. The sartorius muscle is retracted laterally to further expose the superficial femoral artery. The mid-superficial femoral artery and distal superficial femoral artery may be approached via a near vertical incision on the medial thigh near the posterior border of the sartorius muscle.

If neither of these proximal sources are viable options secondary to artherosclеotic burden or concern for infectious involvement, other proximal inflow sources may include an obturator bypass, an axillofemoral graft, or an axillopopliteal graft. For the axillofemoral or axillopopliteal grafts, they may be tunneled along the flank away from the infectious region, and the distal anastomosis may be constructed using an entirely lateral approach. Unilateral axillofemoral bypasses to the profunda femoris

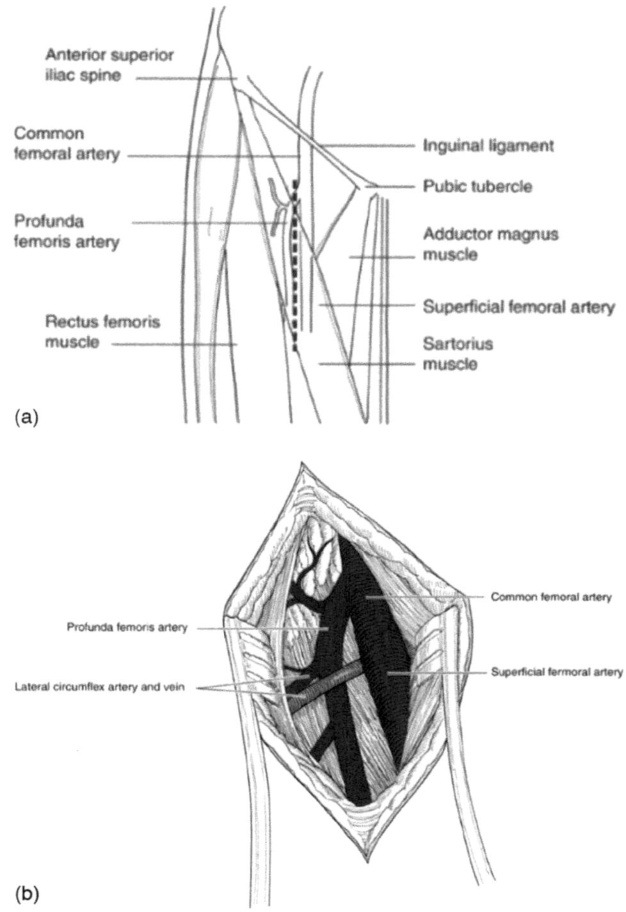

Figure 27.1 (a) The mid and distal profundal femoris artery is exposed through an incision below the regular common femoral artery exposure with dissection lateral to the sartorius muscle (dashed line). (b) The proximal and mid profundal femoris artery has multiple branches which must be controlled on exposure. Care is taken to ligate the circumflex femoral vein to avoid injury.

or superficial femoral artery through an uninfected tissue plane have acceptable patency rates (94% at 6 months), but distal anastomoses to the popliteal artery are prone to early failure (42% at 6 months).[16] For the distal anastomotic site, like the creation of a native bypass, the distal target vessel should bypass all significant atherosclerotic disease to the most proximal limb artery that has at least one runoff artery to the foot. When the initial distal anastomotic site is involved in the graft infection, a new bypass graft tunnel should be created away from the prior tunnel in order to reduce the likelihood of reinfection.

Conduits for revascularization should generally be autologous tissue; the great saphenous vein (GSV) or a superficial upper extremity vein can be used for reconstruction of infrainguinal after excision of an infected graft. Preoperative ultrasonographic vein mapping of the GSV, an arm vein, and the femoral vein can be done in nonurgent scenarios to best match available autologous conduit and repair site diameters. Adequacy of the femoral vein (absence of acute/chronic thrombus, diameter > 5–6 mm) can be confirmed by ultrasound when a small-diameter GSV or arm vein (< 4 mm) is seen. Additionally, for infrainguinal graft infections, in situ prosthetic replacement with PTFE or polyester conduit has been associated with recurrent infection in 10% - 20% of cases, primarily with gram-negative bacteria and MRSA involvement. These results have increased interest in antibiotic-bonded prosthetic grafts to potentially improve results.[17] A third option for in situ replacement is the use of aortic and iliofemoral arterial segments harvested from transplant donors and rendered nonantigenic by cryopreservation. The incidence of limb loss, recurrent infection, and mid-term patient survival compares favorably with that for other methods of in situ replacement. However, allograft dilatation or aneurysm formation (17%) or stenosis/occlusion (20%) occurred during late follow-up (mean of 40 months), especially with the earlier fresh, iliofemoral allograft segments.[18]

Following debridement of subcutaneous and perigraft tissue for infection with potential revascularization, local soft tissue coverage is essential to prevent infection recurrence. As such, transfer or rotation of local soft tissue structures to provide coverage of preserved or new graft material may be needed when surrounding tissue are inadequate or an excessive skin defect exists. Within the inguinal region, the sartorius muscle flap has become the most common technique to assist with graft coverage. The muscle is typically exposed lateral to the femoral vessels and divided at its proximal attachment on the anterior superior iliac spine. The muscle is reflected medially, which reveals the segmental branches of the superficial femoral artery on the underside of the muscle. The muscle is placed so as to cover the femoral vessels and associated grafts as well as obliterate remaining dead space (Figure 27.2). An attempt should be made to interrupt as few segmental feeding vessels as possible to minimize flap ischemia. Usually, a VAC device is placed directly on the muscle flap to allow healing and granulation. The sartorius flap can be used for graft preservation or in situ replacement and has been shown to have good medium, and long-term results for local tissue defects and preventing recurrent infections.[15] Another option for treatment of localized infection in the groin or tissue defect is a rectus femoris rotational flap. Within this flap, the muscle is mobilized from a clean bed based on a pedicle blood supply that is independent from the site of infection. The vascularity of this muscle flap is excellent, and there is minimal evidence that this flap may be an improved option over the sartorius flap.[19] The specific muscle used depends on the patient's arterial anatomy as well as the size and anatomic requirements of the wound that is being treated. A number of muscles may be mobilized to cover a graft in an infected groin, including the rectus abdominis, tensor fasciae latae, and gracilis.

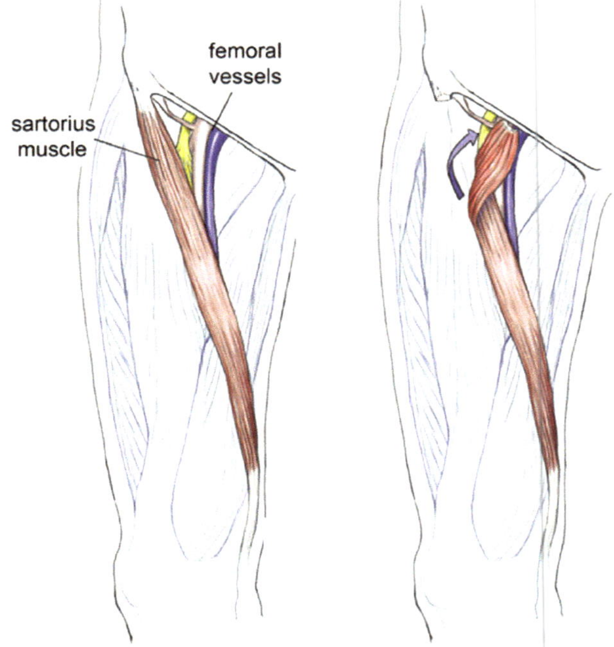

Figure 27.2 For high-risk groins with minimal soft tissue coverage, a sartorius flap is a viable option to improve wound closure. The sartorius muscle is disconnected from its proximal origin and medially rotated over the femoral vessels. Care should be taken to preserve segmental feeding vessels to insure a robustly vascularized flap.

Last, parenteral antibiotics should be selected according to specific perigraft/graft culture results. Antibiotic adjustment should be based on results of cultures performed at each staged procedure to document the success of sterilization or to identify the development of bacterial resistance. Parenteral antibiotics should be continued for a minimum of 2 weeks. Patients with invasive infections or who underwent in situ replacement (prosthetic or allograft) or graft preservation techniques require 4–6 weeks of parenteral antibiotics. Indefinite oral antibiotic therapy as prophylaxis against reinfection is recommended for use in prosthetic grafts, and less commonly with autologous.

Lymphedema and lymphatic fistula

Due to the close proximity of lymph vessels and lymph nodes to the corresponding artery and veins, lymphatic complications following infrainguinal bypass are common. Intraoperative dissection contributes to lymphatic injury and/or transection. Fortunately, lymphatic channels can spontaneously heal; however, interruption of lymphatic vessels can lead to lower extremity edema, lymphatic fistula, or lymphocele.

Lower extremity edema occurs in 50–100% of patients undergoing infrainguinal arterial reconstruction for chronic ischemia. Significant edema can result in impairment in ambulation and local wound complications.

Lymphedema develops when the rate of production of protein-rich interstitial fluid exceeds the capacity of the lymphatic system to remove the increased lymph volume. In an interesting study, patients underwent lymphangiography after infrainguinal bypass; the average number of patent superficial lymph vessels visualized was reduced to 1.7 per patient compared with the normal average of 9.5.[20] Although venous thrombosis has been proposed as a cause of postoperative leg edema, studies have demonstrated a low incidence of deep venous thrombosis in patients with post-bypass edema.[21] In order to minimize the occurrence of lymphedema, lymph-preserving surgical dissection is important. For infrainguinal bypass, a vertical groin incision slightly lateral to the femoral pulse should be made in an attempt to preserve the patency and integrity of the lymph nodes. The inguinal lymphatics should be retracted medially, and a vertical incision should be made in the femoral sheath to dissect the femoral arteries. The lymphatics should be carefully preserved; if they must be divided, they should be ligated or cauterized to avoid leakage of lymph. Attempts should be made to preserve as much lymphatic tissue as possible between the saphenofemoral junction and the femoral artery. Lastly, if a saphenous vein conduit is used, prospective randomized studies have demonstrated that endoscopic versus open vein harvesting results in a reduced rate of lymphatic and infectious wound complications and improvement in cosmesis.[22,23]

For patients who develop lymphedema, leg swelling after femoropopliteal or femorotibial bypass becomes evident with dependency, usually when the patient resumes ambulation. Pitting edema generally subsides within 2-3 months after reconstruction, although it may be persistent in some patients. Lymphedema is frequently unilateral and involves the dorsum of the foot ("buffalo hump") and the toes ("squaring"). The history and physical examination can aid in identifying cellulitis, and duplex scanning of the deep veins is the test of choice for excluding deep venous thrombosis. Postoperatively, mild edema of the extremity should be treated by frequent elevation of the limb and some restriction of ambulation. Moderate to severe post-bypass edema is treated with compression wrapping until the incisions have healed, followed by calf-length, 30-40 mmHg compression stockings. For patients with a below knee, in situ bypass or any bypass to the distal tibial or pedal arteries, management is individualized to avoid direct compression of the subcutaneous vein graft.

Due to the prominent lymphatic network in the femoral triangle, lymphatic fistulas following lower extremity vascular reconstruction occur at an incidence of approximately 1.1%.[24] Important contributing factors to the develop of a lymphatic fistula include failure to ligate or cauterize lymphatic tissue, inadequate closure of layers, and patient factors such as diabetes or concurrent infection. The diagnosis of a lymphatic fistula is made clinically with persistent leakage of clear or yellow fluid from the groin incision. Lymphoscintigraphy is rarely needed, except when the lymphatic leakage occurs in a delayed fashion several months after surgery, at which time a computed tomography and fistulography may be used to exclude a vascular graft infection.

Early diagnosis and management of a lymphatic fistula are important to prevent prolonged hospitalization, delayed wound healing, and readmission. For the first few days, conservative management with antibiotics, local wound care, and bed rest with elevation are warranted to reduce lymph flow. However, conservative management does not have a role when prosthetic material is present due to the risk of infection.

Unfortunately, if the fistula continues to produce large volume despite conservative therapy, then more invasive therapy is necessary. Recently, the widespread use of vacuum-assisted closure (VAC) therapy has been suggested in the use of lymphocutaneous fistulae with an average treatment duration of 16 days and without recurrence.[25] However, if wound VAC therapy fails, then further surgical intervention is warranted. For surgical intervention, isosulfan blue dye is injected into the first and third interdigital spaces of the foot and a sequential compression pump is placed over the affected leg to increase lymphatic and venous drainage. The groin incision is then re-explored in order to identify the lymphatic injury with leakage of blue dye. This area is then oversewn and the wound is closed.

A lymphocele is a localized collection of lymph that develops between two planes of tissues and fails to be reabsorbed. In contrast to a seroma, a lymphocele usually has a well-localized connection with one or more of the lymphatic channels. For this reason, lymphoscintigraphy can readily demonstrate a lymphocele. The infrainguinal region represents the most common location for lymphoceles following vascular reconstruction. Large lymphoceles cause local discomfort, pain, and leg swelling. Hematoma, seroma, and wound infection should be considered in the differential diagnosis. The presence of a soft, fluid-filled cyst and intermittent drainage of clear lymph through a fistula confirms the diagnosis of lymphocele. Ultrasonography is helpful in distinguishing a solid, dense hematoma from a cystic lymphocele. CT is performed when a lymphocele develops several weeks to months after the operation. CT is helpful in excluding graft infection or identifying a retroperitoneal lymphocele extending to the groin. Regarding the management of lymphoceles, small lymphoceles can be monitored with a chance of slow reabsorption over time. In contrast, large lymphoceles or those within the vicinity of prosthetic graft should undergo surgical intervention to reduce the risk of graft infection. Injection of isosulfan blue into the foot is helpful for identifying the lymphatic channels supplying the lymphocele. The lymphocele is excised, and the lymphatic pedicle is ligated or oversewn. Sclerotherapy can also be used for groin lymphoceles but has mixed results.

GRAFT THROMBOSIS

Graft thrombosis remains a significant clinical challenge in the vascular surgery practice. Whether early or delayed, graft thrombosis accounts for significant morbidity, limb loss, and mortality in patients requiring vascular intervention. It is incumbent on the clinician to document graft thrombosis in a timely fashion. The clinical signs/symptoms may be easily detected, such as absence of a palpable pulse or the return of the patient's ischemic symptoms. In less obvious circumstances, noninvasive vascular imaging including the ankle-brachial index and the use of duplex ultrasonography to determine patency and location of occlusion are warranted. Once the diagnosis of graft thrombosis has been confirmed, this is followed by accurate determination of the necessity for and urgency of aggressive intervention, which is driven by the patient's limb status at time of evaluation. If urgent revascularization is warranted, then immediate anticoagulation becomes imperative to minimize or halt thrombus propagation. If there is no neurologic compromise and the degree of tissue ischemia appears minimal, diagnostic or alternative therapeutic maneuvers, including thrombolysis, can be contemplated. Nonetheless, secondary patency after treatment for infrainguinal bypass graft thrombosis is generally poor. If the initial reconstruction was performed for ongoing tissue loss, and the ulcer has subsequently healed, urgent revascularization may not be required. When considering both the timing and etiology of failed arterial reconstructions, two temporal categories should be taken into account: early (within 30 days of placement) and late (after 30 days).

Early graft thrombosis (< 30 days)

Early graft thrombosis has significant prognostic implications in that a failed reconstruction is associated with poor clinical outcomes, particularly when performed for limb salvage indications. Despite improvement in revascularization techniques, 5–10% of grafts will fail within 30 days of placement.[26] Classically, early graft failure has been attributed to a technical error at the time of the operation. However, a recent review demonstrated that technical error accounts for roughly 25% of the early graft failures.[27] This improvement is likely attributed to the increase usage of intraoperative duplex scanning and angiography at the time of the initial surgery. Other factors that contribute to early graft failure include inadequacy of the conduit, as well as low flow or poor distal runoff.

After diagnosis of early graft failure, the treatment options include either surgical thrombectomy or thrombolysis. For open surgical revision, upon returning to the operating room, the distal anastomosis can be inspected first. If the graft hood is pulsatile, an arteriogram can be conducted to identify the point of concern. If the hood is not pulsatile, then it is opened and a distal thrombectomy and graft embolectomy can be performed with balloon catheters of the appropriate caliber. Of note, if the graft is a reversed vein, both proximal and distal anastomoses usually require exploration. Specifically, an uninflated balloon can be passed from proximal to distal; a second catheter can be tied to the first, and then retracted uninflated proximally. The tie is cut, and the second catheter is inflated to thrombectomized the graft from proximal to distal. Heparinized saline is then forcibly irrigated through the graft to flush any residual thrombosis. Both anastomoses are then carefully inspected to identify technical defects. If identified, the graftotomy can be extended in order to repair the defect and closed with a patch angioplasty. Further, if previously unidentified outflow disease is encountered, the graft should be extended beyond the lesion with a jump graft or a different outflow vessel should be chosen. Lastly, if marginal vein conduit is used at the time of the initial procedure and no technical defect is identified, consider replacing the venous conduit or converting to a prosthetic graft.

Late graft thrombosis (> 30 days)

Many of the aforementioned diagnostic and therapeutic decisions remain germane in the setting of delayed or late graft failure. There are, however, several distinctions. In contrast to early graft thrombosis, for grafts that occlude more than 30 days after implantation, technical errors no longer constitute a significant cause of graft pathology. Instead, neointiamal fibroplasia, graft (vein or prosthetic) structural abnormalities, and progressive atherosclerosis contribute to late graft occlusion. Regarding treatment options, late graft occlusion should be treated only if the patient's symptoms are severe enough to warrant intervention based on Rutherford limb ischemia criteria. When vein conduit is limited, thrombolysis, mechanical thrombectomy, or both and treat the underlying lesion responsible for graft failure represents a valuable treatment option. For example, patients with class I or IIa ischemia often have time for angiography and possible thrombolytic therapy in a semi-elective fashion, whereas patients with class IIb and early III typically require immediate revascularization.

Previous investigations have demonstrated that the time interval since arterial reconstruction can act as a positive predictor of the successful application of thrombolytic therapy. Specifically, the longer a graft has been in place, the greater the likelihood that thrombolytic therapy will confer graft patency.[28] If thrombolysis is pursued, after systemic heparinization, the initial diagnostic test in this patient is an aortogram. A hydrophilic 0.035" wire can then be used to select the stump of the proximal anastomosis and is manipulated into the mid-portion of the occluded bypass graft. Percutaneous mechanical thrombectomy with a pulse spray of tissue plasminogen activator (TPA) 10 mg in 50 mL saline is laced throughout the extent of the thrombus. Repeat arteriography will typically show resolution of the thrombus and reveal the underlying culprit stenosis. If a significant amount of thrombus persists despite thrombectomy, an infusion catheter running

TPA 1 mg/h along with systemic unfractionated heparin at 500 U/h may be run overnight. A repeat arteriogram is performed within 24 hours. After restoration of graft patency, it has been well documented that further endovascular or surgical therapy may be required in up to 85% of cases to correct the inciting event for graft thrombosis and achieve sustained patency. Available therapeutic options in this setting include (1) balloon angioplasty of an intragraft or juxta-anastomotic stenosis, (2) open surgical vein patch angioplasty, (3) and interposition bypass reconstruction.

However, the results of thrombolysis remain limited. Instead, if autogenous vein is available, a new bypass with autogenous vein can be performed, which often provides superior results and durability.[29] Lastly, if vein is unavailable and thrombolysis is contraindicated or fails, a repeated bypass with PTFE and a vein patch or cuff is the best option. Ultimately, the optimal therapy for graft occlusion is to prevent its occurrence by identifying graft-threatening stenosis before the onset of graft occlusion through routine postoperative duplex graft surveillance.

BYPASS GRAFT SURVEILLANCE AND MANAGEMENT OF GRAFT STENOSIS

Multicenter prospective data have demonstrated that only 50% of patients with infrainguinal bypasses are free from clinically significant stenosis, revisions, or amputation at 1 year. Progressive loss of primary patency in the 6- to 18 month time frame occurs predominately through intimal hyperplasia developed in the perianastomotic sites (53% incidence) or mid-graft (30% incidence) regions. After 2 years, graft stenosis is reduced to approximately 4% per year resulting from intimal hyperplasia or progressive atherosclerotic disease at the proximal or distal anastomotic sites. In order to detect graft stenoses prior to graft occlusion, long-term vascular laboratory surveillance of infrainguinal bypass graft function has evolved to a recommended standard of care. Postoperative surveillance includes regular visits with physical exams and duplex ultrasound. Measurement of peak systolic velocity should be performed at 1, 3, 6, and 12 months after surgery and then every 12 months thereafter. Duplex surveillance is of the utmost importance in 'high-risk' bypass grafts, whether this relates to conduit type, vein diameter, or poor inflow and outflow considerations. Diagnostic testing of a failing graft involves ultrasound graft imaging combined with measurement of Doppler-derived ankle-brachial indices (Table 27.1). Grafts with focal lesions associated with a peak systolic velocity greater than 300 cm/s or a velocity ratio greater than 3.5 should undergo prophylactic repair to prevent graft stenosis. Grafts that develop low-flow velocities over time (peak systolic velocity < 45 cm/s throughout the graft) or a drop in ankle-brachial index exceeding 0.15 in the absence of detectable graft lesions should undergo arteriography to search for inflow, outflow, or missed graft lesions.[30]

For patients with severe stenosis necessitating an intervention to prevent graft occlusion, a variety of open and endovascular options exist. The tailoring of the surgical approach to optimize the long-term success often depends on factors including: time after implantation, lesion location, and stenotic length. Severe graft stenosis detected < 3 months after implantation is often attributed to technical deficiency at the time of the initial surgical procedure, such as kinking of the graft during tunneling, retained venous valves, constricted anastomosis, or sub-optimal selection of a distal target. Although these lesions represent a variety of etiologies, in aggregate they present a challenge for less invasive endovascular approaches. Next, stenotic length is a well described factor for influencing the long-term durability of endovascular therapy with lesions > 2 cm in length representing a three-fold increased risk of endovascular reintervention in comparison to those < 2 cm. Lastly, the role of endovascular therapy in perianastomotic lesions is less well established. Endovascular repair of lesion extending into the suture line are constrained by the local geometry and are thereby at an increased risk of failure in comparison to mid-graft lesion.

Endovascular repair of critical graft stenosis

The principal technique used in endovascular revision of a stenotic bypass graft involves percutaneous balloon angioplasty. During this procedure access can be achieved

Table 27.1 Ultrasound surveillance after lower extremity bypass

Category	Indication	PSV (cm/s)	Velocity Ratio	GFW (cm/s)	ABI Change
I - Highest risk	> 70% stenosis, low graft flow	> 300	> 3.5	< 45 or staccato graft flow	> 0.15
II - High risk	> 70% stenosis, no change, or normal flow	> 300	> 3.5	> 45	< 0.15
III - Moderate risk	50–70% stenosis, normal graft flow	180–300	> 2.0	> 45	< 0.15
IV - Low risk	Normal bypass or < 50% stenosis, normal graft flow	< 180	< 2.0	> 45	< 0.15

ABI, ankle-brachial index; GFV, graft flow velocity; PSV, peak systolic velocity. (*Source:* Table modified from Idu et al. J Vasc Surg. 1993.)

in a contralateral retrograde or antegrade fashion. A contralateral approach offers a comfortable working length from the arterial entry site to the site of the lesion. A crossover method may not be practical if the patient has a prior placement of a bifurcated aortic graft or if there is insufficient catheter length to reach a distal tibial lesion in the contralateral limb. During such occasions, an antegrade approach or brachial access may be acceptable alternatives depending on patient body habitus.

The angioplasty balloon should be sized based on the apparent normal diameter of the proximal or distal graft. Due to the hyperplastic nature of vein graft lesions, high-pressure balloons with prolonged inflate times may be employed. In addition, recent investigations have demonstrated mixed results with the use of cutting balloon angioplasty as a solution to reduce recurrent stenosis following treatment of hyperplastic vein graft lesions. Although initial studies failed to demonstrate an improvement in primary patency when using cutting balloon in comparison to conventional angioplasty, subsequent reports have presented a contrasting view. Indeed, recent reports have shown marked improved stenosis-free patency with the use of cutting angioplasty versus conventional angioplasty (62% vs 34% at 4 years). Last, stenting and directional atherectomy have also been described in small series as an adjunct for stenotic or failing bypass grafts. However, complication rates associated with atherectomy are relatively high, with major complications reported in approximately 10% of the cases.[31,32]

Open repair of critical graft stenosis

Open surgical procedures for graft stenosis depends on the length, number, and location of the lesions. For patients with < 2 cm in length lesions, often with underlying intimal hyperplasia or a scarred valve, a focal patch angioplasty at the stenotic site serves is a viable option. More extensive mid-graft lesions with diffuse narrowing or tandem lesion are often best treated with interposition grafting. Lastly, hyperplastic lesions at the proximal or distal anastomosis can be treated with a jump graft bypass. Although the optimal conduit for a sequential bypass has not been determined, arm veins, particularly the basilic vein, can be a viable option.

Outcomes

Few studies have provided direct comparison of each treatment modality for graft stenosis. The largest study for which a comparison can be extracted is the PREVENT III investigation in which, of the 1404 patients enrolled, 313 required graft revisions. These data demonstrated that open surgical revision had an improved long-term graft survival over endovascular therapy and endovascular therapy require more frequent procedures to maintain graft patency. However, this is balanced by the increased morbidity and mortality associated with open surgical revision in comparison to endovascular. Interestingly, the hospital length of stay and quality of life did not differ between treatment groups.

Case Example 1

A 58-year-old male with a long-standing history of peripheral arterial disease initially underwent placement of a left popliteal stent at a referring institution that thrombosed. This resulted in a left distal superficial femoral artery to tibial-peroneal trunk bypass with reversed great saphenous vein. He presented 6 months after the procedure for surveillance imaging, which demonstrated a proximal graft velocity of 564 cm/s and mid-graft velocity of 41 cm/s (Figure 27.3a,b). Given the severity of graft stenosis, the patient was admitted to the hospital and placed on anticoagulation. He then underwent an urgent lower extremity diagnostic angiogram revealing a severe flow-limiting stenosis of the proximal graft 4 mm in length (Figure 27.3c). The decision was made to perform a balloon angioplasty. A 2 mm balloon angioplasty was conducted followed by a 4 mm balloon angioplasty with severe wasting of the balloon secondary to stenosis (Figure 27.3d). Completion angiogram demonstrated absent residual stenosis and adequate flow in DP and PT distally (Figure 27.3e,f). The patient continues to have 6-month interval surveillance follow-up and remains free of additional stenosis at 1 year.

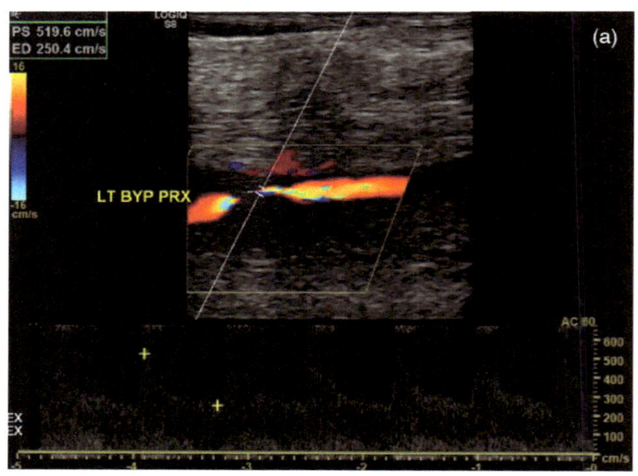

Figure 27.3 (a) Surveillance ultrasonography demonstrates a high risk bypass graft with elevated PSV (519 cm/s) and low flow (EDV 20.1 cm/s) (b) in the graft. (c) Diagnostic angiogram exhibits an occluded popliteal artery stent that was previously placed and severe stenosis at the proximal anastomosis of reversed GSV bypass. (d) Balloon angioplasty (4 mm) with severe narrowing of balloon at region of maximal stenosis. (e) and (f) Completion angiogram with resolution of severe stenosis at proximal anastomosis of bypass and adequate flow in DP and PT distally to supply the foot.

(continued)

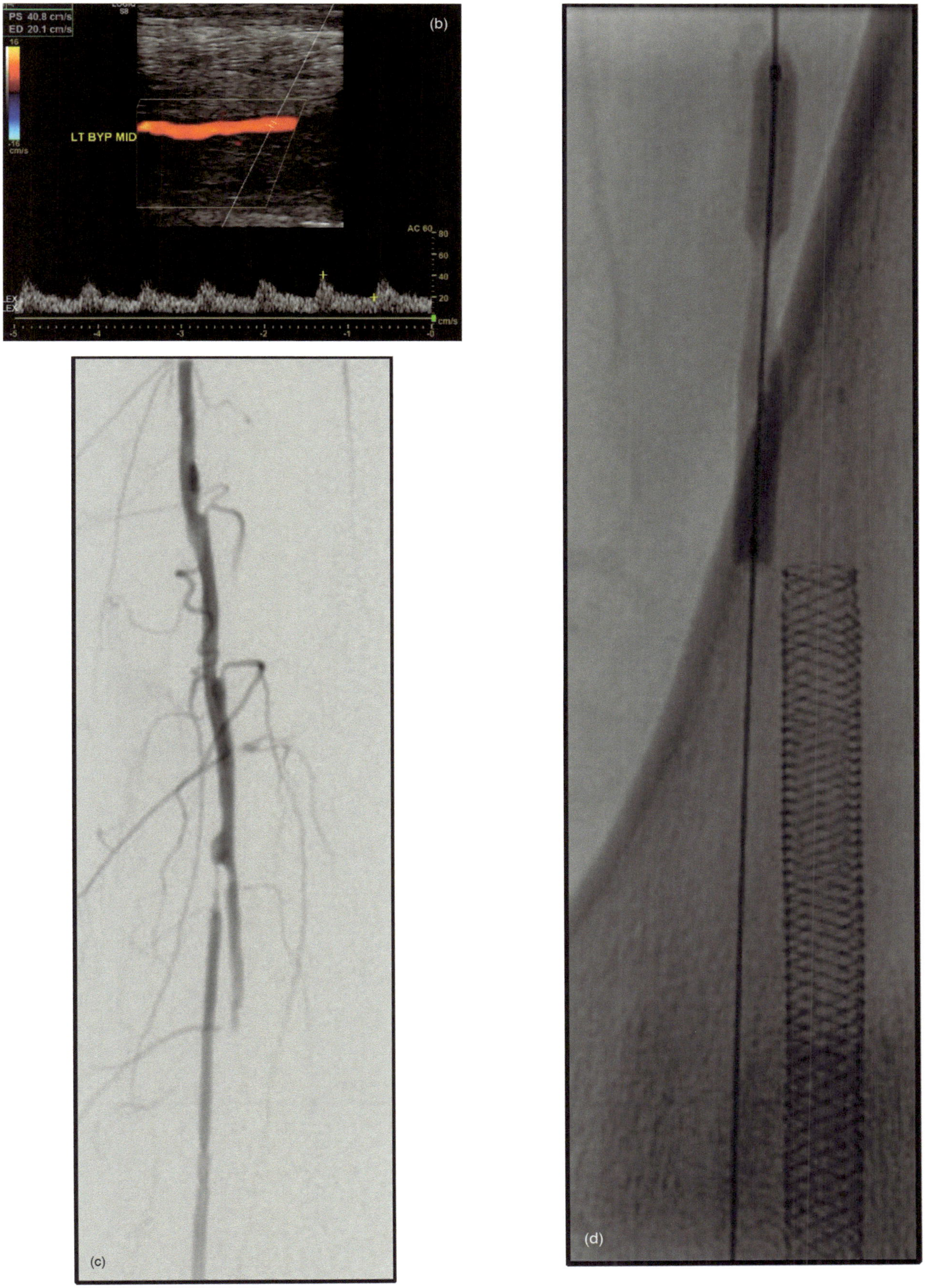

Figure 27.3 *(continued)*

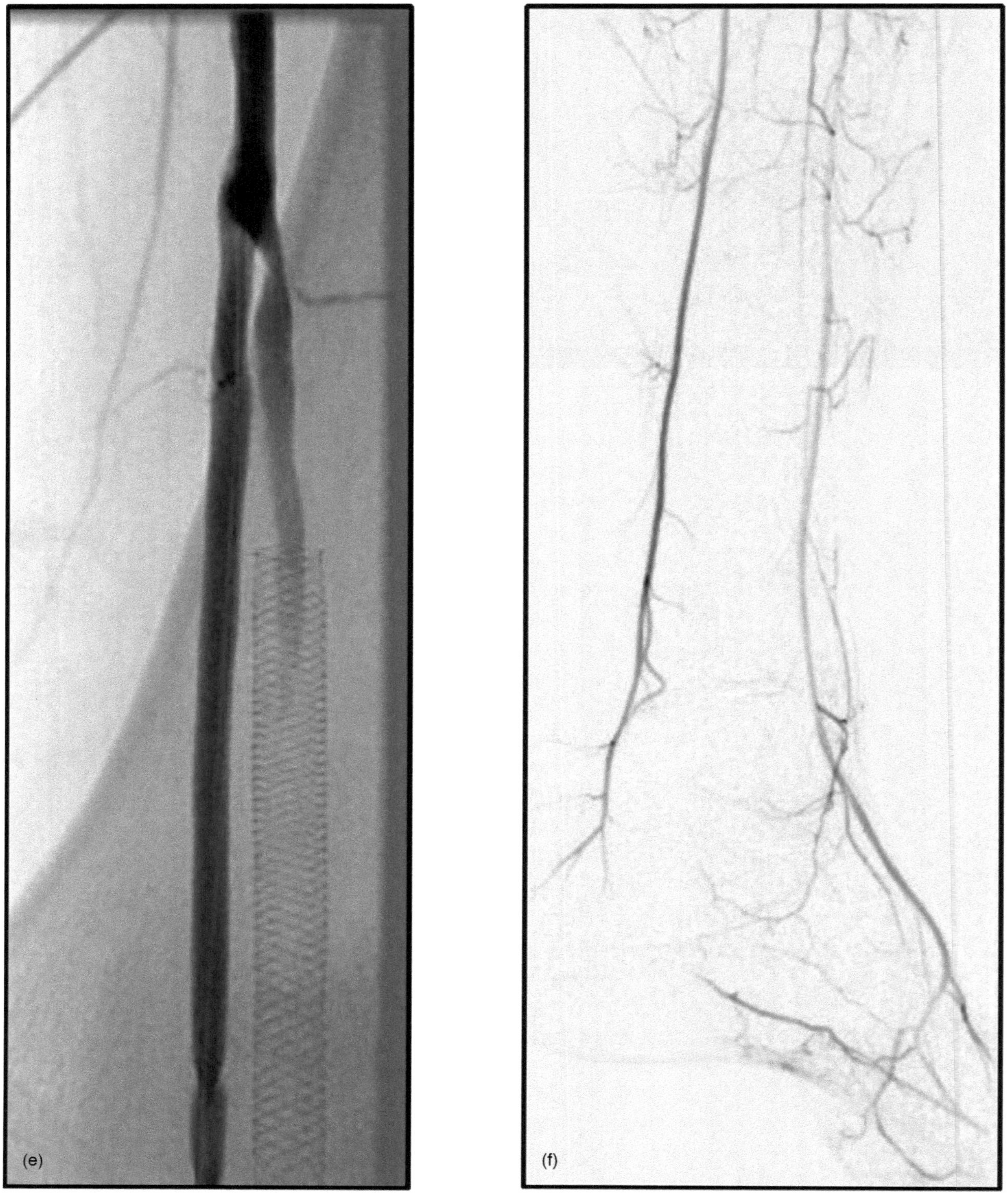

Figure 27.3 *(continued)*

Case Example 2

A 71-year-old male with a history of thrombosed popliteal aneurysm for which he underwent a common femoral patch angioplasty with bovine pericardial patch followed by a common femoral to below-knee popliteal bypass with saphenous vein at a referring institution. He presented to the hospital 5 months later with swelling and erythema of the previously healing groin incision. At the time of his presentation, he had a leukocytosis to 14. A CTA was conducted which demonstrated (Figure 27.4a) a large fluid collection measuring 7.3 × 5.8 × 12.2 cm adjacent to the proximal anastomosis and bypass graft. Given the concern for underlying bovine pericardial patch infection, the patient was taken to the operating room for an explanation of the previous placed patch material and replacement with a saphenous vein patch angioplasty with reimplantation of the previous reversed great saphenous vein bypass. In addition, there was vigorous washout and debridement of the surrounding fluid and necrotic tissue with placement of a sartorius flap. Intraoperative culture demonstrated *Escherichia coli* and *Streptococcus anginosus*. Postoperatively, in collaboration with the infectious disease team the patient was placed on a 2-week course of ceftriaxone. The wound gradually closed with the aid of a vacuum-assisted dressing and adequate granulation of the sartorius flap (Figure 27.4b).

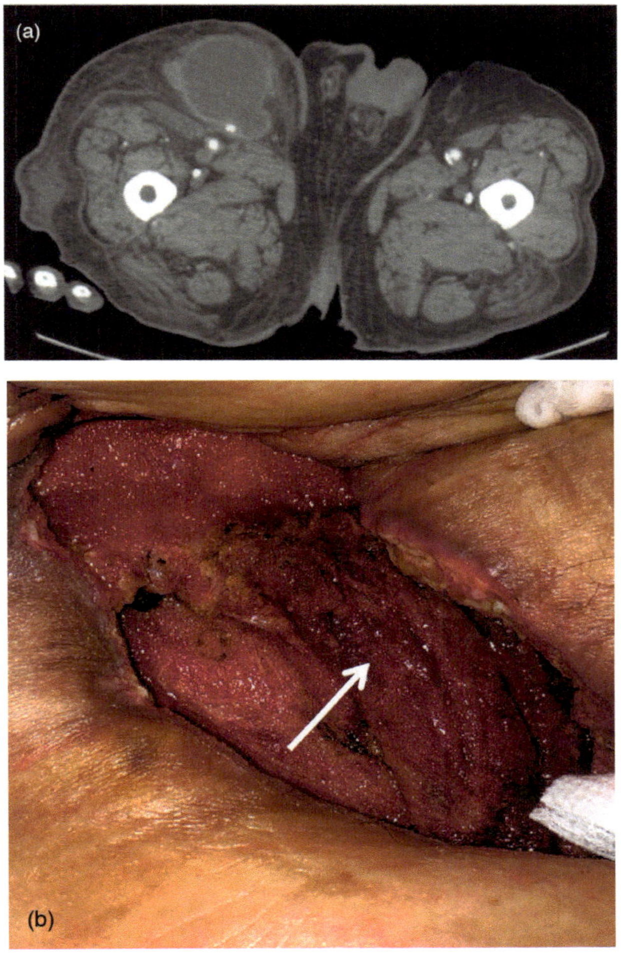

Figure 27.4 (a) Preoperative CTA of patient demonstrating large fluid collection measuring 7.3 × 5.8 × 12.2 cm adjacent to the proximal anastomosis and bypass graft concerning for deep surgical site infection. (b) Day 3 postoperative sartorius flap (arrow denotes sartorius muscle) overlying prior common femoral to popliteal bypass demonstrating well vascularized tissue.

REFERENCES

1. Hirsch AT, Hartman L, Town RJ, Virnig BA. National health care costs of peripheral arterial disease in the Medicare population. Vasc Med. 2008;13(3): 209–15.
2. Wolfe JH, Wyatt MG. Critical and subcritical ischaemia. Eur J Vasc Endovasc Surg. 1997;13(6): 578–82.
3. Norgren L, Hiatt WR, Dormandy JA, Nehler MR, Harris KA, Fowkes FG, et al. Inter-Society Consensus for the Management of Peripheral Arterial Disease (TASC II). Eur J Vasc Endovasc Surg. 2007;33 Suppl 1: S1–75.
4. Klinkert P, Schepers A, Burger DH, van Bockel JH, Breslau PJ. Vein versus polytetrafluoroethylene in above-knee femoropopliteal bypass grafting: 5-year results of a randomized controlled trial. J Vasc Surg. 2003; 37 (1): 149–55.
5. Harris PL, Veith FJ, Shanik GD, Nott D, Wengerter KR, Moore DJ. Prospective randomized comparison of in situ and reversed infrapopliteal vein grafts. Br J Surg. 1993;80(2): 173–6.
6. Johnson WC, Lee KK. A comparative evaluation of polytetrafluoroethylene, umbilical vein, and saphenous vein bypass grafts for femoral-popliteal above-knee revascularization: A prospective randomized Department of Veterans Affairs cooperative study. J Vasc Surg. 2000;32(2): 268–77.
7. Pereira CEA, Albers M, Romiti M, Brochado-Neto FC, Pereira CEA. Meta-analysis of femoropopliteal bypass grafts for lower extremity arterial insufficiency. J Vasc Surg. 2006;44(3): 510–7.
8. Mills Sr. JL. P values may lack power: The choice of conduit for above-knee femoropopliteal bypass graft. J Vasc Surg. 2000;32(2): 402–5.
9. Veith FJ, Gupta SK, Ascer E, White-Flores S, Samson RH, Scher LA, et al. 6-year prospective multicenter randomized comparison of autologous saphenous vein and expanded polytetrafluoroethylene grafts in infrainguinal arterial reconstructions. J Vasc Surg. 1986;3(1): 104–14.

10. Stonebridge PA, Prescott RJ, Ruckley C V. Randomized trial comparing infrainguinal polytetrafluoroethylene bypass grafting with and without vein interposition cuff at the distal anastomosis. The Joint Vascular Research Group. J Vasc Surg. 1997;26(4): 543–50.
11. Darling JD, O'Donnell TFX, Deery SE, Norman AV, Vu GH, Guzman RJ, et al. Outcomes after first-time lower extremity revascularization for chronic limb-threatening ischemia in insulin-dependent diabetic patients. J Vasc Surg. 2018;68(5): 1455–1464.e1.
12. Davis FM, Sutzko DC, Grey SF, Mansour MA, Jain KM, Nypaver TJ, et al. Predictors of surgical site infection after open lower extremity revascularization. J Vasc Surg. 2017;65(6): 1769–1778.e3.
13. Cherry KJ, Roland CF, Pairolero PC, Hallett JW, Meland NB, Naessens JM, et al. Infected femorodistal bypass: Is graft removal mandatory? J Vasc Surg. 1992;15(2): 295-303; discussion 303–5.
14. Bandyk DF, Novotney ML, Back MR, Johnson BL, Schmacht DC. Expanded application of in situ replacement for prosthetic graft infection. J Vasc Surg. 2001;34(3): 411–9; discussion 419–20.
15. Armstrong PA, Back MR, Bandyk DF, Johnson BL, Shames ML. Selective application of sartorius muscle flaps and aggressive staged surgical debridement can influence long-term outcomes of complex prosthetic graft infections. J Vasc Surg. 2007;46(1): 71–8.
16. Seeger JM, Back MR, Albright JL, Carlton LM, Harward TR, Kubulis PS, et al. Influence of patient characteristics and treatment options on outcome of patients with prosthetic aortic graft infection. Ann Vasc Surg. 1999;13(4):413–20.
17. Koshiko S, Sasajima T, Muraki S, Azuma N, Yamazaki K, Chiba K, et al. Limitations in the use of rifampicin-gelatin grafts against virulent organisms. J Vasc Surg. 2002;35(4): 779–85.
18. Zhou W, Lin PH, Bush RL, Terramani TT, Matsuura JH, Cox M, et al. In situ reconstruction with cryopreserved arterial allografts for management of mycotic aneurysms or aortic prosthetic graft infections: A multi-institutional experience. Texas Hear Inst J. 2006;33(1): 14–8.
19. Perler BA, Kolk CA, Manson PM, Williams GM. Rotational muscle flaps to treat localized prosthetic graft infection: Long-term follow-up. J Vasc Surg. 1993;18(3): 358–64; discussion 364–5.
20. Vaughan BF, Slavotinek AH, Jepson RP. Edema of the lower limb after vascular operations. Surg Gynecol Obstet. 1970;131(2): 282–90.
21. Myhre HO, Storen EJ, Ongre A. The incidence of deep venous thrombosis in patients with leg oedema after arterial reconstruction. Scand J Thorac Cardiovasc Surg. 1974;8(1): 73–6.
22. Allen KB, Griffith GL, Heimansohn DA, Robison RJ, Matheny RG, Schier JJ, et al. Endoscopic versus traditional saphenous vein harvesting: A prospective, randomized trial. Ann Thorac Surg. 1998;66(1): 26–31; discussion 31–2.
23. Puskas JD, Wright CE, Miller PK, Anderson TE, Gott JP, Brown WM, et al. A randomized trial of endoscopic versus open saphenous vein harvest in coronary bypass surgery. Ann Thorac Surg. 1999;68(4): 1509–12.
24. Skudder PA, Geary J. Lymphatic drainage from the groin following surgery of the femoral artery. J Cardiovasc Surg (Torino). 1987;28(4): 460–3.
25. Hamed O, Muck PE, Smith JM, Krallman K, Griffith NM. Use of vacuum-assisted closure (VAC) therapy in treating lymphatic complications after vascular procedures: New approach for lymphoceles. J Vasc Surg. 2008;48(6):1520–3, e1-4.
26. Conte MS, Bandyk DF, Clowes AW, Moneta GL, Seely L, Lorenz TJ, et al. Results of PREVENT III: A multicenter, randomized trial of edifoligide for the prevention of vein graft failure in lower extremity bypass surgery. J Vasc Surg. 2006;43(4): 742–751; discussion 751.
27. Walsh DB, Zwolak RM, McDaniel MD, Schneider JR, Cronenwett JL. Intragraft drug infusion as an adjunct to balloon catheter thrombectomy for salvage of thrombosed infragenicular vein grafts: A preliminary report. J Vasc Surg. 1990;11(6): 753–9; discussion 760.
28. Schwierz T, Gschwendtner M, Havlicek W, Schmoeller F, Boehmig HJ, Függer R. Indications for directed thrombolysis or new bypass in treatment of occlusion of lower extremity arterial bypass reconstruction. Ann Vasc Surg. 2001;15(6): 644–52.
29. Edwards JE, Taylor LM, Porter JM. Treatment of failed lower extremity bypass grafts with new autogenous vein bypass grafting. J Vasc Surg. 1990;11(1): 136–44; discussion 144–5.
30. Idu MM, Blankenstein JD, de Gier P, Truyen E, Buth J. Impact of a color-flow duplex surveillance program on infrainguinal vein graft patency: A 5-year experience. J Vasc Surg. 1993;17(1): 42–52; discussion 52–3.
31. Azar Y, DeRubertis B, Baril D, Woo K. Atherectomy-Associated Complications in the Southern California Vascular Outcomes Improvement Collaborative. Ann Vasc Surg. 2018;49: 241–6.
32. Lee MS, Yang T, Adams G. Pooled Analysis of the CONFIRM Registries: Safety Outcomes in Diabetic Patients Treated with Orbital Atherectomy for Peripheral Artery Disease. J Endovasc Ther. 2014;21(2): 258–65.

28

Complications of surgery for thoracic outlet syndrome

ROBERT W. THOMPSON

Thoracic outlet syndrome (TOS) encompasses a group of disorders caused by compression of the neurovascular structures that serve the upper extremity, as they pass through the closely related anatomic spaces of the scalene triangle, the costoclavicular space, and/or the subcoracoid (pectoralis minor) space.[1] The clinical presentation of patients with TOS depends on the specific structures compressed, giving rise to three clinically distinct conditions.[2–4]

Neurogenic TOS (85–95% of all patients with TOS) is characterized by compression of the brachial plexus nerve roots within the scalene triangle and/or subcoracoid space. This may arise as a result of two factors: (a) predisposing variations in anatomy, such as anomalous scalene musculature, aberrant fibrofascial bands, or cervical ribs; and (b) neck or upper extremity injury that has resulted in chronic spasm, fibrosis, and other pathological changes affecting the scalene and pectoralis minor muscles. The symptoms of brachial plexus nerve root compression consist of variable degrees of pain, numbness, and tingling (paresthesias) in the neck, shoulder, arm, and hand, aggravated by arm elevation and activity.[2–5]

Venous TOS (10–15% of all patients with TOS) is characterized by compression of the subclavian vein between the clavicle, subclavius muscle, and first rib. Most patients present with abrupt spontaneous arm swelling, cyanotic discoloration, heaviness, and pain, which form the characteristic features of axillary-subclavian vein "effort thrombosis" (Paget-Schroetter syndrome) occurring in young, active, and otherwise healthy individuals.[2,3,6] The pathogenesis of effort thrombosis involves repetitive extrinsic compression of the subclavian vein during activities involving arm elevation or exertion, leading in time to chronic venous injury and progressive fibrous stenosis of the vein. Despite simultaneous expansion of collateral veins passing around the narrowed subclavian vein, stagnant blood within the narrowed subclavian vein eventually leads to thrombotic occlusion.

Arterial TOS (2–5% of all patients with TOS) is caused by longstanding compression of the subclavian artery within the scalene triangle, almost always occurring in association with a congenital cervical rib or other bony anomaly, leading to the development of subclavian artery occlusion or aneurysmal dilatation.[2,3,7] These lesions are often accompanied by mural thrombus formation, and frequently complicated by distal thromboembolism with hand and/or digital ischemia. Patients with acute thromboembolism present with a sudden onset of hand pain and weakness, numbness and tingling, and cold and pale fingers. Those with more longstanding ischemia may present with chronic arm fatigue or claudication, non-healing wounds, or ulcerations in the fingers. Subclavian artery occlusions or aneurysms may also be asymptomatic. A second form of arterial TOS is observed almost solely in overhead-throwing athletes, associated with occlusive or aneurysmal lesions of the distal axillary artery.[8] These lesions are caused by repetitive trauma from hyperextension during the throwing motion, in which the axillary artery can be compressed by mild humeral head subluxation. The complications of these lesions are similar to those of arterial TOS caused by subclavian artery lesions at the level of the first rib.

Successful surgical treatment for all three types of TOS depends on a sound understanding of the relationships between the musculoskeletal and neurovascular structures in this region, as well as the many anatomic variations and pathologic findings that are likely to be encountered.[1,3] Thoracic outlet decompression may be accomplished by lateral (transaxillary) or anterior (supraclavicular or infraclavicular) approaches, which each have their own advantages and disadvantages.[9–12] The overall mortality risk of these procedures is extremely low, but every few years one hears of a case of intraoperative or postoperative death following a thoracic outlet decompression operation. In almost all such cases, death occurs due to rapid unexpected hemorrhage following injury to the subclavian artery or vein, coupled with delayed or inadequate resuscitation. Another rare occurrence in thoracic outlet decompression operations is inadvertent resection of the second rib during intended first rib resection. This usually occurs during transaxillary or infraclavicular approaches in the setting of unexpectedly difficult anatomic exposure, surgical inexperience, or poor selection of operative approach for the individual anatomy. The remaining risks of thoracic outlet decompression revolve around the potential for nerve or vascular injury that exists for any operation in this area, as well as operative inadequacies that may lead to persistent or recurrent problems. In current practice the risks associated with thoracic outlet decompression are very low in the hands of experienced surgeons.[13–20] Nonetheless, it should be acknowledged that these procedures are technically demanding, and that accomplishing them with acceptably low complication rates requires a considerable amount of training and experience.[21–25]

OPERATIVE STRATEGY IN THORACIC OUTLET DECOMPRESSION

The advantages of transaxillary first rib resection include a hidden incision and sufficient exposure for resection of the first rib, applicable to neurogenic and venous forms of TOS. However, only a limited amount of scalene muscle can be resected from this approach and it is difficult to perform brachial plexus neurolysis above the lower trunk (C8 and T1 nerve roots). The principal advantage of the supraclavicular approach is excellent exposure of all the relevant anatomy, allowing more complete decompression with first rib resection, complete scalenectomy, and thorough brachial plexus neurolysis.[26] This approach is thereby applicable to all three forms of TOS. In addition, coupling the supraclavicular approach with a concomitant infraclavicular incision (paraclavicular approach) for venous TOS allows the surgeon to perform simultaneous subclavian vein reconstruction when appropriate. A similar approach may be used for arterial reconstructions when distal control of the axillary artery is needed.

Based on these considerations, our longstanding preference is for supraclavicular thoracic outlet decompression for all forms of TOS, as described in detail elsewhere.[3,6,7,12,26] To accomplish this approach with the greatest margin of safety, we have defined six "critical views" of the surgical anatomy that should be sequentially obtained during the course of supraclavicular decompression: (1) view of the operative field after lateral reflection of the scalene fat pad, with visualization of the internal jugular vein, anterior scalene muscle, phrenic nerve, brachial plexus, subclavian artery, middle scalene muscle, and long thoracic nerve; (2) view of the lower part of the anterior scalene muscle where it attaches to the first rib, with space sufficient to allow a finger to pass behind the anterior scalene muscle and in front of the brachial plexus and subclavian artery, prior to division of the anterior scalene muscle insertion from the top of the first rib; (3) view of the upper part of the anterior scalene muscle at the level of the transverse process of the cervical spine, in relation to the C5 and C6 nerve roots, prior to division of the origin of the anterior scalene muscle; (4) view of the insertion of the middle scalene muscle on the first rib, with each of the 5 nerve roots of the brachial plexus and the subclavian artery retracted medially and the long thoracic nerve retracted posteriorly, prior to division of the insertion of the middle scalene muscle from the top of the lateral first rib; (5) view of the posterior neck of the first rib, with the T1 nerve root passing from underneath the rib to join the C8 nerve root to form the inferior trunk of the brachial plexus, prior to division of the posterior first rib; and (6) view of the anterior portion of the first rib, with placement of the rib shears medial to the scalene tubercle, prior to division of the anterior first rib.[3,26] The typical anatomic exposure obtained from the supraclavicular approach is illustrated in Figure 28.1.

Early postoperative management is similar for all approaches to thoracic outlet decompression.[27] An upright chest x-ray is performed in the recovery room and for several days after surgery, and any small air or pleural fluid collections are observed with the expectation of spontaneous resolution. Postoperative analgesia is initially provided by patient-controlled intravenous opiates until adequate pain control can be achieved by oral medications. Continuous-infusion local anesthesia may also be used for several days, administered through small-caliber perfusion catheters placed at the time of surgery. Oral narcotics, a muscle relaxant, and a non-steroidal anti-inflammatory agent are routinely prescribed upon hospital discharge and for at least several weeks following surgery. Hospital discharge may be as early as the next day after transaxillary first rib resection, but is typically 3–4 days for supraclavicular operations. Issues prolonging hospital stay may include difficulty achieving satisfactory pain control on oral medications, post-anesthetic nausea, and side effects of opioid medications. The closed-suction drain placed at the time of operation is removed when daily output is less than 50 mL, which is usually 5–7 days after supraclavicular decompression. Gentle range-of-motion physical therapy is resumed the day after surgery and continued upon hospital discharge, with patients advised to avoid excessive reaching overhead, heavy lifting with the affected upper extremity, and any activities that can result in muscle strain, spasm, and significant pain in the trapezius and other neck muscles. A gradual return to use of the upper extremity is encouraged, with the majority of patients permitted cautious light-duty work by 4–6 weeks and full activity by 2–3 months. Those undergoing treatment for venous TOS are maintained on oral anticoagulation until 3 months after operation. Patients are typically seen in follow-up every 3 months in the first year to assess long-term results, and

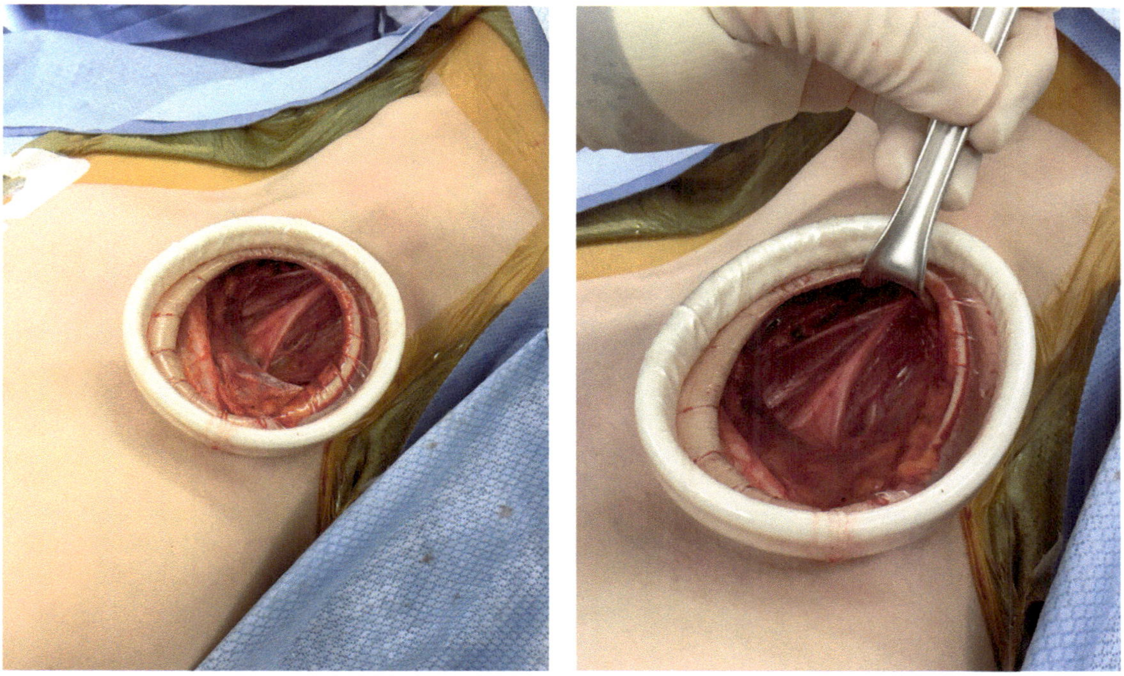

Figure 28.1 Operative exposure during supraclavicular thoracic outlet decompression. Operative photograph of left supraclavicular exposure illustrating critical view #1, viewed from the left side. Structures exposed after lateral mobilization of the scalene fat pad include the internal jugular vein, anterior scalene muscle, phrenic nerve, brachial plexus, subclavian artery, middle scalene muscle, and long thoracic nerve. Use of a self-retaining flexible ring wound protector serves to maintain the optimal exposure. (Kandyce K. Branham, RN.)

physical therapy is continued for as long as necessary to achieve an optimal level of function.

SPECIFIC COMPLICATIONS

BRACHIAL PLEXUS NERVE INJURY

The potential for nerve injury is a primary concern in any operation for TOS, particularly the brachial plexus and its branches.[28–33] The mechanisms of nerve injury may include overt transection or partial laceration, thermal damage from electrocautery, or excessive traction resulting in neuropraxia. The incidence of these complications should be negligible in experienced hands, but several factors may elevate the risk of brachial plexus nerve injury during thoracic outlet decompression, including unexpected anatomic variations, pathological findings, intraoperative bleeding, and reoperative procedures.[28–33] Nerve injury rarely presents as an obvious injury identified in the operating room or as a significant deficit immediately after operation, but more often becomes evident as persistent nerve dysfunction over time. In most of these situations where the affected nerve was observed to be anatomically intact at the time of surgery, full functional recovery can be anticipated after several weeks to months.

Prevention of brachial plexus nerve injury

Careful exposure and meticulous operative technique are critical to avoid injury to the brachial plexus nerve roots by minimizing handling of the nerves, dissecting the perineural tissues under direct vision, and constant awareness of the extent of any retraction being placed on individual nerve roots. The presence of a cervical rib or ligamentous band may displace the brachial plexus more forward than usually expected, and scalene muscle anomalies (e.g., a scalene minimus muscle) and fibrofascial bands may obscure the lower nerve roots. Division of the anterior scalene muscle from the first rib should be done with a finger placed between the muscle and the underlying brachial plexus and subclavian artery, using scissors rather than the electrocautery. Prior to resection of the middle scalene muscle, the brachial plexus should also be mobilized such that all 5 nerve roots are visible and gently retracted medially. Full visualization of the T1 nerve root should also be obtained, where it passes from underneath the first rib to join the C8 nerve root, before dividing the posterior neck of the first rib (Figure 28.2). Although the C8 and T1 nerve roots typically join within 1–2 cm of the first rib, one anomaly that can increase risk of injury is a long T1 nerve root, which may run for 3–4 cm underneath the first rib before passing across the bone to join the C8 nerve root. In this setting,

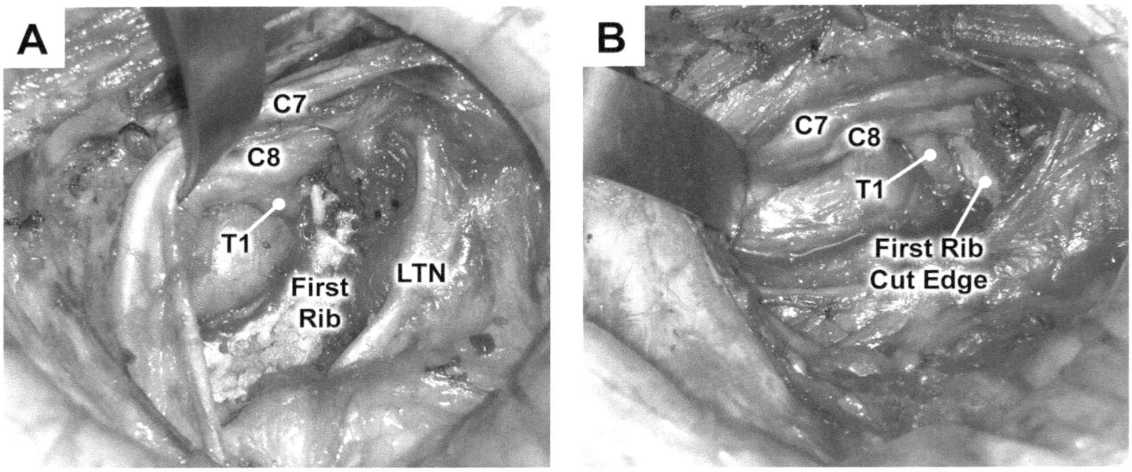

Figure 28.2 Brachial plexus exposure during first rib resection. Operative photographs showing the proximal C8 and T1 nerve roots passing adjacent to the posterior first rib, viewed from the left side after resection of the middle scalene muscle. The junction of C8 and T1 to form the lower trunk of the brachial plexus is seen before (A) and after (B) division of the posterior first rib. LTN, long thoracic nerve. (Robert W. Thompson, MD.)

an unrecognized long T1 nerve root may be injured by the instrument used to divide the rib, reinforcing the need to observe and protect the C8-T1 junction and lower trunk before dividing the posterior first rib.

PLEURAL EFFUSION

Mild-to-moderate pleural fluid collections are often observed on the side of surgery following supraclavicular decompression, consisting of serosanguinous fluid that can be expected to spontaneously resorb within several days to weeks. Although well-tolerated by most patients, some individuals may experience shortness of breath with exertion until the fluid has resolved. Chest radiographs are useful to distinguish the presence of a pleural effusion from diaphragmatic elevation due to phrenic nerve dysfunction and to monitor resolution of the effusion, but thoracentesis or chest tube placement is rarely necessary.

INTRAOPERATIVE AND POSTOPERATIVE BLEEDING

Postoperative bleeding is uncommon but can result in wound hematomas or, when substantial, may lead to hemothorax. Early anticoagulation following operations for the vascular forms of TOS can elevate the risk of bleeding complications. While often self-limited, early re-exploration of the supraclavicular wound allows the operative site to be directly inspected and any specific site of bleeding to be controlled. Evacuation of hemothorax can usually be achieved through this approach as well, through the pleural apex visible through the supraclavicular exposure, avoiding the need for chest tube placement (Figure 28.3).

Prevention of vascular injury

The subclavian artery is directly exposed during supraclavicular decompression and must be protected from injury throughout the procedure. Complete mobilization of the subclavian artery, with ligation and division of small arterial branches that commonly arise from its superior aspect (i.e., the thyrocervical trunk), is helpful to avoid traction and avulsion injuries that can extend onto the main vessel. It is important to keep in mind that intraoperative bleeding from the subclavian artery can rapidly become significant and even life-threatening. The surgeon must have a plan prepared for this contingency in order to obtain prompt proximal control of the vessel if necessary. For this reason, we ensure that instruments needed for median sternotomy or thoracotomy are always available in the operating room during supraclavicular operations, and that the preparation and draping includes a wide sterile field in the event of a vascular emergency.

Although the subclavian vein is not usually directly exposed during supraclavicular decompression for neurogenic TOS, it is susceptible to injury underneath the medial clavicle and where it joins the internal jugular vein. In venous TOS, an increased network of collateral veins is usually encountered throughout the supraclavicular space. Although larger collateral vessels are preserved, such as the external jugular vein, small venous collaterals should be ligated and divided to minimize intraoperative bleeding. Any localized bleeding that may occur during the course of supraclavicular decompression should be meticulously identified and controlled, so that blood does not obscure the operative field and elevate the risk of nerve injury. When intraoperative anticoagulation and direct vascular reconstruction are performed as part of treatment for venous or arterial TOS, suture line hemostasis must be assured with meticulous suture technique and topical agents.

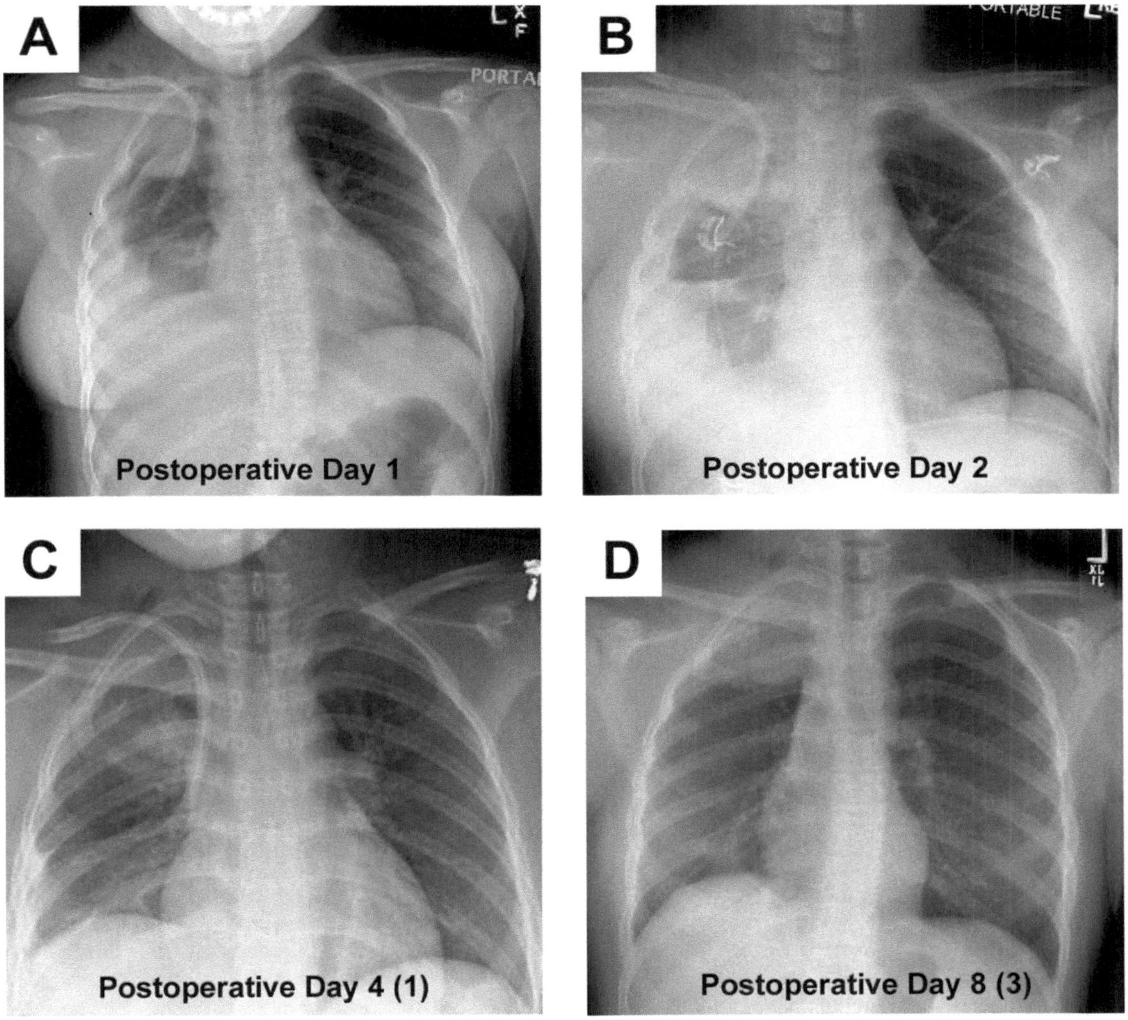

Figure 28.3 Hemothorax after thoracic outlet decompression. Postoperative chest radiographs after right-sided supraclavicular operation, depicting an apical hematoma and right pleural effusion on postoperative day 1 (A) that has increased on postoperative day 2 (B). The patient underwent supraclavicular reexploration on postoperative day 3, with evacuation of the pleural space from the neck alone. The subsequent radiographs demonstrate resolution of the hemothorax (C) and removal of the supraclavicular drain by postoperative day 8 (D).

More common local sources of bleeding include the ends of the divided first rib and the edges of the resected scalene or intercostal muscles. Although bleeding from these sites is typically minimal in amount and is self-limited, effort should be made to diminish fluid accumulation in the operative field. To this end, bone wax is pressed into the divided ends of the first rib, cut muscle edges are often sutured, a topical hemostatic agent is placed along the edges of the resected muscles, and the scalene fat pad is closely reapproximated over the brachial plexus to reduce potential space in the wound. The pleural apex is also purposefully opened to promote dependent drainage away from the operative field, and a closed-suction drain is placed within the supraclavicular space, with its tip extending into the upper chest, upon completion of the procedure. The value of these steps is reinforced by recognition that postoperative accumulation of blood and serum may foster local wound-healing responses that promote fibrosis, thereby contributing to the potential for late neural compression and recurrent symptoms that can follow thoracic outlet decompression.

LYMPH LEAK

The closed-suction drain that is placed at the time of surgery is monitored for the nature and daily volume of fluid output. If there is persistent or increasing drain output of lymphatic fluid > 250 mL/day, particularly when it is chylous in appearance and/or on the left side, a clear liquid diet is maintained. Administration of octreotide is used to reduce the volume of lymph flow, and removal of the closed-suction drain is deferred until the leak has subsided. Early supraclavicular re-exploration is

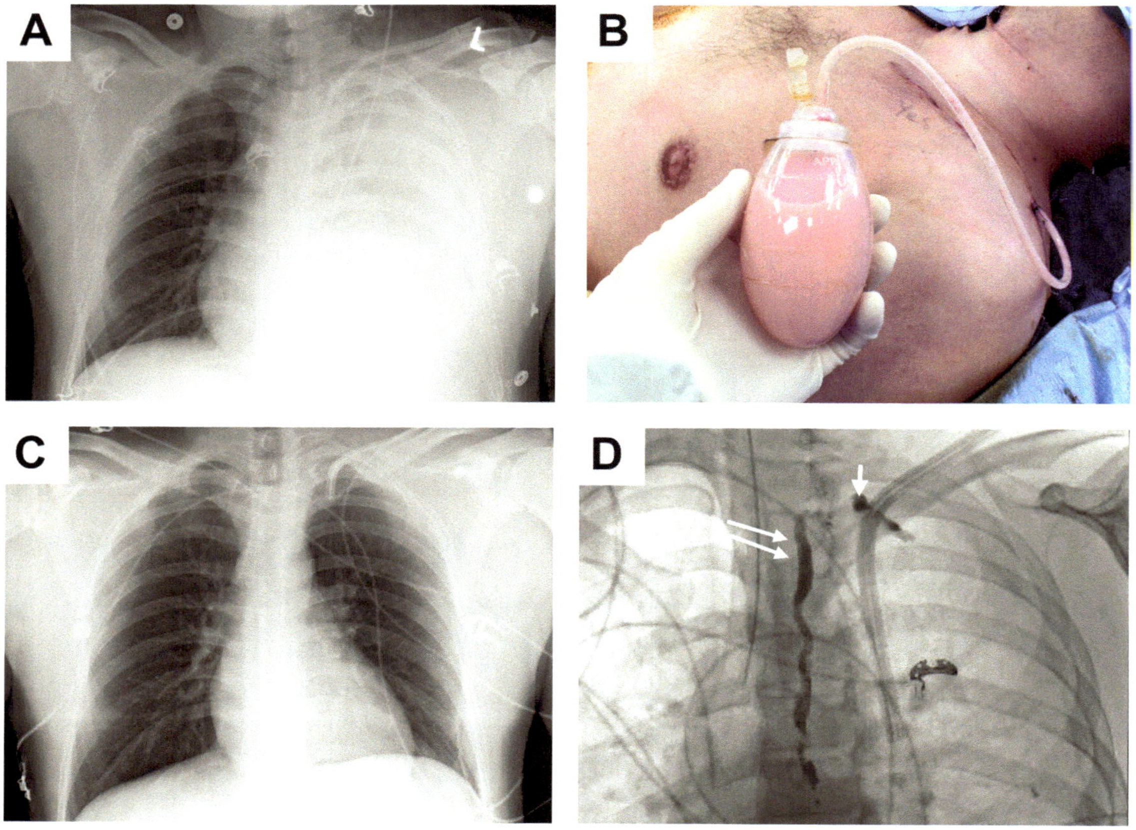

Figure 28.4 Chylothorax after thoracic outlet decompression. Postoperative chest radiograph showing large pleural effusion several days after left-sided supraclavicular operation (A), with high closed-suction drain output characteristic of chylous lymph fluid (B). Chest radiograph after supraclavicular reexploration, local suture control of the lymph leak, and evacuation of the chylothorax (C). Chest radiograph in a separate patient following lymphangiography and embolization of the thoracic duct (D). The site of lymph leak in the neck is depicted by a small contrast blush in the left neck (single arrow) and the main thoracic duct is filled with contrast indicating successful embolization (double arrows). (Robert W. Thompson, MD.)

recommended for persistent high-volume lymph leaks (> 500 mL/day for more than 5 days) or those resulting in chylothorax (Figure 28.4). In extreme cases, surgical ligation of the thoracic duct may be indicated, usually through the right pleural space. In recent years, management of postoperative lymph leaks has been facilitated by the use of lymphangiography and thoracic duct embolization procedures (Figure 28.4D).

Prevention of thoracic duct injury

The thoracic duct joins the venous system near the junction of the internal jugular and subclavian veins. It is susceptible to injury during mobilization of the scalene fat pad, and should therefore be sought out and directly divided between silk ligatures during the early stages of the operation. When a lymphatic leak is observed during the course of the procedure, the site of the leak is identified and oversewn with a pledgeted polypropylene suture, and a topical hemostatic/fibrin tissue sealant is applied to the site before wound closure.

PHRENIC NERVE DYSFUNCTION

Elevation of the ipsilateral diaphragm on postoperative chest x-rays indicates the presence of phrenic nerve dysfunction. This may be associated with shortness of breath on exertion or supine reclining, as well as lower lateral chest discomfort. Most individuals compensate satisfactorily for a unilateral phrenic nerve palsy through increased function of the contralateral diaphragm and intercostal muscles. Many patients will become asymptomatic within a short period of time, but those with severe underlying pulmonary disease may be at risk for significant and persistent disability. Postoperative phrenic nerve dysfunction is usually temporary when it is related to intraoperative mobilization of the nerve or postoperative infusion of local anesthetic, but on occasion phrenic neuropraxia can persist for several weeks. In rare situations, phrenic neuropraxia may be prolonged up to 9–10 months before signs of reinnervation appear. The vast majority of patients are successfully managed expectantly.

Prevention of phrenic nerve injury

The phrenic nerve lies on the surface of the anterior scalene muscle, passing from its lateral to medial edge before descending behind the subclavian vein into the mediastinum. Even with the gentle mobilization of the phrenic nerve necessary to complete resection of the anterior scalene muscle, intraoperative traction or postoperative inflammation around the nerve may result in temporary neuropraxia and ipsilateral diaphragmatic paralysis. Since a phrenic nerve palsy may be asymptomatic and compensated by the other side, it is important to verify normal phrenic nerve function on the side of any previous operation for thoracic outlet syndrome before undertaking a contralateral procedure. An accessory phrenic nerve often arises from the edge of the brachial plexus, where it passes medially to join the primary phrenic nerve near the lower aspect of the anterior scalene muscle. In some cases, the primary or accessory phrenic nerve passes anterior to the subclavian vein, known as a "pre-venous" phrenic nerve. This anomaly can serve as a potential cause of subclavian vein obstruction in venous TOS and is only observed with supraclavicular exposure.

LONG THORACIC NERVE DYSFUNCTION

Postoperative dysfunction of the long thoracic nerve is occasionally observed following thoracic outlet decompression, resulting in a winged scapula defect due to weakness of the serratus anterior muscle. Scapular dysfunction due to this defect is readily detectable by physical examination, and it may interfere with shoulder girdle mechanics and physical therapy, thereby prolonging full recovery from operation. While there is no specific treatment, long thoracic neurpraxia is usually self-limited and recovery can be expected within several months.

Prevention of long thoracic nerve injury

The long thoracic nerve forms within the body of the middle scalene muscle from three separate branches, and then emerges from the muscle to pass over the lateral aspect of the first rib. Protection of the long thoracic nerve is achieved by direct visualization and gentle posterior retraction during middle scalenectomy.

LATE COMPLICATIONS

SPECIFIC TO NEUROGENIC TOS

Residual neurological symptoms of numbness and tingling in the hand or fingers are common early after thoracic outlet decompression, arising as a result of previous neurological damage, intraoperative mobilization of the brachial plexus, and postoperative inflammation and perineural wound healing.[28–33] More pronounced neurological dysfunction including motor deficiencies are rarely observed, particularly arm weakness and loss of handgrip strength, but may represent temporary brachial plexus neuropraxia or pain-limited restrictions in mobility. Spontaneous resolution of such symptoms usually occurs within several days to weeks, but may persist for several months. It is notable that patients with longstanding neurogenic TOS can often display residual symptoms that may not be completely eliminated by thoracic outlet decompression. While these symptoms may be tolerable and are expected to gradually improve, the surgeon must provide continuing support and reassurance during the potentially prolonged period of recovery and rehabilitation.

In some patients, peri-incisional skin hypersensitivity after operation can be quite significant and progressively debilitating. When this is coupled with hypersensitivity symptoms extending into the upper limb, the surgeon must consider the possibility of complex regional pain syndrome (CRPS). This rare and idiopathic condition may be more prevalent in patients with neurogenic TOS than in other patient populations, and must be distinguished from the type of symptoms that can usually be expected in patients undergoing thoracic outlet decompression. Early recognition of CRPS and specific forms of physical therapy, as well as interventions such as stellate ganglion anesthetic blocks, may be useful in symptom management.

Prevention of inadequate decompression and recurrence

The potential for persistent or recurrent symptoms of brachial plexus compression remains one of the most challenging aspects of surgical treatment for neurogenic TOS.[34–39] Persistent symptoms are those that remain despite thoracic outlet decompression and/or progress during the postoperative period and follow-up. Recurrent neurogenic TOS is defined as significant resolution or improvement in symptoms for several months after operation, with development of similar symptoms at a later time interval.[2] Development of recurrent symptoms is often accompanied by an increase in activity or secondary injury.

In patients with persistent or recurrent symptoms, it is first necessary to assess whether the original diagnosis prompting surgical intervention was accurate and, secondly, to evaluate whether the operative strategy that was used in treatment was sufficiently thorough. Utilization of formalized diagnostic and reporting standards for neurogenic TOS, such as those published by the Society for Vascular Surgery, is of great value.[2,5] The surgeon must reassess the surgical approach that was used in the context of the advantages and disadvantages of each operation that might have been performed previously. The incidence of recurrent neurogenic TOS may be as high as 20–25% following transaxillary first rib resection, but is approximately 5% after supraclavicular decompression.[34–39]

FIRST RIB AND CERVICAL RIB RESECTION

There remains some room for debate regarding the necessity for first rib resection during supraclavicular thoracic outlet decompression, with some advocating for routine first rib resection and others for a more selective approach based on intraoperative findings following scalenectomy and brachial plexus neurolysis alone.[40] However, it remains unclear if there are any advantages to retaining the first rib, and incomplete first rib resection is often a factor contributing to recurrent neurogenic TOS.[34–39] It is therefore recommended that first rib resection always be included in supraclavicular decompression for neurogenic TOS, extending posteriorly as far as the level of the T1 nerve root and anteriorly to the costochondral junction (just medial to the scalene tubercle) (Figure 28.5). The first rib is often abnormal in patients with a cervical rib, and may serve as a source of persistent/recurrent nerve compression after isolated cervical rib resection. Thus, first rib resection is also advocated in patients with cervical ribs, along with resection of the cervical rib, in order to ensure the most complete decompression feasible.[41]

EXTENT OF SCALENE MUSCLE RESECTION

Reattachment of the anterior scalene muscle is a well-documented cause of recurrent neurogenic TOS following simple scalenotomy, partial scalenectomy, or transaxillary first rib resection.[34–39] In these circumstances the anterior scalene muscle may reattach to remaining portions of the first rib, to the bed of the resected first rib, to the extrapleural fascia, or directly to the brachial plexus nerve roots. Anomalous scalene muscles and fibrofascial bands may also persist as a source of brachial plexus compression if not previously removed. It is therefore recommended that both the anterior and middle scalene muscles be completely resected, along with any anomalous scalene muscle and fibrofascial bands that might

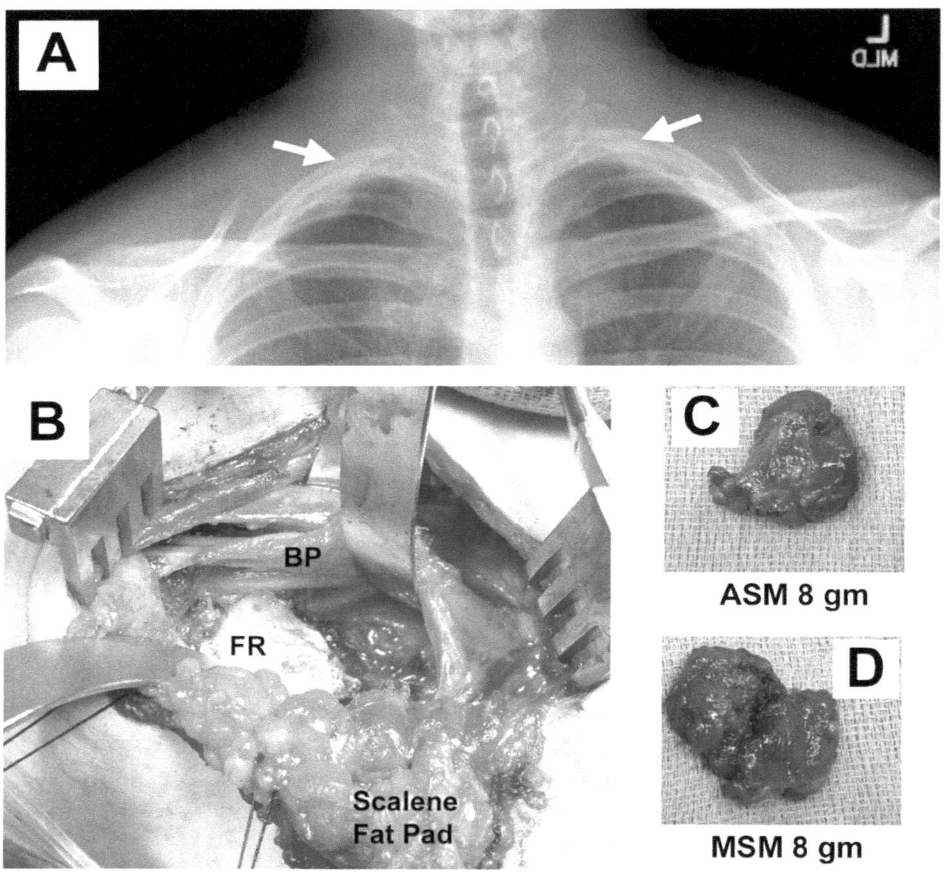

Figure 28.5 Incomplete decompression in neurogenic TOS. Chest radiograph in a patient with recurrent symptoms of neurogenic TOS several months after bilateral first rib resection using a video-assisted thoracoscopic (VATS) approach, demonstrating long posterior first rib remnants (arrows) (A). Operative photograph during supraclavicular re-exploration on the right side, demonstrating exposure of the posterior first rib remnant (FR) and adjacent brachial plexus (BP) (B). Operative specimens of the anterior scalene muscle (ASM, C) and middle scalene muscle (MSM, D). (Robert W. Thompson, MD.)

be encountered, during supraclavicular thoracic outlet decompression (Figure 28.5). It is notable that, due to a limited field of exposure, complete scalene muscle resection is not feasible during thoracic outlet decompression by other approaches.

BRACHIAL PLEXUS NEUROLYSIS

Most patients undergoing surgery for neurogenic TOS exhibit visual evidence of fibrous scar tissue surrounding the brachial plexus nerve roots, a reflection of previous injury and inflammatory tissue healing. This fibrous tissue may contribute to nerve fixation and irritation and, when retained, may be a cause for residual neurogenic symptoms. It is therefore recommended that any perineural fibrous scar tissue be meticulously removed from around each of the brachial plexus nerve roots during the course of thoracic outlet decompression ("external neurolysis"). This step is also facilitated by the exposure obtained with the supraclavicular approach (Figure 28.6).

ABSORBABLE FILM BARRIERS

Postoperative scarring around the brachial plexus nerve roots is inevitable after any operation for TOS, and dense perineural fibrosis is a potential cause of recurrent nerve entrapment and irritation. As in other operations involving direct nerve exposure, it is recommended that the brachial plexus nerve roots be covered with an absorbable anti-adhesion film barrier to decrease the potential for later nerve encasement, using one of several different materials that have been developed for this purpose (Figure 28.6C).

PECTORALIS MINOR TENOTOMY

Brachial plexus compression by the pectoralis minor muscle has become increasingly appreciated as a factor contributing to neurogenic TOS.[42,43] In our experience up to 10% of patients with neurogenic TOS exhibit physical findings that are isolated to the subcoracoid space and 85–90% have findings that co-localize to both the scalene triangle and subcoracoid space. Even in patients with findings predominantly localized to the scalene triangle, residual nerve compression at the site of the pectoralis minor muscle may be a source of persistent or recurrent neurogenic TOS. Simple division of the pectoralis minor muscle tendon immediately below the coracoid process can provide substantial relief of brachial plexus compression while adding little to the operative procedure. Thus, pectoralis minor tenotomy should be included with transaxillary or supraclavicular decompression whenever suggested by preoperative clinical findings.

LATE COMPLICATIONS SPECIFIC TO VENOUS TOS

In venous TOS, the subclavian vein is typically compressed at the point where it passes over the first rib and directly underneath the clavicle. Resection of the

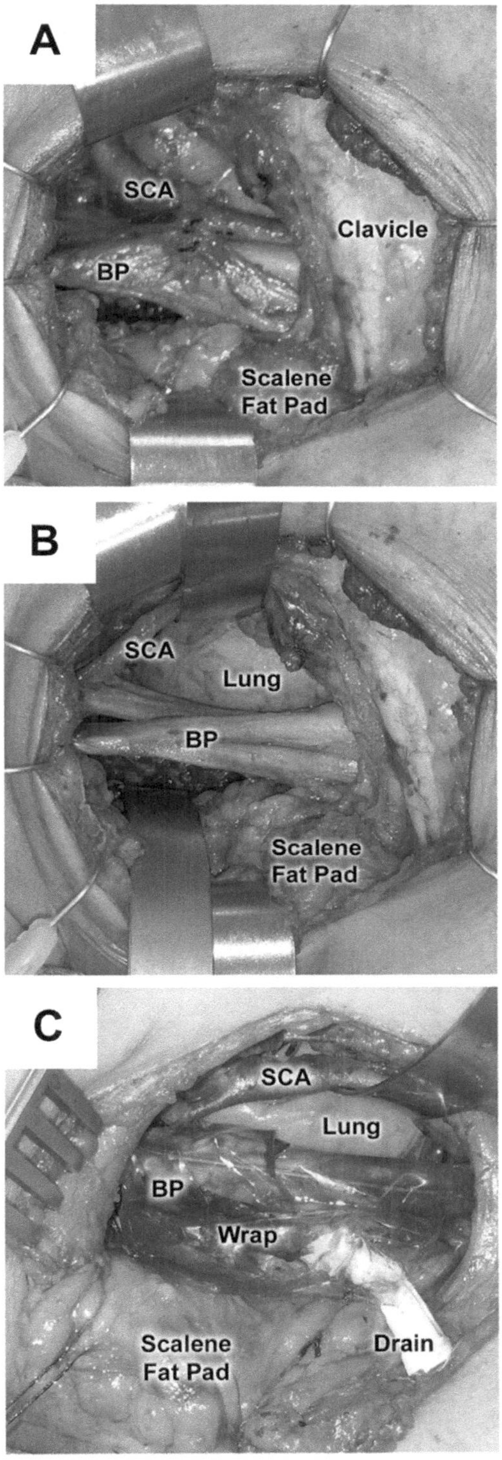

Figure 28.6 Recurrent neurogenic TOS. Operative photographs depicting supraclavicular operation for recurrent right neurogenic TOS, with the brachial plexus (BP) surrounded by dense fibrous scar tissue adjacent to the subclavian artery (SCA) (A). Appearance of the brachial plexus after complete external neurolysis (B). Prior to wound closure, the brachial plexus is loosely wrapped with a bioabsorbable transparent polymer film to help limit perineural adhesions during recovery and wound healing (C). (Robert W. Thompson, MD.)

anterior-most portion of the first rib is therefore considered important in operations for venous TOS to prevent persistent or recurrent subclavian vein obstruction, but this cannot be achieved through the supraclavicular approach alone.[6,44–48] For this reason, as well as to provide more complete access to the axillary-subclavian vein (in the event that direct venous reconstruction is warranted), a medial infraclavicular incision is added to the supraclavicular approach in operations for venous TOS. Operations using an isolated infraclavicular approach are also advocated by some for treatment of venous TOS.[48] While this permits resection of the anterior rib and may allow subclavian vein reconstruction, the remaining posterolateral first rib and unresected scalene muscles may also be a factor in later development of secondary neurogenic TOS.

One of the most common issues with treatment of venous TOS is the management of residual subclavian vein obstruction following decompression.[6] This is addressed in the paraclavicular and infraclavicular approaches by intraoperative venography and direct vein reconstruction at the time of operation. In protocols based on transaxillary first rib resection, venography is usually performed several weeks after surgery and any residual venous obstruction is addressed with endovascular approaches at that time. Unfortunately, up to 25% of patients will have a fixed subclavian vein occlusion that cannot be crossed with a guidewire, for whom long-term anticoagulation is recommended.

In patients having successful operative treatment for venous TOS, subclavian vein obstruction may also arise during follow-up. This may be attributed to persistent compression due to inadequate previous decompression, residual fibrous scar around the vein due to incomplete venolysis, or residual fibrous stenosis in the subclavian vein (Figure 28.7). Re-operation is a feasible option in most patients, unless there is an exceptionally long chronic occlusion of the axillary-subclavian vein beyond the level of the shoulder.

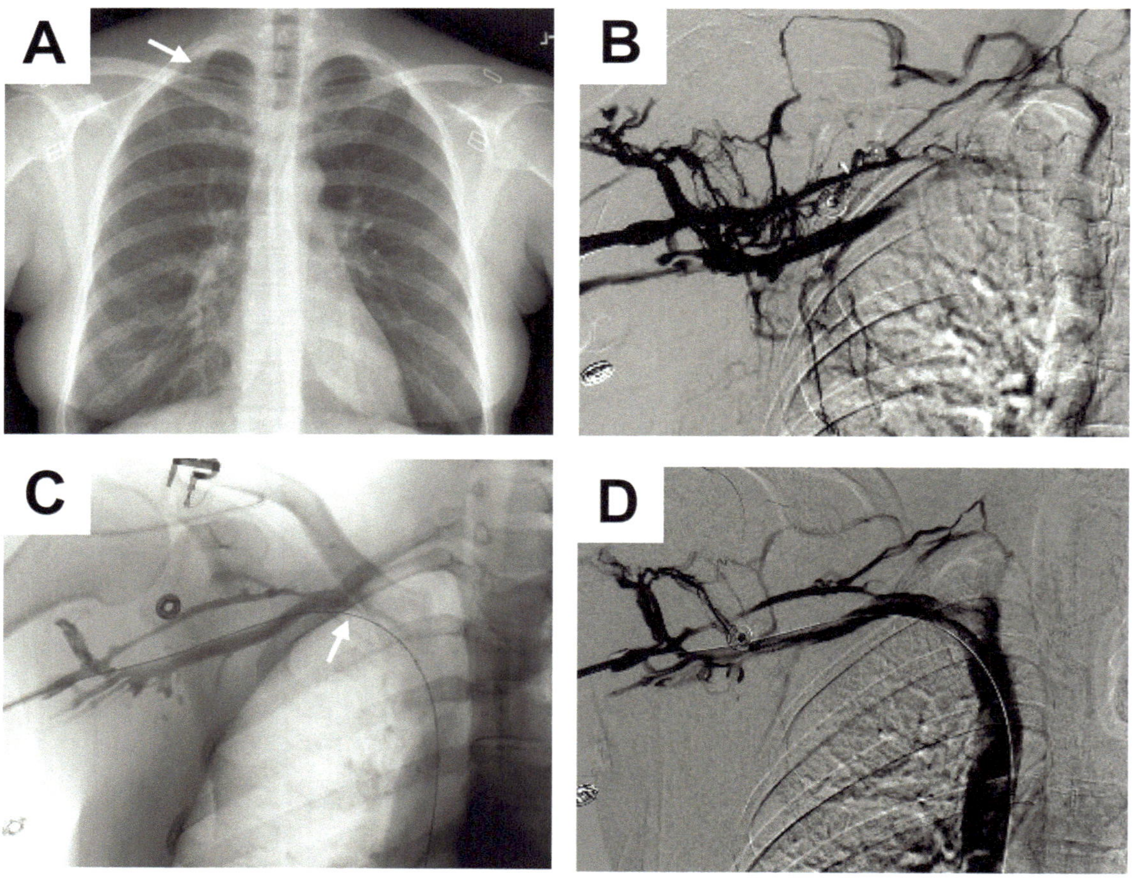

Figure 28.7 Recurrent venous TOS. Chest radiograph in a patient with recurrent right arm selling several months after transaxillary first rib resection for venous TOS, demonstrating an unusually long posterior first rib remnant (arrow) (A). Right upper extremity venogram showing thrombosis of the entire axillary-subclavian vein with extensive collaterals (B). After initial thrombolysis, there is residual focal obstruction in the subclavian vein (arrow) adjacent to the end of the first rib remnant (C). Improvement in venous flow after further thrombolysis and balloon angioplasty, with persistent stenosis in the central subclavian vein (D). Aggressive intervention for postoperative subclavian vein thrombosis can permit more definitive paraclavicular reoperation with resection of the first rib remnant and subclavian vein reconstruction. (Robert W. Thompson, MD.)

LATE COMPLICATIONS SPECIFIC TO ARTERIAL TOS

Arterial TOS is characterized by subclavian artery pathology in the presence of a bony anomaly, most frequently a cervical rib.[7] The typical arterial pathology encountered is post-stenotic dilatation or overt subclavian artery aneurysm formation, frequently complicated by thromboembolism. Operative treatment thereby involves cervical and first rib resection with direct subclavian artery reconstruction, along with simultaneous or staged management of the distal circulation.[7,49] Late complications arising after these procedures may thereby include failure to satisfactorily address distal emboli and/or persistent digital vasospasm.[50] In operations in which a cervical rib was resected but the first rib was retained, recurrent or progressive subclavian artery dilatation may occur due to extrinsic compression by the retained first rib. Like any arterial bypass graft procedure, subclavian artery reconstructions may also be compromised by late restenosis or occlusion due to intimal hyperplasia. This may occur with an increased prevalence in subclavian artery bypass graft reconstructions, where the frequent motion of the arm may place an undue amount of physical strain on the anastomotic suture lines or kinking of bypass grafts. For this reason, it is our preference to use flexible biological conduits in this position rather than prosthetic grafts, such as reversed saphenous vein or cryopreserved femoral artery. While late subclavian artery graft occlusion can be addressed by re-operations, such as carotid-subclavian artery bypass, it is emphasized that these procedures remain a considerable challenge even for surgeons with experience and expertise in this area.

ACKNOWLEDGMENT

This work was supported in part by the Thoracic Outlet Syndrome Research and Education Fund of the Foundation for Barnes Jewish Hospital, BJC Healthcare, St. Louis, Missouri.

REFERENCES

1. Sanders RJ. Anatomy of the thoracic outlet and related structures. In: Illig KA, Thompson RW, Freischlag JA, Donahue DM, Jordan SE, Edgelow PI, eds, Thoracic Outlet Syndrome. London: Springer-Verlag; 2013: 17–24.
2. Illig KA, Donahue D, Duncan A, et al. Reporting standards of the Society for Vascular Surgery for thoracic outlet syndrome. J Vasc Surg 2016;64: e23–e35.
3. Thompson RW. Thoracic outlet syndrome. In: Fischer JE, Ellison EC, Upchurch GR Jr, Galandink S, Gould JC, Klimberg VS, Henke PK, Hochwald SN, Tiao GM, eds, Fischer's Mastery of Surgery, 7th ed. Philadelphia: Wolters Kluwer Health; 2018: 2548–2560.
4. Sanders RJ, Hammond SL, Rao NM. Diagnosis of thoracic outlet syndrome. J Vasc Surg. 2007;46: 601–604.
5. Balderman J, Holzem K, Field BJ, et al. Associations between clinical diagnostic criteria and pretreatment patient-reported outcomes measures in a prospective observational cohort of patients with neurogenic thoracic outlet syndrome. J Vasc Surg. 2017;66: 533–544.
6. Vemuri C, Salehi P, Benarroch-Gampel J, et al. Diagnosis and treatment of effort-induced thrombosis of the axillary subclavian vein due to venous thoracic outlet syndrome. J Vasc Surg Venous Lymphat Disord. 2016;4: 485–500.
7. Vemuri C, McLaughlin LN, Abuirqeba AA, et al. Clinical presentation and management of arterial thoracic outlet syndrome. J Vasc Surg. 2017;65: 1429–1439.
8. Duwayri YM, Emery VB, Driskill MR, et al. Positional compression of the axillary artery causing upper extremity thrombosis and embolism in the elite overhead throwing athlete. J Vasc Surg. 2011;53: 1329–1340.
9. Cikrit DF, Haefner R, Nichols WK, et al. Transaxillary or supraclavicular decompression for the thoracic outlet syndrome: A comparison of the risks and benefits. Am Surg. 1989;55: 347–352.
10. Sanders RJ, Pearce WH. The treatment of thoracic outlet syndrome: a comparison of different operations. J Vasc Surg 1989;10:626–634.
11. Green RM. Controversies in NTOS: Transaxillary or supraclavicular first rib resection in NTOS? In: Illig KA, Thompson RW, Freischlag JA, Donahue DM, Jordan SE, Edgelow PI, eds, Thoracic Outlet Syndrome. London: Springer-Verlag; 2013: 315–317.
12. Thompson RW. Surgical approaches to thoracic outlet syndrome: Supraclavicular versus transaxillary. In: Eskandari MK, Pearce WH, Yao JST, eds, Current Vascular Surgery: Northwestern Vascular Symposium. Raleigh: People's Medical Publishing House-USA; 2017: 375–381.
13. Athanassiadi K, Kalavrouziotis G, Karydakis K. Treatment of thoracic outlet syndrome: Long-term results. World J Surg. 2001;25: 553–557.
14. Degeorges R, Reynaud C, Becquemin J-P. Thoracic outlet syndrome surgery: Long-term functional results. Ann Vasc Surg. 2004;18: 558–565.
15. Povlsen B, Hansson T, Povlsen SD. Treatment for thoracic outlet syndrome. Cochrane Database Syst Rev. 2014;(11): CD007218.
16. Peek J, Vos CG, Unlu C, et al. Outcome of surgical treatment for thoracic outlet syndrome: Systematic review and meta-analysis. Ann Vasc Surg. 2017;40: 303–326.

17. Rinehardt EK, Scarborough JE, Bennett KM. Current practice of thoracic outlet decompression surgery in the United States. J Vasc Surg. 2017;66: 858–865.
18. Nejim B, Alshaikh HN, Arhuidese I, et al. Perioperative outcomes of thoracic outlet syndrome surgical repair in a nationally validated database. Angiology 2017;68: 502–507.
19. Maqbool T, Novak CB, Jackson T, et al. Thirty-day outcomes following surgical decompression of thoracic outlet syndrome. Hand. 2019;14: 107–113.
20. Morel J, Pirvu A, Elie A, et al. Functional results of cervical rib resection for thoracic outlet syndrome: impact on professional activity. Ann Vasc Surg. 2019;56: 233–239.
21. Desai SS, Toliyat M, Dua A, et al. Outcomes of surgical paraclavicular thoracic outlet decompression. Ann Vasc Surg. 2014;28: 457–464.
22. Shutze W, Richardson B, Shutze R, et al. Midterm and long-term follow-up in competitive athletes undergoing thoracic outlet decompression for neurogenic thoracic outlet syndrome. J Vasc Surg. 2017;66: 1798–1805.
23. Hosseinian MA, Loran AG, Soleimanifard Y. Evaluation of complications after surgical treatment of thoracic outlet syndrome. Korean J Thorac Cardiovasc Surg. 2017;50: 36–40.
24. Gelabert HA, Rigberg DA, O'Connell JB, et al. Transaxillary decompression of thoracic outlet syndrome patients presenting with cervical ribs. J Vasc Surg. 2018;68: 1143–1149.
25. White JM, Soo Hoo AJ, Golarz SR. Supraclavicular thoracic outlet decompression in the high-performance military population. Mil Med. 2018;183: e90–e94.
26. Duwayri YM, Thompson RW, Supraclavicular approach for surgical treatment of thoracic outlet syndrome. In: Chaikof EL, Cambria RP, eds, Atlas of Vascular Surgery and Endovascular Therapy. Philadelphia: Elsevier Saunders; 2014: 172–192.
27. Annest SJ, Sanders RJ, Becher M, et al. NTOS: Postoperative care. In: Illig KA, Thompson RW, Freischlag JA, Donahue DM, Jordan SE, Edgelow PI, eds, Thoracic Outlet Syndrome. London: Springer-Verlag; 2013: 239–246.
28. Chang DC, Lidor AO, Matsen SL. Reported in-hospital complications following rib resections for neurogenic thoracic outlet syndrome. Ann Vasc Surg. 2007;21: 564–570.
29. Hong J, Pisapia JM, Ali ZS, et al. Long-term outcomes after surgical treatment of pediatric neurogenic thoracic outlet syndrome. J Neurosurg Pediatr. 2018;21: 54–64.
30. Caputo FJ, Wittenberg AM, Vemuri C, et al. Supraclavicular decompression for neurogenic thoracic outlet syndrome in adolescent and adult populations. J Vasc Surg. 2013;57: 149–157.
31. Rochlin DH, Gilson MM, Likes KC, et al. Quality-of-life scores in neurogenic thoracic outlet syndrome patients undergoing first rib resection and scalenectomy. J Vasc Surg. 2013;57: 436–443.
32. Ohman JW, Abuirqeba AA, Jayarajan SN, et al. Influence of body weight on surgical treatment for neurogenic thoracic outlet syndrome. Ann Vasc Surg. 2018;49: 80–90.
33. Balderman J, Abuirqeba AA, Pate C, et al. Physical therapy management, surgical treatment, and patient-reported outcomes measures in a prospective observational cohort of patients with neurogenic thoracic outlet syndrome. J Vasc Surg. 2019;70: 832–841.
34. Cheng SW, Stoney RJ. Supraclavicular reoperation for neurogenic thoracic outlet syndrome. J Vasc Surg. 1994;19: 565–572.
35. Ambrad-Chalela E, Thomas GI, Johansen KH. Recurrent neurogenic thoracic outlet syndrome. Am J Surg. 2004;187: 505–510.
36. Altobelli GG, Kudo T, Haas BT, et al. Thoracic outlet syndrome: Pattern of clinical success after operative decompression. J Vasc Surg. 2005;42: 122–128.
37. Rochlin DH, Likes KC, Gilson MM, et al. Management of unresolved, recurrent, and/or contralateral neurogenic symptoms in patients following first rib resection and scalenectomy. J Vasc Surg. 2012;56: 1061–1067.
38. Likes K, Dapash T, Rochlin DH, Freischlag JA. Remaining or residual first ribs are the cause of recurrent thoracic outlet syndrome. Ann Vasc Surg. 2014;28: 939–945.
39. Greenberg JI, Alix K, Nehler MR, et al. Computed tomography-guided reoperation for neurogenic thoracic outlet syndrome. J Vasc Surg. 2015;61: 469–474.
40. Cheng SW, Reilly LM, Nelken NA. Neurogenic thoracic outlet decompression: rationale for sparing the first rib. Cardiovasc Surg 1995;3: 617–623.
41. Sanders RJ, Hammond SL. Management of cervical ribs and anomalous first ribs causing neurogenic thoracic outlet syndrome. J Vasc Surg. 2002;36: 51–56.
42. Vemuri C, Wittenberg AM, Caputo FJ, et al. Early effectiveness of isolated pectoralis minor tenotomy in selected patients with neurogenic thoracic outlet syndrome. J Vasc Surg. 2013;57: 1345–1352.
43. Ammi M, Peret M, Henni S, et al. Frequency of the pectoralis minor compression syndrome in patients treated for thoracic outlet syndrome. Ann Vasc Surg. 2018;47: 253–259.
44. Thompson RW. Assessment and treatment of recurrent VTOS. In: Illig KA, Thompson RW, Freischlag JA, Donahue DM, Jordan SE, Edgelow PI, eds, Thoracic Outlet Syndrome. London: Springer-Verlag; 2013: 493–502.

45. Siracuse JJ, Johnston PC, Jones DW, et al. Infraclavicular first rib resection for the treatment of acute venous thoracic outlet syndrome. J Vasc Surg Venous Lymphat Disord. 2015;3: 397–400.
46. Archie MM, Rollo JC, Gelabert HA. Surgical missteps in the management of venous thoracic outlet syndrome which lead to reoperation. Ann Vasc Surg. 2018;49: 261–267.
47. Edwards JB, Brooks JD, Wooster MD, et al. Outcomes of venous bypass combined with thoracic outlet decompression for treatment of upper extremity central venous occlusion. J Vasc Surg Venous Lymphat Disord. 2019;7: 660–664.
48. Wooster M, Fernandez B, Summers KL, et al. Surgical and endovascular central venous reconstruction combined with thoracic outlet decompression in highly symptomatic patients. J Vasc Surg Venous Lymphat Disord. 2019;7: 106–112.
49. Archie MM, Gelabert HA. Endovascular reconstruction of subclavian artery aneurysms in patients with arterial thoracic outlet syndrome. Ann Vasc Surg. 2019;57: 10–15.
50. Thompson RW. Management of digital emboli, vasospasm, and ischemia in arterial thoracic outlet syndrome. In: Illig KA, Thompson RW, Freischlag JA, Donahue DM, Jordan SE, Edgelow PI, eds, Thoracic Outlet Syndrome. London: Springer-Verlag; 2013: 557–563.

29

Complications of hemodialysis access

MIA MILLER, PRAKASH JAYANTHI, AND WILLIAM OPPAT

The incidence of end-stage renal disease (ESRD) continues to rise at an alarming rate. As of December 2016, 0.7 million patients (726,331) were being treated for ESRD in the United States.[1] Historically, a large population initiate dialysis with central venous catheters (CVC) insertion rather than creation of permanent vascular access. Due to the significant issues associated with prolonged catheter use, the National Kidney Foundation Kidney Disease Outcomes Quality Initiative (NKF-KDOQI) developed the Fistula First Initiative in 2003, recommending initiation of dialysis through early creation of arteriovenous fistulas or grafts. As a result of this statement, fistula and graft placement dramatically increased.[2] Of the patients currently on dialysis, approximately 62.5% are arteriovenous fistula (AVF) dependent, 18.4% are arteriovenous graft (AVG) dependent, and 19.2% undergo dialysis by CVC.[3]

With increased prevalence of ESRD, the associated healthcare expenditure also continues to increase. Medicare fee-for-service spending for ESRD beneficiaries has steadily increased yearly, with over 30 billion in 2013 accounting for 7.1% of the overall Medicare paid claims costs.[3] These costs include cardiovascular issues, infection, and, importantly, vascular access-related costs, which include complications and maintenance. Given the substantial representation of vascular access-related costs, it becomes ever more important to gain earlier recognition of the complications to prevent further depletion of Medicare resources. Here, we discuss complications associated with hemodialysis access creation, with appropriate diagnosis and management. We hope to provide education to healthcare providers to improve expertise and optimize management of vascular access, thereby decreasing complications.

STENOSIS

A venous outflow obstruction from stenosis, either peripherally or centrally, accounts for the most common reason of failure of fistulas and shunts.[4] The development of venous stenosis likely results from exposure of the outflow vein to the stress of significantly high arterial flow velocities and turbulent blood flow. Venous outflow stenosis causes gradual decrease in blood flow proximal to the narrowing, which eventually leads to stasis and thrombosis of the vascular access. Neointimal hyperplasia (NIH) remains the most common cause of stenosis.[4] Arteries and veins are composed of three layers: the intima, media, and adventitia. In veins, a single layer of squamous endothelium rests atop an elastic basement membrane. The healthy and thin venous intima overlays the media, which is composed of smooth muscle cells and structural proteins such as collagen and elastin. In neointimal hyperplasia, fibroblasts, smooth muscle cells, and extracellular matrix (ECM) accumulate in the intima and narrow the vessel lumen. Studies that collected tissue samples of stenotic graft-vein anastomoses encountered during surgical revision revealed venous neointimal hyperplasia characterized by presence of smooth muscle cells, ECM and multiple growth factors like platelet-derived growth factor (PDGF), basic fibroblast growth factor (bFGF), and vascular endothelial growth factor (VEGF) expressed by macrophages. However, NIH can be accelerated by circulating inflammatory markers in uremic states, and repeated injury to the graft via large-bore needlesticks during dialysis. It is likely that other metabolic derangements play a role in contributing to the development of NIH as well.[4–7]

Stenoses exist throughout the dialysis circuit. Common sites of NIH include within the venous outflow tract, juxta-anastomotic, needling sites, central outflow tract, arterial inflow tract, and venous valvular scarring. Most commonly, the stenoses involve the venous outflow tract or occur adjacent to the anastomosis.[8] These stenoses can cause an issue both in the newly created fistula, causing thrombosis or failure to mature, or in the well-used fistula. When hemodynamically significant, patients with peripheral or central venous stenosis usually present due to either problems undergoing dialysis or concerns with the affected extremity. The problems with dialysis manifest in many ways such as increased venous pressures, difficulty of access, and prolonged bleeding after removal. Extremity complaints include pain, swelling and decreased fistula flow.

Physical examination is an important modality of diagnosis and also allows for differentiation between inflow and outflow disease. Findings including presence of a water-hammer pulse (hyper-pulsation), systolic thrill (bruit), and abnormal arm elevation test (failure of fistula to collapse on elevation) are suspicious for a peripheral venous outflow stenosis. These signs are secondary to the stasis of blood unable to pass the stenotic lesion and drain into the venous outflow tract.

If the obstruction is due to central venous stenosis, clinical features may include edema including arm, shoulder, breast, supraclavicular region, neck, and face depending on the location and extent of the venous stenosis. When investigating the accuracy of physical examination in the detection of stenosis in an AVF, Asif et al. found a strong correlation between physical examination and angiography in the diagnosis of outflow and inflow stenosis. The sensitivity and specificity for the outflow and inflow stenosis were 92% and 86%, and 85% and 71%, respectively.[9] The physical exam tests used are the arm elevation test and pulse augmentation test. In the arm elevation test, elevation of the arm in a patient with venous outlet stenosis reveals no venous collapse, indicating stasis of blood flow impeded by the obstruction. In the pulse augmentation test, the access is occluded distally, and a normal fistula will show augmentation of the arterial pulse. However, in the presence of inflow stenosis, there is no augmentation.

Imaging studies will confirm the diagnosis of a stenotic lesion in the hemodialysis circuit. When surveying a vascular access, a physician may perform a duplex ultrasound to assess fistula or graft function. The sonographic variables that best reflect fistula function are volume flow in the brachial artery and the caliber of and presence of stenosis in the efferent vein. Volume flows in the brachial artery in successfully functioning AVFs range from 500 to 1500 mL/min, with flow rates less than 500 mL/min associated with significant risk of thrombosis.[10] However, on many occasions physical examination with clinical history of associated problems with undergoing dialysis or extremity swelling is enough to warrant intervention without the additional step of a duplex.

The gold standard for the diagnosis of a stenosis in the hemodialysis circuit is a fistulogram. Additionally, a diagnostic fistulogram provides the ability to intervene if indicated. The basic indication for percutaneous transluminal angioplasty is stenosis > 50% or thrombosis of the AVF or graft. Primary patency within the first year after angioplasty is > 50%, while primary-assisted patency is

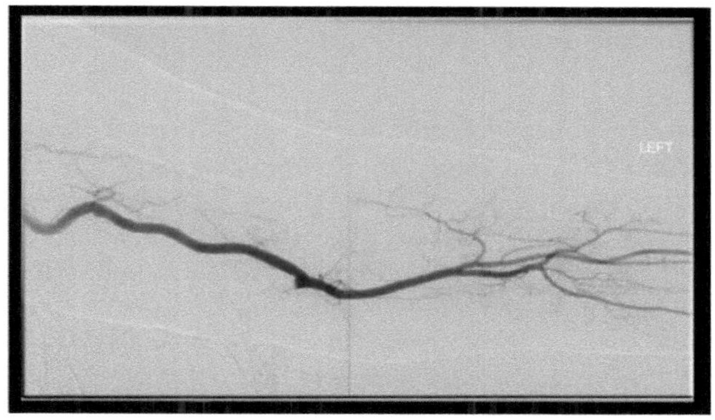

Figure 29.1 Angiography of a basilic vein fistula revealing stenosis of the outflow tract.

80–90% in the same time period. An example of a fistulogram revealing an outflow stenosis and subsequent angioplasty can be seen in Figures 29.1 and 29.2. A cutting balloon can be used as a second-line method, and stents and covered stents are reserved for the management of complications and central outflow stenosis.[11] According to a study by Mohjuddin et al., fistula flow rate change was significantly better in native AVFs after fistuloplasty (percent flow increase 88.4%) than that in AVGs (percent flow increase 9.2%). Increase in fistula flow was greatest for valvular lesions (percent increase in flow: 42.6%), followed by lesions at the needling site (40.1%), peripheral outflow vein stenosis (29%), central outflow vein stenosis (25.9%), and at the anastomosis (19.9%).[7]

Graft surveillance with duplex ultrasound is most frequently performed within first 2 years of surgery, as this is the most prevalent time of NIH formation. Early detection of developing stenoses before manifestation as a thrombosed fistula or graft allows the possibility of early intervention.[7,12]

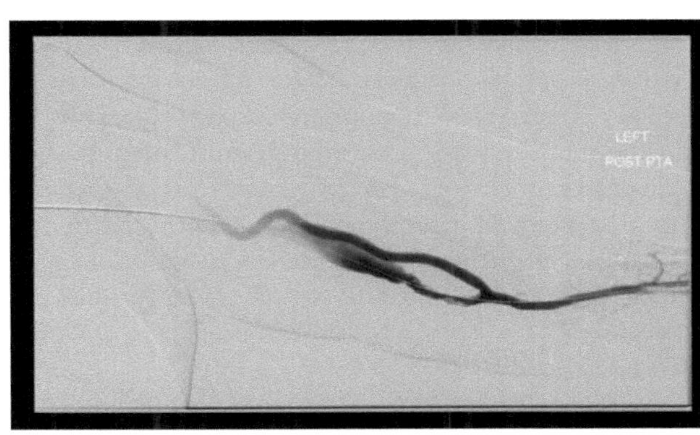

Figure 29.2 Angiography of a basilic vein fistula revealing reconstitution of flow after balloon angioplasty of the stenosis of the basilic vein, performed by radial artery approach.

THROMBOSIS

Hemodynamically significant stenoses secondary to NIH causes flow disturbances and changes, beginning the cascade that results in access thrombosis in 85% of cases. Virchow's triad, including hypercoagulability, hemodynamic changes like stasis or turbulence, and vessel injury resulting in endothelial dysfunction, define common causes of thrombosis.[5] Significant factors cited for early failure include prior history of access surgery, and absence of a good intraoperative thrill within the fistula or shunt.[13] Early thrombosis, defined as the loss of flow within the hemodialysis circuit, was found to be associated with female gender, forearm AVF, and smaller arterial size. Paradoxically, diabetes and stiff, noncompliant feeding arteries were associated with a lower frequency of early thrombosis but likely have a lower rate of maturation.[14] Other factors have a noted effect on risk of thrombosis including preoperative aspirin use and intraoperative protamine use decrease and increase the odds of thrombosis, respectively. Additionally, vein diameters 2–3 mm have been found to affect early thrombosis rates as cited by Farber et al.[14]

Antiplatelet and anticoagulant use to prevent thrombosis has been controversial. In a clinical trial including 567 patients by Irish et al., the occurrence of fistula failure within 12 months of surgery was high and not reduced by fish oil supplementation or aspirin use.[15] Patients with uremia appear to possess dysfunctional platelets which may explain variations in long-term patency.[16] Conversely, hemodialysis patients are also noted to have hypercoagulable disorders due to elevated factor VIII and fibrinogen concentrations and may benefit from systemic anticoagulation. However, these benefits must be compared to the increased risk of hemorrhagic complications.[17] In a recent randomized controlled trial of 877 participants, Dember et al. demonstrated that clopidogrel reduced early thrombosis rates at 6 weeks from 19.5% to 12.2%; however, there was no significant difference in the number of successfully matured fistulas prepared to undergo dialysis.[18] Other findings, such as a study by Dixon et al. including 649 patients receiving dipyridamole plus aspirin, showed a significant but modest effect in reducing the risk of stenosis and improving the duration of primary-unassisted patency of newly created grafts.[19] The literature remains conflicted in the role of antiplatelet and anti-coagulant therapy for thrombosis prevention, and no specific conclusions or recommendations can be made at this time.

A lack of palpable thrill and audible bruit of a graft leads to the diagnosis of a thrombosed shunt. If simple physical examination is equivocal, a duplex may be performed to demonstrate a lack of flow. Treatment of a thrombosed fistula or graft is thrombectomy, via open versus percutaneous methods. Generally, open thrombectomies are performed under local or general anesthesia with an overlying incision and isolation of the vessel. Subsequently, a venotomy is performed followed by insertion of Fogarty balloon embolectomy catheters to assist in removing the clot. Typically, a fistulogram is obtained after clot evacuation to reveal the cause of thrombosis. If an outflow stenosis or needle-site thrombus are the underlying causes, balloon thrombectomy is then followed by any indicated angioplasty of the obstruction. If inflow stenosis identified at the arterial anastomosis or feeding artery is the underlying cause, simple balloon angioplasty or anastomotic revision, by either patch angioplasty or proximalization of the arterial anastomosis, is usually warranted. For percutaneous mechanical dissolution thrombectomies, ultrasound guidance sheath placement using modified Seldinger technique is used to achieve proximal and distal access in dialysis circuit, to allow utilization of the entire length of the shunt. Catheters, such as the AngioJet, Solent Omni Catheter, or Rotarex, are introduced into the thrombosis and drawn back slowly. Following completion of percutaneous thrombectomy, venography is performed to identify any residual thrombus load and potential causes of stenoses that may benefit from angioplasty. A study by Lambert et al. showed that interventional radiological thrombectomies have better outcomes in terms of a lower re-thrombosis rate and better assisted primary patency than surgical thrombectomies. However, percutaneous thrombectomies have a lower intervention-free patency and more frequently need additional procedures to main patency. Therefore, surgical revision procedures significantly increase success rate of access thrombectomies.[20,21]

A recent publication by Brooke et al. examined the cost effectiveness of repeated interventions on failing AVFs. The study reviewed 720 fully matured upper extremity AVFs of which 56% underwent at least one intervention to maintain functional patency, with a mean time to first reintervention of 12.6 months. While the clinical effectiveness of performing percutaneous interventions on failing AVFs decreases after each reintervention, the study found this more cost-effective than the creation of a new AVF. Conversely for open thrombectomies, it was more cost-effective to create a new AVF after the second open reintervention procedure. In the setting of burgeoning healthcare costs for ESRD patients, especially in regards to maintenance of vascular access, this study suggests the benefits of continued percutaneous interventions over open thrombectomies or new AVF creations.[22]

PSEUDOANEURYSM/ANEURYSMS

Two types of aneurysms occur in hemodialysis access circuits: aneurysms and pseudoaneurysms. Aneurysms are defined as dilation involving all vessel layers, whereas pseudoaneurysms typically are fibrous cavities in continuity with the circulatory system that exist within the subcutaneous tissues. While pseudoaneurysms can occur both in arteriovenous grafts and fistulas, true aneurysms only occur in fistula vein downstream of an obstruction. The major concern with the development of any kind of aneurysm is the risk of rupture with resulting catastrophic hemorrhage. Most clinically significant aneurysms are false or 'pseudo'-aneurysms that commonly occur at the site of needling/puncture or at the anastomoses. Pseudoaneurysms are simply hematomas formed by extravasation of blood from the access that eventually develop a surrounding fibrotic sac lacking endothelium or vascular wall structure. These pseudoaneurysms can be thrombosed or continue to experience some flow. Pseudoaneurysms at the anastomosis site reflect leaking of blood outside a lumen because of poor surgical technique with inadequate depth of suture bites or excessive tension. Breakdown of an anastomosis is commonly due to an infectious complication, which must always be suspected.[23,24] The incidence of aneurysm development in hemodialysis circuits is highly variable, with reports of 5% to over 60%, and likely results from a lack of standardized reporting. It is known, however, that the incidence is higher in both proximal AVFs and AVFs involving the cephalic vein rather than basilic vein.[25] In the setting of AV grafts, pseudoaneurysm may develop from eventual breakdown of the graft wall, which may be indirectly caused by the presence of outflow stenosis. The presence of downstream lesions may induce high pressures within an AVG during dialysis, and the resulting increased pressure, along with the concomitant trauma from cannulation, leads to loss of graft integrity.[26]

Valentini et al. recently proposed a classification system based on fistula morphology. Types 1–3 are characterized as being true aneurysms and Type 4 as pseudoaneurysms. Type 1 aneurysms are subdivided into Type 1a involving the entire length of the vein, and Type 1b defined as proximal vein dilatation occurring < 5 cm from anastomosis. Type 1 aneurysms were most common on created fistulas in patients with low creatinine clearance who were not currently undergoing dialyzed. Type 2 aneurysms are localized and are subdivided into 2a being at least 1 localized pseudoaneurysm, but can be more and 2b including post-anastomotic dilatation with localized dilatations. Type 3 are classified as complex and heterogenous, bearing no resemblance to other subtypes. The overall incidence of aneurysms amongst patients was 43.5%, with the large majority of dialyzed patients being Type 2, likely secondary to needle puncture. They noted the highest risk of rupture was amongst Type 2 aneurysms. They also noted Type 1a fistulas should be monitored due to increased risk for high-output cardiac failure, but that the risk of thrombosis was low. Hence, Type 1a and 2 fistulas should be monitored, but for differing reasons.[27]

The principles of treatment for both true and false aneurysms are similar. Intervention should only be considered for clinically significant aneurysms, with risk of rupture as the most concerning outcome. Traditionally, clinically significant aneurysms considered for repair include those that are rapidly enlarging, involving the anastomosis, overlying skin compromise, or association with outflow vein stenosis.[27] In the setting of known aneurysmal disease, monitoring prior to each dialysis session with frequent follow-up can help identify access issues and help determine treatment plans. Assessment for venous outflow obstruction is routinely evaluated and corrected if present. Asymptomatic aneurysms can be followed, but patients undergoing issues with dialysis, progressive enlargement, and/or with skin thinning/ulceration/bleeding are patients who benefit from intervention.[26] Regardless of clinical significance, awareness of the presence of aneurysms and education of dialysis staff to avoid those areas for future puncture sites should comprise the universal plan of care.

The method of true aneurysmal repair varies and usually is reserved for compromised or dysfunctional access. If the aneurysm is localized (Type 2), it may be possible to excise and directly anastomose end-to-end after mobilization. An illustration of excision of a true aneurysm is seen in Figures 29.3–29.6. One may consider plication (RITS) and interposition 8 mm grafts for more complex reconstructions, which becomes especially necessary with any skin compromise.[28]

Treatment of pseudoaneurysms is also multimodal. As with true aneurysms, surgical excision plays a role; however, more minimally invasive techniques are available. Small saccular pseudoaneurysms with narrow necks have been shown to be amenable to thrombin injection or ultrasound compression with good results in small series.[29,30] Endovascular techniques using covered stents or stent grafts to exclude the sac or aneurysm are trending; however, this creates issues with access due to the now thick layer that the needle must traverse during dialysis. If a stent graft were to be used, it is advisable to notify dialysis staff to exclude that area from puncture unless absolutely necessary, which may cause loss of access length necessary for effective clearance.[31] Particularly in the setting of a graft, there is always the concern for infection, with prior studies demonstrating an increased risk of infection with direct-graft cannulation.[32,33] Therefore, the preferred treatment choice for AVG pseudoaneurysm is surgical repair. Much like true aneurysms, a bypass interposition graft can be used to divert flow around the aneurysmal portion.[26]

The presence of aneurysms should also entail the performance of a shuntogram. Angiographic evaluation of the shunt allows for diagnostic examination of anastomotic site(s) and outflow vein, identification of ideal sites for cannulation, and performance of therapeutic measures as well. For significant aneurysmal disease, if the circuit is inappropriate for attempted revision or bypass, ligation and creation of a new access should be considered as well.

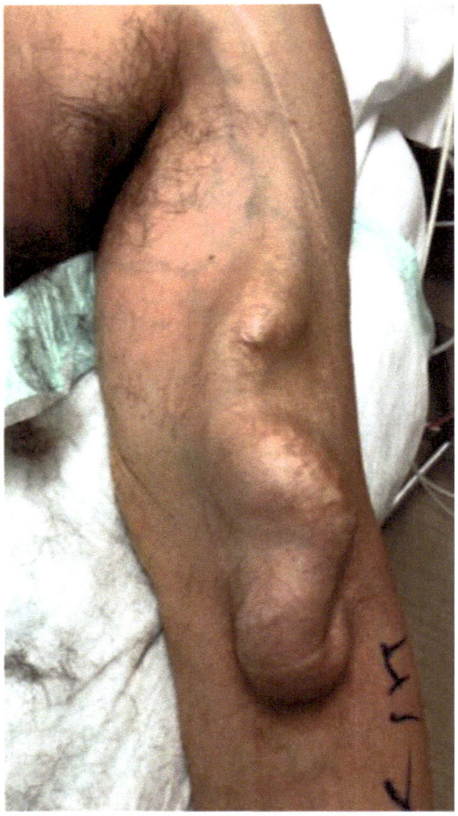

Figure 29.3 Large AV fistula constructed many years ago for hemodialysis access (prior to resection).

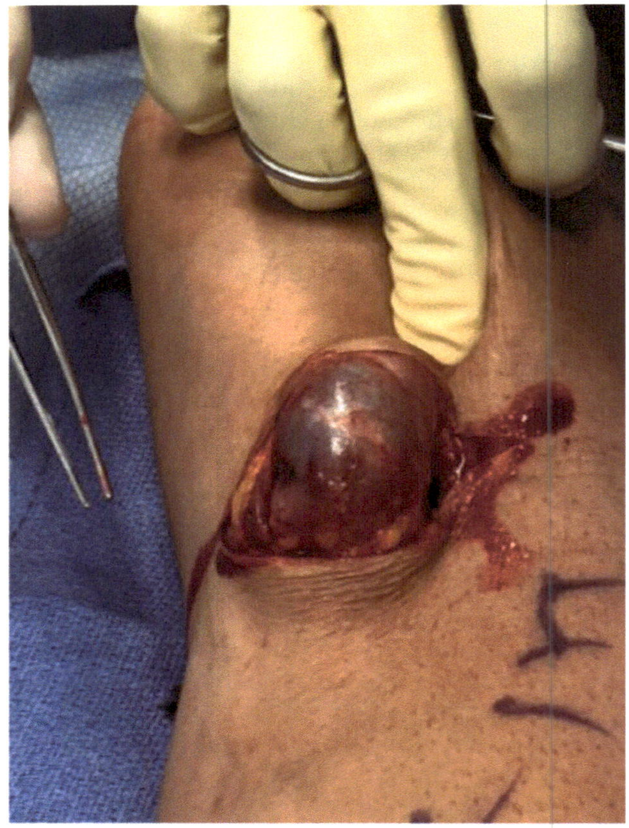

Figure 29.4 Exposed AV fistula.

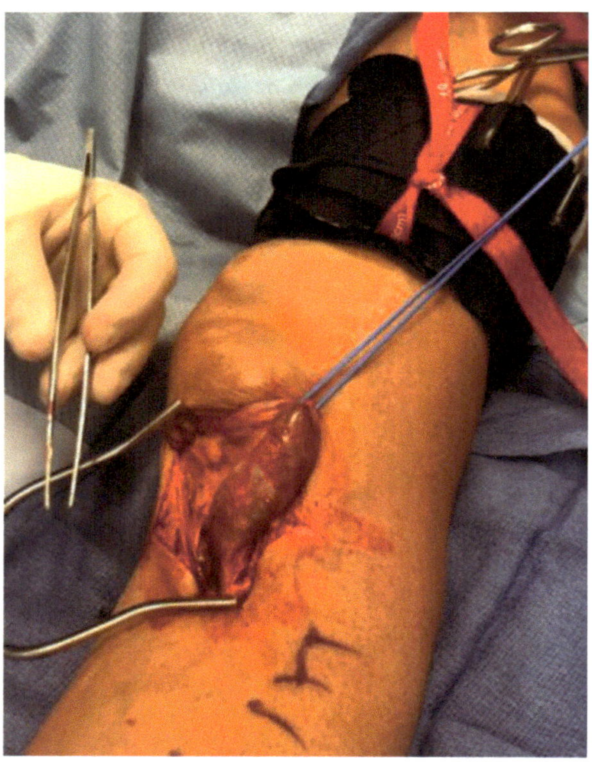

Figure 29.5 Proximal control using silastic vessel loop.

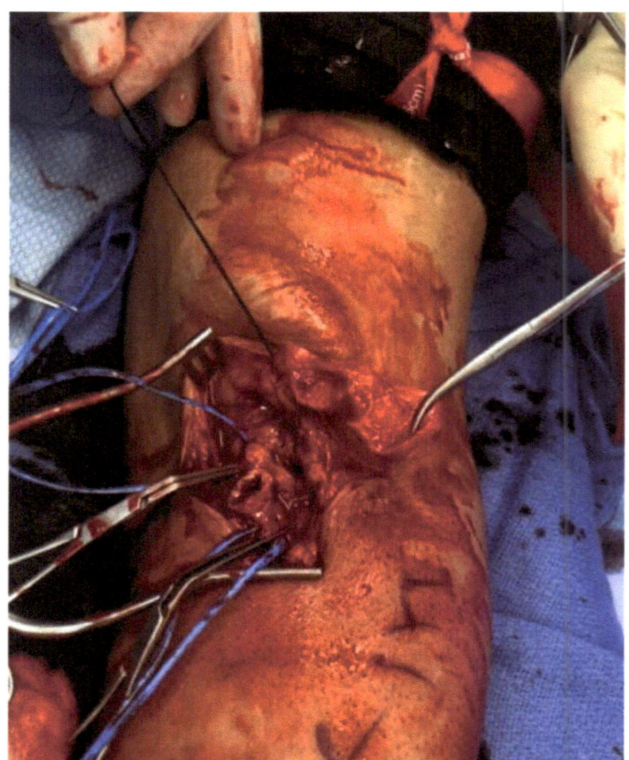

Figure 29.6 Resection AV fistula.

INFECTION

Access infection accounts for roughly 20% of hemodialysis circuit complications and is an important cause of failure of AVFs and PTFE grafts. The incidence of infection of autogenous AVFs is approximately 0.56–5%, and 4–20% of prosthetic AV grafts. *Staphylococcus* species account for 30–50% of infections, while infection with *Enterococci* and coagulase-negative *Staphylococcus* occur in 20–30% cases. Polymicrobial infections with gram-negative bacteria account for 10–20%. *Staphylococcus* and *Pseudomonas* may both be highly destructive and likely to incur anastomotic disruption.[34]

Without question, infection is more commonly encountered with a prosthetic AV graft rather than an autologous AVF, which is thought to be secondary to foreign body insertion. Typical symptoms of graft infection include erythema, induration, drainage with sinus tracts, and systemic signs like fevers, chills, and malaise. AV graft infections typically present with localized symptoms as opposed to catheter-related infections, which present with systemic symptoms.[34] In the septic patient, it is of utmost importance to distinguish access infection from other sources like pneumonia, osteomyelitis, endocarditis, urinary tract infections, decubitus ulcers, septic arthritis, and intra-abdominal sources. Patients with ESRD are more prone to infections from uremia-induced immunologic dysfunction, including impaired lymphocyte-mediated cellular immunity, neutrophil chemotaxis, phagocytosis, bacterial killing, and metabolic dysfunction. Other mechanisms of altered polymorphonuclear neutrophil function include malnutrition, iron overload, increased intracellular calcium, the dialysis treatment, and circulating plasma factors.[35]

Diagnosis of dialysis access infection remains largely clinical. There is conflicting literature regarding the actual utility of a tagged leukocyte scan. While it can provide information, reasons for a false-negative scan include chronic infection and antibiotic therapy, which most patients begin at first clinical suspicion.[36,37] Additional to the difficulty in obtaining the scan, interpretation by radiologists remains variable due to the decreased familiarity. Combined with conflicting reports in the literature of the tests sensitivity and specificity, we are not able to strongly recommend its use as a first-line diagnostic tool.[37] Computed tomography (CT) scans have low sensitivity in differentiating between prosthetic infection and postoperative changes in the acute setting. Moreover, contrast-enhanced CT may produce false-negative results in chronic low-grade and very late infection, and more than 80% of cases show inconclusive findings. Duplex ultrasound and magnetic resonance angiography (MRI) have not been proven superior to CT either.[34,38,39]

The treatment of infected grafts and fistulas varies based on level of infection and the condition of the overlying skin. For localized infections, initial treatment includes antibiotics for 4–6 weeks tailored by cultures when attempting to salvage the dialysis access. Without question, careful follow-up is mandatory. If at any point antibiotics fail to control the infection, surgical resection should be performed. Autogenous AV access infections are usually localized to the access site and will respond to antibiotics when the overlying skin is healthy. Prosthetic AV graft infections usually require surgical management because antibiotics alone will not sterilize the implanted graft. Truly localized prosthetic graft infections can be managed with segmental excision and jump graft reconstruction, and partial excision without excising the arterial or venous anastomoses while leaving a small cuff of prosthetic attached to the artery can decrease the morbidity of extensive dissection in dense scar adjacent to the neurovascular structures. Total excision is required for removal of infections involving the anastomoses, and those infections involving particularly virulent organisms.[34]

The differential diagnosis of a fistula or peri-graft fluid collection must include infection, but the collection of fluid could also be a hematoma, seroma, or lymphocele. Hematoma incidence is approximately 0.073–0.2 per patient without regard to type of access.[34] Treatment for a non-expanding, non-pulsatile hematoma usually includes conservative management with elevation, compression, and warm compresses. CTA can reveal a blush or active extravasation that may require surgical hemostasis, however most active bleeding halts with tamponade within the involved compartment. Monitoring with serial exams and hemoglobin measurements must occur to ensure the patient remains stable for non-operative management. Seroma incidence ranges from 0.48% to 4.2% and preferred treatment is observation.[38] Serial aspirations of the fluid collections is controversial as needle aspiration can result in bacterial seeding and subsequent infection. In chronic seromas, surgical excision with debridement and replacement of the graft is necessary, and this strategy is reserved for severe cases and chronic infection. An interestingly novel idea introduced by Gargiulo et al. describes intra-graft stent deployment for the management of seromas with success.[40] This case series described two patients who failed percutaneous and open therapy, and subsequent Wallgraft stent insertion revealed gratifying results. Lymph leaks must also be considered in the differential. Characterized by the hallmark clear fluid of extremity lymph fluid, lymph leaks generally occur secondary to incomplete ligation of lymphatic drainage around the surgical site, and can present as lymphoceles, lymphedema, and lymphorrhea. The treatment of small lymphoceles mirrors the management of a seroma, with the first-line therapy being observation and control of symptomatic swelling with compression. Edema is usually improved with elevation, with refractory cases treated with careful compression. Lymphorrhea or lymphocele connection to access can be ligated surgically for definitive management.[35]

ISCHEMIA

Ischemia remains a serious complication of AV access creation. Connecting an artery to a vein creates a short circuit that decreases the distal extremity capillary circulation of the hand. Both fistulas and shunts create a large arterial-venous pressure gradient that augments blood flow into the venous outflow circulation. Because AVFs and AVGs cause shunting of a high volume of blood from arterial into venous system, distal ischemia can occur as blood ceases to reach distal capillaries. By definition, physiologic steal results with AV access creation; pathologic steal occurs when the patient experiences ischemic signs and symptoms of the hand.

The incidence of upper extremity ischemia in dialysis patients is up to 5%, with increased incidence in upper arm shunts compared to forearm shunts. Symptomatic ischemia may develop in 10–25% brachiocephalic and basilic AVF, 4.3–6% in forearm grafts, and 1–1.8% in radiocephalic AVFs. The larger the caliber of artery, the higher the flow velocity and blood flow through the AV access, with more blood flow shunted due to the large artery, the more likely the patient is to experience symptomatic distal ischemia. Flow velocities and volumes through upper arm shunts may be 2–3 times that of a radiocephalic fistula, which explains the above findings. However, with adequate collateral circulation, most patients should maintain appropriate digital pressures, which illustrates why many patients remain asymptomatic.[41] Collateral flow from the ulnar circulation assists in preventing significant ischemia for forearm access creations. An Allen's test with Doppler of the palmar arch preoperatively assists in confirmation of compensatory ulnar flow. This is especially significant in occlusive upper extremity arterial ulnar disease, or radial-dominant flow.[42] The incidence of steal syndrome is approximately 6.2% per Davison et al. and is most commonly found in brachial artery-based AV shunts, females, diabetics, and smokers with significant atherosclerosis.[41,43,44]

Steal syndrome is a graded complication, with stages to classify symptomatology and assist in directing management (see Table 29.1). Symptoms can occur within days to months of creation of the fistula or graft. The timing for development can separated into two categories: prior to and after 30 days. Approximately 50–66% of patients who develop steal occur within 30 days postoperatively. Steal syndrome can occur immediately; or may declare itself over time, often worsened by dialysis.[35]

Table 29.1 Grades (staging) of steal syndrome

Stage	Symptoms
I	Pale, blue, or cold hand without pain
II	Pain during exercise or hemodialysis
III	Rest pain
IV	Ulcers, necrosis or gangrene

Steal syndrome remains predominantly clinical diagnosis, and a thorough history and physical is mandatory for its recognition. Confirmatory diagnosis is obtained by unilateral neurologic complaints associated with digital tissue necrosis, pallor/cyanosis of distal extremity, reduced arterial flow distal to anastomotic site, and distal artery flow reversal.[35] In this regard, arterial duplex ultrasonography, digital pressures, and arteriography become essential modalities, as they can measure blood flow through the fistula or graft, locate collateral vessels, and help differentiate dialysis-associated steal syndrome (DASS) from other causes, such as stenoses or obstructions that may require possible intervention. Digital pressures of less than 50 mmHg, digit/brachial index (DBI) less than 0.6, and $TcPO_2$ less than 20–30 mmHg are noninvasive markers of steal physiology.[41]

To intraoperatively predict likelihood of steal, Tynan-Cuisinier et al. found a DBI of 0.45 rather than 0.5 as a more accurate predictor in their data set, with 80% sensitivity and 70% specificity. However, there was a low positive predictive value, as there is wide variability in the ability of patients to tolerate objectively decreased finger perfusion without becoming symptomatic and must be applied by individual clinical basis. A low DBI at time of construction may raise concern for subsequent DASS, especially in conjunction with other risk factors. The authors recommend two pathways based on postoperative dopplerable wrist signals. If signals are present, one may observe the patient closely and intervene as indicated. If no signals can be obtained after optimization of patient's hemodynamics, one must attempt reconstruction with a goal of DBI > 0.45.[45]

Treatment varies by underlying cause of the arterial steal. If arterial stenosis exists proximal to the AVF, percutaneous transluminal angioplasty (PTA) is the initial treatment of choice. Banding, which has fallen out of favor due to high complication rate of fistula thrombosis, involves suturing a small piece of Teflon/Dacron around the AVF 2 cm distally from the anastomosis, and tightened to a lumen reduction of 4mm.[25,46] With banding, blood flow and/or digital blood pressure should be measured intraoperatively in order to precisely control the degree of reduced flow obtained.[47] The minimally invasive limited ligation endoluminal-assisted revision (MILLER) procedure is a new modified banding technique. This procedure requires a small 1–2 cm skin incision for placement of a ligature, while utilizing a 4–5 mm diameter endoluminal balloon to achieve and standardize the desired reduction of inflow size.[48] The balloon is passed retrograde to the area of dissection, and inflated. The ligature is placed around the artery. Using fluoroscopy, the tightness of the ligature can be measured by visualization of the waist. In several series, Miller et al. noted significant improvement in both steal syndrome and high-flow patients, with 89% of steal patients achieving clinical success with a single procedure. Primary access patency was 52% at 3 months, with 90% secondary patency rate at 24 months. However, subsequent studies by other authors have shown variable outcomes.[49]

Distal revascularization and interval ligation (DRIL) procedure was first reported by Schanzer et al. in 1988. The two-step procedure consists of ligation of the artery just distal to the anastomosis with creation of an arterial bypass from the artery proximal to the anastomosis to the artery distal to the ligation using PTFE or reversed saphenous vein. This procedure theoretically blocks retrograde blood flow to access while increasing distal extremity perfusion.[50] Studies have shown symptomatic relief in 83–100% of patients with steal syndrome, with secondary access patency in 73–98% of patients. Complications ranged up to 17% and were mostly surgical site infections and thrombosis.[49] DRIL continues to be a frequently used modality for treatment of dialysis-associated steal syndrome and has been very successful at both maintaining access and alleviating steal symptoms. Long-term data regarding durability demonstrate 90% patients showing significant or complete symptomatic improvement. They also noted complete or current healing of all patients with tissue loss. Primary patency rate at 12 months was 80% for AVF, and 40–50% for prosthetic grafts. No reports of ischemic limb complications from bypass failure were noted.[45]

There are multiple other surgical techniques described in the literature to revise AVFs to decrease or eliminate steal syndrome. Revision using distal inflow (RUDI), described in 2005, is accomplished by ligating the original upper arm AV outflow near the anastomosis and creating a new anastomosis to a smaller-caliber, more distal artery such as proximal radial or ulnar artery for the inflow, using a graft.[51] Outflow is accomplished by reconstruction of this newly anastomosed graft to the original venous outflow. For successful RUDI, a minimum 2 mm radial or ulnar target, with intact secondary flow to the hand is mandated.[49] Another procedure referred to as proximalization of arterial inflow (PAI) entails moving the arterial supply to a more proximal brachial artery level, or axillary artery, using an interposition graft.[52] In severe cases of steal, ligation of the AVF may be warranted to restore blood flow to the distal extremity emergently, with the obvious caveat of loss of access.

Interestingly, in the preoperative setting of dominant radial flow or inadequate ulnar flow to the hand, there has been discussion for the creation of a proximal ulnar AVF creation. In small series, they have been shown to have primary and cumulative patency rates of 80% and 94% at 12 months, 55% and 81% at 36 months.[42]

NEUROPATHY

There are several causes of neuropathy in the dialysis patient, with 70% of dialysis patients experiencing it in some form.[35] These include entrapment causing peripheral nerve compression, uremic neuropathy, diabetic polyneuropathy, and most devastatingly of all, ischemic monomelic neuropathy (IMN). IMN is a rare and specific type of ischemia affecting only nerves. This complication was first described by Wilbourn et al. in 1983 as a condition with arterial insufficiency involving a single extremity (monomelic) and causing selective dysfunction (neuropathy) of multiple peripheral nerves.[53] Immediately after surgery, there is steal that results in hypoperfusion of the vasa nervosum, as described by Kelly et al. using electron microscopy.[54] This causes damage to distal nerve fibers initiating severe acute neurologic symptoms including pain, paresthesias, numbness in median, radial, and/or ulnar nerves distally, as well as motor weakness or paralysis. This devastating complication can result in permanent disability, even if the fistula or graft is ligated immediately after surgery. IMN differs from steal syndrome in that it is irreversible, exhibits no tissue necrosis, and the hand is usually warm with a palpable pulse or audible Doppler signal. The differential diagnosis of IMN includes vascular steal, complications of axillary block anesthesia, patient positioning, carpal tunnel syndrome, and postoperative pain or swelling.[55,56] Risk factors include female gender, long-standing diabetes with prior peripheral neuropathy, and peripheral vascular disease.

Diagnosis of IMN involves good clinical suspicion with a thorough physical exam. Clinically, sensory findings are more prominent, and these patients often present with a continuous deep, burning discomfort in the distal extremity. There can also be sensory impairment distally, with numbness, paresthesias, and pain in the radicular distribution of all three forearm nerves. Motor compromise includes weakness of muscles innervated by the forearm nerves; with a result of claw-hand deformity, significant loss of function, and severe neurogenic pain.[35] Electromyography (EMG) can confirm the diagnosis, especially in the presence of other confounding etiologies. EMG typically shows axonal loss, and low-amplitude or absent responses to sensory and motor nerve stimulation with relatively preserved conduction velocities.[57] Treatment includes surgical intervention urgently upon diagnosis, with immediate arterial reconstruction or ligation as previously mentioned. Additional nonsurgical measures include medications for neuropathic pain with aggressive physical therapy to aid in recovery.

IMN is not the only neuropathy to occur in patients with renal dysfunction, and therefore, it is important to differentiate IMN from other etiologies. Uremic polyneuropathy progresses over months and has been estimated to be present in 60–100% of patients on dialysis.[57] Typically, uremic polyneuropathy targets large-diameter axons in most distal nerve trunks causing distal segmental demyelination and axonal degeneration, with proximal nerve sparing. Nerve biopsies establish these patterns.[58] The nerves of uremic patients have been shown to exist in a chronically depolarized state prior to dialysis, with subsequent improvement and normalization of resting membrane potential after dialysis. The degree of depolarization correlates with serum potassium, suggesting that chronic hyperkalemic depolarization plays an important role in the development of nerve dysfunction in ESRD. This, in turn, encourages strict maintenance of serum potassium between periods of dialysis to reduce the incidence and severity of uremic neuropathy, rather than simple avoidance of hyperkalemia.[54] Neuropathy generally only develops at glomerular filtration rates of less than 12mL/min.[58,59]

Diabetic polyneuropathy is like uremic polyneuropathy as it correlates with chronicity of disease and appears bilaterally. However, in diabetic polyneuropathy, the most common presenting abnormality is a reduction or absence of vibration sense in the toes and a sensory loss in a "stocking and glove" distribution. Other associated symptoms in diabetic polyneuropathy include gastroparesis, impotence, and loss of sphincter control.[60]

VENOUS HYPERTENSION

Venous hypertension most commonly occurs secondary to central outflow stenosis or occlusion. In patients with central venous stenosis (CVS), most cases are subclinical due to adequate collateral flow allowing the patient to remain asymptomatic. However, CVS has been identified in 17–26% of patients undergoing venography for failing access and edema.[61] CVS or occlusion is often asymptomatic in the preoperative setting; however, patients may demonstrate symptoms after an AV access is placed. The presumed etiology of CVS is secondary to chronic endothelial trauma during cardiac and respiratory cycles, caused most likely by previous catheter placement. When specimens were resected and observed under the microscope, fibrous tissue and NIH were discovered.[62] Central venous catheters (CVC), peripherally inserted central catheters (PICC), pacemakers, defibrillators, and temporary or permanent dialysis catheters include the majority of instigators. Approximately 50% of patients had a previously catheterized subclavian, and 50% of those had significant stenoses.[61] History and physical examination prior to AV access creation should include inquiring about previous catheter usage and inspecting for scars. Central venous catheters and dialysis catheters are placed in the jugular or subclavian veins, whereas PICCs are placed directly into cephalic and basilic veins and later traverse the central veins. In a study with 150 patients undergoing PICC line placement, venography before and after insertion found a 7% incidence of stenosis or occlusion centrally, especially in those with a longer catheter dwell time.[63] However, not all stenoses or occlusions are centrally located. Sources of peripheral venous stenosis include NIH in the outflow anastomosis or outflow vein in prosthetic AV access, cephalic arch vein stenosis, incompetent valves, or feeding branches. Peripheral stenoses do not produce venous hypertension as much as central lesions, with symptomatology more evident with increased venous pressures during dialysis, recirculation, and thrombosis. However, more proximal vein outflow stenosis may show similar symptoms to central venous stenosis.[35]

Symptoms of venous hypertension include unilateral pigmentation, induration, dermatosclerosis, and even ulceration. Bilateral edema can occur if the superior vena cava (SVC) is stenosed or occluded, as seen in SVC syndrome. However, in chronic SVC obstruction, alternative drainage into the azygous system can confound symptoms and stenosis is recognized on angiogram.[64] Diagnosis by physical exam reveals a strong pulse with decreased thrill on palpation, or a color flow duplex ultrasound can detect the absence of respiratory variations in vessel diameter, a lack of polyphasic atrial wavers, or the presence of collateral vessels.[65]

Treatment for symptomatic venous hypertension secondary to central venous stenosis includes endovascular angioplasty and stenting versus open surgical management. Endovascular approach harvests concern that angioplasty may not be as effective in vessels with increased elasticity and recoil. Angioplasty has even been shown to accelerate restenosis, with recurrent lesions showing a more aggressive neointimal hyperplasia.[66] Therefore, close follow-up for non- or mildly symptomatic CVS is recommended, with judicious use of PTA as needed. However, when requiring treatment, PTA is the first-line approach recommended by KDOQI, with stenting reserved for angioplasty failure.[67] The caveat with angioplasty alone is an excellent early technical result but a poor long-term primary patency with patency outcomes of 50% at 6 months and 25% at 12 months. There are significant variabilities, however, in the reporting of the nature and severity of lesion, outcomes, patient populations, instruments, and techniques used. Secondary patency can be significantly better with repeated angioplasty, even without use of stent.[66]

Stenting is an attractive option for this disease, but caution must be maintained. The KDOQI recommends it in the setting of failed or recurrent CVS with angioplasty.[67] In Figures 29.7 and 29.8, we illustrate a brachiocephalic vein stenosis treated with angioplasty and stenting. It is inadvisable to stent the thoracic outlet, where it will be exposed to the compressive forces of the clavicle and first rib and may result in extrinsic compression and stent fracture.[35,67] Stent grafts have shown improved outcomes over bare metal stents, with improved primary and assisted patency rates. This may allow for immediate salvage for accesses in difficult cases.[66] A covered stent may unintentionally occlude important collaterals of other central veins, posing complications for the future.[67] Post-procedural monitoring should also consider the possibility of edge stent stenosis. In the setting of pacers, it may be easier to place a contralateral access, due to the refractory nature of stenotic lesions from pacer wires.[67] However, if relocating the wires is not deemed possible, the pacer

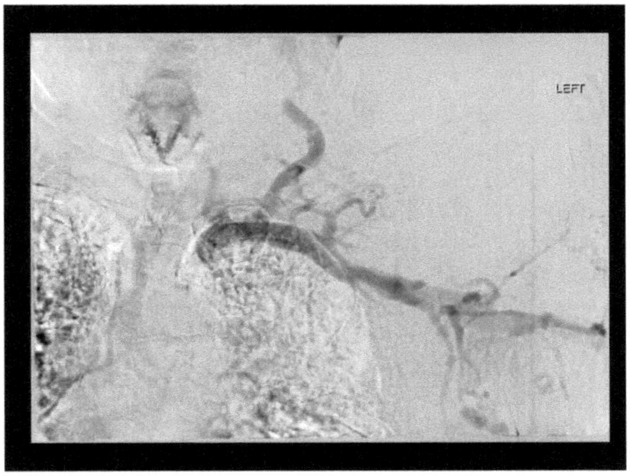

Figure 29.7 Angiography revealing a brachiocephalic vein central occlusion.

wires should be removed and the pacer moved to a different site, to allow for intraluminal stenting without crushing of the wire. Angioplasty alone is possible but has the added risk of injury to the wires.

Open surgical techniques are considered in the setting of recurrent or failed endovascular options. Surgical interventions are not first-line treatment choices, and are reserved for failure of endovascular management. These open surgical techniques typically include options such as jugular vein transposition, axillary-jugular bypass and axillary-axillary crossover bypass, axillary-femoral bypass, and axillary-atrial bypass. Venous hypertension may also be reduced by limiting AV flow using a banding or flow-limiting procedure of some kind, as previously described.[67] With refractory and/or recurrent lesions, hybrid alternatives can be used, such as the Hemoaccess Reliable Outflow (HeRO) vascular access device (Hemosphere, Inc., Minneapolis, Minn.).[68,69] This will allow for combination with an existing shunt to provide unimpeded central venous flow, as long as the catheter is distal to the lesion. Other alternatives include a new AV access creation on another extremity, or conversion to peritoneal dialysis.[64,68]

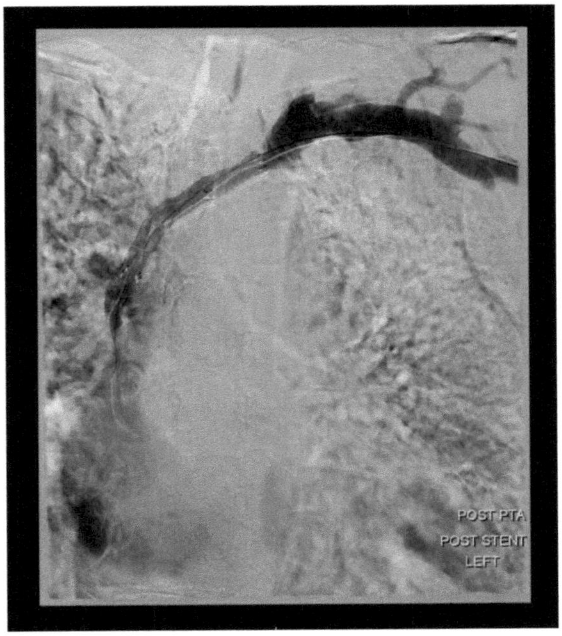

Figure 29.8 Post-angioplasty and stenting across the brachiocephalic vein occlusion with reconstitution of flow.

BLEEDING

Several factors contribute to the increased risk of bleeding in the dialysis patient, like coagulopathies, anemia, uremia, usage of blood thinners, and trauma from needle punctures. A common etiology is anemia of chronic disease secondary to ESRD. As hematocrit declines, there is a reduced clearance of nitric oxide causing platelet inhibition and vasodilation, ultimately causing coagulopathy. Maintenance of hematocrit > 30% is key, with an inverse relationship between packed red cells and bleeding times noted.[35] Hypothetically, increased red cell mass redirects platelets toward vessel walls, increasing platelet-endothelial interaction. Another described cause is uremia-induced platelet dysfunction, which interferes with intrinsic function and interaction with the vessel wall. Mechanisms include ineffective adhesion to the sub-endothelium from reduced expression of Gp1b receptions and reduced affinity for von Willebrand factor (vWF), as well as conformational changes in fibrinogen receptors causing platelet aggregation.[69] To combat platelet dysfunction, treatment with 0.3 μg/kg desmopressin (DDAVP) immediately acts on endothelial vasopressin receptors and cAMP-mediated signaling leading to exocytosis of vWF, thereby decreasing bleeding time. Maximal effect is seen at 1 hour, lasting 4–6 hours, with repeated infusions noted to be less efficacious.[70,71] Infusion of other blood products to replenish clotting factors and vWF may be used such as cryoprecipitate (rich in vWF, factor VIII, and fibrinogen), platelets, red blood cells, and tranexamic acid.[69,72]

Along with coagulopathies due to underlying dysfunction, other causes of bleeding exist. Most ESRD patients do not have kidney failure in isolation, with associated comorbidities requiring antiplatelet or anticoagulant therapy being quite common, such as peripheral arterial disease, venous thrombosis, atrial fibrillation, and coronary artery disease. This medication use increases bleeding risk in a patient population already predisposed toward coagulopathy.

Physical trauma endured during dialysis is a continuous risk of bleeding. With serial dialysis needle punctures occurring multiple times per week, hematomas/bleeding often occur. Rapidly expanding hematomas should be temporarily controlled with constant, direct pressure to the bleeding site for at least 30–40 minutes, or until bleeding resolves. If this bleeding persists despite pressure, a stitch may be placed through the skin and subcutaneous tissue, with care not to involve the underlying shunt. Proximal and distal control with digital pressure aids in reducing blood flow to the area of concern to enhance visualization. Persistent pulsatile bleeding is concerning for a variety of issues, including venous outflow stenosis, graft infection, and pseudoaneurysm. Therefore, this requires at least a shuntogram, and possible duplex, for further evaluation. If there is noted skin compromise including thinning, ulceration, exposed shunt, the patient requires surgical therapy similar to an infected access. Reconstruction should be performed with an interposition graft through healthy tissue to uninvolved portions of the AV circuit.[35]

HIGH-OUTPUT CARDIAC FAILURE

Development of high-output heart failure is an underappreciated complication in patients. As a fistula shunts blood from the arterial circulation to venous circulation bypassing capillary resistance, there is increased preload, as well as decreased systemic arterial flow. Fistula flow in a well-functioning fistula is approximately 700–1500 mL/min.[73] Over time, this leads to left ventricular hypertrophy, reduced ejection fraction, and heart failure. Symptoms include tachycardia, elevated pulse pressure, dyspnea on exertion, fluid retention, and jugular venous distension.[74] On physical examination, the fistula appears large with rapid flow and aneurysmal growth, often times referred to as a "mega-fistula".[75] Workup begins with an echocardiogram to document left ventricular function, and investigation to rule out other etiologies of high-output heart failure. Elevated levels of biochemical assays such as ANP and BNP confirm volume expansion. To determine high-output heart failure as the definitive cause, a right heart catheterization is required. Characteristic findings include pulmonary hypertension with normal pulmonary vascular resistance and high cardiac output with low-normal systemic vascular resistance.[74]

The burden remains to prove that the high cardiac output failure is secondary to the AV shunt. If deemed secondary to the shunt, intraoperative access flow monitoring demonstrates blood flows > 2000 mL/min. Unsurprisingly, as in steal syndrome, this is more common with proximal shunts. Diagnostic measures include the Nicoladoni-Branham sign, which shows immediate increase in blood pressure and decrease in heart rate with compression of the fistula. This is due to the immediate restoration of normal systemic flow.[74] As the issue is one of flow rate, treatment involves inflow reduction with the previous techniques described for steal syndrome, such as banding of the arterial inflow with intraoperative flow measurements to confirm reduction of output, RUDI, and the MILLER technique.[74,75]

CONCLUSION

ESRD remains a growing burden for both patients and the healthcare system. For successful long-term hemodialysis, AV access creation is necessary. However, numerous issues affect the maintenance of these accesses, with concomitant increase in spending to ensure their continued functioning. Prolongation of the life-span of an AV access requires close monitoring, appropriate medical therapy, and well-timed surgical intervention. In this regard, proper diagnosis of complications is essential and will lead to efficient care of patients dependent upon hemodialysis.

REFERENCES

1. Centers for Disease Control and Prevention. Chronic Kidney Disease Surveillance System—United States website. http://www.cdc.gov/ckd. Accessed October 8, 2019.
2. Daugirdas JT, et al. KDOQI Clinical Practice Guideline for Hemodialysis Adequacy: 2015 Update. American Journal of Kidney Diseases. 2015;66: pp. 884–930.
3. Saran R, et al. US Renal Data System 2017 Annual Data Report: epidemiology of kidney disease in the United States. American Journal of Kidney Diseases. 2018;71: pp. 1–672.
4. Reyna A, Anaizza M. Hemodialysis Vascular Access Complications. Journal of Hospital Medicine Clinics. 2014;3: pp. 504–530.
5. Roy-Chaudhury P, et al. Venous Neointimal Hyperplasia in Polytetrafluoroethylene Dialysis Grafts. Kidney International. 2001; 59: 2325–34.
6. Padberg F, et al. Complications of arteriovenous hemodialysis access: Recognition and management. Journal of Vascular Surgery. 2008;48: pp. 55–80.
7. Mohiuddin K, et al. Predicting Technical Success after Fistuloplasty: An Analysis of 176 Procedures. Annals of Vascular Surgery. 2018;51: pp. 141–146.
8. Collins MJ, et al. Therapeutic Strategies to Combat Neointimal Hyperplasia in Vascular Grafts. Expert Review of Cardiovascular Therapy. 2012;10: pp. 635–47.
9. Asif A, et al. Accuracy of Physical Examination in the Detection of Arteriovenous. Clinical Journal of American Society of Nephrology. 2007; 2: 1191–1194.
10. Pietura R, et al. Doppler ultrasound assessment of well-functioning mature arteriovenous fistulas for haemodialysis access. European Journal of Radiology. 2005;55: pp. 113–119.
11. Bountouris I, et al. A Review of Percutaneous Transluminal Angioplasty in Hemodialysis Fistula. International Journal of Vascular Medicine. 2018.

12. Mauro R, et al. Impact of duplex ultrasound surveillance program on patency of prosthetic arteriovenous graft for hemodialysis: A single-center experience. Annals of Vascular Surgery. 2015;29: pp. 1211–1217.
13. Korn A, et al. Factors Associated with Early Thrombosis after Arteriovenous Fistula Creation. Annals of Vascular Surgery. 2018; 49; pp. 281–284.
14. Farber A, et al. Multiple preoperative and intraoperative factors predict early fistula thrombosis in the hemodialysis fistula maturation study. Journal of Vascular Surgery. 2016;63: pp. 163–170.
15. Irish AB, Viecelli AK,Hawley CM, et al. Effect of fish oil supplementation and aspirin use on arteriovenous fistula failure in patients requiring hemodialysis: a randomized clinical trial. Journal of American Medical Association Internal Medicine. 2017; 177: pp. 184–193.
16. Brahmbhatt, A, Misra S. The Biology of Hemodialysis Vascular Access Failure. Seminars in Interventional Radiology. 2016; 33: pp. 15–20.
17. O'Shea SI, et al. Hypercoagulable states and antithrombotic strategies in recurrent vascular access site thrombosis. Journal of Vascular Surgery. 2003; 38: pp 541–548.
18. Dember LM, et al. Effect of clopidogrel on early failure of arteriovenous fistulas for hemodialysis: a randomized controlled trial. Journal of American Medical Association. 2008; 299: pp. 2164–2171.
19. Dixon, BMD, et al: Effect of Dipyridamole Plus Aspirin on Hemodialysis Graft Patency. The New England Journal of Medicine. 2009; 360: 2191–201.
20. Vascular Access Work Group. Clinical practice guidelines for vascular access. American Journal of Kidney Diseases. 2006; 48: pp. 176–247.
21. Lambert G, et al. Comparison of surgical and radiological interventions for thrombosed arteriovenous access. The Journal of Vascular Access. 2018; 19: pp. 555–560.
22. Brooke BS, Griffin CL, Kraiss LW, Kim J, Nelson R. Cost-effectiveness of repeated interventions on failing arteriovenous fistulas. Journal of Vascular Surgery. 2019;70(5): 1620–1628. doi:10.1016/j.jvs.2019.01.085.
23. Mudoni, A, et al. Aneurysms and pseudoaneurysms in dialysis access. Clinical Kidney Journal. 2015;4: pp. 363–367.
24. Lazarides MK, et al. Aneurysm formation and infection in AV prosthesis. Journal of Vascular Access. 2014; 15: pp. 120–124.
25. Pasklinsky G, et al. Management of true aneurysms of hemodialysis access fistulas. Journal of Vascular Surgery. 2011; 53: pp. 1291–1297.
26. Patel DV, Vaccharajani TJ. Principles of treating enlarging pseudoaneurysm in a dialysis arteriovenous graft. Hemodialysis International. 2017;22(1). doi:10.1111/hdi.12588.
27. Valenti D, et al. A novel classification system for autogenous arteriovenous fistula aneurysms in renal access patients. Vascular and Endovascular Surgery. 2014; 48: pp. 491–496.
28. Almehmi A, Wang S. Partial aneurysmectomy is effective in managing aneurysm-associated complications of arteriovenous fistulae for hemodialysis: Case series and literature review. Seminars in Dialysis. 2012; 25: pp. 357–364.
29. Clark TW, Abraham RJ. Thrombin injection for treatment of brachial artery pseudoaneurysm at the site of a hemodialysis fistula: Report of two patients. Cardiovascular and Interventional Radiology. 2000; 23: pp. 396–400.
30. Witz M, et al. Ultrasound-guided compression repair of pseudoaneurysms complicating a forearm dialysis arteriovenous fistula. Nephrology Dialysis Transplantation. 2000; 15: pp. 1453–1454.
31. Keeling AN, Naughton PA, McGrath FP, et al. Successful endovascular treatment of a hemodialysis graft pseudoaneurysm by covered stent and direct percutaneous thrombin injection. Seminars in Dialysis. 2008; 21: pp. 553–556.
32. Asif A, Gadalean F, Eid N, Merrill D, Salman L. Stent graft infection and protrusion through the skin: Clinical considerations and potential medicolegal ramifications. Seminars in Dialysis. 2010; 23:540–542.
33. Niyyar VD, Moossavi S, Vachharajani TJ. Cannulating the hemodialysis access through a stent graft – is it advisable? Clinical Nephrology. 2012; 77:409–412.
34. Padberg Jr FT, Calligaro KD, Sidawy AN. Complications of arteriovenous hemodialysis access: Recognition and management. Journal of Vascular Surgery. 2008;48(5): pp. 555–580.
35. Cohen GM, et al. Immune dysfunction in uremia. Kidney International Supplements. 1997;62: pp. 79–82.
36. Palestro, C., Vega, A., Kim, C., Vallabhajosula, S, Goldsmith, S. (1990). Indium-i 11-Labeled Leukocyte Scintigraphy in Hemodialysis Access-Site Infection. Journal of Nuclear Medicine. 1990;31(3): pp. 319–324.
37. Lewis SS, Cox GM, Stout JE. Clinical Utility of Indium 111-Labeled White Blood Cell Scintigraphy for Evaluation of Suspected Infection. Open Forum Infectious Diseases. 2014;1(2). doi:10.1093/ofid/ofu089.
38. Yoo JR, et al. Arteriovenous Fistula Stent Infection Diagnosed with Radiolabelled Leucocyte Scintigraphy. Infectious Diseases (London, England). 2015; 47: pp. 510–514.
39. Erba P, et al. Radiolabelled leucocyte scintigraphy versus conventional radiological imaging for the management of late, lowgrade vascular prosthesis infections. European Journal Nuclear Medicine and Molecular Imaging. 2014; 41: pp. 357–68.

40. Gargiulo NJ, et al. Experience with covered stents for the management of hemodialysis polytetrafluoroethylene graft seromas. Journal of Vascular Surgery. 2008; 48: pp. 216–7.
41. Tordoir JHM, et al. Upper extremity ischemia and hemodialysis vascular access. European Journal Vascular of Endovascular Surgery. 2004; 27: pp. 1–5.
42. Jennings WC, Mallios A. Proximal ulnar artery arteriovenous fistula inflow is an uncommon but useful vascular access option. Journal of Vascular Access. 2017 DOI: 10.5301/jva.5000783
43. Davidson D, et al. Steal syndrome complicating upper extremity hemoaccess procedures: Incidence and risk factors. Canadian Journal of Surgery. 2003;46: pp. 408–412.
44. Rutherford RB. The value of noninvasive testing before and after hemodialysis access in the prevention and management of complications. Seminars in Vascular Surgery. 1997; 10: pp. 157–161.
45. Tynan-Cuisinier GS, Berman SS. Strategies for Predicting and Treating Access Induced Ischemic Steal Syndrome. European Journal of Vascular and Endovascular Surgery. 2006; 32(3): pp. 309–315. https://doi.org/10.1016/j.ejvs.2006.01.003
46. Ebeid A, Saranchak HJ. Banding of a PTFE hemodialysis fistula in the treatment of steal syndrome. Clinical and Experimental Dialysis and Apheresis. 1981; 5: pp. 251–257.
47. Zanow J, et al. Flow reduction in high-flow arteriovenous access using intraoperative flow monitoring. Journal of Vascular Surgery. 2006;44: pp. 1273–1278.
48. Goel N, et al. Minimally Invasive Limited Ligation Endoluminal-assisted Revision (MILLER) for treatment of dialysis access-associated steal syndrome. Kidney International. 2006; 70: pp. 765–770.
49. Sheaffer WW, et al. Minimally Invasive Limited Ligation Endoluminal-Assisted Revision (MILLER): A Review of the Available Literature and Brief Overview of Alternate Therapies in Dialysis Associated Steal Syndrome. Journal of Clinical Medicine. 2018;7(6): 128. doi: 10.339/jcm7060128
50. Davidson I, et al. The DRIL procedure for arteriovenous access ischemic steal: A controversial approach. Journal of Vascular Access. 2017;18: pp. 1–2.
51. Minion DJ, et al. Revision using distal inflow: A novel approach to dialysis-associated steal syndrome. Annals of Vascular Surgery. 2005; 19: pp. 625–628.
52. Zanow J, et al. Proximalization of the arterial in-flow: A new technique to treat access-related ischemia. Journal of Vascular Surgery. 2006; 43: pp. 1216–1221.
53. Wilbourn AJ, et al. Ischemic monomelic neuropathy. Neurology. 1983;33: pp. 447–451.
54. Kelly CJ, et al. An investigation of the pathophysiology of ischaemic neuropathy. European Journal of Vascular Surgery. 1991;5: pp. 535–539.
55. Sheetal S, et al. Ischemic monomelic neuropathy. Journal of postgraduate medicine. 2017;63: pp. 42–43.
56. Thimmisetty RK, et al. Ischemic Monomelic Neuropathy: Diagnosis, Pathophysiology, and Management. Kidney International Reports. 2017;2: pp. 76–79.
57. Krishnan AV, Kiernan MC. Uremic neuropathy: Clinical features and new pathophysiologica insights. Muscle Nerve. 2007;35: pp 273–290.
58. Asbury AK, et al. Uremic polyneuropathy. Archives of Neurology & Psychiatry. 1963;8: pp. 413–428.
59. Brouns R, et al. Neurological complications in renal failure: A review. Clinical Neurology Neurosurgery. 2004; 107: pp 1–16.
60. Tesfaye S, and Boulton A. Diabetic neuropathy. New York: Oxford University Press; 2009.
61. Schwab SJ, et al. Hemodialysis-associated subclavian vein stenosis. Kidney International. 1988;33: pp. 1156–1159.
62. Gray RJ, et al. Directional atherectomy treatment for hemodialysis access: Early results. Journal of Vascular and Interventional Radiology. 1992;3: pp. 497–503.
63. Gonsalves CF, et al. Incidence of central vein stenosis and occlusion following upper extremity PICC and port placement. Cardiovascular and Interventional Radiology. 2003;26: pp. 123–127.
64. Dammers R, et al. Central vein obstruction in hemodialysis patients: Results of radiological and surgical intervention. European Journal of Vascular and Endovascular Surgery. 2003;26: pp. 317–321.
65. Rose SC et al. Importance of Doppler analysis of transmitted atrial waveforms prior to placement of central venous access catheters. Journal of Vascular and Interventional Radiology. 1998;9: pp. 927–934.
66. Agarwal AK. Endovascular interventions for central vein stenosis. Kidney Research and Clinical Practice. 2015;34(4): 228–232. doi: 10.1016/j.krcp.2015.10.005
67. National Kidney Foundation Guideline 26. KDOQI Clinical Practice Guideline for Vascular Access: 2018. https://www.kidney.org/sites/default/files/kdoqi_vasc-access-review2019_v2.pdf Accessed 11/10/2019
68. Agarwal, AK. Central Vein Stenosis: Current Concepts. Advances in Chronic Kidney Disease. 2009;16: pp. 360–370.
69. Pavord S and Myers B. Bleeding and thrombotic complications of kidney disease. Blood Reviews. 2011;25: pp. 271–278.

70. Manucci PM, et al. Deamino-8-D-Arginine vasopressin shortens the bleeding time in uremia. New England Journal of Medicine. 1983;308: 8–12.
71. Canavese C, et al. Reduced response of uraemic bleeding time to repeated doses of desmopressin. Lancet. 1985;1: 867–868.
72. Köhler M, et al. Subcutaneous Injection of Desmopressin (DDAVP): Evaluation of a New, More Concentrated Preparation. Pathophysiology of Haemostasis and Thrombosis. 1989;19: pp. 38–44.
73. Zamboli P, et al. Color-Doppler imaging and arteriovenous fistula: Preoperative evaluation and surveillance. Italian Journal of Nephrology. 2012;29: pp. 36–46.
74. Stern AB, Klemmer PJ. High-output heart failure secondary to arteriovenous fistula. Hemodialysis International. 2011;15: pp. 104–107.
75. Miller G. Challenges and Management of High-Flow AVFs. Endovascular Today. 2012.

30

Open central and peripheral venous reconstruction

Complications and strategies for managing these complications

GLORIA Y. KIM, DAWN M. COLEMAN, AND THOMAS W. WAKEFIELD

In the current era of endovascular therapies, open surgical venous reconstruction is primarily utilized for select cases of central reconstruction and those peripheral cases that have failed endovascular strategies. Operative planning decisions should be made with the etiology in mind and the goal of a durable repair. Patient selection is an important aspect of operative planning as this has implications for long-term patency and the durability of treatment. This chapter will focus on the perioperative, early, and late complications of open venous reconstruction and will discuss the management of these complications. We hope to shed light on the importance of surveillance and describe appropriate salvage procedures to preserve primary and secondary patency in the event a complication should arise. Furthermore, a summary of existing data on anticoagulation and/or antiplatelet therapy will be included.

Flow dynamics and physiology are important considerations in open venous operations as grafts placed in the venous system tend to undergo thrombosis more frequently than those placed in the arterial system. The reason for this difference is attributed to a general tendency for lower flow in the venous graft compared to an arterial graft placed in the same location, particularly in cases where the obstruction is chronic and has led to the development of a robust collateral venous circulation. Furthermore, it is possible for venous grafts to collapse due to the low pressure within the venous system coupled with increased abdominal pressure or the confinement of tight spaces (e.g., under the inguinal ligament, in the retrohepatic space, tunneling through the diaphragm). We cannot ignore the thrombogenic surface of prosthetic graft material and its associated increased risks for graft failure. And finally, patients with chronic obstruction have decreased circulating anticoagulants, including protein C, protein S, and antithrombin III, putting them at higher risk for graft failure.[1]

CENTRAL VENOUS RECONSTRUCTION

ILIOCAVAL RECONSTRUCTIONS

Major inferior vena cava (IVC) reconstructions are indicated in select cases of retroperitoneal malignancies, trauma, and iatrogenic complications related to IVC filter placement. The most commonly encountered retroperitoneal malignancies are renal cell carcinoma and sarcomas.[2] Both blunt and penetrating trauma may produce a large enough defect that requires reconstruction of the IVC. Controversy exists when it comes to the optimal management of the IVC in any of the clinical scenarios mentioned above. While some advocate for ligation,[3,4] others either selectively[11] or routinely reconstruct the IVC.[5–7] Patient selection is an important consideration as this has implications for long-term patency as thrombosis can lead to significant chronic venous stasis, including lower extremity edema, pain, varicosities, and venous claudication, and acute sequalae such as pulmonary embolism and other thromboembolic events. However, ligation can always be an option in a life-threatening situation.

In general, we advocate for the use of primary IVC repair when < 50% of the patent lumen is narrowed as a result of the repair, liberal use of a patch (native or bovine) if > 50% of the lumen is narrowed, and use of ringed polytetrafluoroethylene (PTFE) graft for graft replacement when circumferential replacement of the IVC is necessary. A smaller diameter ringed PTFE graft, in comparison to the native IVC, is advocated (i.e., 12–14 mm) to promote faster velocities through the graft segment and decrease the risk of thrombosis.[1] Autogenous conduit should be considered when bowel resection is required for an oncological resection or trauma operation. Consideration should be given to reimplantation of the right renal vein when there is a lack of collateral venous outflow (i.e., when the left gonadal and left adrenal veins have been ligated as part of the resection).

It may be necessary to employ cardiopulmonary bypass or veno-venous bypass in patients who are at risk for hemodynamic instability.[2–4,6,7] In particular, these adjunctive techniques should be considered in patients who have suprahepatic extension of the thrombus (level III) or supradiaphragmatic involvement and extension of thrombus into the right atrial thrombus (level IV). Some groups advocate that extent of the IV thrombus in the IVC necessitates cardiopulmonary bypass.[5–9] It should be noted that the use of cardiopulmonary bypass (CPB) in the setting of IVC reconstruction is associated with more complex IVC reconstructions (both supra- and infrarenal IVC) and longer disease-free survival (in the case of IVC reconstruction for oncological pathology), but more overall perioperative complications when compared to cases without CPB use. Additionally, although the rate of perioperative complications was higher, the morbidity and mortality rates were similar to those of cross clamp application alone.[6] Despite these statistics, the need for cardiopulmonary bypass or cross clamp should not preclude a patient from an IVC reconstruction, as tumor resection and IVC reconstruction has the potential for oncological control and significant reduction of disease burden, even in the setting of metastatic disease, which can greatly improve the patient's quality of life.

IVC reconstruction is generally associated with acceptable morbidity, low mortality, and excellent long-term outcomes. In a series of 62 patients at Johns Hopkins who underwent IVC reconstruction after tumor resection, the overall perioperative complication rate was 39%, with reports of the following specific complications: death (3%), bleeding (9.7%), ascites (1.6%), atrial fibrillation (4.8%), surgical site infection (9.7%), VTE (including first time DVT/PE) (27%), and renal injury (acute kidney injury (9.7%), renal failure (4.8%), and ESRD (4.8%)).[6] Another single-center experience of 47 patients who underwent IVC reconstruction for retroperitoneal malignancy at UCLA reports an overall perioperative complication rate of 13%, including bowel obstruction requiring surgery, bleeding requiring re-exploration and ligation, renal failure, chyle leak that resolved with medical therapy, and early (< 30 days) graft thrombosis with associated scrotal and lower extremity edema that resolved with anticoagulation.[3]

Although no large-scale or multi-institutional studies exist, which may limit our understanding of all possible complications associated with IVC reconstruction, it appears that the most common perioperative complication is venous thromboembolic events, including DVT and PE. These should be treated conservatively with anticoagulation, particularly if the patient was not already on systemic anticoagulation following the original reconstruction. If the patient presents with PE and signs of right heart strain, the usual practice of treating these patients with catheter-directed thrombectomy should be strongly considered given the potentially life-threatening nature of clinically significant pulmonary embolism.

Late complications (> 30 days postoperative) of IVC reconstruction are associated with graft thrombosis. Based on the previously mentioned single-institutional study reports, these events are rare (approximately 0.2%) and related to either infection or a hypotensive event.[3,6] This highlights the importance of considering systemic anticoagulation postoperatively. No formal guidelines exist for the role of postoperative systemic anticoagulation following IVC reconstruction, but some centers advocate for routine anticoagulation in all patients.[2,7,9–11] Based on the limited data and absence of clinical guidelines, it may be worth considering in cases of replaced graft (or complete reconstruction versus patch or primary repair) and in cases of large tumor burden witnessed during primary reconstruction intervention.[2]

Overall, graft thrombosis in the setting of IVC reconstruction is rare and conservative management helps to alleviate symptoms. However, if the patient develops graft thrombosis with significant symptoms that are not alleviated with conservative management and systemic anticoagulation, reintervention with either catheter-directed thrombolysis or open thrombectomy should be considered. Alternatively, in the case of infection-related thrombosis, resection and reconstruction with interposition vein graft should be considered. Percutaneous transluminal balloon angioplasty should be considered for cases with flow-limiting (late) stenosis; and if the suprahepatic inferior vena cava is bleeding or requires revision due to stenosis, a cavoatrial bypass with PTFE or spiral vein graft can be considered.

Iliac venous injuries are relatively uncommon and can be technically more challenging to manage than arterial injuries in the setting of trauma, secondary to posterior positioning and resulting difficulties with exposure and visualization. While a transverse suture line is preferred, lateral venorrhaphy should be considered only if it can be performed without significant stenosis; alternatively, reconstruction with patch venoplasty or PTFE may yield acceptable results.[12] Ligation is often favored in cases of trauma, as leg edema is typically well tolerated and transient. Ligation is certainly preferred to a repair that yields venous stenosis and risks thrombosis and pulmonary embolism, and complex reconstructions that require spiral grafts or prosthetic in the critically ill patient, especially one with concurrent arterial injury and hemorrhagic shock, are to be avoided.[13] A contemporary retrospective review of prospectively collected data of the National Trauma Data Bank reported a mortality rate of 16.5% for isolated iliac vein injuries, that increased to 48.7% for combined iliac arterial and venous injuries. These authors identified that ligation of isolated vein injury was associated with a 2.2 odds ratio for mortality when compared to primary repair with similar rates (14%) of DVT, PE (0.5% vs 1.8%), and acute kidney injury (4.7% vs 5.8%) and propose repair in this clinical setting whenever feasible.[14]

Iliocaval reconstructions may be considered for chronic occlusive disease that have failed endovascular attempts at revascularization. Contralateral saphenous vein used in a straight, panel, or spiral graft fashion should be considered first line for conduit deep vein, procurement of such which may be a source of significant morbidity especially for those patients with a history of DVT. Expanded polytetrafluoroethylene (ePTFE) is the most frequently used prosthetic conduit for the replacement of large veins given its large diameter, immediate availability, and external ring or spiral support associated with relatively low thrombogenicity. In a published case series, where the majority of conduits (n = 12, 71%) were autogenous vein (contralateral great saphenous vein), the primary patency rate was 79% at both 2 and 5 years.[5] Another case series where most of the venous reconstruction was done with ring-sustained expanded polytetrafluoroethylene (ePTFE) (n = 10, 83%), primary patency of the venous reconstructions was 55% at 2 and 5 years.[15] Proper patient selection is important, as patients with severe infrainguinal postthrombotic disease and valvular incompetence have added risk of graft thrombosis and decreased likelihood of clinical success.[16,17]

The creation of an arteriovenous fistula may improve the patency of venous graft by increasing flow and decreasing platelet and fibrin deposition in the prosthetic graft, and is recommended for elective prosthetic grafts anastomosed to the femoral vein and all longer (> 10 cm) iliocaval grafts.[17,18] The optimal ratio between the diameter of the fistula and the graft should not exceed 0.3, to avoid additional risks of high fistula flow and elevated cardiac output. Patency is improved with perioperative intermittent pneumatic compression, leg elevation, elastic bandages, and early ambulation, followed by graduated elastic compression stockings at the time of discharge.[19] Therapeutic anticoagulation for at least 3 months postoperatively is recommended for prosthetic grafts, and judicious surveillance is imperative with venous duplex.

The most commonly encountered complication associated with iliocaval reconstruction is venous graft occlusion and associated unilateral or bilateral lower extremity edema. Pulmonary embolism is a potentially life-threatening complication that is also associated with iliocaval reconstruction. Venous hypertension is a rare complication that may, in extreme cases, compromise arterial flow. Additional nonvascular complications to consider include: surgical site infection, hematoma, neurological injury, late infection (as above) with secondary venoenteric fistula, and chylous ascites.

Graft occlusion, when associated with bilateral lower extremity edema, is often managed nonoperatively. Manual lymphatic massage and inelastic bandaging followed by elastic compression after the condition stabilizes offer symptomatic relief to patients without preoperative lymphedema.[5] Patients with significant morbidity associated with the thrombosed iliocaval reconstruction may benefit from catheter-directed thrombolysis or mechanical thrombectomy.[20,21]

NUTCRACKER SYNDROME (LEFT RENAL VEIN COMPRESSION) TREATMENT

Nutcracker syndrome (NS) describes a phenomenon that occurs when the left renal vein is compressed between the aorta and the superior mesenteric artery (SMA). Posterior nutcracker syndrome is another variant of this condition, which occurs when a retro aortic left renal vein is compressed between the aorta and the vertebral body. The prevalence of nutcracker syndrome is unknown, but is thought to be a rare entity as much of the literature is composed of case reports and small case series.[8] This syndrome may present without clinical symptoms and signs, and in these cases, it is considered a normal anatomic variant. If the syndrome is associated with signs and symptoms, most commonly hematuria, it is thought to be secondary to left renal venous congestion. It is hypothesized that the increased intraluminal pressure within the left renal vein contributes to the development of hilar varices around the renal pelvis and ureter, and the rupture of the thin-walled veins within the collecting system lead to both macroscopic and microscopic hematuria.[22] The most common symptom associated with this syndrome is flank pain, with other less common signs and symptoms of renal venous hypertension including orthostatic proteinuria, pain of the left flank or the left upper quadrant of the abdomen, left-sided varicocele, and fatigue.[9,23]

Conservative management of nutcracker syndrome emphasizes weight gain as this is believed to increase the retroperitoneal fat and consequently decrease the tension on the left renal vein; additionally the development of venous collaterals may help to relieve the renal vein hypertension.[24,25] Conservative management is recommended for patients who are young and/or present with mild hematuria or other mild or tolerable symptoms and is associated with success rates up to 30%.[24,26] For patients with more severe or persistent symptoms, many experts advocate open repair, particularly with distal transposition of the left renal vein directly into the IVC, to be the mainstay for treating NS with other open surgical options including gonadal vein reimplantation, orthotopic kidney transplantation, and nephrectomy to name a few.[8,9,27] While endovascular stenting is gaining traction, there is a paucity of long-term outcomes data, making it difficult to determine the true durability of an endovascular repair.

The preferred open technique for treating NS is left renal vein transposition approximately 3–5 cm below the formal opening of the left renal vein with adjunct vein patch or cuff in selected cases.[9] Adjunct procedures using great saphenous vein (GSV) should be considered in select cases to prohibit narrowing of the left renal vein and to decrease tension between the left renal vein and IVC when the length of the left renal vein is too short to reach the new site on the IVC. A contemporary and relatively large series of NS includes 37 patients, of whom 36 (97%) underwent open surgery while 1 (3%) underwent endovascular treatment.[9] Of those who were treated with the open approach, 31 (84%) patients underwent distal transposition of the LRV to the IVC, 3 (8%) patients underwent patch angioplasty with GSV, and 2 (5%) patients had transposition of the left gonadal vein (LGV) to the IVC. Primary patency was 74% at 2 years. Three (10%) patients required re-intervention within 30 days of the original open venous procedure for recurrence of symptoms and confirmed stenosis ($n = 2$) or occlusion ($n = 1$). After the initial 30 days, 8 (26%) patients needed re-intervention for left renal vein stenosis ($n = 7$) or occlusion ($n = 1$).

Complications that require re-intervention include stenosis and occlusion that are associated with symptom recurrence. Angioplasty and stenting can be attempted to treat these complications when they occur in the early postoperative period, within 30 days. Thrombosis may require mechanical thrombolysis with subsequent angioplasty and stenting with self-expanding Wallstents (Boston Scientific, Natick, MA). Nonvascular complications include retroperitoneal hematoma, ileus, DVT, and chylous ascites.[8]

PERIPHERAL VENOUS RECONSTRUCTION

SAPHENOPOPLITEAL VEIN BYPASS

Saphenopopliteal bypass (or May-Husni) is used to treat unilateral occlusion of the femoral vein, particularly when the profundal femoris vein (PFV) is an inadequate collateral or conduit. The PFV normally provides compensatory flow when the femoral vein is occluded. However, when both the femoral vein and PFV are occluded, consideration of a saphenopopliteal bypass may be indicated.[28,29] The saphenopopliteal bypass requires transplantation of the ipsilateral great saphenous vein (GSV) to usually the popliteal vein in order to bypass the occluded segment of the femoral vein into the iliac vein. This procedure should only be considered if the inflow (i.e., patent popliteal vein, GSV) and outflow (i.e., patent SFJ, proximal iliocaval vein) are deemed adequate. If this is not the case, endovascular adjuncts or AVF creation may be required to improve inflow and outflow to ensure success of the saphenopopliteal vein bypass.

Complications from the saphenopopliteal vein bypass include: surgical site infection, hematoma, and early graft occlusion/failure. The clinical presentation of these complications may manifest as chronic lower extremity edema and venous claudication that is refractory to medical and surgical treatment. Early postoperative complications benefit most from operative intervention, so it is imperative to maintain close surveillance to detect hematomas or signs of early graft occlusion/failure. This includes the use of venous duplex scan for bypass surveillance. Hematomas may cause external compression and subsequent early graft occlusion, and as such early surgical decompression is recommended.[30] Open thrombectomy of the occluded vein bypass may be warranted in the scenario where the hematoma has already caused graft thrombosis. Early graft occlusion or failure, defined to occur within 30 days of initial bypass surgery, without concomitant hematoma also requires intervention depending on the etiology. Graft patency does not seem to be associated with severity of disease (CEAP score).[30] Graft revision should always be considered to restore secondary patency. Some causes of early graft occlusion include, but are not limited to, kinking and twisting of the graft, inadequate inflow or outflow, and inadequate anticoagulation. Following the additional intervention, good venous health practices should continue as described above.

PALMA PROCEDURE (PALMA/CROSS-FEMOROFEMORAL VENOUS BYPASS) FOR UNILATERAL OCCLUSION OF ILIAC VEINS

The cross-femorofemoral venous bypass, also known as the Palma procedure, is used to treat unilateral occlusions of the iliac vein when the occlusion is refractory to or the patient is not a candidate for an endovascular approach. The procedure was first described by Palma and Esperon in 1960 and consists of transposing the contralateral GSV to the ipsilateral common femoral vein (CFV).[29,31] An adjunct arteriovenous fistula may be created with a side branch or distal segment of the GSV interposition graft from the common femoral artery to the transposed GSV during the index operation to help augment inflow if there is concern for poor inflow intraoperatively. All patients are started postoperatively on anticoagulation. For patients who have an AVF, it is recommended that they are seen 8–12 weeks postoperative for venography and coil embolization of the AVF. Although the procedure has been described with prosthetic material (ePTFE), it is generally felt that an autologous conduit provides better long-term results.

The Palma procedure is an effective procedure for relieving unilateral iliac vein obstruction. A contemporary series of 25 patients at the Mayo Clinic reported a 70% primary patency and 78% secondary patency at 5 years.[32] Reported complications of the Palma procedure are surgical site infection, hematoma, and early graft occlusion. Surgical site infection should be treated aggressively as with any surgical site overlying a vascular graft. Hematomas should also be treated early and aggressively as they may impact patency of vein conduit. Additionally, although there has been concern about these bypass in patients of childbearing potential, we have had multiple patients undergo successful pregnancy without loss of the autologous crossover graft.

POPLITEAL VEIN ANEURYSM REPAIR

Venous aneurysms are rare and the etiology is poorly understood. Much of what we know about venous aneurysms is based on single-institution series. A known primary risk factor for venous aneurysms is venous stasis. Up to 71% of patients with venous aneurysms develop venous thromboembolism (VTE).[33] Although there are few reports of VTE associated with venous aneurysms in the literature, it is recommended that these aneurysms be treated because of the risk for thromboembolic event, including deep venous thrombosis (DVT) and pulmonary embolism (PE). And unlike arterial aneurysms, there is no risk of rupture.

Popliteal vein aneurysms (PVA), in particular, are most likely to be associated with PE (24%–51%) when compared to other venous aneurysms.[34–37] The presenting symptoms commonly found with PVAs range from asymptomatic or incidental finding to include pain, DVT, PE, and death. There is no consensus on treating PVAs when considering the broad spectrum of symptomatology associated with the disease, but all vascular experts agree that symptomatic PVAs should be surgically treated.[38] Anticoagulation alone is not sufficient for preventing PE in this group.

Open surgical repair with tangential aneurysmectomy with lateral venorrhaphy is the most commonly described technique.[35,39,40] Another method of repair would be to resect the venous aneurysm with an end-to-end anastomosis of the proximal and distal segments of the vein. Furthermore, if thrombus is present, an open thrombectomy should be performed. We have a unique experience with closed plication of these venous aneurysms when there is no thrombus in the aneurysm. The main advantage of this approach is the lack of need for perioperative and postoperative anticoagulation, as the aneurysm is not opened and the endothelial surface disrupted. No endovascular approaches are described in the literature.[37]

The largest single-institution series of PVA cases to date consists of 25 patients who underwent surgical repair, 57% (n = 19) of which were repaired with tangential aneurysmectomy and lateral aneurysmorrhaphy, with no recurrence of PE after repair.[35] In addition, no re-intervention was required in the mean follow-up period of 63 months (range 11–168 months). The reported complications were: 8% hematoma, 8% nerve injury (transient peroneal nerve palsy), 4% local infection, and 12% early thrombosis. A recent meta-analysis summarizes the complications reported in the literature over a recent decade reveals that 20% (5/25) of cases had early thrombosis from the procedure, 4% (1/25) had late thrombosis from the procedure, and 12% (3/25) had aneurysm recurrence.[40]

The varying rates of early thrombosis likely reflect differing practice patterns in anticoagulation, ranging from using low-molecular-weight heparins for a limited time to varying treatment lengths of oral anticoagulation ranging from 3 months to lifetime. In the setting of thrombosis and recurrence of PE, open thrombectomy with an adjunct procedure to correct the cause of nidus for thrombus formation should be considered. If, however, aneurysm relapse or recurrence of aneurysm occurs, it may be worth considering a redo interposition vein graft using autologous tissue. The GSV or femoral vein are good conduits to consider for this. Alternatively, the spiral vein graft, a technique first described by Rheinlander in 1969, may be employed.[41]

REFERENCES

1. Neglén P, Raju S. Iliocaval Obstruction: Endovascular Treatment. In: Cronenwett JL, Johnston KW., editor. Rutherford's Vascular Surgery. 8th ed. Philadelphia, PA: Elsevier Saunders; 2014. p. 928–54.
2. Hicks CW, Glebova NO, Piazza KM, Orion K, Pierorazio PM, Lum YW, et al. Risk of venous thromboembolic events following inferior vena cava resection and reconstruction. J Vasc Surg. 2016;63(4): 1004–10.
3. Quinones-Baldrich W, Alktaifi A, Eilber F, Eilber F. Inferior vena cava resection and reconstruction for retroperitoneal tumor excision. J Vasc Surg. 2012;55(5): 1386–93; discussion 93.
4. Kuehnl A, Schmidt M, Hornung HM, Graser A, Jauch KW, Kopp R. Resection of malignant tumors invading the vena cava: Perioperative complications and long-term follow-up. J Vasc Surg. 2007;46(3): 533–40.
5. Nishinari K, Wolosker N, Yazbek G, Zerati AE, Nishimoto IN. Venous reconstructions in lower limbs associated with resection of malignancies. J Vasc Surg. 2006;44(5): 1046–50.
6. Glebova NO, Hicks CW, Piazza KM, Lum YW, Abularrage CJ, Black JH 3rd. Outcomes of Bypass Support Use during Inferior Vena Cava Resection and Reconstruction. Ann Vasc Surg. 2016;30: 12–21.

7. Obi AT, Kim GY, Coleman DM, Osborne NH, Rectenwald JE, Gallagher KA, et al. Aggressive Phenotype of Intravascular Lymphoma Relative to Other Malignant Intraabdominal Tumors Requiring Vascular Reconstruction. Ann Vasc Surg. 2019;54: 72–83.
8. Velasquez CA, Saeyeldin A, Zafar MA, Brownstein AJ, Erben Y. A systematic review on management of nutcracker syndrome. J Vasc Surg Venous Lymphat Disord. 2018;6(2): 271–8.
9. Erben Y, Gloviczki P, Kalra M, Bjarnason H, Reed NR, Duncan AA, et al. Treatment of nutcracker syndrome with open and endovascular interventions. J Vasc Surg Venous Lymphat Disord. 2015;3(4): 389–96.
10. Hollenbeck ST, Grobmyer SR, Kent KC, Brennan MF. Surgical treatment and outcomes of patients with primary inferior vena cava leiomyosarcoma. J Am Coll Surg. 2003;197(4): 575–9.
11. Fiore M, Colombo C, Locati P, Berselli M, Radaelli S, Morosi C, et al. Surgical technique, morbidity, and outcome of primary retroperitoneal sarcoma involving inferior vena cava. Ann Surg Oncol. 2012;19(2): 511–8.
12. Lee JT, Bongard FS. Iliac vessel injuries. Surg Clin North Am. 2002;82(1): 21–48, xix.
13. Demetriades D. Iliac Vessel Injuries. In: Rich N, editor. Vascular Trauma. Philadelphia, PA: WB Saunders; 2004. p. 339–51.
14. Magee GA, Cho J, Matsushima K, Strumwasser A, Inaba K, Jazaeri O, et al. Isolated iliac vascular injuries and outcome of repair versus ligation of isolated iliac vein injury. J Vasc Surg. 2018;67(1): 254–61.
15. Schwarzbach MH, Schumacher H, Bockler D, Furstenberger S, Thomas F, Seelos R, et al. Surgical thrombectomy followed by intraoperative endovascular reconstruction for symptomatic iliofemoral venous thrombosis. Eur J Vasc Endovasc Surg. 2005;29(1): 58–66.
16. Gloviczki P, Pairolero PC, Toomey BJ, Bower TC, Rooke TW, Stanson AW, et al. Reconstruction of large veins for nonmalignant venous occlusive disease. J Vasc Surg. 1992;16(5): 750–61.
17. Menawat SS, Gloviczki P, Mozes G, Whitley D, Anding WJ, Serry RD. Effect of a femoral arteriovenous fistula on lower extremity venous hemodynamics after femorocaval reconstruction. J Vasc Surg. 1996;24(5): 793–9.
18. Gloviczki P, Hollier LH, Dewanjee MK, Trastek VF, Hoffman EA, Kaye MP. Experimental replacement of the inferior vena cava: factors affecting patency. Surgery. 1984;95(6): 657–66.
19. Hobson RW, 2nd, Lee BC, Lynch TG, Jain K, Yeager R, Jamil Z, et al. Use of intermittent pneumatic compression of the calf in femoral venous reconstruction. Surg Gynecol Obstet. 1984;159(3): 284–6.
20. Hage AN, Srinivasa RN, Abramowitz SD, Cooper KJ, Khaja MS, Barnes GD, et al. Endovascular iliocaval reconstruction for the treatment of iliocaval thrombosis: From imaging to intervention. Vasc Med. 2018;23(3): 267–75.
21. Williams DM. Iliocaval reconstruction in chronic deep vein thrombosis. Tech Vasc Interv Radiol. 2014;17(2): 109–13.
22. Li H, Sun X, Liu G, Zhang Y, Chu J, Deng C, et al. Endovascular stent placement for nutcracker phenomenon. J Xray Sci Technol. 2013;21(1): 95–102.
23. Coolsaet BL. The varicocele syndrome: venography determining the optimal level for surgical management. J Urol. 1980;124(6): 833–9.
24. Reed NR, Kalra M, Bower TC, Vrtiska TJ, Ricotta JJ, 2nd, Gloviczki P. Left renal vein transposition for nutcracker syndrome. J Vasc Surg. 2009;49(2): 386–93; discussion 93–4.
25. He Y, Wu Z, Chen S, Tian L, Li D, Li M, et al. Nutcracker syndrome–how well do we know it? Urology. 2014;83(1): 12–7.
26. Ananthan K, Onida S, Davies AH. Nutcracker Syndrome: An Update on Current Diagnostic Criteria and Management Guidelines. Eur J Vasc Endovasc Surg. 2017;53(6):886–94.
27. Markovic J, Shortell C. Right gonadal vein transposition for the treatment of anterior nutcracker syndrome in a patient with left-sided inferior vena cava. J Vasc Surg Venous Lymphat Disord. 2016;4(3): 340–2.
28. Husni EA. In situ saphenopopliteal bypass graft for incompetence of the femoral and popliteal veins. Surg Gynecol Obstet. 1970;130(2): 279–84.
29. Frileux C, Pillot-Bienayme P, Gillot C. Bypass of segmental obliterations of ilio-femoral venous axis by transposition of saphenous vein. J Cardiovasc Surg (Torino). 1972;13(5): 409–14.
30. Coleman DM, Rectenwald JE, Vandy FC, Wakefield TW. Contemporary results after sapheno-popliteal bypass for chronic femoral vein occlusion. J Vasc Surg Venous Lymphat Disord. 2013;1(1): 45–51.
31. Palma EC, Esperon R. Vein transplants and grafts in the surgical treatment of the postphlebitic syndrome. J Cardiovasc Surg (Torino). 1960;1:94–107.
32. Garg N, Gloviczki P, Karimi KM, Duncan AA, Bjarnason H, Kalra M, et al. Factors affecting outcome of open and hybrid reconstructions for nonmalignant obstruction of iliofemoral veins and inferior vena cava. J Vasc Surg. 2011;53(2): 383–93.
33. Calligaro KD, Ahmad S, Dandora R, Dougherty MJ, Savarese RP, Doerr KJ, et al. Venous aneurysms: surgical indications and review of the literature. Surgery. 1995;117(1): 1–6.
34. Dahl JR, Freed TA, Burke MF. Popliteal vein aneurysm with recurrent pulmonary thromboemboli. JAMA. 1976;236(22): 2531–2.

35. Sessa C, Nicolini P, Perrin M, Farah I, Magne JL, Guidicelli H. Management of symptomatic and asymptomatic popliteal venous aneurysms: a retrospective analysis of 25 patients and review of the literature. J Vasc Surg. 2000;32(5):902–12.
36. Maggiore C, Rizzo L, Capotondi C, Dito R, Taurino M. Pulmonary embolism due to popliteal vein aneurysm: approach and surgical treatment - a case report. Phlebology. 2014;29(5): 325–7.
37. Teter KA, Maldonado TM, Adelman MA. A systematic review of venous aneurysms by anatomic location. J Vasc Surg Venous Lymphat Disord. 2018;6(3): 408–13.
38. Johnstone JK, Fleming MD, Gloviczki P, Stone W, Kalra M, Oderich GS, et al. Surgical treatment of popliteal venous aneurysms. Ann Vasc Surg. 2015;29(6): 1084–9.
39. Aldridge SC, Comerota AJ, Katz ML, Wolk JH, Goldman BI, White JV. Popliteal venous aneurysm: report of two cases and review of the world literature. J Vasc Surg. 1993;18(4): 708–15.
40. Maldonado-Fernandez N, Lopez-Espada C, Martinez-Gamez FJ, Galan-Zafra M, Sanchez-Maestre ML, Herrero-Martinez E, et al. Popliteal venous aneurysms: results of surgical treatment. Ann Vasc Surg. 2013;27(4): 501–9.
41. Rheinlander HF. Superior vena cava replacement. Report of a successful autogenous composite vein graft. J Thorac Cardiovasc Surg. 1969;57(6): 774–7.

31

Complications of iliofemoral venous recanalization and stent placement

MAHMOOD K. RAZAVI

Correlation between venous obstructive lesions (VOL) and chronic venous disease, as well as deep vein thrombosis, has been established.[1–4] With the enhanced recognition of the physiologic role of VOL and demonstrated effectiveness of stents in the treatment of symptomatic lesions,[2–3] there has been a steady increase in the number of patients undergoing endovascular recanalization and stenting of iliocaval and iliofemoral venous segments. While stenting of symptomatic VOL is highly effective, the revascularization procedure is not without associated complications.

In this chapter, complications of endovascular management of VOL are reviewed and strategies to minimize such are discussed. While the list of potential complications is long, their risk of occurrence is low. In a meta-analysis and systemic review of literature, overall 30-day serious complications were reported to be in the range of 6–8%.[3] For the sake of brevity, complications related to general angiographic procedures such as allergic reactions and nephrotoxicity are not discussed.

LOCAL PAIN AND PRESSURE

Transient back or groin pain and pressure are very common and self-limiting. This is related to dilation pressure on the vessel wall and should not be considered a complication per se. Management is usually conservative with anti-inflammatory medication. Narcotics are rarely necessary and should be avoided when possible.

DEATH AND PULMONARY EMBOLISM

Death and pulmonary embolism (PE) are rare but the most serious complications of deep venous interventions. 30-day mortality after iliofemoral venous stent placement has been reported to be between 0.1% and 0.7%.[3] This mortality rate is generally comparable to that of an age-matched population with deep venous disease and hence unlikely to be directly related to the procedure of venous stent placement itself.

Pulmonary embolism has been reported to occur in 0.2–0.9% of patients within 30-days of venous stent procedures. Given the low rate of clinically significant PE, we do not routinely use prophylactic inferior vena cava (IVC) filtration during our venous recanalization procedures, even in the setting of acute iliofemoral DVT.

ACCESS SITE COMPLICATIONS

Unlike arterial interventions, access site bleeding and hematoma appear to be uncommon complications of endovenous stent procedures, likely due to the low-pressure environment of venous channels. Although the majority are not considered serious, complications requiring intervention or prolonging hospitalization have been reported, with most of the reported bleeding complications related to concomitant thrombolytic therapy. In the VIRTUS trial, the only reported 30-day safety events were access site arteriovenous fistulae (AVF). In this trial, 2 of 170 patients enrolled in the pivotal arm developed AVF, requiring endovascular interventions.[4] Conversely, in the study by Neglén and colleagues, no serious access site bleeding or AVF were reported.[5] Vascular injury and hematoma as well as access site thrombosis appear to be a function of the size of the introducer sheath and associated use of thrombolytic agents. Arterial injury appears to be a function of the site of access and can occur with mid femoral vein access. Neglén et.al reported 4 injuries to the superficial femoral artery related to venous access in the femoral vein.[5] Ultrasound-guided access can substantially reduce the risk of access site injury and hence familiarity with such is of paramount importance in reducing this complication.

BLEEDING AND VESSEL INJURY

Clinically significant bleeding or venous rupture are rare complications of iliofemoral venous procedures. The reported rates of 0.3–1.1% are mostly related to either the thrombolytic or anticoagulant drugs used during the procedure, with majority being at the puncture site (see access site complications above). Rupture of chronically occluded venous channels or balloon dilation of inadvertently crossed venous collaterals may occur. Kollbel and colleague reported venous perforation in 2 of their 59 patients with chronic total occlusions of iliofemoral veins who required blood transfusion.[6]

Over-enthusiastic dilation with grossly over-sized balloons or stents may also cause local rupture and bleeding. Due to the generally low-pressure environment of venous channels, such interruptions of vessel integrity may not lead to disastrous clinical sequela. Prolonged balloon inflation at the site of injury or use of covered stents is usually sufficient to control the bleed.

A potentially disastrous bleed could occur as a result of inadvertent passage of wire and or catheter into the epidural space via the epidural venous plexus. There is commonly a rich network of veins in and around the vertebral canal which are in direct communication with iliac veins and IVC. These connections are frequently used during diagnostic and therapeutic maneuvers for venous malformations of the spine and the cord. In an acute or chronic occlusion of the iliocaval segments, it is possible to inadvertently enter these collateral veins and puncture through into the epidural space. Awareness of this pitfall and frequent venography in orthogonal projections can avoid this rare but devastating complication that may lead to serious neurologic injury.

EARLY AND LATE THROMBOSIS

Occlusion or in-stent stenosis in the deep venous system is usually related to thrombosis rather than a cellular hyperplastic reaction such as seen in the arteries. As such, conditions that predispose to thrombosis are the main risk factors for early occlusion of stents. In a meta-analysis of the literature, early (30-day) stent thrombosis has been reported to occur in 6.5% of patients with acute thrombotic conditions and 6.8% of patients with chronic post-thrombotic lesions.[3] The risk of DVT after stent placement in patients with nonthrombotic VOL has been reported to be 1.5% at 30 days.[5] Raju reported a 30-day DVT rate of 7%,[7] which is comparable to that reported by O'Sullivan[8] and within the range of the meta-analysis referenced above.

It has long been postulated that poor quality of inflow and/or outflow predispose patients to early thrombosis (Figure 31.1). Hence, stenting of a chronic iliofemoral occlusion in absence of good flow from either femoral or profunda femoris veins is not likely to yield effective results. Leaving a diseased inflow or outflow segment may lead to loss of stent patency. Stents should hence be extended into venous segments with good flow. Similarly, establishment of inadequate flow channel through the stent as may occur with acute recoil or use of under-sized stents with low radial force/crush resistance may lead to early thrombosis. Placement of a stent in a difficult to

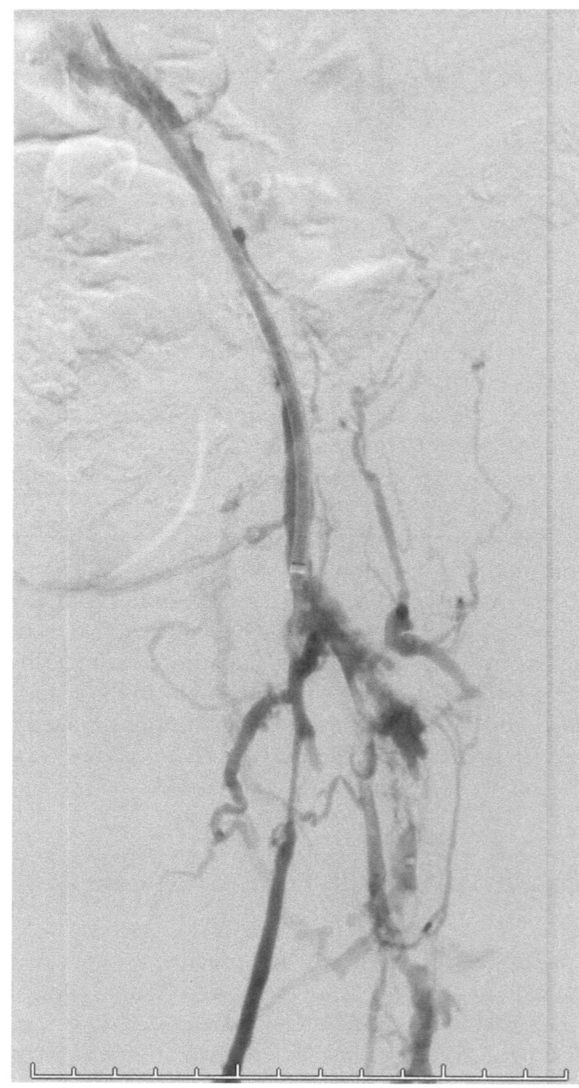

Figure 31.1 Venogram of an 80-year-old female with history of LLE DVT and chronic left limb swelling and pressure. Venogram after retrograde recanalization of a chronically occluded external iliac and common femoral veins reveals subacute thrombosis of profunda femoris vein and chronic occlusion of the femoral vein. Reflux into the greater saphenous vein is seen. Placement of stent in the external iliac and CFV will likely not remain patent due to poor inflow.

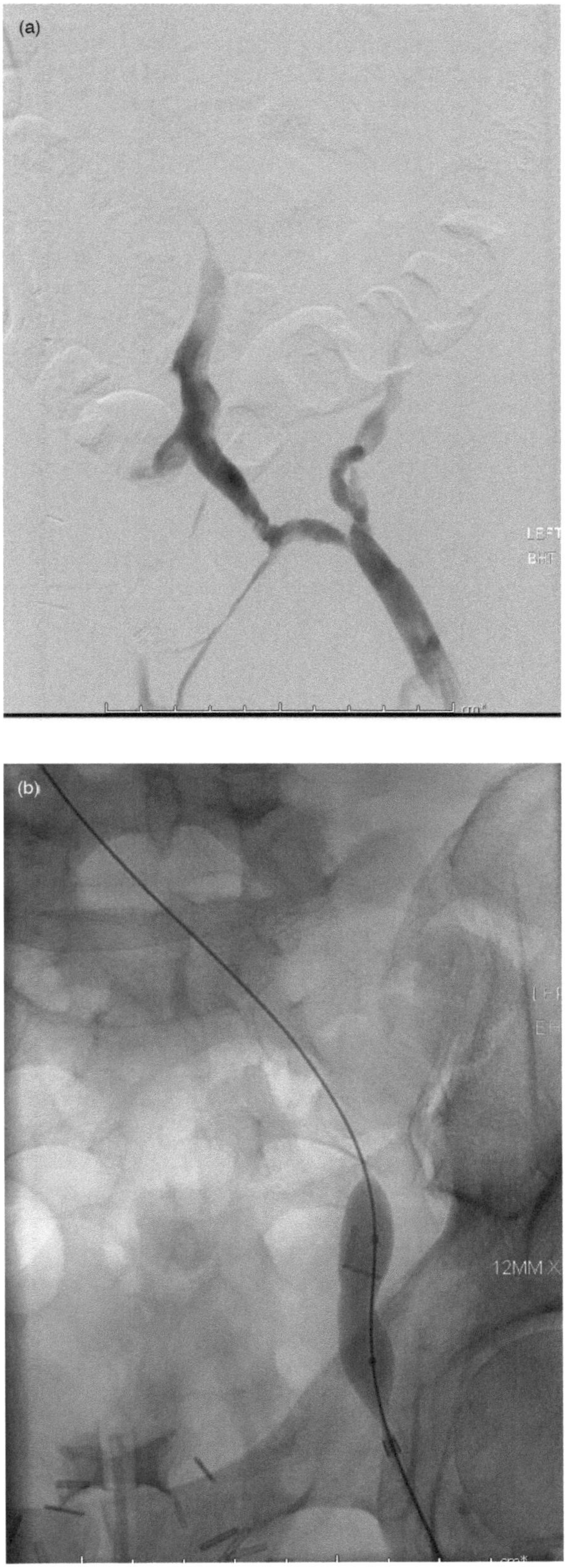

dilate venous lesion will likely lead to suboptimal stent expansion and flow restriction (Figure 31.2). In such cases use of cutting balloons or serial high-pressure balloon dilation may be indicated prior to stent placement.

Suboptimal anticoagulation regimen or patient non-compliance may also predispose to early stent thrombosis. While anticoagulation does not appear to be necessary in non-thrombotic venous lesions (nonthrombotic iliac vein compression for example), it is mandatory after recanalization of chronic postthrombotic occlusions

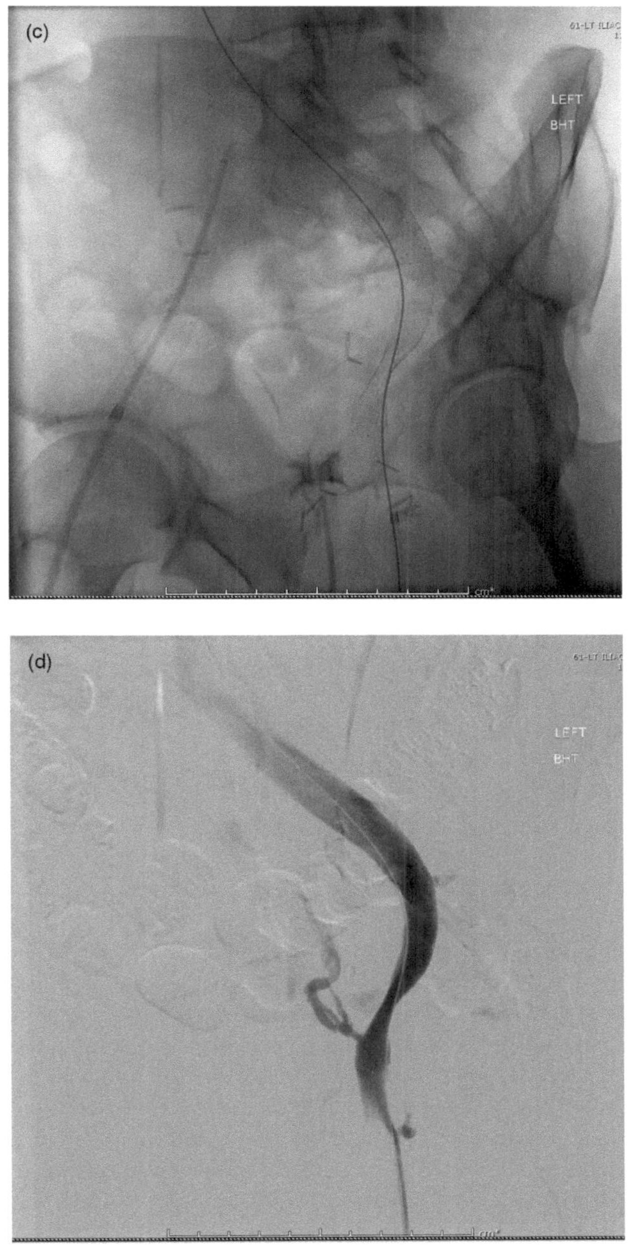

Figure 31.2 (a) Iliac venogram in a 57-year-old male with history of pelvic radiation for stage-IV prostate cancer resulting in chronic occlusion of his external iliac veins. (b) After recanalization, there is focal balloon-resistant lesion which did not resolve with high-pressure balloon inflation. (c and d) Residual stenosis after stent placement predisposing to reocclusion. The external iliac vein thrombosed on the follow-up duplex at 6 months.

and postthrombolysis/thrombectomy patients. The duration and type of anticoagulation in such patients should be determined by the etiology of thrombosis, and patient condition. In our practice, younger patients with hypercoagulable conditions are initially treated with heparinoids for 1–3 months before switching to oral direct thrombin inhibitors while recurrent malignant thromboses are treated with warfarin at supra-therapeutic INR levels.

Unexplained early stent thrombosis is usually a poor prognostic sign. Rethrombosis in such patients is high after reintervention attempts.

Risk factors for late loss of patency include etiology of disease with chronic postthrombotic occlusions posing the highest risk followed by stenting after thrombolysis in acute thrombotic conditions. Nonthrombotic obstruction is associated with a 12-month patency > 96% in pivotal trials of venous stent placement.[4,9] Presence of residual thrombus in flow channels is another risk factor for late loss of stent patency and suboptimal clinical outcome.[10]

In a subgroup analysis of the VIRTUS trial, factors associated with better clinical outcome (change in Venous Clinical Severity Score (VCSS) of ≥ 3 points) included degree of pre-procedural symptoms as measured by VCSS, change in luminal area, and ASPECT ratio (a measure of lumen morphology).[4] Lesion length and stent extending into the common femoral vein were found to correlate with lower stent patency.

STENT FRACTURE

Fracture of stents in the arterial system has been well-studied and its incidence, predisposing factors, and sequelae are much better understood. None of these have been studied in depth nor reported in the iliofemoral venous segments. Gutzeit reported stent fracture in the iliac vein of one patient which had remained patent.[11] Anecdotal reports of stent fractures have been talked about at various international meetings, but the incidence has not been documented as of this writing.

Studies on stent fractures in the arterial system reveal a direct correlation between fracture rate and the biomechanical forces exerted on the stents. Finite element analysis shows areas of increased stress on stent struts during many physiologic body motions such as walking and bending of the knee and hip joints. These motions create axial compression and elongation, segmental bending, and repetitive compression of the stents, which predispose to strut fracture. Further in-depth finite element analysis has shown that stress on the stent material during cyclic bending is proportional to the acuity of the radius of the bend; the smaller the radius of the bend, the higher the stress. Focal compression of the stent (as with residual narrowing of the stent after deployment) appears to increase the stress, especially during cyclic compression and bending (Figure 31.2c). These findings suggest that stents should be fully dilated when deployed at locations subject to cyclic bending such as the common femoral vein.

In addition to the stent location in the body, stent material, surface finish, and geometric design have also been implicated in stent fracture. Similar forces would likely be in action in the veins, although to variable degrees. While iliac veins are not as mobile as the superficial femoral artery, they are subject to repetitive cyclic compression by the adjacent artery. Extension of stents into the common femoral vein, however, may predispose the stent to similar stress forces as described above. As alluded to above, residual narrowing in the stent in the CFV may further increase stress and hence the risk of fracture.

Results of the ongoing pivotal studies in venous stents should provide a clearer picture of the risks, consequences, and etiologies of venous stent fracture in the iliofemoral segments.

STENT MIGRATION AND EMBOLIZATION

Stent migration is an uncommon problem with majority of studies reporting no migration or movement of stent. Hartung reported 2 stent migrations in their study of 89 patients with iliofemoral venous stents.[12] Similarly, Ye and colleagues observed 3 local stent migration among their 224 patients undergoing venous stent placement.[13]

In general, stent migration is a function of stent location, sizing, type of stent, deployment mechanism, and the familiarity of the operator with all of the above. Wallstent (Boston Scientific, Natick, MA) has been the most commonly used stent platform in the iliofemoral veins. Ironically, its braided design and deployment system predisposes it to migration if not sized and deployed correctly. Many authors have advocated using large and long stents in the venous circuits due to the design shortcomings of the Wallstent. It can slide forward or backward after deployment if not centered and sized properly. This has been referred to as "watermelon seeding" of the stent.

Stent embolization is an extremely rare phenomenon and is likely related to mis-sizing of the stent. An exhaustive review of rescue maneuvers in case of stent embolization is beyond the scope of this chapter, and readers are referred to the article by Slonim et al. for a more comprehensive review.[14] Operator familiarity with performance characteristics of the stent and appropriate sizing and matching of stent to location and pathology usually avoids unnecessary stent migration and embolization.

REFERENCES

1. Mewissen MW, Seabrook GR, Meissner MH, Cynamon J, Labropoulos N, Haughton SH. Catheter-directed thrombolysis for lower extremity deep venous thrombosis: report of a national multicenter registry. Radiology. 1999;211: 39–49.
2. Raju S, Darcey R, Neglén P. Unexpected major role for venous stenting in deep reflux disease. J Vasc Surg. 2010 Feb; 51(2): 401–8.
3. Razavi MK, Jaff MR, Miller LE. Safety and effectiveness of stent placement for iliofemoral venous outflow obstruction: a systematic review and meta-analysis. Circ Cardiovasc Interv. 2015 Oct; 8(10).
4. Razavi MK, Marsten W. Predictors of clinical outcome after venous stenting. J Vasc Interv Radiol. 2019; Feb (Suppl).
5. Neglan P, Hollis KC, Olivvier J, Raju S. Stenting of venous outflow in chronic venous disease: Long-term stent-related outcome, clinical, and hemodynamic results. J Vasc Surg. 2007;46:979–90.
6. Kolbel T Lindh M, Akesson, et al. Chronic iliac vein occlusion: Mid term results of endovascular recanalization. J Endovasc Ther. 2009:16: 483–91.
7. Raju S, Neglén P. Percutaneous recanalization of total occlusions of the iliac vein. J Vasc Surg. 2009;50: 360–8.
8. O'Sullivan G, Semba C, Bittner CA, Kee ST, Razavi MK, Sze DY, Dake MDD. Endovascular management of iliac vein compression syndrome. J Vasc Interv Radiol. 2000;11: 823–36.
9. Dake M, O'Sullivan G. 12-month results of the VENACULAR venous stent system. J Vasc Interv Radiol. 2019; Feb (Suppl).
10. Enden T, Haig Y, Klow N, et al. Long-term outcome after additional catheter-directed thrombolysis versus standard treatment for acute iliofemoral deep vein thrombosis (the CaVenT study): a randomized trial. Lancet. 2012;379: 31–8.
11. Gutzeit A, Zollikofer C, Dettling-Pizzolato M, et al. Endovascular stent treatment for symptomatic benign Iliofemoral venous occlusive disease. Cardiovasc Interv Radiol. 2011;34: 542–9.
12. Hartung O, Loundou AD, Barthelemy P, et al. Endovascular managementof chronic Disabling chronic Ilio-caval Obstructive Lesions; Long term results. J Vasc Endovasc Surg. 2009;38: 118–24.
13. Ye K, Lu X, Li W, et al. Long-term outcome of stent placement for symptomatic non-thrombotic iliac vein compression lesions in chronic venous disease. J Vasc Interv Radiol. 2012;23: 497–502.
14. Slonim S, Dake M, Razavi MK, Kee S, Samuels S, Rhee J, Semba C. Management of misplaced or migrated endovascular stents. J Vasc Interv Radiol. 1999 Jul-Aug; 10(7): 851–9.

32

Complications of endovenous ablation of varicose veins

DANIYAL ABBAS AND JUDITH C. LIN

Endovenous thermal ablation (EVTA) of the great saphenous vein (GSV) or small saphenous vein (SSV) has replaced surgical ligation and stripping as the procedure of choice for the treatment of incompetent saphenous vein.[1] EVTA is a vein procedure that uses radiofrequency or laser energy to treat varicose veins. The mechanism of action is reported to be vein wall injury mediated directly via absorption of photon energy. The vein wall receives direct thermal radiation, thermal conduction from heated blood, and indirect thermal convection from steam bubbles.[2]

Indications for vein ablation include presence of reflux in a truncal vein of a duration greater than 500 ms with associated patient symptoms, edema, skin changes, or venous ulceration. Measurement of the vein diameter should be carried out during the course of preoperative ultrasound. The duplex ultrasound inclusion criteria for truncal veins are greater than 3 mm and a treatable length of at least 10 cm. The course of the saphenous vein, from the saphenofemoral or saphenopopliteal junction to the insertion site, is mapped by ultrasound. A marking pen is used to mark incompetent sources of venous reflux under duplex ultrasound guidance before the procedure.

Complications of EVTA can be categorized as minor or serious. Minor complications include bruising (51%), hematoma (2.3%), temporary numbness (3.8%), phlebitis (7.4%), induration (46.7%), and a sensation of tightness (24.8%).[3] More serious complications include skin burns (0.5%), deep venous thrombosis (0.4%), pulmonary embolism (0.1%), and nerve injury (0.8%).[2,3] The complications discussed in this chapter include superficial burns, nerve injury, arteriovenous fistula (AVF), deep venous thrombosis (DVT), endothermal heat-induced thrombosis (EHIT), and recurrence.

SUPERFICIAL BURNS

During EVTA, there can be a significant amount of heat dispersed around the vein intended for treatment. The majority of heat generated remains within the venous lumen. When the vein becomes epifascial or close to the skin surface, the patient can suffer a full thickness burn to the skin. Superficial burns have been extensively reported in the literature after endovenous ablation with incidence ranging from 0.2–3.7% in the literature.[2] While cutaneous skin burns can be painful and unsightly, they appear to be self-limited and do not appear to be associated with any other significant complications. They can be treated with local wound care and followed clinically to evaluate for skin infection. If the burn is apparent immediately at the time of ablation, it can be excised with primary wound closure. The incidence of skin burns is low, and most can be prevented by appropriate tumescent anesthesia and avoiding treatment of veins that are close to the skin surface. Correct energy dose, stopping laser activation at entry site, and caution at extrafascial part are other means of prevention that can be implemented to avoid skin burns.

NERVE INJURY

Nerve injury is a common cause for litigation after endovenous laser ablation.[4] Reasons of nerve injury during EVTA include needle stick injury during vein cannulation, needle stick injury during administration of tumescent anesthesia, and heat transfer during EVLA.

The risk of nerve injury during EVTA is directly related to the relative proximity of several nerves to the most commonly ablated veins. The **saphenous nerve**, the largest cutaneous branch of the femoral nerve, travels along the path of the superficial femoral artery from the groin to the knee. It innervates the skin of the medial surface of the calf and the medial surface of the foot. Hence, damage to the saphenous nerve usually causes sensory loss on the medial aspect of the calf, above the medial malleolus. The main saphenous nerve pierces the deep fascia just

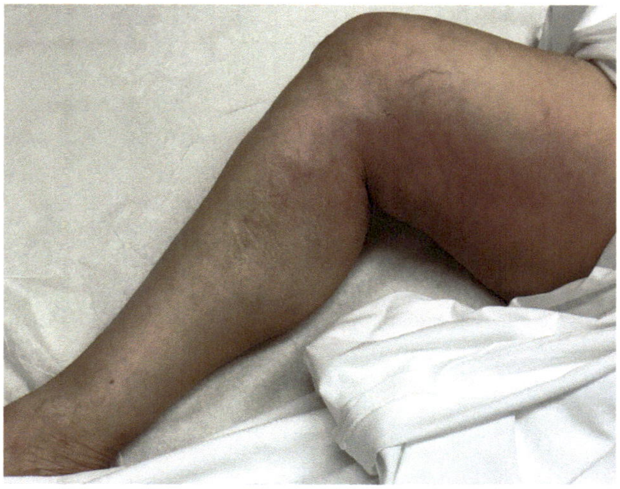

Figure 32.1 Skin burns.

above the knee and becomes superficial at the level of the knee between sartorius and gracilis muscles. It becomes more superficial below the knee and runs alongside the long saphenous vein. At the popliteal fossa, it travels medially and approximates the GSV at the level of the upper calf to the level of the ankle, where it splits into two branches. It is at greatest risk of injury in the mid- to distal calf. EVTA is thus usually performed up to the level of the knee excluding patients with significant venous reflux in the below-knee saphenous vein. Injury to the saphenous nerve causes a cutaneous paresthesia, which is usually transient.

The **sural nerve** is a cutaneous nerve that originates from the tibial nerve in the mid-posterior calf that travels alongside the SSV down to the lateral malleolus. The sural nerve innervates the skin of the lower half of the posterior aspect of the leg, the lateral part of the dorsum of the foot, and the lateral side of the fifth toe. The greatest risk of injury is located in the distal calf where it is in close proximity to the SSV. Damage to the sural nerve due to thermal ablation can cause numbness or significant burning and pain in the heel and lateral aspect of the foot.

The **common peroneal nerve** is a motor and sensory cutaneous nerve that descends within the lateral popliteal fossa, posterior to the head of the fibula. It lies in close proximity to the saphenopopliteal junction. The most common nerve injured during EVLA is the common peroneal nerve with incidence ranging from 2–4.7%.[5] It can lead to foot drop as it contains both motor and sensory fibers. The common peroneal nerve is relatively superficial and remains unprotected as it traverses the lateral aspect of the head of the fibula, and it is easily compressed at this site. While it is not at risk of direct needle injury during EVLA, it is at risk of being injured from heat transfer from the laser while treating the saphenopopliteal junction. All of these injuries were self-limited and had completely resolved within 3 weeks. Using endovenous radiofrequency catheter, the paresthesia rate with the addition of tumescence dropped from 15% to 9%.[6] Many of these nerve injuries can be avoided by careful needle entry under ultrasound guidance, large volume tumescence, and avoidance or judicious use of ablation in areas at high risk of nerve injury.

ENDOTHERMAL HEAT-INDUCED THROMBOSIS AND DEEP VENOUS THROMBOSIS

Endothermal heat-induced thrombosis (EHIT) is defined as the propagation of thrombus from the superficial vein into a more central deep vein. The incidence of EHIT was 1.4% after EVTA of the GSV.[7] The complications can range from deep venous thrombosis to pulmonary embolism. In a review of the literature, the incidence of DVT after EVTA ranges between 0% and 5.7%.[8] Risk factors include a large diameter at the SFJ or SPJ, presence of reflux at the junction, oral contraceptive use, tobacco use, advanced body mass index (BMI), prior intervention, prior DVT, family history of DVT, hypercoagulable state, clinical classification greater than C3, male sex, and increased Caprini risk assessment model. In a study by Lin et al., patients with valvular insufficiency of the SFJ and a large proximal GSV diameter had a significantly higher risk of developing heat-induced thrombosis after endovenous catheter ablation.[9]

Diagnosis of patients with EHIT includes venous duplex imaging for follow-up to assess for resolution or propagation of thrombus. The thrombus produced by thermal injury has a different echogenicity on duplex ultrasound than de novo DVT. EHIT are more echogenic as compared to de novo thrombus; thus, EHIT is more stable and do regress or disappear completely.

Based on the classification divided into 4 classes, a treatment algorithm is suggested:[10] If EHIT is found in class 1, the patient is advised serial duplex ultrasound, every month until clot regresses. If EHIT 2 is found, LMWH is advised for 2 weeks, and duplex ultrasound is done after 2 weeks. If clot regression is found, LMWH treatment is discontinued. If clot still persists, LMWH is continued until clot disappears on duplex ultrasound which is performed every week. If EHIT 3 and EHIT 4 are found, it should be treated like any other provoked DVT as per guidelines with full-dose anticoagulation. In a study, patients presenting with EHIT level more than or equal to 2 or DVT after EVTA, therapeutic anticoagulation with rivaroxaban or fondaparinux was initiated until complete recanalization on ultrasound imaging was documented.[11] They observed that rivaroxaban offered an oral medication approach showing no difference in preventing EHIT and DVT compared with fondaparinux, without increased bleeding risk.

RECURRENCE

Residual varicosities that persist after EVTA should be differentiated from recurrent varicose veins. The extent of residual varicosities depends on the pre-treatment anatomical distribution of varicosities and their hemodynamic relationship with the incompetent axial vein. Varicosities that are directly connected to the incompetent axial vein tend to shrink when this is ablated both below and above their origin. In contrast, varicosities that cross-communicate with other "feeding" veins tend to remain as residual varicosities.[12] Recanalization occurs in up to 4% of axial veins after EVLA, although most are not associated with recurrent varicose veins unless it occurs within 6 weeks of treatment (primary treatment failure due to thrombus dissolution).[13] It is thought to occur due to treatment with low-energy densities less than or equal to 60 Joules per centimeter.

ARTERIOVENOUS FISTULA

Concomitant venous and arterial injuries during administration of tumescent anesthesia, as well as transmission of thermal energy across the venous wall into the neighboring artery, can lead to late vascular wall degradation and formation of an arteriovenous fistula (AVF). Creation of AVF during venous ablation is extremely rare with an incidence of 0.15%.[14] Potential anatomical pitfalls include deep external pudendal artery branches coursing posterior to the proximal GSV and sural artery branches in close proximity to the SSV or perforators.

Potential serious sequelae of post-ablation AVFs include severe limb edema, steal syndrome with claudication, and distal ischemia. The literature also supports a conservative approach to management of AVF associated with EVLA. Five patients required further intervention including open repair, embolization, and stent grafting. While only 3 of 11 closed spontaneously, 3 were persistent in long-term follow-up and remained asymptomatic. The literature appears to support nonoperative management and observation of the majority of AVF associated with EVLA. These patients can be followed with serial clinical exams and duplex ultrasound. Invasive imaging and surgical or endovascular treatment should be reserved for patients who become symptomatic.

Overall rates of complications with endovenous techniques appear to be lower than those for conventional surgery. Endothermal ablation carries very low risks of pulmonary embolism, deep venous thrombosis, wound infection, and hematoma. This change has likely taken place due to the minimally invasive nature and acceptable safety of endovenous ablation while remaining as efficacious and more acceptable than high saphenous ligation and stripping.

REFERENCES

1. Gloviczki P, Comerota AJ, Dalsing MC, Eklof BG, Gillespie DL, Gloviczki ML, Lohr JM, McLafferty RB, Meissner MH, Murad MH, Pdberg FT, Pappas PJ, Passman MA, Raffetto JD, Vasquez MA, Wakefield TW. Society for Vascular Surgery; American Venous Forum. The care of patients with varicose veins and associated chronic venous diseases: Clinical practice guidelines of the Society for Vascular Surgery and the America Venous Forum. J Vasc Surg. 2011 May; 53(5 Suppl): 2S–48S. doi: 10.1016/j.jvs.2011.01.079.
2. Kheirelseid EAH, Crowe G, Sehgal R, Liakopoulos D, Bela H, Mulkern E, McDonnell C, O'Donohoe M. Systematic review and meta-analysis of randomized controlled trials evaluating long-term outcomes of endovenous management of lower extremity varicose veins. J Vasc Surg Venous Lymph Disorders. 2018;6 (2): 256–270.
3. Wikipedia, the Free Encyclopedia. Endovenous laser treatment. https://en.wikipedia.org/wiki/Endovenous_laser_treatment Downloaded on 3/1/2019.
4. Campbell WB, France F, Goodwin HM. Medicolegal claims in vascular surgery. Ann R Coll Surg Engl. 2002;84: 181–4.
5. Atkin GK, Round T, Vattipally VR, Das SK. Common peroneal nerve injury as a complication of short saphenous vein surgery. Phlebology. 2007;22(1): 3–7.
6. Merchant RF, Pichot O, for the Closure Study Group. Long-term outcomes of endovenous radiofrequency obliteration of saphenous reflux as a treatment of superficial venous insufficiency. J Vasc Surg. 2005;42: 502–9.
7. Healy DA, Kimura S, Power D, et al. A systematic review and meta-analysis of thrombotic events following endovenous thermal ablation of the great saphenous vein. Eur J Vasc Endovasc Surg. 2018 Sep; 56(3): 410–424. doi: 10.1016/j.ejvs.2018.05.008. Epub 2018 Jun 9. Review.
8. Van Den Bos RR, Neumann M, De Roos KP, et al. Endovenous laser ablation-induced complications: Review of the literature and new cases. Dermatol Surg. 2009;35: 1206–14.
9. Lin JC, Peterson EL, Rivera ML, et al. Vein mapping prior to endovenous catheter ablation of great saphenous vein predicts risk of endovenous heat-induced thrombus formation. Vasc Endovasc Surg. 2012 Jul; 46(5): 378–383.
10. Lawrence PF, Chandra A, Wu M, Rigberg D, DeRubertis B, Gelabert H, Jimenez JC, Carter V. Classification of proximal endovenous closure levels and treatment algorithm. J Vasc Surg. 2010 Aug; 52(2): 388–93. doi: 10.1016/j.jvs.2010.02.263. Epub 2010 Jun 19.

11. Keo, HH, Baumann F, Diehm N, Regli C, Staub D. Rivaroxaban versus fondaparinux for thromboprophylaxis after endovenous laser ablation. J Vasc Surg. 5(6): 817–823. doi:10.1016/j.jvsv.2017.04.017.
12. Theivacumar NS, Beale RJ, Dellagrammaticas D, Mavor AI, Gough MJ. Factors influencing the effectiveness of endovenous laser ablation (EVLA) in the treatment of great saphenous vein reflux. Eur J Vasc Endovasc Surg. 2008;35: 119e23.
13. Theivacumar NS, Dellagrammaticas D, Beale RJ, Mavor AI, Gough MJ. Fate of the great saphenous vein following endovenous laser ablation: Does re-canalisation mean recurrence? Eur J Vasc Surg. 2008;36: 211e5.
14. Rudarakanchana N, Berland T, Chasin C, Sadek M, Kabnick L. Arteriovenous fistula after endovenous ablation for varicose veins. J Vasc Surg, 2011, 55(5):1492–1494.

33

Complications of cervical, thoracic, and abdominal interventions for trauma

KARA HESSEL AND MOUNIR HAURANI

CERVICAL TRAUMA

Cervical trauma involving the vascular structures of the neck is a highly feared complication of both penetrating and blunt trauma. Morbidity and mortality associated with both blunt and penetrating trauma to the carotid and vertebral arteries is high. Complications of carotid injury are not limited to local tissue damage, but extend further to stroke risk and permanent neurological deficit. Surgical or endovascular access to the vertebral arteries is also challenging and leads to limited options for management.

COMPLICATIONS OF INTERVENTION

Carotid injury—Penetrating

Penetrating carotid injuries are more likely to involve the common carotid artery, due to the relatively protected position of the internal carotid artery behind the jaw and skull. Blunt mechanisms, however, are more likely to involve the internal carotid due to its relatively fixed positions at the bifurcation and skull base. Interventions for carotid injury for both blunt and penetrating trauma range from open exploration to endovascular angioplasty and stent placement. Exposure of the common carotid artery is typically via an incision along the medial border of the sternocleidomastoid. This incision is preferred over a transverse incision because it can extended from the base of the skull through the chest wall using a median sternotomy. Proximal control on the left common carotid or subclavian arteries can alternatively be obtained through a left posterolateral thoracotomy via the fourth rib space.

Adjacent structures that may be injured in the course of carotid dissection include major veins, nerves, and airway structures. As the incision is planned, it is important to understand the potential for incisional paresthesia from transection of cutaneous cervical nerves. For example, the greater auricular and transverse cervical nerves course along and then superior to the sternocleidomastoid muscles. While these are sensory nerves, traction or bruising may lead to hyperparesthesias. As the dissection continues deep to the platysma and sternocleidomastoid, the most prominent vein that runs adjacent to the carotid artery is the internal jugular vein. This is often involved with penetrating injuries given its relatively close position to the carotid artery. More typically injured as part of the dissection however is the facial vein and superior thyroid veins. These tributaries empty from medial to lateral where they enter the internal jugular vein, crossing over the carotid (Figure 33.1). The facial and superior thyroid veins are routinely ligated in order to better expose the carotid artery. Careful ligature of these vessels will prevent postoperative hematoma, as there is significant increase in venous pressure as the patients emerge from anesthesia and may cough or otherwise bear down. Additionally, care must be taken when encircling the facial vein to avoid injuring the hypoglossal nerve, and similarly when encircling the superior thyroid vein, not to injure the vagus nerve.

The vagus and hypoglossal nerves are routinely identified and protected during carotid artery dissection, but there are other cranial nerves and their branches which must be protected as well. The marginal mandibular (branch of the facial nerve), spinal accessory, and glossopharyngeal nerves may be injured during the course of carotid dissection. Nerve injury is a potentially devastating complication of carotid exposure with the morbidity of

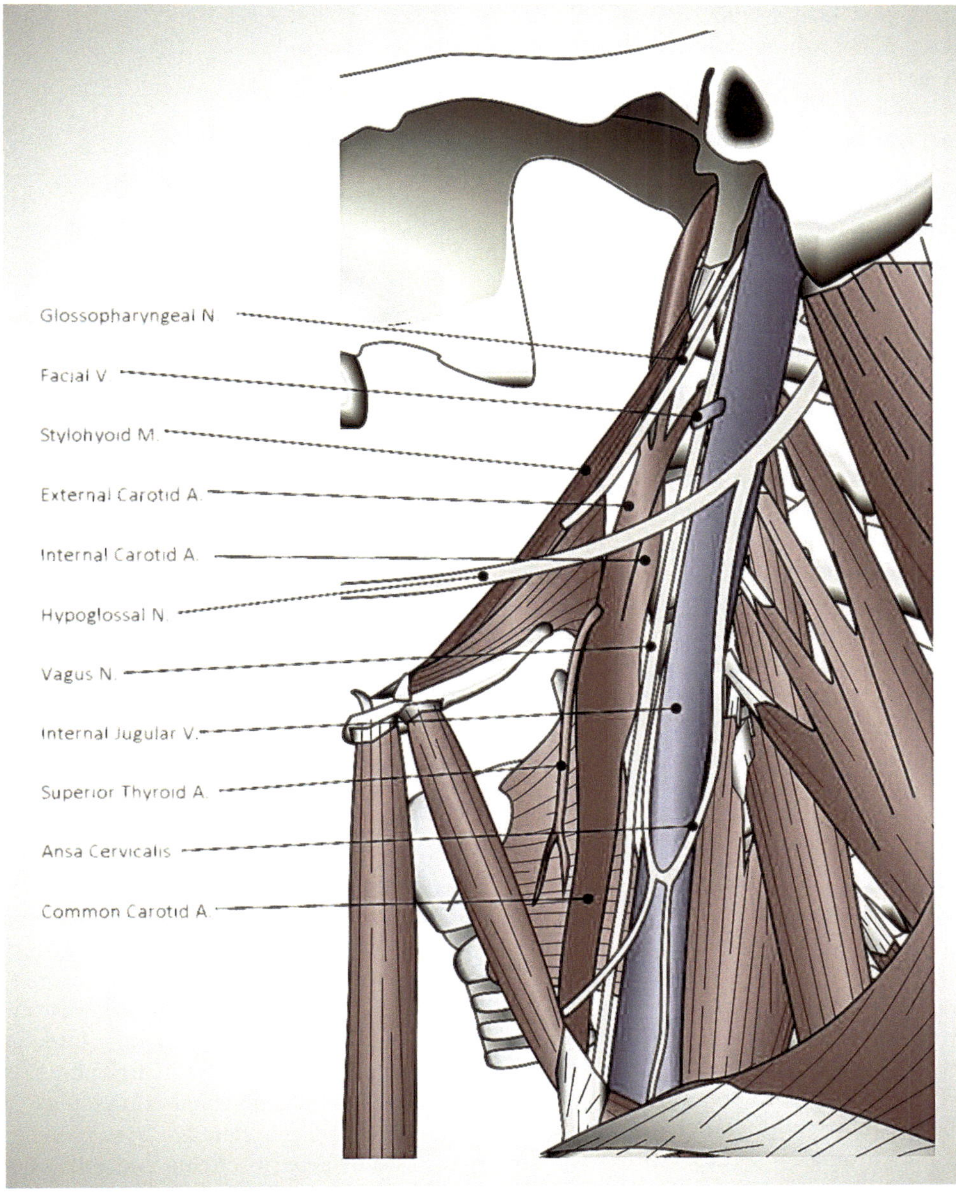

Figure 33.1 Anatomy of the common carotid artery and its associated neurovascular structures.

the injury contingent upon the nerve damaged. Therefore, knowing their anatomic course and possible variants is necessary before performing any neck exploration. The vagus nerve courses between the internal jugular and the carotid, usually just posterior to the structures. Injury to the vagus nerve will result in downstream effects on the recurrent laryngeal nerve and vocal fold innervation. This might occur during mobilization of the common carotid for circumferential control or can be injured during placement of the common carotid clamp. The hypoglossal nerve typically courses from lateral to medial, just distal and superficial to the carotid bifurcation. It can be identified by tracing the ansa cervicalis superiorly. As dissection of the internal carotid artery progress more distally, the hypoglossal nerve will be encountered running over the internal carotid artery and may need further mobilization in order to fully expose the artery. This is typically done by careful dissection of its lateral border with division and ligation of venous tributaries. Damage to the hypoglossal results in diminished tongue mobility. The marginal mandibular nerve courses from lateral to medial along the angle of the mandible. Careful placement of retractors to ensure they are pulling along the incision and not under the angle of the mandible is essential in avoiding injury to this nerve. The glossopharyngeal nerve can be damaged if distal control on the internal carotid is necessary for control or intervention. The glossopharyngeal nerve courses from medial to lateral posterior to the digastric muscles. This nerve is most often damaged during division of the digastric muscles and has devastating effects on swallow function. Lastly, the spinal accessory nerve, which courses medial to lateral in the posterior triangle, can be injured from retraction on the sternocleidomastoid.

Once the artery has been exposed, it should be carefully inspected to determine if the extent of the injury necessitates ligation or repair. If the patient is neurologically intact and unstable, ligation may be the safer option over repair. Primary repair can be performed if a sharp injury with a diameter of injury less than 50% of the full circumference of the vessel can be performed, especially on the common carotid. However, if the injury is secondary to a gunshot, the devitalized tissues must be debrided. This often results in the need for a patch angioplasty or interposition bypass. Given the structures that are in close proximity to a penetrating carotid injury (i.e., the esophagus and the trachea), the risk of patch infection and the potential development of patch aneurysm and rupture may be prohibitively high, and many surgeons may opt for a different repair option. The type of patch to be utilized has been long debated, without a truly favorable option between autologous vein, bovine pericardium, and Dacron or PTFE. In a grossly infected field, the best option is generally a vein patch or interposition bypass. One option that may readily be available in the operative field would be the external or internal jugular, facial, or superior thyroid veins. However, in the setting of a grossly unstable patient, there may not be time for a vein harvest, and another conduit, such as bovine pericardium, Dacron or PTFE, may be necessary.

Carotid injury—Blunt

Blunt carotid injury is present in 0.1% of all trauma patients and 0.67% of motor vehicle accidents.[3] The mortality rate is high (28%) and a high proportion of patients have a permanent neurological deficit (58%).[1] Clearly identification and early intervention on these injuries are paramount. Pseudoaneurysm formation, thrombosis, and embolization may result from unidentified injuries and may result in the aforementioned neurologic deficit. Screening for these injuries is based on the Denver or Memphis criteria for blunt cerebrovascular injury and intervention is based on grade of injury on the Denver scale (Figures 33.2 and 33.3).

Grade	Injury
I	Intimal irregularity or hematoma <25% stenosis of vessel diameter
II	Intimal disruption or hematoma >25% stenosis of vessel diameter
III	Pseudoaneurysm
IV	Occlusion
V	Transection

Figure 33.2a Grades of blunt cerebrovascular injury by Denver criteria.

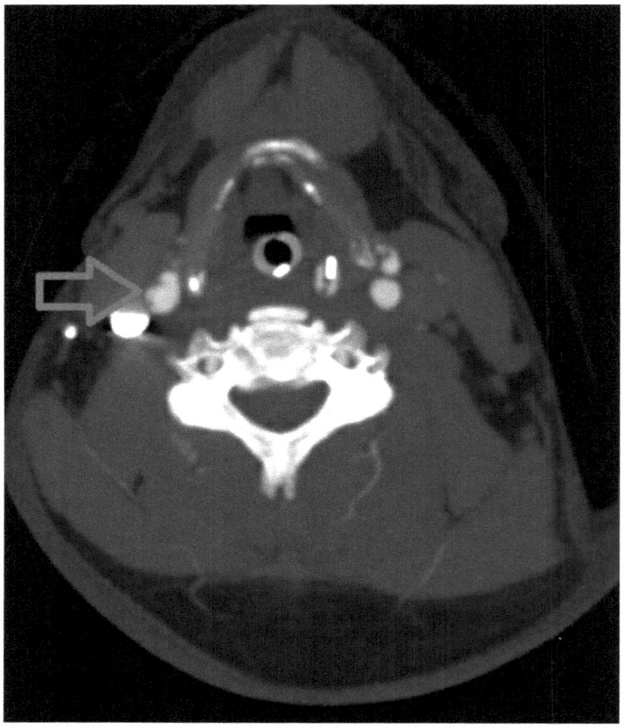

Figure 33.2b Traumatic right common carotid dissection following hanging injury. The right common carotid artery is noted to have a small dissection (arrow).

Generally, a grade III injury or greater would warrant intervention, whether endovascular or open. In regards to endovascular intervention, both balloon expandable and self-expanding, bare metal and covered stents have been utilized. The type of stent used varies based on surgeon preference and the indication for intervention. Regardless of the stent type, in-stent thrombosis is a highly feared complication, and dual antiplatelet therapy is often employed when a stent has been placed.

Use of heparin during and following these repairs is controversial in the setting of additional injuries, such as intracranial or intraabdominal hemorrhage. Either aspirin or heparin anticoagulation is the recommended treatment in the patient who is to have only medical management for a blunt carotid injury. Biffl et al. found a stroke risk of 3% in grade I patients, 11% in grade II,

Risk Factors	Signs/Symptoms
LeForte II or III fracture	Active hemorrhage, expanding hematoma
Basilar skull fracture	Carotid bruit
Cervical vertebral body or transverse foramen fracture, subluxation or ligamentous injury	Focal deficit
Closed head injury, diffuse axonal injury, Glasgow coma scale<6	Ischemic stroke on CT or MRI
Near hanging with anoxic brain injury	Neurologic deficit not consistent with CT or MRI
Clothesline injury/ seatbelt sign	

Figure 33.3 Indications for screening for blunt cerebrovascular injury by Denver criteria.

33% in grade III, and 44% in grade IV, if anticoagulation/antiplatelet therapy was not started.[1] When it can be used, anticoagulation has also demonstrated trends toward improved neurologic recovery.[1] However, heparin use is not without risk, as there have also been reports of increased bleeding risk in heparinized trauma patients.

Vertebral injury

Penetrating vertebral artery injury is relatively uncommon outside of the iatrogenic setting, owing to its relatively protected position as it courses through the vertebral bodies. Conversely, blunt vertebral injury is relatively common. In the absence of a cervical spine injury, vertebral artery contusion or dissection may go unnoticed (Figure 33.4). An unfortunate consequence of missed vertebral artery injury is vessel thrombosis and embolization and subsequent cerebellar infarction. This may occur days to weeks after a missed injury. Grading of vertebral artery injury and recommendations for intervention are again based on the Denver scale. Many vertebral artery injuries require only anticoagulation or antiplatelet administration and neurologic monitoring. Higher-grade injuries may require endovascular or open repair. Exposure of the vertebral artery may be beneficial for injuries to the V1 or V3 segments. The V2 and V4 segments are within bony confines and require an endovascular approach.[2]

Open exposure of the proximal vertebral artery requires attention to the surrounding structures, including the thoracic duct, phrenic nerve, and spinal accessory nerve. The thoracic duct is found in the left neck, where

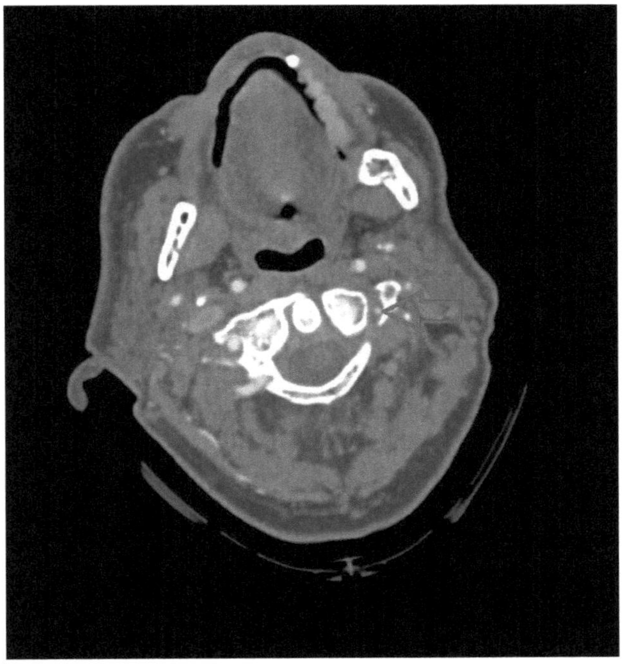

Figure 33.4 Traumatic left vertebral artery compression without associated hematoma or dissection due to transverse foramen fracture.

it terminates at the junction between the left subclavian and left internal jugular veins. Injury to the thoracic duct during proximal subclavian and vertebral exposure could result in a chyle leak. Depending on the volume of output, this may require transition to a short- and medium-chain fatty acid diet, with exclusion of long-chain fatty acids. Persistent chyle leaks at times require re-exploration for ligation or lymphangiogram with use of sclerosing agents.

The thoracic duct is only one structure that can potentially be injured when attempting to dissect out the proximal vertebral artery. The phrenic nerve runs along the anterior surface of the anterior scalene muscle. The anterior scalene is divided in order to better expose the origin of the vertebral and proximal subclavian arteries. Injury to the phrenic nerve results in hemiplegia of the diaphragm and decreased respiratory excursion. Injury to the spinal accessory nerve can occur with more distal exposure on the artery. Spinal accessory damage results in disfiguring and debilitating motor deficits to the trapezius and sternocleidomastoid. Winging of the scapula may also occur.

Due to its proximity to the cervical transverse foramina and the skull base, the vertebral artery can be difficult to control proximally and distally, especially in the setting of laceration and hemorrhage. However, proximal ligation in an attempt to control hemorrhage is unlikely to result in complete resolution of bleeding.[10] Persistent hemorrhage may occur as a result of retrograde flow via the contralateral vertebral and the communication with the basilar artery. In addition, ligation of the dominant proximal vertebral artery may result in thrombosis of the basilar artery and subsequent stroke.[9] Basilar occlusion has a higher mortality (80%) than carotid occlusion, as the basilar artery supplies the brainstem, which regulates autonomic function.[10]

Endovascular intervention for vertebrobasilar injury is also not without risk. Distal embolization, stent thrombosis due to poor compliance/inability to take antiplatelet agents, or stent thrombosis due to undersizing may result. Additionally, there are no readily available stent grafts in the smaller diameters needed to treat the vertebral arteries.

TORSO TRAUMA

Vascular trauma to the chest and abdomen has a high morbidity and mortality, with a large number of patients expiring in the field. In patients that do make it to the hospital, long-term outcomes with major vascular injury are still dismal.

THORACIC VASCULAR TRAUMA

Thoracic aortic injury in blunt trauma affords the most likely opportunity for intervention, compared to penetrating thoracic aortic injury, which often results in unrecoverable hemorrhage in the field. Blunt aortic injury is graded by the degree of injury—grade I is an intimal injury, grade II is an intramural hematoma, grade III is a pseudoaneurysm, and grade IV is an aortic transection. The grade of injury dictates whether intervention is offered. Grade I and II injuries are monitored, with repeat imaging to document stability. Grade III and IV injuries are most commonly managed with thoracic endovascular aortic aneurysm repair (TEVAR) (Figure 33.5). However, there is limited long-term data regarding the usage of TEVAR in trauma patients, without aneurysmal pathology.

In the trauma patient, the complications of TEVAR placement are similar to those of the aneurysm patient. There are, however, complications that are more likely in the trauma patient than in the aneurysm patient. Sizing of a TEVAR in the trauma patient is difficult, as the aortic pathology is not the same as in an aneurysm, there is rarely baseline aortic dilation. The average aortic diameter in trauma patients was 22 mm.[4] TEVAR was originally designed for aneurysmal disease, so the original devices were not made for smaller diameter aortas. The majority of devices are oversized by 20–30% in the trauma setting. Thus, the aorta undergoes modeling when the TEVAR is placed. This can result in degeneration of the aortic wall over time. In fact, one study found that a 10% increase in oversizing lead to a 3.4% proximal aortic diameter increase.[4] Most concerning is that oversizing of 25–30% is associated with graft collapse in multiple studies.[5,7] Graft collapse was a relatively early complication, most commonly occurring in the first 2–4 weeks following placement, but has been described as a long term complication as well. Newer models of grafts have smaller diameters to address this issue; however, there have been reports of graft thrombosis with smaller diameter stent grafts.[11]

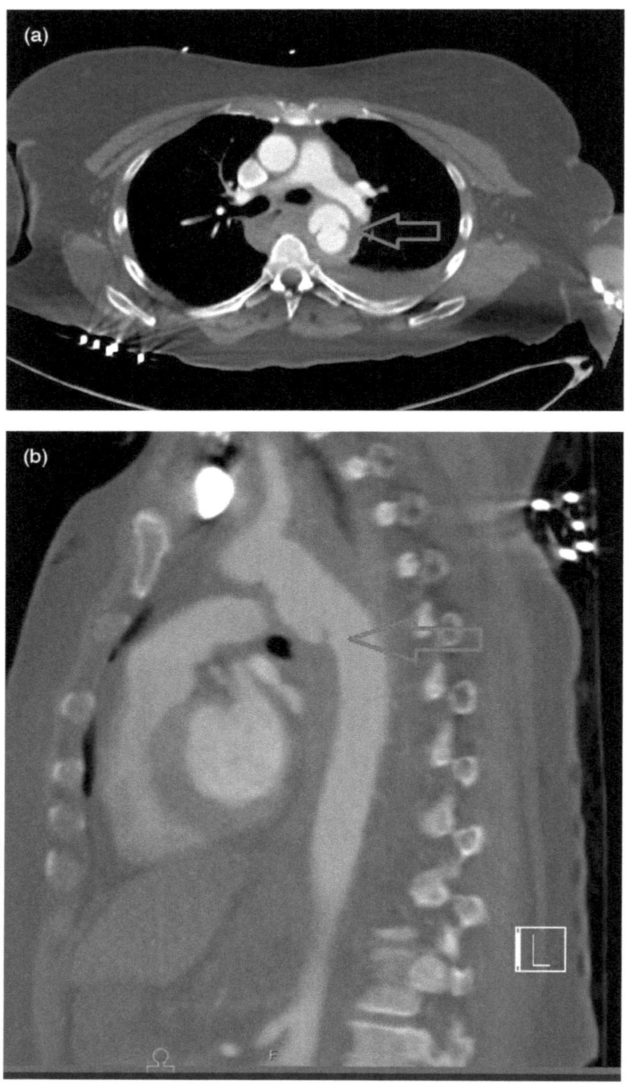

Figure 33.5 Traumatic thoracic aortic dissection at the isthmus. (a) AP view. (b) Sagittal view.

Another commonly described pathology following placement of an oversized TEVAR in the setting of thoracic aortic injury is poor apposition of the stent graft along the lesser curve of the aortic arch resulting in a bird-beak configuration. This poor apposition along the lesser curve has been seen in as many of 65% of patients undergoing TEVAR for traumatic indications, but the implications of this are unclear.[7] Some patients with the bird-beak configuration go on to develop type I endoleak and graft collapse, but this cannot be directly attributed to the configuration itself. There is also some development of in-stent thrombosis due to the angulation of the proximal potion of the stent graft. This may also result in complete thrombosis and graft collapse, but again, it has not been proven that incomplete apposition to the aortic arch is the cause.

Coverage of the left subclavian artery can often be avoided when placing a TEVAR for a traumatic aortic injury, as 90% of blunt aortic injuries occur at the isthmus. The seal zone is often long enough to not necessitate coverage of the left subclavian (Figure 33.6). If there is not an adequate seal zone, then a stent graft with a bare metal portion proximally may be used to maintain the antegrade subclavian flow or the subclavian can be covered, with reliance on the vertebral artery to provide retrograde flow to the arm. The obvious concern with this is left upper extremity ischemia, but this is an uncommon occurrence. If the opportunity for operative planning is afforded, one can determine whether the left vertebral artery is dominant and perform a carotid-subclavian bypass in select patients.

An additional concern with covering the left subclavian is that it provides important collateral flow via the internal mammary artery to the intercostal arteries. This collateral flow limits spinal cord ischemia. TEVARs for traumatic injuries are generally short-segment stent-grafts (11 cm), which decreases the risk of spinal cord ischemia, but this should be considered if a longer stent-graft is utilized. Plugging, coiling, or ligation of the subclavian artery may be necessary, and in these cases, carotid subclavian bypass may be considered to restore retrograde

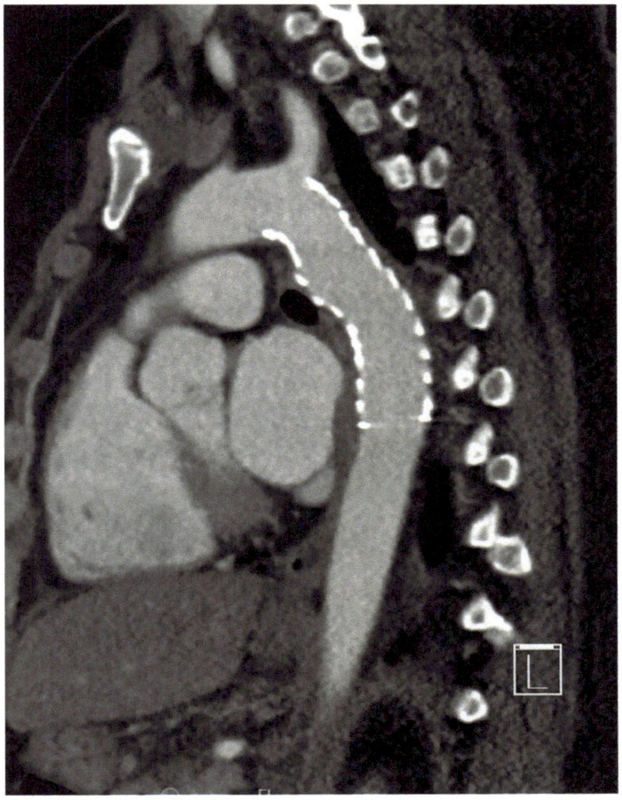

Figure 33.6 TEVAR of traumatic aortic dissection with placement of stent-graft just distal to left subclavian artery, preserving left subclavian flow.

flow to the internal mammary, vertebral, and their collateral branches.

Lastly, TEVAR has the potential of causing a retrograde dissection into the arch and ascending aorta. This can result in cardiac tamponade and cardiac arrest, or devastating cerebral ischemia secondary to extension into or exclusion of the arch vasculature. To combat the likelihood of retrograde dissection, as well as to avoid mal-positioning, the patient's blood pressure is decreased during deployment of the device. However, there is a higher risk of retrograde dissection in patients undergoing TEVAR for dissection versus aneurysm, so this complication should be discussed with patient preoperatively whenever possible.

ABDOMINAL VASCULAR TRAUMA

Management of abdominal vascular trauma is defined by the mechanism and zone of injury. There are three zones within the abdomen and pelvis. Zone 1 is the central portion of the abdomen and contains the aorta, mesenteric vasculature, and IVC. Zone 2 involves the bilateral flanks and involves the renal vasculature. Zone 3 involves the pelvis, containing the iliac arteries and veins.

Mechanism of injury also defines whether intervention is pursued. Blunt abdominal trauma in the absence of instability and/or expanding hematoma does not necessitate operative intervention, while all penetrating trauma warrants operative exploration.

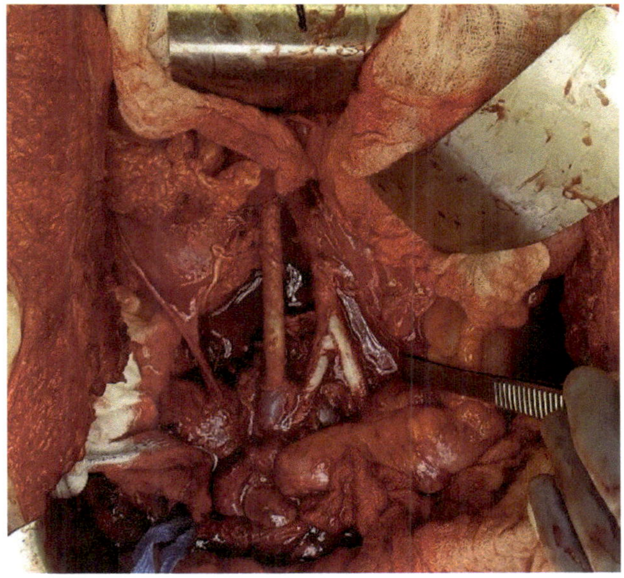

Figure 33.7 Traumatic aortic injury with concomitant IVC injury following motor vehicle collision. Aorta repaired with bovine pericardial patch angioplasty. IVC repaired with bovine carotid graft due to contaminated field.

Zone 1 injury is primarily managed by open operative intervention with aortic repair or replacement. Repair, either primary or with patch angioplasty, should be performed if the vessel in question involves < 50% diameter and the injury is sharp (Figure 33.7). Replacement should be performed if the diameter of the injury is greater than 50% or the length of the injury does not allow for primary repair. Sharp injuries can be primarily repaired without debridement, but gunshot wounds require debridement prior to repair. If replacement is necessary, then the surgeon must consider the entire field, as gross contamination within the abdomen makes synthetic repair a less than desirable option. For this reason, surgeons must widely prep and be prepared to harvest saphenous or deep femoral vein for replacement. The saphenous vein may serve as a conduit if the vessel to be replaced is of small diameter (a mesenteric vessel) or a patch can be performed. However, if the segment to be replaced involves the aorta or the IVC, then deep femoral vein harvest may be necessary due to the diameter of the vessel. The vein to be harvested deserves consideration in regards to concomitant injuries, as one would not want to harvest a deep femoral vein if there is an ipsilateral venous or arterial injury distally. Other options for aortic replacement in the setting of gross contamination include replacement with rifampin-soaked graft or cryopreserved vein. Rifampin-soaked graft has been shown to have adequate patency and resistance to recurrent infection when compared to aortic ligation and extra-anatomic bypass, though this comes with the addition of lifelong antibiotics in most cases.[6]

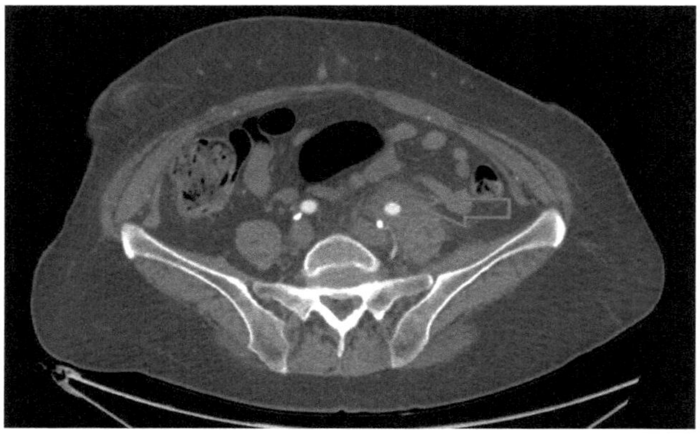

Figure 33.8 Infected aortobifemoral bypass graft with associated left iliac limb fluid collection.

Graft infection is the most feared complication following aortic replacement in the setting of trauma and gross contamination, as formation of pseudoaneurysm and hemorrhage may follow (Figure 33.8). At this juncture, graft explant with aortic ligation and extraanatomic bypass may be necessary. Graft explant with repeat replacement with cryopreserved vein or rifampin-soaked is a second option. There are risks associated with either attempt at repair, primarily of repeat graft infection, but additionally renal failure, lower extremity ischemia, and ultimately limb loss may result. Aortic stump rupture is an additional concern described in the literature, with an incidence of approximately 2% in one study.[8] Concern for these complications should dictate the surgeon's choice for initial repair and strong consideration for long-term antibiotics should be employed.

REFERENCES

1. Biffl WL. Blunt carotid arterial injuries: implications of a new grading scale. Journal of Trauma. 1999;47: 845–53.
2. Conenwett JL, Johnston KW. Rutherford's Vascular Surgery. Philadelphia, Pennsylvania. Saunders. 2014.
3. Fabian T, et al. Blunt carotid injury. Importance of early diagnosis and anticoagulant therapy. Annals of Surgery. 1996;223(5): 513–25.
4. Gennai S, et al. Influence of thoracic endovascular repair on aortic morphology in patients treated for blunt traumatic aortic injuries: long term outcomes in a multicentre study. European Journal of Vascular and Endovascular Surgery. 2020;59(3): 428–36.
5. Jonker F, et al. Endograft collapse after thoracic endovascular aortic repair. Journal of Endovascular Therapy. 2010;17: 725–34.
6. Oderich GS, et al. In situ rifampin-soaked grafts with omental coverage and antibiotic suppression are durable with low reinfection rates in patients with aortic graft enteric erosion or fistula. Journal of Vascular Surgery. 2011;53(1): 99–107.
7. Reyes M, et al. Long-term outcomes of thoracic endovascular aortic repair focused on bird beak and oversizing in blunt traumatic thoracic aortic injury. Annals of Vascular Surgery. 2018;50: 140–7.
8. Seeger J, et al. Long-term outcome after treatment of aortic graft infection with staged extra-anatomic bypass grafting and aortic graft removal. Journal of Vascular Surgery. 2000;32(3): 451–61.
9. Shintani A, Zervas NT. Consequence of ligation of the vertebral artery. Journal of Neurosurgery. 1972;36: 447–50.
10. Stanley JC, Veith F, Wakefield TW. Current Therapy in Vascular and Endovascular Surgery. Philadelphia, Pennsylvania. Saunders. 2014.
11. U.S. Food and Drug Administration. Cook Medical Inc. recalls Zenith Alpha thoracic endovascular graft for the treatment of blunt traumatic aortic injury (BTAI) due to the potential formation of thrombus inside the device after implantation. https://www.fda.gov/medical-devices/medical-device-recalls/cook-medical-inc-recalls-zenith-alpha-thoracic-endovascular-graft-treatment-blunt-traumatic-aortic

34

Management of vascular complications during nonvascular operations

KUSH SHARMA AND M. ASHRAF MANSOUR

As surgical disciplines have evolved to favor a multidisciplinary approach, a vascular surgeon's role is becoming critical within a hospital environment.[1] Intraoperative vascular surgery assistance is typically required for hemorrhage control with repair of vascular injury, assistance with anatomic exposure, or oncologic resection.[2,3] The involvement of vascular surgeons in nonvascular procedures is generally during unplanned surgical situations that require immediate assistance to prevent a potential morbidity or even the death of the patient.[1] Some series have shown that over 80% of vascular surgery consultations requested were unexpected, while other series have demonstrated the opposite, that intraoperative vascular surgery assistance was coordinated ahead of time.[2,3] Regardless of whether vascular surgery assistance is requested in advance to a procedure, timely availability of vascular surgery expertise is crucial in large medical centers, as most cases needing vascular repair are intraoperative emergent consultations.[2] Additionally, nonoperative vascular complications outside of the operating room after cardiac catheterizations and iatrogenic trauma further support the value of having vascular surgery expertise readily available.[2] As the number of vascular surgery consults by other specialties, vascular trainees will need to learn a full breadth of anatomic exposures.[2] The aim of this chapter is to review the common complications leading to vascular consultations and how to manage them. We also review the types of cases requiring vascular assistance for exposure or help in resecting important vascular structures.

VASCULAR INJURIES OF THE NECK

CENTRAL LINE INJURIES

Overview

Accessing the internal jugular vein (IJV) in the neck for the purpose of inserting a temporary central venous access or a long-term port for the delivery of total parental nutrition or chemotherapy is a common procedure in the hospital for adults and children. The most serious complications with this procedure are vascular injury or CLABSI (central line-associated blood stream infection).[4] Many efforts have been spent to decrease CLABSI in hospitals; however, despite the use of new technology (ultrasound guidance), iatrogenic vascular injuries from central venous cannulation (CVC) attempts are still fairly common complications.[4,5] Puncturing the pleura with any size needle may lead to a pneumothorax or hemothorax. The most serious complication with central venous injury is pericardial tamponade, which, if not treated immediately, can lead to arrhythmia and death.[5]

The incidence of arterial puncture in large studies has been reported to range from 4.2–9.3%. Early recognition of injury from a smaller gauge needle should prompt withdrawal and manual pressure; however, arterial puncture with a large bore catheter (> 7 Fr) include hematoma, pseudoaneurysm, arteriovenous fistula (AVF), dissection, bleeding, limb ischemia, stroke, and death.[5,6] Risk factors that predispose patients to iatrogenic arterial injury include obesity, previous radiation therapy or surgical field in the region of catheter placement, multiple needle passes, and operator inexperience.[7] Current American Society of Anesthesiologists Task Force guidelines on central venous access recommend that misplaced CVCs should be left in place and have a vascular or general surgery consultation for further evaluation.[6]

Clinical presentation

ARTERIAL INJURIES

- Arterial puncture during attempted CVC access has been reported more frequently with the jugular approach (3%) compared to subclavian (0.5%).[8] Despite the use of ultrasound guidance, these injuries may occur, even in experienced hands.

VENOUS INJURIES

- Even though we are focusing on arterial injuries associated with CVC placement, life-threatening injuries of intrathoracic veins may also occur. Pericardial tamponade from a stiff wire or catheter injury has been reported. While the latter is uncommon, it is believed to occur if a guidewire becomes trapped against the vein wall and the vein is then torn when a dilator, sheath, or catheter is advanced.[5]

DIAGNOSIS OF INJURY

- Clinical exam
- Duplex ultrasound
- CT angiography
- MR angiography
- Catheter-based angiography

Management

NONSURGICAL

- Noninvasive management of inadvertent carotid artery or subclavian artery cannulation for CVCs has been the "pull-and-pressure" technique. This is only feasible if the injury is immediately recognized, caused by a small gauge needle, and the patient is not on anticoagulants. In a series of injuries to the carotids, the morbidity and mortality of patients has been significant including stroke, arteriovenous fistula, hemothorax, hematoma, or death.[5]
- For the subclavian artery, manual compression is ineffective because the artery cannot be compressed against a bony structure, like the femoral artery in the groin. With the carotid artery, prolonged pressure may be effective, however there is risk of an ischemic stroke or precipitating a vasovagal attack.[9]

ENDOVASCULAR

- Open surgical repair is the gold standard for iatrogenic arterial injuries during CVC placement. Currently, there are many endovascular alternatives, especially when dealing with a hemodynamically unstable or critically ill patient.[7]

Covered stents

- The placement of a covered stent to repair a subclavian artery injury can be considered in some cases, especially if patients are unstable, have multiple injuries from trauma, or have been subjected to prior radiation. The stent can be delivered either from the ipsilateral brachial approach or from a groin approach.[10]
- Case series of subclavian or carotid pseudoaneurysms treated with covered stents have shown favorable outcomes compared to surgery with additional benefits of decreased morbidity and enhanced recovery.[10]
- Limitations compared to an open surgical approach include coverage of arterial side branches such as the vertebral artery in an iatrogenic subclavian injury, risk of stent collapse if arterial injury site at thoracic inlet/outlet, or in patients who have sepsis with evidence of bacteremia.[7,10]

Arterial closure devices

- Arterial closure devices were designed for use in the femoral artery. When these devices are utilized to close, an inadvertent arterial cannulation during the attempted CVC is possible but considered an off-label use. It may be an alternative for patients who remain critically ill where a surgical operation is not ideal.[9] It presupposes that the injury is immediately recognized and the vessel in question is still accessed with a wire.
- Different devices that can be used include suture-mediated devices, plug-mediated designs, or Boomerang devices. Arterial closure device choice is dependent on location of vessel injury, anticoagulation, arteriotomy size, and operator experience.[9]

SURGICAL

- Based on 11,870 attempted IJV cannulations in a series, 20 arterial cannulations were recognized. Based on the size of cannula, the authors recommended direct surgical repair of the arterial injury caused by large bore (> 7 Fr) catheters.[5]
- Open surgical repair is favored in the setting of large diameter catheter cannulation, complex arteriovenous fistula or pseudoaneurysm, or when an excessive

bleeding risk and coagulopathy is anticipated. When endovascular repair is not effective or anatomically feasible, open repair is an alternative definitive method for repair.[6]

- Carotid artery injuries should preferentially be treated with an open approach in order to allow for distal clamping, and thrombectomy and to protect from a possible risk of embolism.[6]

Injury prevention

ULTRASOUND GUIDANCE

- Meta-analyses of ultrasound guidance for central venous cannulation demonstrated their utility. A higher rate of first time successful venous access was seen for internal jugular vein (IJV) access when used with ultrasound guidance.[5]
- The use of ultrasonography was not found to be beneficial for subclavian vein access as the clavicle interferes with ultrasound-guided catheter placement.[5]
- Ultrasound guidance is better than following anatomic landmarks for a higher success rate on the first attempt; however, its use does not rule out arterial cannulation.[5]

PRESSURE MONITORING PRIOR TO CATHETER INSERTION

- Measurement of back pressure in the needle via column manometry or pressure transducer can help recognize inadvertent arterial cannulation.[5]
- Data from 11,804 patients demonstrated that pressure monitoring can be useful in preventing arterial injury, compared to reliance on color/pulsatility alone, which would have resulted in 0.8% arterial cannulation rate.[5]

TRACHEOINNOMINATE ARTERY FISTULA

Overview

Tracheo-innominate artery fistula (TIF) is a potentially life-threating iatrogenic complication that is typically associated with percutaneous or surgical placement of a tracheostomy tube and has also been described in cases of tracheal resection and tracheal stenting (Figure 34.1).[11,12] The incidence after surgical tracheostomy has been reported to be 0.1–1% with a peak incidence typically seen 7–14 days after the procedure.[12] Risk factors for fistula development include high cuff pressure necrosis, mucosal trauma from mal-positioned cannula, low tracheal incision, excessive neck motion, or radiotherapy.[12] This condition is typically fatal unless

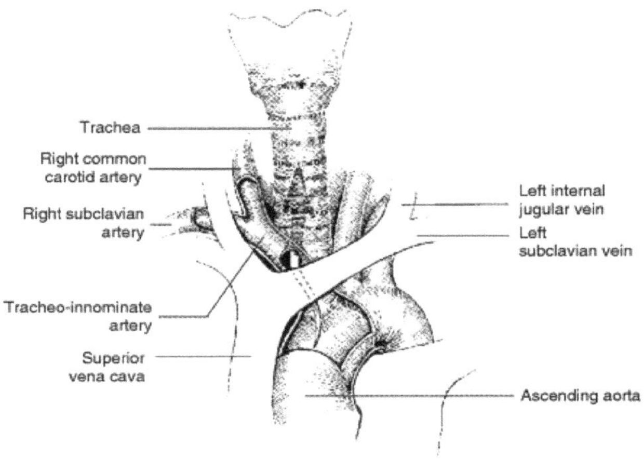

Figure 34.1 Tracheo-innominate artery fisula.[12]

the problem is immediately recognized and patients have immediate definitive surgical treatment; however, more recently endovascular stent grafts have helped in reducing the morbidity and mortality associated with invasive repair.[13]

Clinical presentation/diagnosis of injury

Any peristomal hemorrhage or hemoptysis in the setting of tracheostomy placement should be further investigated with a high index of suspicion for TIF.[12] The timeline for presentation can give some insight to the etiology. Hemorrhage within 48 hours of tracheostomy placement is usually due to anterior jugular or thyroid vein tear, coagulopathic state, tracheal suction, or bronchopneumonia.[12] The peak incident of TIF is between the first and second weeks after tracheostomy.[14] Hemorrhage after this time up to 6 weeks from tracheostomy placement should be considered a TIF until proven otherwise and warrant further clinical evaluation.[12] If patients are stable, arteriography is an option. Patients with bleeding can be diagnosed via bronchoscopy. When the source of bleeding cannot be ascertained via bronchoscopy, thoracotomy is the next step in management.[15]

Management

NONSURGICAL

- If TIF is suspected, the Utley maneuver, placement of a finger in the stoma to compress the innominate, is the first thing to do. Temporizing measures can be used for patients who present with TIF until definitive repair is performed. This can be achieved by over-inflating the cuff of the tracheostomy tube and placing a pressure dressing on the neck.[13] Suction may be necessary to prevent blood trickling down the trachea and causing the patient to drown in blood.

ENDOVASCULAR

- There have been a handful of reported cases where endovascular treatment has offered a less morbid alternative to open surgical management. The endovascular approach may afford a faster hemorrhage control than a thoracotomy, however there is a potential for stent graft infection.[16] Stent graft insertion has been performed by accessing the brachial, axillary, or femoral arteries with placement of a covered stent at the fistula site for rapid control of bleeding.

SURGICAL

- Open surgical repair is associated with significant mortality rates estimated to be approximately around 50%.[16] Management includes a median sternotomy to expose the great vessels and trachea with repair using sutured pericardial pledgets.[16] Innominate artery exclusion and extraanatomic bypass graft such as carotid-carotid, axillo-axillo, or femoroaxillo bypass graft may offer a less morbid option than direct reconstruction.[13]

VASCULAR INJURIES OF THE CHEST

Overview

Major vascular injuries within the thorax are generally a result of blunt or penetrating trauma; however, iatrogenic vascular injuries have been described and appear to be the most troublesome and dangerous complications of video-assisted thoracoscopic surgery.[17] Even though injuries within the chest are typically within the expertise of cardiothoracic surgery, a brief overview of potential complications may be useful if vascular surgery assistance if required.

VIDEO-ASSISTED THORACOSCOPIC SURGERY (VATS)

VATS was introduced in the early 1990s and has gained increasing popularity secondary to the treatment of benign or malignant lung cancers. The most feared vascular injury during VATS lobectomy is to the pulmonary artery, most commonly seen during left upper lobectomy, and may be one of the main deterrents for widespread acceptance.[18] Injury to pulmonary artery branches/veins has been widely described in the literature, however descending aortic injury is a rare complication within the realm of vascular injuries.[19]

Management

Initial management includes pressure with rolled-up sponges with some series reporting a minimum of 7 minutes of pressure held.[18] If the injury cannot be repaired thoracospically, open thoracotomy is recommended. The specific details are not within the scope of this chapter.

VASCULAR INJURIES OF THE BACK

VASCULAR COMPLICATIONS OF ANTERIOR LUMBAR DISC SURGERY

Overview

The anterior approach to the lumbar spine for treatment of Pott's disease was initially described in 1934. Since then, advances in spinal instrumentation and the creation of small metal cages for disc fusion have popularized this approach.[20] Anterior lumbar spine interbody fusion (ALIF) is done through a paramedian fascial/retroperitoneal exposure where the peritoneal contents and ureter are mobilized medially and away from the quadratus lumborum and psoas muscles. The aorta, inferior vena cava (IVC), iliac vein, and iliac artery all can be easily mobilized, depending on the disc space(s) of interest.[21] Ligation of middle sacral vessels, iliolumbar vein, and segmental lumbar veins is often required.[21] Abdominal vascular injury following operation for a herniated lumbar disc is a major complication secondary to close anatomic relationship between lumbar vertebrae and major vessels.[22] Because of these complications and the need for adequate exposure of vertebral bodies for a successful operation, vascular surgeons are now functioning as co-surgeons with both neurosurgeons and orthopedic spine surgeons for anterior disc space exposure.[20]

Vascular manipulation for lumbar exposure for ALIF

L1-L2, L2-L3, AND L3-L4 DISC SPACE

- Requires little to no aortic/iliac mobilization as the approach is usually the lateral retroperitoneal one.[23]

L4-L5 DISC SPACE

- Exposure can be above (lateral to) the left common iliac artery (CIA), between the left CIA and common iliac vein (CIV), or below (medial to) the left CIV, this is likely the most complicated one and also the one fraught with potential complications.[23]
- For exposure at the L4 level or above, the iliolumbar vein should be identified and ligated for proper spinal exposure.[21]

L5-S1 DISC SPACE

- Blunt and sharp dissections assist with iliac vessel mobilization from the spine.[21] Single exposure at this level requires mobilization between left CIA and CIV, while some exposure between the left and right iliac vessels beyond the bifurcation allows for visualization of the middle sacral artery/vein that are ligated and divided.[21,23]

Factors contributing to vascular injuries and management

Vascular injuries have been reported at various time intervals from intraoperative, postoperative, and at 30-day follow-up. There is a wide range of vascular injuries reported in the literature, from 1–24%, and the risk of DVT from 0.7–5%, and retrograde ejaculation from 0–50%.[20] Arterial injuries to major vessels generally present as thrombosis or vasospasm. Thrombosis is generally seen with clinical symptoms in the postoperative phase, but lacerations are immediately encountered and can be repaired primarily with Prolene sutures.[21] Venous injuries typically manifest as bleeding from lacerations or avulsions and generally occur when mobilizing the iliac vein.[21] Most venous injuries in studies have shown to be encountered with the L4-L5 exposure and most commonly related to avulsion of the ilio-lumbar vein.[21] Occasionally, iliac vein lacerations can be caused by the spikes in the delivery tube which is used with some ALIF kits. Venous lacerations can be controlled with suture repair, but small lacerations (< 4 mm) can be managed with hemostatic agents.[21] Minor vascular injury has been defined as the need for monofilament suture repair and major vascular injury defined as anything more than a simple suture (i.e., lateral venorrhaphy, venous/arterial reconstruction, or suture ligation of a major venous structure).[23] Minor vascular injuries have been reported as being more common in the L4-L5 disc space and related to iliac vessel exposure as space between left CIA/CIV has been shown to have a high rate of minor injury.[23] Major vascular injuries have been reported to be most common to the left common iliac vein in series and the level of spinal exposure was shown to have no influence on incidence of vascular injuries.[23]

Measures to decrease incidence of intraoperative vascular injury

Intraoperative vascular injury is largely dependent on vessel mobilization required for lumbosacral vertebral exposure. In exposing the anterior surface of the lumbar spine, small lumbosacral vessels may be encountered and either clipped or cauterized. If these vessels are ignored, they may cause vexing and persistent bleeding. Preoperative review of history for atherosclerotic risk factors and appropriate physical exam of peripheral pulses is crucial in all patients. Major abdominal vasculature can be seen on preoperative MRI obtained by the spine surgeons, but when expected mobilization may be greater depending on implant required, computed tomography angiogram (CTA) may help with preoperative planning.[24] A series of 76 patients who underwent anterior lumbar spine procedure with preoperative CTA had surgical decision making impacted in 21% of patients, findings of prevertebral anatomic anomalies in 11.8% of patients, and discovery of atherosclerotic disease in 17% of patients.[25] CTA has helped with identifying pertinent anatomy and may impact surgical decision making preoperatively, however has not been validated for measuring outcomes.[24] Some studies have suggested that the rate of vascular injury may be associated with the surgical approach. Pooled rate of injury with laparoscopic or thoracoscopic procedure has been shown to be 4.2% vs 2.2% in open and 2.0% in mini-open procedure respectively.[24] Also, transperitoneal approach has shown a higher incidence of vascular injury compared to retroperitoneal exposure (3.6% vs 1.9%).[24]

Based on a systematic review of literature looking at vascular injury in elective anterior lumbosacral surgery, there have been no studies directly comparing the effect of patient positioning on the operating room table (supine vs lateral), type of incision (paramedian vs flank), or abdominal muscle treatment (muscle cutting vs muscle-splitting).[24] Additionally, even though a vascular access surgeon is mentioned in many of the large series, there have been no studies to show that this practice guarantees an improved outcome.[24]

There have been several case reports of aortic and iliac vascular injury with the posterior approach for lumbar laminectomy by the overzealous use of the rongeur or other sharp instruments. This injury should be suspected immediately with excessive bleeding and hypotension. In many cases, a delayed presentation with an iatrogenic arteriovenous fistula, pseudoaneurym, or even iliac deep venous thrombosis have been reported.

VASCULAR INJURIES OF THE ABDOMEN

VASCULAR INJURY DURING LAPAROSCOPIC SURGERY

Overview

Laparoscopy is one of the most common procedures performed by abdominal surgeons and has been further expanded by the development of robotic surgery.[26] Vascular injuries are relatively rare with reported incidence of 0.22–1.1%, however when they occur, they may be associated with an increased mortality rate between 8–17%.[27] Even though laceration to a major artery/vein by either the Veress needle or primary trocar can result in exsanguination as a major complication, additional complications such as peritoneal insufflation into a vein can result in gas embolism.[26] Some cases of vascular injury can be clearly evident requiring assistance from a vascular surgeon; however venous insufflation or minor needle injury to a retroperitoneal vessel can have difficult visualization.[26]

Clinical presentation

Vascular injuries to arteries and veins can occur with laparoscopy. In a series of laparoscopic vessel injuries reported to the US Food and Drug Administration (FDA), injuries were most commonly seen in the distal abdominal aorta, right/left common iliac artery, and vena cava. Less frequently, injury was seen with the internal/external iliac artery and veins.

Diagnosis of injury

Initial access to the abdomen with a needle (Veress) or trocar is usually blind, as the course of entry cannot be observed with the laparoscope. Safe and effective management of a major vessel injury starts with early recognition. The most likely signs of injury to a major vessel are immediate hemoperitoneum or poor visualization of the peritoneal cavity due to blood that cannot be attributed to bleeding from anterior abdominal wall.[26] Hemodynamic changes from bleeding would first be seen in the form of sinus tachycardia. When bleeding is present, any degree of insufflation can result in a possible gas embolism.[26] When this is suspected, the anesthesiologist should be alerted. It is possible with a venous injury that the gas used for insufflation gains access to the central circulation causing an "air lock" and preventing blood from circulating to the lungs.[28] If this occurs, it can cause sudden severe hypotension. With "Durant's maneuver," the patient is placed in the left lateral decubitus position in an attempt to displace the air bubble away from the pulmonary circulation.[28]

Management

Initial management of patients with an unexpected surgical hemorrhage should be to establish adequate vascular access, increase intravenous hydration, notify the blood bank for blood products, and finally call for assistance from a vascular surgeon.[26] A few methods can be used to decrease blood loss prior to definitive repair. For venous injuries, increasing the insufflation pressure to 20 mmHg once the port is out of the blood vessel can limit hemorrhage as central venous pressure is normally 8 mm Hg.[26] Additionally, pressure should be applied with a laparoscopic Kitner, blunt grasper, or suction cannula once the area of hemorrhage is identified. Generally, laparoscopic repair of retroperitoneal arterial/venous injuries is not possible and will require conversion to an emergency laparotomy.[26]

A midline laparotomy is preferred for retroperitoneal major vessel injury as it enables better surgical exposure of the aortic bifurcation and vena cava.[26] After exposure has been obtained, blood loss can be minimized through manual compression of the aorta at the esophageal hiatus. By having an assistant on the left side of the patient, placing the right hand above the lesser curve of the stomach and feeling for a pulse will allow to compress the aorta against the vertebral bodies.[26] Otherwise, once the site of hemorrhage is visualized, the most effective way to prevent further blood loss is to place either direct finger/sponge pressure over the laceration until the patient can be stabilized by anesthesia.[26] After obtaining proximal and distal control, vessels can be closed primarily, with a patch, or interposition graft depending on the degree of vessel injury.

ARTERIAL INJURY DURING LAPAROSCOPIC MEDIAN ARCUATE LIGAMENT DECOMPRESSION

Overview

The median arcuate ligament is a fibrous band of the diaphragmatic crus surrounding the celiac artery origin and the insertion at the celiac axis can cause extrinsic compression of the celiac access.[29] Since first described in 1963, median arcuate ligament syndrome (MALS), also known as celiac artery compression (Dunbar's syndrome), has been controversial due to the poor understanding of its pathophysiology and patient variability with presentation and treatment.[30] The gold standard traditional therapy has been open surgical decompression, but since 2000 there has been an increased incidence of laparoscopic or robotic decompression.[31] Laparoscopic approach has been increasingly favorable due to faster recovery and less morbidity; however, there is reported increased risk of significant arterial bleeding reported in some series to 7.4%.[29] More recently, small series of robot-assisted decompression for MALS have shown fewer incidences of bleeding and conversion to open surgery.[29] Despite these findings, the risk of arterial injury during decompression is still present and vascular surgeons should be prepared to step in, if needed.

Clinical presentation

The most common finding from median arcuate ligament decompression is injury directly to the celiac artery; however, injury to surrounding arterial branches or paraceliac aortic injury has been described with laparoscopy.[31] Dissection around the aorta results in increased bleeding risk and difficult to control as demonstrated in a series of patients who had arterial injury.[31]

Management

Conversion from laparoscopic to an open exploratory laparotomy to gain access to the supraceliac aorta can be performed in a transperitoneal approach as patients will already be in a supine position. Repair of the celiac artery has been performed with patch angioplasty or aortoceliac bypass if intrinsic stenosis is found in addition to celiac artery injury.[31] Depending on size of aortic branch injuries, they may be able to be repaired primarily or ligated to prevent further hemorrhage. If an injury is present during robotic-assisted decompression, a third robotic arm can apply pressure or occlude bleeding while the suture is passed to the remaining two arms for celiac/inferior phrenic artery repair.[29]

VASCULAR RECONSTRUCTION DURING ONCOLOGIC RESECTIONS

Overview

Intraabdominal malignancies, most notably pancreatic tumors and sarcomas, have a tendency to invade adjacent blood vessels as they grow. Vascular invasion is not necessarily a contraindication to resection, and with adjuvant chemotherapy and radiation, many oncologic surgeons attempt tumor shrinkage before surgical extirpation. Vascular surgeons will be asked for intraoperative assistance with vessel reconstruction for iatrogenic injury or if there is tumor invasion in surrounding vascular structures.[32] In some cases, iatrogenic injury to surrounding structures can be possible without tumor invasion requiring vascular surgery assistance in an emergent setting. The following malignancies are common intraabdominal pathologies that may require a vascular surgeon to be available during surgical resection in a planned or urgent setting.

Clinical presentation

PANCREATIC ADENOCARCINOMA

Pancreatic adenocarcinoma can commonly manifest with invasion into the portal vein or superior mesenteric vein when a tumor is locally advanced.[33,34] In some cases, a replaced right hepatic artery may necessitate arterial resection due to tumor involvement.[35] Invasion of the portal vein or superior mesenteric vein is not a contraindication to oncologic resection as long as venous patency is maintained.[36] Some studies have demonstrated survival after pancreaticoduodenectomy for pancreatic cancer with portal vein/superior mesenteric vein reconstruction similar to patients undergoing the same procedure who had no vascular involvement.[36] Based on this evidence, the National Comprehensive Cancer Network classifies a diagnosis of pancreatic adenocarcinoma with tumor invasion to SMV/PV as borderline resectable after neoadjuvant therapy.[37]

RETROPERITONEAL SARCOMA

Retroperitoneal sarcoma is a common malignant neoplasm that can involve the IVC through invasion arising from mesenchymal tissue or primarily arising from IVC wall itself.[33,38] When evaluating soft tissue sarcomas, long-term survival is not affected by vascular resection or reconstruction, making complex reconstruction more likely to eliminate local tumor extension.[39]

RENAL CELL CARCINOMA

Primary renal cell carcinomas (RCC) are one of the most common tumors that are associated with vascular invasion and have propensity for tumor thrombus extending into the renal vein or inferior vena cava.[33]

Diagnosis

The degree of venous involvement may be diagnosed preoperatively with contrast-induced CT scan demonstrating wall irregularity, vessel narrowing, or circumferential involvement of venous structures.[36] In some cases, endoscopic ultrasound (EUS) scan has also been described for helping identify portal vein (PV) involvement.[36] Both studies have poor sensitivities, making intraoperative unplanned vascular surgery consultation for surgical resection a possibility.[36]

Management

PANCREATIC ADENOCARCINOMA

Several methods of portal vein reconstruction are possible if tumor invasion is present (Figure 34.2).[34] Primary venorrhaphy is acceptable if there is not any risk of luminal narrowing > 30%.[33,34] Otherwise, autologous vein or bovine pericardial patch can be used to maintain portal vein circumference.[33] Autologous vein conduit is preferentially the internal jugular vein compared to a saphenous vein due to size mismatch.[33] Additional graft options that have been described include femoral vein, gonadal vein, left renal vein, external iliac vein, or synthetic graft

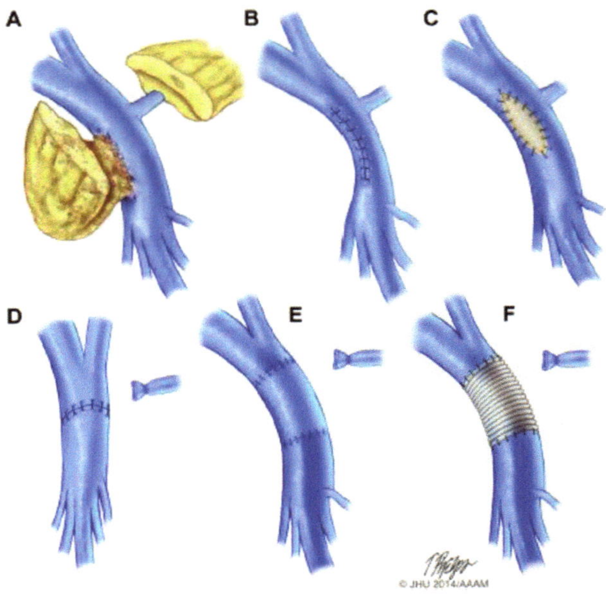

Figure 34.2 (A) Demonstrates involvement of portal vein with pancreatic head tumor (B) Primary repair with lateral venorrhaphy (C) Patch repair (D) End-to-end anastomosis (E) Vein interposition (F) Prosthetic graft interposition.[34]

(PTFE or Dacron).[34] Other techniques include primary end to end repair if there is risk of > 30% intraluminal narrowing or circumferential resection.[34] In some series, postoperative management of patients who undergo vascular reconstruction involves venous thromboembolism chemoprophylaxis and aspirin.[37]

RETROPERITONEAL SARCOMA

The typical management for sarcomas with IVC invasion includes *en bloc* resection and IVC reconstruction; however, if < 50% of the IVC circumference is involved, primary repair with prolene sutures is possible without narrowing the vein too much. Venous reconstruction has been performed with bovine patch to address narrowing the IVC.[33] *En bloc* resection with complete venous excision and reconstruction with PTFE interposition graft is popular, though Dacron graft, superficial femoral vein, cryopreserved vena cava, or aortic homograft have all been reported. The advantage of using externally reinforced PTFE is the avoidance of kinking and compression of the neo-IVC by the viscera. In some cases, primary IVC ligation has been reported; however, patients can develop massive lower extremity edema, renal dysfunction, and abdominal ascites, so this has to be discouraged.[33,38]

RENAL CELL CARCINOMA

In addition to nephrectomy, caval thrombectomy has been shown to improve patient outcomes for renal cell carcinoma.[33] With disease extending to intrahepatic IVC or higher, liver mobilization allows for clamping to at the diaphragmatic cava.[33]

VASCULAR INJURIES OF THE EXTREMITIES

VASCULAR INJURY ASSOCIATED WITH RADIAL ARTERIAL LINE PLACEMENT

Overview

The radial artery is a convenient location for cannula placement when close hemodynamic monitoring is required.[40] Given that the ulnar artery provides dominant flow to the hand in most patients, radial artery cannulation complications such as thrombosis are either unrecognized or well tolerated resulting in nonoperative management.[40] Furthermore, the radial artery is frequently the preferred access vessel for diagnostic coronary angiography. Studies have demonstrated decreased flow or thrombosis after radial artery decannulation in 25–33% of patients, but hand ischemia is seen in < 1% of cases.[41] Given the frequency of arterial line placement, it is important for a vascular surgeon to be aware of these complications. Of course, the "Allen test" should be performed prior to using the radial artery as an access vessel for angiography or monitoring.

Clinical presentation

In patients who have non-dominant flow, cannulation can lead to serious complications including hand ischemia due to thrombosis, pseudoaneurysm, hematoma, or perforation requiring surgical management.[40] If hand ischemia is present, the risk of amputation is significantly increased.[40]

Diagnosis

ISCHEMIC COMPLICATIONS

Digital pulse oximetry can be used to monitor hand ischemia; however, continuous Doppler examination of the radial artery/palmar arch can give further information on limb-threatening ischemia.[40] Other options include duplex ultrasound imaging or arteriography in rare cases.[40] However, the ultimate decision to pursue an operative intervention would be clinical examination looking for motor/sensory changes and skin discoloration indicating an ischemic complication of radial arterial line placement.[40]

NONISCHEMIC COMPLICATIONS

Radial artery pseudoaneurysms are most commonly seen as nonischemic complication of cannulation where it is possible secondary to removal with inadequate compression. Clinical diagnosis demonstrating a pulsatile wrist mass/expanding hematoma can be with a duplex ultrasound.[40]

Management

ISCHEMIC COMPLICATIONS

Treatment of digital thromboemolization from atherosclerotic or catheter-related debris with a patent radial artery would be catheter removal, anticoagulation/antiplatelet, or both if clinically appropriate.[40] Lytic agents for digital emboli is appealing, but insufficient experience with these agents in the setting of hand ischemia makes widespread application difficult.[41] For patients who presented with thrombotic radial artery occlusion, patients may undergo radial artery exploration and thromboembolectomy, followed patch angioplasty.[40]

NONISCHEMIC COMPLICATIONS

Pseudoaneurysm is the most common nonischemic complication where patients can either undergo primary repair, vein patch angioplasty, or radial artery ligation in the setting of ruptured pseudoaneurysm.[40] Patients may also have thrombin injection to the radial artery pseudoaneurysm, which appears to be safe and effective for iatrogenic injury.[42] Patients can also have infections with severe infectious arteritis. Management would be antibiotics, excision and wide debridement, and/or irrigation with debridement of abscess.[40]

VASCULAR INJURY ASSOCIATED WITH KNEE ARTHROPLASTY

Overview

Total knee arthroplasty is a commonly performed operation. Iatrogenic arterial injury is reported to be less than 1%.[43] Delayed diagnosis and improper management can result in significant morbidity with the risk for limb loss.[43] Most commonly, popliteal artery injury is possible and would require prompt response by a vascular surgeon to avoid hemodynamic collapse and complications of acute limb ischemia.

Clinical presentation

Recognizing acute arterial injury can be difficult especially if the surgeon did not specifically check for pulses or perform an ABI (ankle brachial index) preoperatively. Furthermore, many orthopedists routinely use tourniquets to decrease bleeding, another potential contributor to vascular problems, whether an arterial injury or compartment syndrome. Mechanisms of injury during knee arthroplasty can be both direct (i.e., instrument injury, heat injury) or indirect (i.e., arterial stretch during retraction).[43] Patients with associated risk factors for complications include history of lower extremity arterial insufficiency with preexisting superficial femoral/popliteal artery calcification.[44]

Diagnosis

Patients should not leave the operating room after knee arthroplasty until vascular checks have been performed. A change in exam from preoperative evaluation should prompt vascular surgery evaluation. Diagnostic testing may be done with CT angiography if a patient is outside of the operating room and stable or arteriography from contralateral femoral artery with patients who are in the operating room/unstable.[43]

Management

Patients who present with a popliteal artery injury can undergo either an endovascular or open approach. The endovascular approach with a covered balloon-expandable stent is possible with minor injury; however, in the setting of thrombosis/laceration, an open surgical approach will be required. In general, exposure of the popliteal artery is done either through a medial approach or a direct posterior approach. If the injury is suspected in the operating room, the patients can be left supine and have the popliteal artery exposed from a medial approach. The drawback of this approach is the relative inaccessibility of the middle portion of the popliteal artery, which is directly behind the knee.[43] If the injury is discovered after the patient has left the operating room, an emergent operation can be done via the posterior approach, for either direct repair with vein patch angioplasty or interposition vein graft.[43] Popliteal artery thrombosis with preexisting vascular disease may require a short segment bypass with PTFE or ideally autogenous conduit. Additionally, depending on the duration of ischemic time, the patient may also need a lower extremity four-compartment fasciotomy to decompress the swollen leg and avoid permanent nerve or vascular damage.

CONCLUSION

Vascular surgeons are called upon to manage complications occurring during a wide variety of procedures, whether these procedures are minimally invasive or open. The most common type of injury is iatrogenic arterial or venous injury requiring repair. Another occurrence, with more aggressive oncologic resections, is the replacement of important structures, planned or unplanned, such as the portal vein, inferior vena cava, or other main arteries and veins. Therefore, the vascular surgeon has to be prepared to step in to repair vascular structures and to avoid severe morbidity or potential mortality associated with these intraoperative complications.

REFERENCES

1. Manzur MF, Ham SW, Elsayed RS, et al. Vascular surgery: An essential hospital resource in modern health care. Journal of vascular surgery. 2016 Aug 1;64 (2): 543.
2. Tomita TM, Rodriguez HE, Hoel AW, et al. Implications of intraoperative vascular surgery assistance for hospitals and vascular surgery trainees. JAMA surgery. 2016 Nov 1;151(11): 1032–8.
3. Danczyk RC, Coleman J, Allensworth J, et al. Incidence and outcomes of intraoperative vascular surgery consultations. Journal of vascular surgery. 2015 Jul 1;62(1): 177–82.
4. Pronovost P, Needham D, Berenholtz S, et al. An intervention to decrease catheter-related bloodstream infections in the ICU. New England Journal of Medicine. 2006 Dec 28;355(26): 2725–32.
5. Bowdle A. Vascular complications of central venous catheter placement: Evidence-based methods for prevention and treatment. Journal of cardiothoracic and vascular anesthesia. 2014 Apr 1;28(2): 358–68.
6. Yoon DY, Annambhotla S, Resnick SA, et al. Inadvertent arterial placement of central venous catheters: Diagnostic and therapeutic strategies. Annals of vascular surgery. 2015 Nov 1;29(8): 1567–74.
7. Abi-Jaoudeh N, Turba UC, Arslan B, et al. Management of subclavian arterial injuries following inadvertent arterial puncture during central

venous catheter placement. Journal of Vascular and Interventional Radiology. 2009 Mar 1;20(3): 396–402.
8. Ruesch S, Walder B, Tramèr MR. Complications of central venous catheters: Internal jugular versus subclavian access—a systematic review. Critical care medicine. 2002 Feb 1;30(2): 454–60.
9. Kirkwood ML, Wahlgren CM, Desai TR. The use of arterial closure devices for incidental arterial injury. Vascular and endovascular surgery. 2008 Oct;42(5): 471–6.
10. Kapadia S, Parakh R, Grover T, et al. Endovascular covered stent for management of arterial pseudo-aneurysms after central venous access. Journal of cardiothoracic and vascular anesthesia. 2007 Feb 1;21(1): 99–102.
11. Allan JS, Wright CD. Tracheoinnominate fistula: Diagnosis and management. Chest Surgery Clinics. 2003 May 1;13(2): 331–41.
12. Grant CA, Dempsey G, Harrison J, et al. Tracheo-innominate artery fistula after percutaneous tracheostomy: Three case reports and a clinical review. British journal of anaesthesia. 2005 Nov 18;96(1): 127–31.
13. Deguchi JO, Furuya T, Tanaka N, et al. Successful management of tracheo-innominate artery fistula with endovascular stent graft repair. Journal of vascular surgery. 2001 Jun 1;33(6): 1280–2.
14. Hamaguchi S, Nakajima Y. Two cases of tracheoinnominate artery fistula following tracheostomy treated successfully by endovascular embolization of the innominate artery. Journal of vascular surgery. 2012 Feb 1;55(2): 545–7.
15. Courcy PA, Rodriguez A, Garrett HE. Operative technique for repair of tracheoinnominate artery fistula. Journal of vascular surgery. 1985 Mar 1;2(2): 332–4.
16. Woerner A, Koo KS, Monroe EJ. Endovascular Stent Graft Exclusion of an Iatrogenic Tracheoinnominate Fistula after Unsuccessful Surgical Repair. Journal of Clinical Interventional Radiology ISVIR. 2018 Aug;2(02): 106–9.
17. Mei J, Pu Q, Liao H, et al. A novel method for troubleshooting vascular injury during anatomic thoracoscopic pulmonary resection without conversion to thoracotomy. Surgical endoscopy. 2013 Feb 1;27(2): 530–7.
18. Cerfolio RJ, Bess KM, Wei B, et al. Incidence, results, and our current intraoperative technique to control major vascular injuries during minimally invasive robotic thoracic surgery. The Annals of thoracic surgery. 2016 Aug 1;102(2): 394–9.
19. Solli P, Pardolesi A, Spaggiari L, et al. Case Presentation: Aortic Injury during VATS Lobectomy. CTSNet. 2015 Feb 16.
20. Garg J, Woo K, Hirsch J, et al. Vascular complications of exposure for anterior lumbar interbody fusion. Journal of vascular surgery. 2010 Apr 1;51(4): 946–50.
21. Hamdan AD, Malek JY, Schermerhorn ML, et al. Vascular injury during anterior exposure of the spine. Journal of vascular surgery. 2008 Sep 1;48(3): 650–4.
22. Jung HS, Kim DJ, Kim HS, et al. Vascular complications related to posterior lumbar disc surgery. Vascular specialist international. 2017 Dec; 33(4): 160.
23. Chiriano J, Abou-Zamzam Jr AM, Urayeneza C, et al. The role of the vascular surgeon in anterior retroperitoneal spine exposure: preservation of open surgical training. Journal of vascular surgery. 2009 Jul 1;50(1): 148–51.
24. Wood KB, DeVine J, Fischer D, et al. Vascular injury in elective anterior lumbosacral surgery. Spine. 2010 Apr 20;35(9S): S66–75.
25. Datta JC, Janssen ME, Beckham R, Ponce C. The use of computed tomography angiography to define the prevertebral vascular anatomy prior to anterior lumbar procedures. Spine. 2007 Jan 1;32(1): 113–9.
26. Sandadi S, Johannigman JA, Wong VL, et al. Recognition and management of major vessel injury during laparoscopy. Journal of minimally invasive gynecology. 2010 Nov 1;17(6): 692–702.
27. Jafari MD, Pigazzi A. Techniques for laparoscopic repair of major intraoperative vascular injury: Case reports and review of literature. Surgical endoscopy. 2013 Aug 1;27(8): 3021–7.
28. Mirski MA, Lele AV, Fitzsimmons L, et al. Diagnosis and treatment of vascular air embolism. Anesthesiology. 2007 Jan 1;106(1): 164–77.
29. Thoolen SJ, van der Vliet WJ, Kent TS, et al. Technique and outcomes of robot-assisted median arcuate ligament release for celiac artery compression syndrome. Journal of vascular surgery. 2015 May 1;61(5): 1278–84.
30. Jimenez JC, Harlander-Locke M, Dutson EP. Open and laparoscopic treatment of median arcuate ligament syndrome. Journal of vascular surgery. 2012 Sep 1;56(3): 869–73.
31. Roseborough GS. Laparoscopic management of celiac artery compression syndrome. Journal of vascular surgery. 2009 Jul 1;50(1): 124–33.
32. Oderich GS, Panneton JM, Hofer J, Bower TC, Cherry Jr KJ, Sullivan T, Noel AA, Kalra M, Gloviczki P. Iatrogenic operative injuries of abdominal and pelvic veins: A potentially lethal complication. Journal of vascular surgery. 2004 May 1;39(5): 931–6.

33. Etkin Y, Foley PJ, Wang GJ, et al. Successful venous repair and reconstruction for oncologic resections. Journal of Vascular Surgery. 2016 Jan 1;4(1): 57–63.
34. Glebova NO, Hicks CW, Piazza KM, et al. Technical risk factors for portal vein reconstruction thrombosis in pancreatic resection. Journal of vascular surgery. 2015 Aug 1;62(2):424–33.
35. Sgroi MD, Narayan RR, Lane JS, et al. Vascular reconstruction plays an important role in the treatment of pancreatic adenocarcinoma. Journal of vascular surgery. 2015 Feb 1;61(2): 475–80.
36. Lee DY, Mitchell EL, Jones MA, et al. Techniques and results of portal vein/superior mesenteric vein reconstruction using femoral and saphenous vein during pancreaticoduodenectomy. Journal of vascular surgery. 2010 Mar 1;51(3): 662–6.
37. Turley RS, Peterson K, Barbas AS, et al. Vascular surgery collaboration during pancreaticoduodenectomy with vascular reconstruction. Annals of vascular surgery. 2012 Jul 1;26(5): 685–92.
38. Obi AT, Kim GY, Coleman DM, et al. Aggressive Phenotype of Intravascular Lymphoma Relative to Other Malignant Intraabdominal Tumors Requiring Vascular Reconstruction. Annals of vascular surgery. 2019 Jan 1;54: 72–83.
39. Krutman M, Nishinari K, Pignataro BS, et al. 20 years of experience in vascular reconstructions associated with resection of malignant neoplasms in a single cancer center. Journal of vascular surgery. 2018 Dec 24.
40. Garg K, Howell BW, Saltzberg SS, et al. Open surgical management of complications from indwelling radial artery catheters. Journal of vascular surgery. 2013 Nov 1;58(5): 1325–30.
41. Valentine RJ, Modrall JG, Clagett GP. Hand ischemia after radial artery cannulation. Journal of the American College of Surgeons. 2005 Jul 1;201(1): 18–22.
42. Garvin RP, Ryer EJ, Yoon HR, et al. Ultrasound-guided percutaneous thrombin injection of iatrogenic upper extremity pseudoaneurysms. Journal of vascular surgery. 2014 Jun 1;59(6): 1664–9.
43. Hans SS, Shepard AD, Reddy P, et al. Iatrogenic arterial injuries of spine and orthopedic operations. Journal of vascular surgery. 2011 Feb 1;53(2): 407–13.
44. Calligaro KD, DeLaurentis DA, Booth RE, et al. Acute arterial thrombosis associated with total knee arthroplasty. Journal of vascular surgery. 1994 Dec 1;20(6): 927–32.

35

Endovascular removal of foreign bodies (catheter wires and sheaths) from the vascular system

MICHAEL TRPKOVSKI AND ROBERT ACHO

Intravascular foreign bodies (IFB) are a rare but serious complication. Multiple therapeutic interventions such as placement of stents, inferior vena cava filters, venous catheters, and coil embolization, can lead to fragmentation of the instrument, with subsequent embolization, migration, or deployment of the fragment into an undesired location. Although extremely rare, the complications of this are serious and sometimes fatal. Embolization of foreign body fragments can lead to sepsis, bacterial endocarditis, cardiac arrhythmias, or myocardial damage, all carrying a reported mortality rate ranging from 24–60%. Due to this high mortality rate, removal of a foreign body is almost always recommended, even in asymptomatic patients. Over the years, retrieval of IFBs has shifted away from traditional open techniques and toward endovascular approaches, which carry excellent success rates along with minimal complications, according to the studies. With the development of multiple instruments and techniques, the percutaneous approach has become the gold standard for IFB retrieval.

SOURCES OF INTRAVASCULAR FOREIGN BODIES

CENTRAL VENOUS CATHETER

Central venous catheter (CVC) placement has become one of the most commonly performed procedures. The overall complication rate associated with this procedure is approximately 15% and is mainly due to hematoma formation, pneumothorax, infection, or arterial injury. Embolization of the catheter or a fragment of the catheter is a rare but serious complication. It comprises roughly 1% of all complications, but has an associated mortality rate as high as 71%, hence the need for retrieval.

Diagnosis can be challenging, as some patients may not manifest any symptoms. Surov et al. reported the signs associated with fragment embolization, which include the following in order of decreasing incidence: catheter malfunction, cardiac arrhythmia, shortness of breath, and signs of sepsis. If clinical suspicion is high, an upright chest x-ray should be obtained to confirm the location of the catheter, ensure the catheter is in its' entirety, and to rule out any embolized fragments (Figure 35.1).

The location of the fractured or migrated catheter is dependent on the following: the original vein it was placed in, catheter flexibility and length, patient positioning, and blood flow within the vessel and/or heart. Common locations of embolized material include the right atrium, pulmonary artery, right ventricle, superior vena cava, and subclavian vein.

WIRES

Wires can both splinter and embolize, or the entire wire can be lost in the vascular system. The evolution of percutaneous interventions over the past decade has led to an increasing incidence of guide-wire fracturing, making it one of the more common sources of IFBs. Wires are subjected to stress with repetitive attempts to cross a narrowed, heavily calcified lesion, leading to weakening and eventual fracturing. This is a well-known phenomenon seen with percutaneous coronary intervention with a reported incidence of 0.1–0.8%. Although less commonly reported in the literature, the same theory applies for broken wires during peripheral vascular interventions.

A foreign body in the arterial system can lead to thrombosis, ischemia, and/or infection. Therefore, patients may present with signs of ischemia and infection, or they may remain asymptomatic. If identified during an intervention, it should be addressed immediately. Compared to

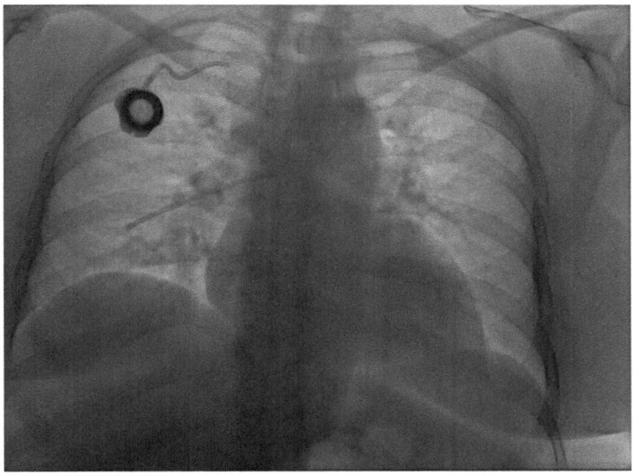

Figure 35.1 A patient with a fragmented mediport lodged in the right pulmonary artery.

venous foreign bodies, those located in the arterial system can be managed conservatively. Situations in which conservative management can be employed include the following: 1) a small fragment lodged in an artery with chronic occlusive disease, and 2) low probability of embolization in an asymptomatic patient. If these criteria are not met, endovascular retrieval should be performed. Although extremely rare, control of the wire can be lost during insertion of CVCs or peripheral interventions, allowing the entire wire to enter the vessel.

INSTRUMENTATION AND TECHNIQUE

LOOP SNARE

The rapid growth of endovascular interventions has led to the development of multiple devices used for retrieval of IFBs. The loop snare is the most widely used and versatile device when it comes to foreign body retrieval. It is designed to be flexible, facilitating navigation through the vasculature to reach the right atrium or pulmonary arteries. A disadvantage to its use is its weak grip strength, making chronic, adherent IFBs difficult to remove. The snare can be a single loop, also referred to as the Amplatz Gooseneck Nitinol Snare (Ev3 Inc., Plymouth, MN), or multiple loops such as the EN Snare (Merrit Medical, Jordan, UT). When deployed, the loop emerges perpendicular to the catheter at a 90-degree angle, making placement of the loop around the IFB much more feasible. The loop snare's design permits its use for removing a variety of IFBs, including fragmented CVCs, wires, stents, and IVF filters.

Various techniques using the loop snare device have been described. The proximal capture technique is the most basic of the approaches. In order to use this method, there must be a free end of the IFB accessible (Figure 35.2). The vascular system is accessed through one of the major vessels, most commonly the right common femoral vein.

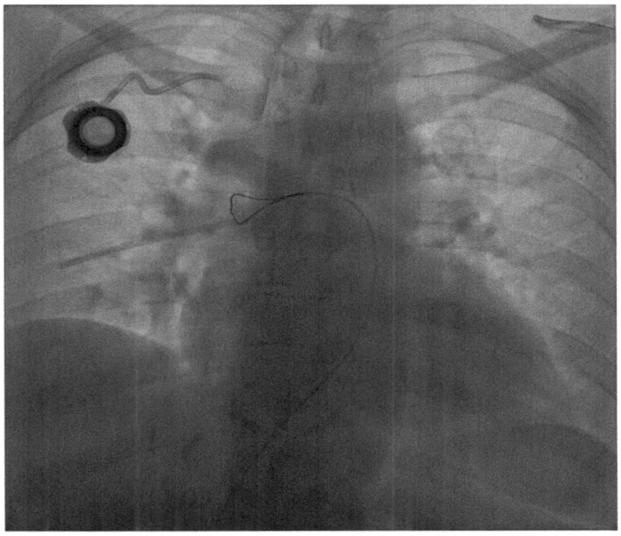

Figure 35.2 The gooseneck snare being used to retrieve an IFB. Note that the operator is attempting to grab the IFB at one of its free ends.

In certain situations, such as patients with IVC filters or bilateral iliac thrombus, the internal jugular vein or subclavian vein is the preferred access site. The catheter is advanced under fluoroscopic guidance into the desired vessel to a point just before the IFB. Once in position, the outer catheter is withdrawn, deploying the snare. The entire system is advanced until the loop is around the free end of IFB. Once the loop encompasses the IFB, the snare is tightened around the IFB by advancing the catheter. After the snare is tightened, the IFB should be oriented parallel to the vessel, which reduces the likelihood of vessel damage during removal (Figure 35.3). The entire

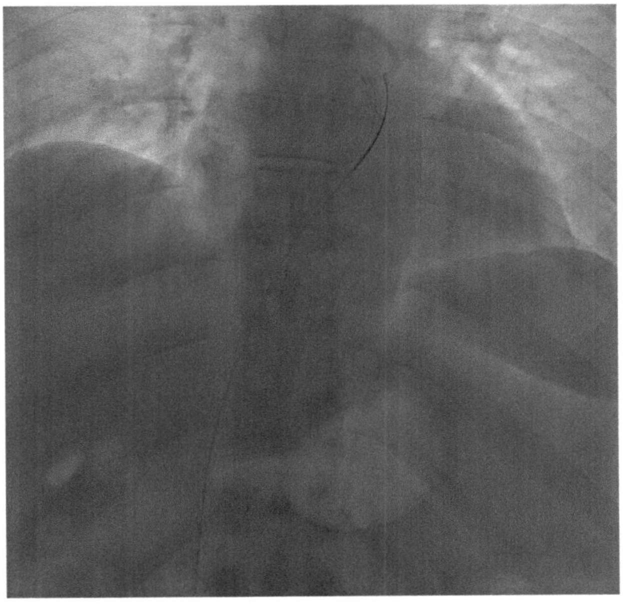

Figure 35.3 The IFB is grasped at its distal end and slowly removed. Note that the IFB is parallel to the vessel that it is traveling in.

system, including the IFB, is then removed through an eight French sheath. Care must be taken to ensure that the loop is around the free end of the IFB. If the loop is in the middle, tightening of the snare will orient the IFB perpendicular to the catheter and vessel, which can ultimately lead to vessel wall damage and, in severe instances, laceration of the vessel wall. Using this technique, success rates have been reported to be in excess of 92%. Other techniques using the loop snare are primarily reserved for stent removal.

ENDOVASCULAR RETRIEVAL FORCEPS

Endovascular forceps are not used as much as the loop snare for foreign body retrieval. Their design typically employs side-opening jaws which allow for greater grip strength. Typically it requires access through the internal jugular or femoral vein. They come in a variety of sizes ranging from 3Fr to 12Fr and can be passed through a guiding catheter. The vascular retrieval forceps (Cook Medical) are used in larger vessels and can be used to retrieve IFBs from central veins and the right atrium. The Alligator retrieval device (Covidien, Mansfield, MA) can be used in small vessels and is used to remove coils from the cerebral circulation. Perhaps the greatest advantage of endovascular forceps is the ability to remove IFBs without having a free end. Drawbacks to using the forceps are their high risk of iatrogenic injuries and rigid design, leading to difficult navigation. Endovascular forceps have been used to facilitate the removal of stents, coils, and IFBs that are adherent to the endothelium of the vessel. Caution should be used with the endovascular forceps given their risk for complications. IFBs which have been intravascular for more than 24 hours usually have some adherence to the vessel. If excessive force is used, the operator runs the risk of damaging the vessel lining and, in severe cases, perforating the vessel.

Once access is obtained, the guiding catheter is then directed to the desired location. Next, the forceps are passed through the catheter and gently advanced until the jaws emerge. The catheter and forceps are then manipulated to grasp the IFB. Once the IFB is in the jaws of the forceps, the guiding catheter and forceps are gently removed as a unit. Excessive force should be avoided to limit trauma to the vessel.

CONCLUSION

Endovascular retrieval has been proven to be a safe and effective technique for removal of intravascular foreign bodies. Multiple instruments have been designed over the years. The loop snare is the most commonly used and has the lowest complication rates. Intravascular graspers are reserved for difficult cases and carry the highest risk of iatrogenic injury. The advancement of endovascular therapy has decreased the morbidity associated with intravascular foreign bodies.

36

Tissue coverage for exposed vascular reconstructions (grafts)

KAITLYN ROUNTREE, VIKRAM REDDY, AND SACHINDER SINGH HANS

Occurring in 5–10% of extracavitary cases, surgical site infections and wound dehiscences after vascular reconstruction can leave patients with exposed vessels or conduits such as polytetrafluoroethylene (PTFE) grafts and occasionally autogenous vein grafts.[1] Extracavitary vascular graft infections carry a mortality of 17%, and a major amputation rate of up to 70%. Intracavitary aortic graft infections occur in 0.2%–5.0% of cases and carry a mortality rate of 24%–75%.[2] The optimal treatment is graft removal, wide debridement, and extraanatomic bypass to bring the vascular conduit away from the infected field while supplying the distal vascular beds.

Standard treatment of extracavitary graft infection is associated with mortality of 10%–30% and major amputation rates of up to 70%.[3] With the use of tailored antibiotics in combination with debridement, vacuum-assisted closure devices, and muscle flap coverage, graft salvage is possible in selected patients. Patients at high risk for wound complication or conduit infection may benefit from prophylactic measures such as local tissue coverage flaps or vacuum-assisted closure devices in prevention of surgical site infection at the index surgery.[1]

Historically, *Staphylococcus aureus* was the leading pathogen isolated from infected vascular wounds; however, *Staphylococcus epidermis* is now the most common isolate. *Pseudomonas* species are the most common gram-negative bacteria responsible for vascular graft infection.[2,4] Infection with *Staphylococcus aureus* is more likely to be identified in cases with anastomotic disruption between graft and native vessel.[5] Predictors of surgical site infections after vascular bypass include obesity, diabetes, poor preoperative functional status, female gender, smoking, active infection at time of index surgery, and redo bypass. Siracuse et al. in a 10 year review of prosthetic graft infection observed no change in incidence of femoral artery graft infection despite changes in preoperative skin preparation, clipper versus razor use, preoperative scrub solution (Betadine vs chlorhexidine), perioperative antibiotic regimen, and conduit choice (vein vs Dacron vs PTFE) over the period of review.[4]

There are two peaks in incidence of vascular graft infection. The first peak occurs early in the postoperative period, up to 4 months from index surgery, with most occurring within the first 2 months. Early vascular graft infections are associated with contamination at the time of surgery or by direct extension from a superficial infection to the graft. These infections are usually more apparent clinically with the surrounding tissues demonstrating signs of infection such as erythema, warmth, or purulent drainage. Risk factors include distal infection where infected lymphatics are injured in the index surgery, and patient body habitus can lead to intertriginous skin folds or gapping in the skin closure, especially in the groin. Contamination from the skin of the groin is the most frequent cause of graft infection.[2]

Late vascular graft infections occur at least 4 months from the index surgery, and are thought to be due to seeding of the graft from bacteremia either from a new infection or reactivation of subclinical infection. Grafts remain susceptible to infection for up to 1 year from implantation while the pseudointimal lining is developing. When vascular grafts are infected, the infection is likely to spread to the native vessel, causing inflammation and subsequent aneurysm formation, hemorrhage, or occlusion.[2] In cases where an anastomosis is involved in the infected field, the authors recommend lifelong antibiotics, where as in cases without an involved suture line 6 weeks of therapy is felt to be adequate. If the vascular anastomosis is involved with infection, removal of graft is mandatory as muscle or myocutaneous flap alone will not be sufficient in managing graft infections.

Tissue Coverage Techniques			
Tissue Flap	**Dependent Artery**	**Area of Coverage**	**Morbidity**
Sartorius Muscle Rotational Flap	Superficial Femoral Artery	Groin	Minimal - decrease in hip flexicn
Gracilis Muscle Retroflexed Flap	Medial Circumflex Femoral Artery	Groin	Minimal - decrease in internal rotation of leg
Gastrocnemius Muscle Flap	Medial Head - Surales Medialis from Popliteal Artery Lateral Head - Surales Lateralis from Popliteal Artery	Circumferential knee, medial, and lateral lower leg	Minimal - decrease in flexion of knee
Omental Pedicle Flap	Anterior - Right Omental Artery Posterior - Left Omental Artery	Anywhere intra- or extracavitary	Minimal, largest source of morbidity from accompanied laparotomy or laparoscopic harvest
Sternocleidomastoid Muscle Rotational Flap	Superior - Occipital Artery Middle - Superior Thyroid Artery/External Carotid Artery Inferior - Variable	Anterolateral neck	Minimal - decrease rotation of head to same side
Pectoralis Major Myocutaneous Flap	Pectoral branch of the Thoracoacromial Artery	Anterolateral neck	Minimal - decrease range of shoulder motion and weakness of the shoulder

TISSUE COVERAGE TECHNIQUES: GROIN

SARTORIUS MUSCLE FLAP

The sartorius muscle is the longest muscle in the human body. It originates on the anterior superior iliac spine (ASIS) and runs superficial to insert on the medial surface of the tibia just inferomedial to the tibial tuberosity. Innervated by the femoral nerve, contraction of the sartorius muscle assists with flexion of the thigh at the hip and flexion of the leg at the knee. As a synergistic muscle, use of the sartorius muscle results in minimal loss of function. The sartorius muscle receives segmental blood supply from the superficial femoral artery (SFA).

The proximity of the sartorius muscle to the standard groin incision makes it an ideal muscle for a local rotational flap in cases requiring tissue coverage of Femoral artery and graft (both prosthetic and autogenous). Use of the rotational sartorius muscle flap to treat a postop groin infection was first reported by Mendez Fernandez et al. in 1980 and has since been used both prophylactically and as a salvage procedure for groin wound infection requiring debridement.[6] Brewer et al. demonstrated an 89% success rate for salvage of prosthetic material in the setting of vascular groin wound complication using sartorius muscle rotational flaps. Interestingly, the presence of significant SFA disease did not impact the viability of the sartorius flap despite a segmental arterial supply from the SFA.[7]

Surgical technique of the sartorius muscle flap comprises lateral-to-medial mobilization of the sartorius muscle within the groin wound, with care to preserve the medial blood supply. The sartorius muscle is mobilized on the lateral side superiorly to the level of its origin on the ASIS, detached at the most proximal portion with electrocautery, and twisted on the long access medially to provide coverage of the femoral vessels or graft. The muscle is twisted, allowing the anterior portion to come in close contact with the femoral vessels. The sartorius muscle twist is useful to prevent necrosis of the muscle flap.[8]

The muscle can be secured to the inguinal ligament and surrounding tissues with interrupted absorbable sutures. The wound can either be closed in layers primarily, or the skin and subcutaneous tissue left open with application of vacuum-assisted closure device. A drain is reccomended in the sartorius muscle bed to prevent seroma formation.

GRACILIS MUSCLE FLAP

The gracilis muscle is a long, slender muscle seated superficially on the inner thigh. It functions as an adductor of the thigh, and assists with flexion of the knee and hip. It receives segmental blood supply from the medial circumflex femoral artery (a branch of the deep femoral artery), usually encountered about 10 cm inferior from its origin at the pubic symphysis, and innervation from the obturator nerve. The gracilis muscle flap has long been a work horse of reconstructive surgery in both pedicle and free flap form. Its proximity to the groin makes it a valuable option for native tissue coverage in vascular patients with complicated groin wounds with little residual morbidity.

Likewise, its blood supply does not rely on the SFA, which is commonly occluded or compromised in vascular patients with arterial occlusive disease.

Retroflexed gracilis flap is preferred in cases where either the sartorius muscle has previously been utilized or is no longer available and a small amount of tissue coverage is required. The retroflexed muscular flap can be performed in conjunction with immediate split thickness skin graft and vacuum-assisted closure device application to the groin wound in cases where no native tissue exists for primary closure.

The gracilis muscle originates from the lower portion of the pubic symphysis and runs vertically and superficially along the inner thigh. The rounded tendon flattens out as it passes behind the medial condyle of the femur and around the medial condyle of the tibia to join the pes anserinus or "goose foot" just deep to the tendon of the sartorius. As the most superficial muscle in the medial thigh, the gracilis muscle can be identified with relative ease through a longitudinal incision over the lower medial thigh by identifying its characteristically rope-like distal portion. Dua et al. described the use of ultrasound to identify the rope-like structure of the gracilis tendon in the distal inner thigh prior to incision.[9]

A vertical incision is made along the distal inner thigh overlying the gracilis muscle and dissection carried down through the subcutaneous tissue to identify the rope-like tendon of the gracilis. Skip incisions are used to decrease the morbidity of the harvest site, with the next incision made more proximally overlying the belly of the gracilis muscle, taking care not to injure the greater saphenous vein. By touching the electrocautery tip to the tendinous portion of the gracilis, the surgeon confirms that the two sites are dissecting the same muscle. The fascial sheath is entered sharply and the anterior and medial edges of the gracilis muscle belly bluntly dissected free with care to preserve perforating vascular bundles on the anterior aspect. The muscle is placed on superior tension and the distal tendon is transected with electrocautery. At this point blood flow to the muscle belly is checked with handheld Doppler as demonstrated in Figure 36.1. A tunnel is created with digital manipulation from the groin wound to the medial incision; it is important to make the tunnel wide enough to accommodate the retroflexed gracilis muscle without risk of compression of its vascular supply. A simple silk suture to the free end of the gracilis muscle and guiding it through the newly created tunnel with a hemostat is recommended. The vascular supply is checked with handheld Doppler and the muscle belly observed to ensure that there is no overt venous congestion. The free end of the gracilis rotational flap can be secured to the inguinal ligament if it is readily available in the groin wound, or to the surrounding tissues with 3-0 absorbable monofilament. A partial thickness skin grafting over top of the rotational muscle flap is recommended, with vacuum-assisted closure device application for 3–5 days opposed to primary skin closure over the tissue flap. Ali et al. demonstrated 85% of patients with complete healing with primary closure,[10] while Dua et al. demonstrated a 100% complete healing rate in 2 months following skin graft application. [9]

The contralateral anterior thigh is a suitable and convenient skin graft donor location. This is harvested in usual fashion with a microplaner and dressed with bacitracin ointment and an occlusive dressing to minimize pain at the site. The dressing is left in place for 48 hours, then changed as needed.

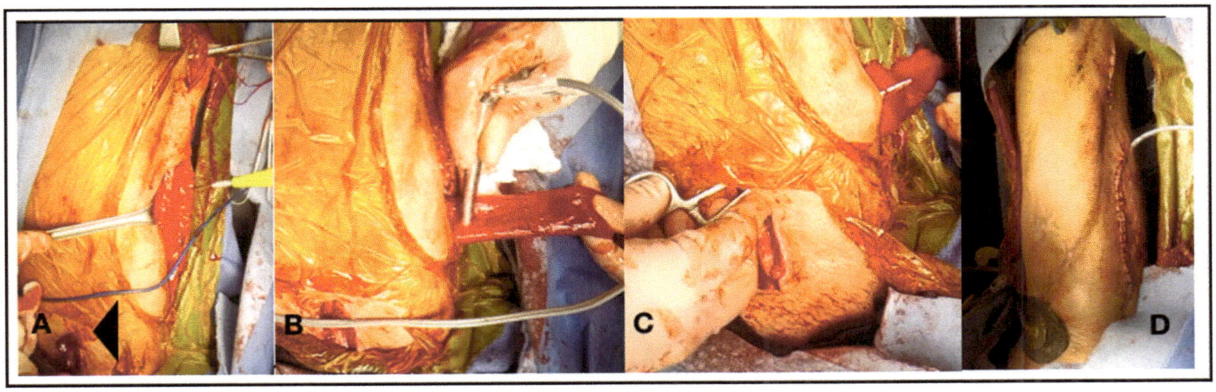

Figure 36.1 Left medial thigh with knee superior and groin inferior. (A) Metzembaum scissors passed behind the isolated tendon of the gracilis muscle, Bovie tip indicating belly of the gracilis muscle and arrow head indicating location of wound to be covered. (B) Muscled belly of the gracilis flap after division of the distal tendon, Doppler signal checked prior to rotation of gracilis flap. (C) A hemostat is passed through the tunnel connecting the groin wound site (handle) and the proximal donor incision, and using a suture affixed to the tendon the gracilis muscle is gently rotated through the tunnel to cover the groin wound. (D) Distal and proximal donor incisions closed with vertical mattress sutures and drain in proximal donor bed. Wound vac applied over the split thickness skjn graft covered gracilis flap site in the groin.

TISSUE COVERAGE TECHNIQUES: NECK

STERNOCLEIDOMASTOID MUSCLE FLAP

The two heads of the sternocleidomastoid muscle (SCM) originate from the manubrium of the sternum and the medial clavicle; as they ascend superiorly, the fibers of the two heads blend together to insert on the mastoid process of the temporal bone. The major function of the SCM is rotation of the head and flexion of the neck. Motor innervation is supplied from the accessory nerve which perforates the muscle at the level of the carotid bifurcation.[11] The blood supply to the SCM is segmental and variable with the exception of the superior segment. Cadaveric dissections and latex injection studies have consistently reported a reliable blood supply to the superior aspect of the muscle from the occipital artery derived from the external carotid artery (ECA). The middle portion of the muscle belly is variably supplied by branches from the superior thyroid artery (STA) or, in 20–27% of cases, directly by branches of the ECA. The lower portion of the sternocleidomastoid muscle belly is variably supplied by either the transverse cervical artery, the Thyrocervical trunk and or the superficial cervical artery.[12]

The superiorly based rotational flap is the most commonly used variation. The ability to rely on the consistent vascular supply of the occipital artery allows for a greater rotational arc for the superiorly based flap as the STA branches may be ligated if necessary without undue risk of flap failure; the inferior based flap requires preservation of both the inferior and middle blood supply. Either a SCM muscle flap or a SMC myocutaneous flap can be performed depending on coverage needs.[11,13]

As described by Yugueros et al., it is recommended to limit the skin island to that directly over the underlying muscle to prevent undue risk of skin paddle necrosis. A key technical point is gently tacking the skin island to the underlying muscle tissue to prevent shearing of the small, tenuous blood vessels running perpendicularly between the skin and underlying muscle.[11,14]

The SCM myocutaneous flap follows an imaginary line overlying the SCM in the direction of its fibers. Should a skin paddle be necessary, a suitable site is chosen on the distal end of the SCM to allow the greatest arc of rotation, keeping in mind the need to preserve the middle blood supply for inferiorly based flaps. The skin paddle and subcutaneous tissue are sutured gently to the underlying muscle to avoid shearing of the underlying perpendicular blood vessels and avulsion during flap manipulation. The skin paddle should be limited to tissue overlying the muscle to reduce risk of skin flap necrosis. Once the desired skin paddle is incised and subcutaneous tissue secured, dissection is sharply carried down to the underlying SCM muscle and the muscle belly is carefully freed of its attachments with care to preserve the accessory nerve and medial blood supply. The flap is then swung to cover the intended site without tension, and the muscle pedicle is sutured into place. The SCM muscle must be securely anchored in place to avoid postoperative traction on the skin paddle with patient head movement. The SCM flap generally allows for closure of the donor site defect.[11,14]

PECTORALIS MAJOR MYOCUTANEOUS FLAP

Larger defects of the neck may require a more extensive reconstructive effort than available within the rotation arch of the SCM flap. The pectoralis major myocutaneous flap was described in a small case series as a viable option with broad coverage capability by Aryian et al. in 1979. Since then, experience with the flap has expanded to include such procedures as reconstruction of the tongue, reconstruction of the hypo pharynx and soft tissue coverage of the great vessels of the neck, and correction of wound breakdown in the neck and oral cavity in both immediate and delayed fashion.[15–17] The use of the pectoralis major myocutaneous pedicle flap will be discussed here in use of soft tissue coverage of the great vessels of the neck.

The pectoralis major muscle originates from the anterior aspect of the medial half of the clavicle; muscle fibers arising from here pass transversely and are often separated from the rest of the muscle by a slight gap. Additional muscle fibers originate from the anterior surface of the sternum, from the cartilages of all the true ribs, and from the aponeurosis of the abdominal external oblique muscle. These muscle fibers converge toward its insertion on the humerus and travel in a superolateral direction. It is the largest and most superficial muscle of the anterior chest wall. There is generous blood supply to the pectoralis major, with the myocutaneous flap based upon the thoracoacromial artery, a branch directly off the axillary artery. Additional blood supply arises medially from the internal mammary artery and laterally from the long thoracic artery, branches of which are generally sacrificed during elevation of the flap to secure adequate pedicle length.[18]

The pectoralis major pedicle flap can be utilized either as a myocutaneous or myofascial flap depending on surgeon needs and patient body habitus. In morbidly obese patients, the skin paddle may be nonviable due to shearing forces on small perforating vessels. Patients with a history of subclavian central lines, prior chest surgery, breast augmentation, or mastectomy may also be at increased risk for skin paddle necrosis or increased difficulty of performance of the pectoralis major flap. Poland syndrome, or congenital absence of the pectoralis muscle, is a contraindication.

The patient should be positioned with the recipient site exposed in association with the ipsilateral chest, shoulder, and axilla. The borders of the pectoralis muscle on the lateral sternum, clavicle, xiphoid, and humeral insertion should be identified. The course of the pectoral branch of the thoracoacromial artery can be identified by drawing a line from the xyphoid to the acromion. A second line perpendicular to this line is drawn that bisects the clavicle. The course of the thoracoacromial artery corresponds to the line drawn from the midpoint of the clavicle continuing to the medial portion of the acromion to xyphoid line. The standard skin paddle is located at the inferomedial border of the pectoralis major muscle that is inserting on the lateral border of the sternum and the second to sixth costal cartilage and should be overlying the identified course of the thoracoacromial artery to ensure reliable blood supply. It is recommended to take a slightly larger-than-needed skin paddle to increase the likelihood the skin will survive the transfer due to the increased number of myocutaneous perforators. The skin paddle should be temporarily secured to the underlying fascia with interrupted sutures to minimize shearing forces to myocutaneous perforators.[15,18]

Initial incision is made from the lateral edge of the designed skin paddle toward the anterior axillary line. Usually this incision is above the nipple in the male patient and below the breast in the female patient to preserve cosmetic outcome and decreases undesired bulk from breast tissue. The incision is carried down to the pectoralis major muscle. This allows for identification of the medial and inferior extents of the muscle, after which the design of the skin paddle can be moved inferiorly or superiorly so as to rest above muscle tissue. The skin and subcutaneous tissues are incised quickly and sharply with either blade or electrocautery with caution not to cone-down to the underlying muscle The subcutaneous tissues are raised from the superior extent of the muscle fibers to the level of the clavicle in similar fashion. At this point the skin paddle should be seated as an island over the inferomedial aspect of the in situ pectoralis major muscle.

The muscle flap is then elevated inferior to superior off the chest wall deep to the pectoralis major fascia with care to elevate the vascular pedicle attached posteriorly to the muscle belly. This can largely be done with blunt finger dissection. As the flap is elevated superiorly, great care must be taken to control branches of the internal mammary artery along the sternal border and other muscular perforators as these can retract into the chest and lead to hemothorax. The lateral muscle attaches to the humerous. A generously wide subcutaneous tunnel is fashioned overlying the clavicle for future delivery of the flap and skin paddle, there must be room enough to prevent kinking or compression of the vascular pedicle as demonstrated in Figure 36.2.

After passing the flap into the neck, the pedicle is carefully checked for any evidence of torsion or kink. In cases where additional length is needed, maneuvers to gain additional centimeters of cephalic coverage can be performed. The first is to transect the pectoralis muscle just below the clavicle, taking great care not to include the vascular pedicle. Another maneuver is resecting a portion of the infra-clavicular pectoralis major. This places the pedicle in immediate contact with the periosteum of the clavicle without interposed muscle and decreases cosmetic bulk over the clavicle.

Sew the pectoral fascia into place within the neck wound independent of the skin paddle. The donor site is usually able to be closed primarily over a closed suction drain with local tissue rearrangement and lifting of cutaneous flaps to facilitate closure. Independently drain the donor and recipient sites; do not place a drain through the tunnel. In cases where a myofascial flap is used,

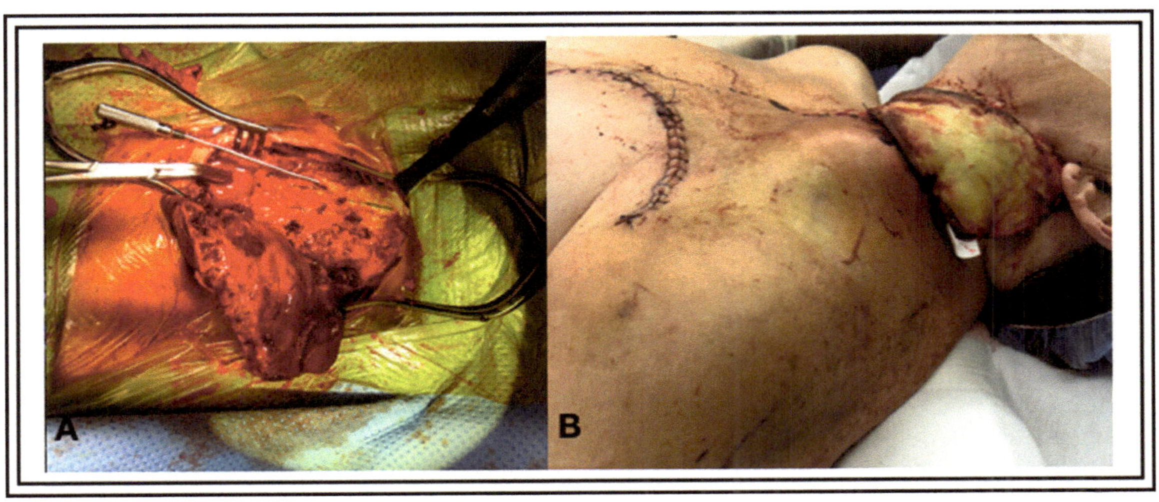

Figure 36.2 (A) Left Pectoralis Major flap within left cervical wound following tunneling over the clavicle. Dilator is indicating the common carotid artery interposition PTFE graft. (B) Immediate postoperative appearance of left Pectoralis Major rotaional flap covering the left anterolateral neck.

immediate split thickness skin grafting is recommended over the completed flap.

Morbidity resulting from the use of the pectoralis major has been reported as minimal. Merve et al. described limited or no additional shoulder morbidity resulting from pectoralis major flap reconstruction than from major head and neck surgery alone. Others have demonstrated an objective decrease in range of motion, specifically abduction, and limited decreased in shoulder strength.[19,20]

TISSUE COVERAGE TECHNIQUES: INTRAABDOMINAL AORTA

OMENTAL FLAP

The omentum is more than a visceral deposit of adipose tissue. Draping like a curtain over the intraperitoneal organs, the greater omentum provides a layer of physical cushion from external trauma. The omentum is recognized as an organ in its own right with many diverse functions including its ability to attenuate the spread of sepsis in cases of peritonitis, to act as a source of angiogenic and hemostatic factors involved in tissue healing and repair, and to serve inflammatory and lymphatic functions with drainage of the peritoneal cavity.[21]

The greater omentum is a double sheet of peritoneum that descends from the greater curvature of the stomach, overlying the small intestine, and then folds back on itself to fuse with the peritoneum on the anterior surface of the transverse colon. The blood supply of the omentum is from the right, left, and middle omental arteries, which originate from the right and left gastroepiploic arteries, respectively. The anterior fold of the greater omentum is supplied by the larger right omental artery, while the smaller left omental artery supplies the posterior surface. The delicate and robust network of vessels transversing the omentum allow it to be crafted into the surgeon's desired size and shape while preserving one or both of the main vascular pedicles for intra-abdominal uses.[22]

The interplay of adipose-rich areas and thin, translucent areas is grossly visible. The translucent areas are thought to function in adhesion formation and the ability of the omentum to 'wall off' areas of inflammation and perforation. The adipose-rich portions are home to the milk spots, so dubbed for their whitish appearance against the yellow adipose tissue. Milk spots are lymphoid aggregates, and while their function and development are not completely understood, they appear to be in large part the reason for the impressive immunologic properties of the greater omentum.[21,23]

Due to its versatility, mobility, and inherent healing and immune properties, use of omental flaps and grafts have been reported by nearly every surgical specialty with descriptions of uses for the omentum in nearly every anatomical location.[22] The omentum is very well vascularized and can be easily divided with energy devices to fit any configuration, and in most cases reach any corner of the abdomen including the pelvis and retroperitoneum as a pedicled flap for tissue coverage. Pedicled flaps have even been described as native tissue treatment for and prevention of lower extremity lymphedema from inguinal lymphadenectomy. Through laparotomy or laparoscopy, the omentum is fashioned into either a single, or dual for bilateral procedure, long strip with continuous pedicled blood supply and drawn through the femoral canal and into the groin extending the desired length down the medial thigh. Authors have reported acceptable success in treatment of severe secondary lymphedema with good long-term results.[22,24,25] Others have reported use of similar technique in cases of infected vascular wounds of the groin requiring extra anatomic bypass via the obturator canal combined with omental flap for wound healing.[26]

In cases of intracavitary vascular reconstructions, the pedicled omental flap is a very reliable source of native tissue coverage with the added benefits inherent to the omentum. For in situ reconstruction after excision of mycotic aortic or aortoiliac aneurysm, pedicled omental flaps are recommended to facilitate delivery of the immune system and phagocytosis of residual infectious particles and for the physical native tissue bolster between the intraperitoneal organs and the new vascular conduit and anastomoses.[27] In patients undergoing open repair of aortoenteric fistulae, either with direct suture repair or excision and in situ reconstruction, pedicled omental flap coverage of the repair is recommended.[28]

TISSUE COVERAGE TECHNIQUES: LOWER LEG

GASTROCNEMIUS MUSCLE FLAP

Tissue healing in the lower extremity can be particularly problematic. Surgical wounds can leave patients with exposed vein graft on the medial or lateral lower leg or around the knee and pose life- and limb-threatening complications. Exposed vein graft is at risk for desiccation and blow out. Native tissue coverage is paramount for adequate wound healing, resolution or control of infection, and prevention of further morbidity and mortality. Wounds about the knee can be particularly challenging due to the scant and unforgiving tissue surrounding the joint with the added demands of joint mobility and preservation of function.

The gastrocnemius muscle is the most superficial muscle of the posterior lower leg. It is responsible for flexion of the knee and plantar flexion of the foot. Comprised of two heads, the medial head originates from the posterior surface of the distal femur just superior to the medial condyle and the lateral head arises from the upper posterolateral surface of the lateral femoral condyle. The muscle fibers converge distally and merge with fibers of the deeper soleus muscle, and insert on the calcaneus as the Achilles tendon. The lateral and medial sural arteries supply their respective heads of the gastrocnemius muscle, entering superiorly as branches from the popliteal artery. The unique vascular supply allows for independently pedicled flaps without the need for microvascular anastomosis.[29]

Knee flexion is minimally affected in patients, with a slight decrease in strength, due to the preserved function of the posterior thigh muscles. It is important that the soleus muscle be protected and intact as it will be the dominant source of plantar flexion following dual gastrocnemius head harvest.[30] Borrowing from orthopedic literature, the gastrocnemius muscle can be used in a generous arc of rotation for coverage of anterior knee wounds, and popliteal fossa coverage, with exposed hardware with salvage rates of 87% in some series.[31,32]

The rotational gastrocnemius flap is a suitable source of viable tissue coverage of below-knee vascular bypasses, and is considered well within the capability of a vascular surgeon. More extensive or re-do flaps may necessitate the expertise and assistance of a plastic surgeon. As the most superficial muscle in the posterior compartment of the lower leg, the bellies of the gastrocnemius are readily identifiable and usually lie within the existing surgical field or wound. The medial head of the gastrocnemius is the traditional work horse of anterior knee and proximal tibial coverage; it is longer than its lateral counterpart and can be harvested without risk to the superficial peroneal nerve. The gastrocnemius can be harvested to suit the needs of the surgeon, with either the medial or lateral heads independently or together.

The gastrocnemius muscle is harvested through an incision made along the medial tibia just posterior to the pes anserinus and carried to 10 cm superior to the medial maleoulus.[32] The fascia of the superficial posterior compartment of the leg is opened sharply with either knife or electrocautery throughout the length of the compartment. The gastrocnemius muscle is separated with gently blunt dissection from the underlying soleus, keeping in mind that the distal tendon fibers become intimately jointed to form the Achilles tendon. Dissection in the proximal incision reveals the two distinct heads of the gastrocnemius muscle with the sural nerve reliably located between their heads. It is important to identify the sural nerve and protect it and the accompanying vascular pedicles entering the muscle heads superiorly. Distally the two heads become confluent, making the distinction between them difficult. Begin separation of the heads of the gastrocnemius muscle proximally and continue distally by following the raphe of the investing fascial envelopes and developing the plane sharply. The flap is then released distally, with or without a portion of tendon depending on coverage needs, taking care to separate the fibers of the gastrocnemius from the deeper fibers of the soleus muscle. Again, either muscle belly can be harvested independently or together. Figure 36.3 demonstrates use of the medial head of the gastrocnemius muscle for coverage of an autologous vein bypass conduit.

If needed for additional rotation above the level of the knee, or additional length is required, dissection can be continued proximally and the origin of the gastrocnemius can be released with great care to preserve the neuromuscular bundle. Great care must be exercised not to induce excessive tension or kinking of the neuromuscular bundle. The fascial envelope of the gastrocnemius can be removed or sequentially scored to increase the length available.

The gastrocnemius muscle flap is not recommended as a myocutaneous flap due to the difficulty in closure of the donor site. Instead split thickness skin grafting over the muscle flap is recommended with wound vac left in place over the sutured sting graft for 3–5 days. For small arc rotational flaps, drainage of the donor site can be omitted, while for larger arcs of rotation or for island flaps, a drain is recommended in the donor site.

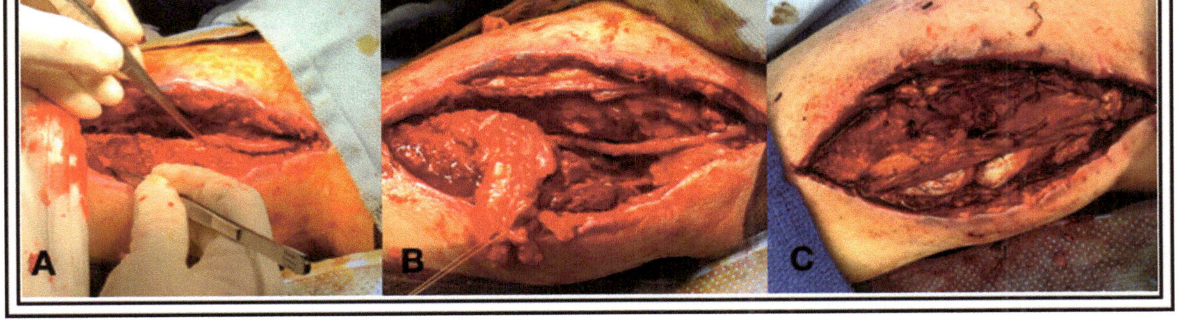

Figure 36.3 (A) Exposed in situ greater saphenous vein bypass on the medial aspect of the knee. (B) Suture through the distal end if the medial head of the gastrocnemius muscle. (C) Rotational flap of the medial head of the gastrocnemius muscle sutured in place covering the previously exposed vein graft.

Case Example 1

A 64-year-old male presented to outpatient clinic in early June 2017, with exposed left femoral graft following a recent (3-week-old) crossover right femoral to left popliteal (8 mm INTERING PTFE – W.L. Gore, Newark, DE) graft. The patient had undergone multiple arterial reconstructions in the past 15 years. In 2002 the patient underwent bilateral iliac stenting; on the left common iliac stent (39 mm × 7 mm), right common iliac stent (29 mm × 7 mm) PALMAZ GENESIS™ balloon-expandable stents (Cardinal Health, Dublin, OH). By 2003, the stenting had failed, and the patient underwent an aortobifemoral bypass graft using a 16 × 8 mm knitted Dacron graft for symptomatic iliac artery occlusive disease. In 2009, the patient developed thrombosis of the left limb of the graft requiring revision. In 2015, patient underwent thrombectomy of the left limb of the aortobifemoral bypass graft extending to superficial and deep femoral arteries. Patient was seen again in June 2016 with a cold left leg and underwent left femoral to popliteal nonreversed great saphenous vein bypass secondary to superficial femoral artery thrombosis and a poor outflow from branches of the deep femoral artery.

In August 2016, patient was found to have superficial left groin wound dehiscence with a small amount of serosanguinous drainage. The seroma was drained; cultures were positive for *Staphylococcus aureus*, coagulase negative, and *Streptococcus viridans*. The following day the patient presented with bleeding from the left groin wound. He was noted to have a 2 cm opening without exposed graft, with no active bleeding. However, there was surrounding induration. The patient was started on intravenous antibiotics Vancomycin and Zosyn, and a CTA was performed. The CTA demonstrated a patent aortobifemoral, bilateral femoropopliteal bypasses, and left groin inflammatory changes with aneurysmal dilatation of the distal aortic limb graft without extravasation.

The patient was scheduled for a debridement on the left groin with sartorius muscle flap on hospital day four; however, on hospital day 3 patient developed secondary hemorrhage in the left groin. He underwent emergent debridement of the skin and soft tissue, and revision of the left femoropopliteal bypass with takedown of the proximal anastomosis with a new anastomosis extending into the proximal superficial femoral artery, with sartorius muscle flap and a wound-vac therapy. At this time, cultures did not show any growth of microorganisms. On hospital day ten, patient was discharged with stable hemoglobin and hematocrit, continued negative-pressure therapy, and oral rifampin with intravenous Ancef for 6 weeks per recommendation of the infectious disease consultant.

Seven days later, the patient presented again with active hemorrhage from the left groin. He was hypotensive with acute blood loss, anemia, and stage III hemorrhagic shock. He was taken to the operating room where bleeding was noted from the anastomotic suture line of the distal left limb of the aortobifemoral bypass graft. The patient underwent removal of the left infected unilateral limb of the aortobifemoral bypass graft with suture ligation of the proximal graft and placement of wound-vac. Cultures at this time grew vancomycin resistant *Enterococcus faecalis* (VRE) and *Candida parapsilosis*.

Following a performance of a left axillopopliteal bypass 2 weeks later with an 8 mm INTERING PTFE graft, the patient regained posterior tibial Doppler signals. During his hospital stay he was continued on intravenous antibiotics. A repeat CTA was performed on postoperative day nine showing a patent left axillopopliteal bypass. He was discharged on postoperative day 14 with continued negative-pressure therapy to his left groin, intravenous Daptomycin and PO Diflucan for an additional 4 weeks. Patient was ambulating and continued to do well until his follow-up visit with palpable dorsalis pedis pulses.

On May 23, 2017, a patient presented to the emergency room with cold, pulseless left lower extremity. Doppler arterial study and CTA of the chest/abdomen showed occluded axillopopliteal bypass with no Doppler flow in the left foot. Patient underwent crossover femoral-popliteal (proximal) graft with 8 mm INTERING PTFE graft. A tunnel was made in the supra-pubic space with 8 mm tunneler.

Patient presented to the clinic 3 weeks later with exposed PTFE graft in the left groin. Since sartorius muscle had already been used, patient underwent gracilis muscle flap with a split thickness skin graft and application of wound vac on June 13, 2017. Complete healing and coverage of the graft in the subsequent 3 weeks occurred. Vascular lab study in May 2018 revealed an ankle brachial index of 0.85 on the right and 0.69 on the left. He subsequently underwent left above-knee amputation on March 13, 2019, due to thrombosis of the crossover femoral-popliteal graft, but his left groin had healed well.

REFERENCES

1. Inui, T, Bandyk DF. Vascular surgical site infection: Risk factors and preventive measures. Semin Vasc Surg. 2015;28(3-4): 201–7.
2. Gharamti A, Kanafani ZA. Vascular Graft Infections: An update. Infect Dis Clin North Am. 2018.
3. Herrera FA, et al., Management of vascular graft infections with soft tissue flap coverage: improving limb salvage rates–a veterans affairs experience. Am Surg. 2009;75(10): 877–81.

4. Siracuse JJ, et al. Prosthetic graft infections involving the femoral artery. J Vasc Surg. 2013;57(3): 700–5.
5. Pounds LL, et al. A changing pattern of infection after major vascular reconstructions. Vasc Endovascular Surg. 2005;39(6): 511–7.
6. Mendez Fernandez MA, et al. Distally based sartorius muscle flap in the treatment of infected femoral arterial prostheses. J Cardiovasc Surg (Torino). 1980;21(5): 628–31.
7. Brewer MB, et al. Sartorius Muscle Flaps for Vascular Groin Wound Complications. Am Surg. 2015;81(11): 1163–9.
8. Khalil IM, Sudarsky L. Sartorius muscle "twist" rotation flap: an answer to flap necrosis. J Vasc Surg. 1987;6(1): 93–4.
9. Dua A, et al. Outcomes of Gracilis Muscle Flaps in the Management of Groin Complications after Arterial Bypass with Prosthetic Graft. Ann Vasc Surg. 2018;51: 113–118.
10. Ali AT, et al. Outcomes after retroflexed gracilis muscle flap for vascular infections in the groin. J Vasc Surg. 2016;64(2): 452–457.
11. Yugueros P, Woods JE. The sternocleidomastoid myocutaneous flap: A reappraisal. Br J Plast Surg. 1996;49(2): 93–6.
12. Leclere FM, Vacher C, Benchaa T. Blood supply to the human sternocleidomastoid muscle and its clinical implications for mandible reconstruction. Laryngoscope. 2012;122(11): 2402–6.
13. Kierner AC, Zelenka I, Gstoettner W. The sternocleidomastoid flap–its indications and limitations. Laryngoscope. 2001;111(12): 2201–4.
14. Ariyan S. Further experience with the sternocleidomastoid myocutaneous flap. Plast Reconstr Surg. 2003;111(1): 381–2.
15. Ariyan S. The pectoralis major myocutaneous flap. A versatile flap for reconstruction in the head and neck. Plast Reconstr Surg. 1979;63(1): 73–81.
16. Wadwongtham W, Isipradit P, Supanakorn S. The pectoralis major myocutaneous flap: Applications and complications in head and neck reconstruction. J Med Assoc Thai. 2004;87 Suppl 2: S95–9.
17. Gonzalez-Garcia R, et al. Straightforward Method for Coverage of Major Vessels after Modified Radical Neck Dissection. J Oral Maxillofac Surg. 2017;75(6): 1299.e1–1299.e4.
18. Fagan J. *The Pectoralis Major Flap.* Open Access Atlas of Otolaryngology, Head and Neck Operative Surgery, 2019.
19. Merve A, et al. Shoulder morbidity after pectoralis major flap reconstruction for head and neck cancer. Head Neck. 2009;31(11): 1470–6.
20. Refos JW, et al. Shoulder morbidity after pectoralis major flap reconstruction. Head Neck. 2016; 38 (8): 1221–8.
21. Meza-Perez S, Randall TD. Immunological Functions of the Omentum. Trends Immunol. 2017;38(7): 526–536.
22. Mazzaferro D, et al. The Omental Free Flap-A Review of Usage and Physiology. J Reconstr Microsurg. 2018. 34(3): 151–169.
23. Collins D, et al. The omentum: Anatomical, metabolic, and surgical aspects. J Gastrointest Surg. 2009;13(6): 1138–46.
24. Piano G, et al. Omental transfer for salvage of the moribund lower extremity. Am Surg. 1998;64(5): 424–7.
25. Benoit L, et al. Preventing lymphedema and morbidity with an omentum flap after ilioinguinal lymph node dissection. Ann Surg Oncol. 2005;12(10): 793–9.
26. Kretschmer G, et al. Groin infections following vascular surgery: Obturator bypass (BYP) versus "biologic coverage" (TRP)–a comparative analysis. Eur J Vasc Surg. 1989;3(1): 25–9.
27. Nemoto Y, et al. In Situ Reconstruction with Extended Debridement in Patients with Mycotic Abdominal Aortic Aneurysms. Ann Vasc Dis. 2017;10(2): 159–163.
28. Chopra A, et al. 20-Year Experience with Aorto-Enteric Fistula Repair: Gastrointestinal Complications Predict Mortality. J Am Coll Surg. 2017;225(1): 9–18.
29. El-Sherbiny M. Pedicled gastrocnemius flap: clinical application in limb sparing surgical resection of sarcoma around the knee region and popliteal fossa. J Egypt Natl Canc Inst. 2008;20(2): 196–207.
30. Jordan DJ, et al. Flap decisions and options in soft tissue coverage of the lower limb. Open Orthop J. 2014;8: 423–32.
31. Moebius B, Scheller EE. The pediculated gastrocnemius muscle flap as a treatment for soft tissue problems of the knee - indication, placement and results. GMS Interdiscip Plast Reconstr Surg DGPW. 2012;1: Doc07.
32. Walton Z, et al. Pedicled Rotational Medial and Lateral Gastrocnemius Flaps: Surgical Technique. J Am Acad Orthop Surg. 2017;25(11): 744–751.

SUGGESTED READING

Mathes SJ and Nahai F. Classification of Vascular Anatomy of Muscles Experimental and Clinical Correlation. *Plastic and Reconstructive Surgery,* 1981;67: 177–87.

Index

Note: Page numbers in *italics* indicate figures and **bold** indicates tables.

A

B

F

G

N

O

P

T